THE NON-HODGKIN'S LYMPHOMAS

THE NON-HODGKIN'S LYMPHOMAS

edited by
Ian T Magrath

MB FRCP FRCPath
Chief, Lymphoma Biology Section
National Cancer Institute – Pediatric Branch
Bethesda, Maryland

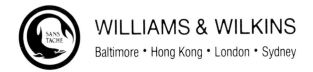

WILLIAMS & WILKINS
Baltimore • Hong Kong • London • Sydney

First published in Great Britain 1990 by
Edward Arnold, the educational, academic and medical publishing
division of Hodder and Stoughton Limited,
Mill Road, Dunton Green, Sevenoaks, Kent

Distributed in North America by
Williams & Wilkins
428 East Preston Street
Baltimore, MD 21202

Library of Congress Cataloging-in-Publication Data

Non-Hodgkin's lymphomas/edited by Ian T. Magrath,
     p.   cm.
  ISBN 0–683–05895–9
  1. Lymphomas. I. Magrath, Ian.
  [DNLM: 1. Lymphoma, Non-Hodgkin's   WH 525 N8119]
  RC280.L9N659   1989
  616.99'442—dc20
  DNLM/DLC   89-14692
  for Library of Congress   CIP

Whilst the advice and information in this book is believed to be true and
accurate at the date of going to press, neither the authors nor the
publisher can accept any legal responsibility or liability for any error or
omissions made.

Typeset in 10/11 pt Palatino by Anneset, Weston-super-Mare
Printed and bound in Great Britain by
Butler & Tanner Ltd, London and Frome

CONTRIBUTORS

Dharam V Ablashi
Laboratory of Tumor Cell Biology, Division of
Cancer Etiology, National Cancer Institute,
Bethesda, Maryland, USA

Francisco Barriga
Departamento de Pediatria, Centenario Pontificia
Universidad Catolica de Chile, Santiago, Chile

Paul A Bunn Jr
Division of Medical Oncology, University of
Colorado Cancer Center and Health Sciences
Center, Denver, Colorado, USA

Fernando Cabanillas
Section of Lymphomas, MD Anderson Cancer
Center, Houston, Texas, USA

Paul J Cohen
Department of Pathology, Hartford Hospital,
Hartford, Connecticut, USA

Carlo M Croce
Fels Institute for Cancer Research and Molecular
Biology, Temple University, Philadelphia,
Pennsylvania, USA

Riccardo Dalla-Favera
Department of Pathology, College of Physicians
and Surgeons, Columbia University, New York,
USA

A H Filipovich
Immunodeficiency Cancer Registry, University of
Minnesota Hospitals, Minneapolis, Minnesota,
USA

Richard I Fisher
Hematology/Oncology Section, Loyola University
School of Medicine, Maywood, Illinois and Hines
Veterans Administration Hospital, Hines, Illinois,
USA

Kenneth A Foon
Division of Hematology/Oncology, Roswell Park
Memorial Institute, Buffalo, New York, USA

Arnold S Freedman
Division of Tumor Immunology, Dana Farber
Cancer Institute, Boston, Massachusetts, USA

G Frizzera
Department of Pediatric Immunology, University
of Minnesota Hospital, Minneapolis, Minnesota,
USA

Ellen R Gaynor
Hematology/Oncology Section, Loyola University
School of Medicine, Maywood, Illinois, USA

Eli Glatstein
Radiation Oncology Branch, Department of
Radiation, National Cancer Institute, Bethesda,
Maryland, USA

Jane Grayson
Department of Radiation Oncology, Alexandria
Hospital, Alexandria, Virginia, USA

Frank G Haluska
Department of Medicine, Massachusetts General
Hospital, Boston, Massachusetts, USA

Sandra J Horning
Division of Oncology, Stanford University School of Medicine, Stanford, California, USA

Klara Horvath
Radiology Department, Diagnostic Medical Imaging, Holy Cross Hospital, Silver Spring, Maryland, USA

Elaine S Jaffe
Laboratory of Pathology, Division of Cancer Biology and Diagnosis, National Cancer Institute, Bethesda, Maryland, USA

Sundar Jagannath
Department of Hematology Bone Marrow Transplantation, MD Anderson Cancer Center, Houston, Texas, USA

Marshall Kadin
Department of Pathology, Beth Israel Hospital, Boston, Massacusetts, USA

Mark Kaminski
Division of Hematology and Oncology, University of Michigan Hospitals, Ann Arbor, Michigan, USA

Daniel M Knowles
Department of Pathology, Columbia University, New York, New York, USA

Ray Lamb
Department of Hematology/Oncology, McLeod Cancer and Blood Center, Johnson City, Tennessee, USA

Elaine C Lee
Medicine Branch, Division of Cancer Treatment, National Cancer Institute, Bethesda, Maryland, USA

Dan L Longo
Biological Response Modifiers Program, NCI Frederick Cancer Research Facility, National Cancer Institute, Frederick, Maryland, USA

Ian Magrath
Pediatric Branch, Division of Cancer Treatment, National Cancer Institute, Bethesda, Maryland, USA

Michael S McGrath
Department of Medicine, San Francisco General Hospital, San Francisco, California, USA

A Mertens
Department of Pediatric Immunology, University of Minnesota Hospital, Minneapolis, Minnesota, USA

Lee M Nadler
Division of Tumor Immunology, Dana Farber Cancer Institute, Boston, Massachusetts, USA

Antonino Neri
Department of Pathology, College of Physicians and Surgeons, Columbia University, New York, New York, USA

Ronald Neumann
Clinical Center, Nuclear Medicine Department, National Cancer Institute, Bethesda, USA

Augusto Pedrazzini
Serbizio Oncologico, Ospedale san Giovanni, Bellinzonr, Switzerland

Thierry Philip
Centre Leon Berard, Lyon, France

B Ramot
Institute of Hematology, The Chaim Sheba Medical Center, Tel-Hashomer, Israel

G Rechavi
Institute of Hematology, The Chaim Sheba Medical Center, Tel-Hashomer, Israel

L Robison
Department of Pediatrics, University of Minnesota Hospital, Minneapolis, USA

Mark S Roth
Department of Hematology/Oncology, University of Michigan, Ann Arbor, Michigan, USA

S Zaki Salahuddin
Laboratory of Tumor Cell Biology, Division of Cancer Etiology, National Cancer Institute, Bethesda, Maryland, USA

John Sandlund
Department of Hematology/Oncology, St. Jude Children's Research Hospital, Memphis, Tennessee, USA

R Shapiro
Department of Pediatric Immunology, University of Minnesota Hospital, Minneapolis, Minnesota, USA

Yoshihide Tsujimoto
Department of Pathology, The Wistar Institute,
Philadelphia, Pennsylvania, USA

Jacqueline Whang-Peng
Medical Branch, National Cancer Institute,
Bethesda, Maryland, USA

Wyndham Wilson
Medicine Branch, Division of Cancer Treatment,
National Cancer Institute, Bethesda, Maryland,
USA

Dennis H Wright
Department of Pathology, Southampton General
Hospital, Southampton, UK

John L Ziegler
School of Medicine, VA Medical Center, University
of California, San Francisco, California, USA

PREFACE

The exponential increase in scientific knowledge which has occurred throughout this century has dramatically changed the face of medicine. While the treatment of bacterial infections provides one of the most dramatic success stories, the broad compass of scientific progress can have had no greater impact than it has in the field of cancer.

Modern diagnostic methods include the use of computerized tomography, magnetic resonance imaging, radionuclide scanning, immunophenotyping, cytogenetics and, increasingly, molecular biology. Conventional treatment currently includes an array of the most sophisticated surgical, radiotherapeutic and pharmacological techniques, while experimental therapy is designed to explore the utility of a broad range of 'biological response modifiers' (BRMs), i.e. molecules which have an effect on cell differentiation or proliferation either by influencing host cellular regulatory mechanisms, or by acting directly on tumour cells via pathways which are utilized by normal cells. Such BRMs include monoclonal antibodies and various cytokines such as interleukin-2 and interferons, the latter frequently produced by means of recombinant DNA technology. In the laboratory, progress towards understanding the pathogenesis of cancer has been made with the help of a wide variety of advanced technologies encompassing the fields of biochemistry, immunology and molecular genetics.

One of the groups of tumours which has benefited the most, or, perhaps more accurately, which has provided the most fertile soil for progress, has been the non-Hodgkin's lymphomas. Yet paradoxically, the current therapeutic success which has been achieved with malignant non-Hodgkin's lymphomas is the result of empirical studies carried out over the last 25 years, and so far, little therapeutic benefit has been gained from recent progress in understanding the genetic and biochemical abnormalities of the tumour cell. Similarly, knowledge of the mechanisms of drug-induced cytotoxicity or drug resistance and of the regulation of cellular growth and differentiation has yet to provide tangible benefit to the patient. It seems highly probable, however, that in the near future this burgeoning growth of the science of oncology will have developed to the point where it will begin to have considerable impact upon the management of patients with malignant lymphomas. Moreover it is likely that therapeutic advances of considerable magnitude will be seen, whereby more specific biochemical targets will be utilized with a resultant increase in therapeutic efficacy and decrease in toxicity. At the same time, we must accept that our present concepts of disease entities are likely to change considerably. New tools will enable us to perceive similarities and differences hitherto unrecognized. Yet the old, as always, will continue to exist beside the new, and the transition will be gradual.

Nomenclature is likely, for the foreseeable future, to continue to be confusing, since it will derive from an increasing number of perspectives and disciplines and, in the absence of international agreement, multiple terms will coexist with varying degrees of synonymity. This process has occurred throughout history, although at markedly different rates in different eras. We live in the most rapidly changing era that mankind has ever experienced, and as such must be more willing than our forebears to give up outmoded concepts, and replace, where necessary, the familiar with the unfamiliar. But this is a small price to pay for the rewards of witnessing, in the course of a professional lifetime, the transition from a purely descriptive morphological view of lymphomas to one which encompasses an understanding of the precise nature of the cell of origin and of the genetic and biochemical changes which lead to malignant behaviour.

This book attempts to convey something of the excitement of the era in which we live, and to deal with the malignant non-Hodgkin's lymphomas, wherever possible, from a biological perspective rather than from a purely clinical and therapeutic one. As a consequence, a large proportion of the book is devoted to the nature of the diseases themselves, and their pathogenesis, representing the foundation upon which future diagnostic and treatment approaches will be built. As such, the practicing oncologist, and even more, the clinical researcher responsible for the design and analysis of clinical trials, will need to become familiar with the broad range of techniques currently available for the characterization of the non-Hodgkin's lymphomas.

I Magrath

1989

CONTENTS

CHAPTER 1

THE NON-HODGKIN'S LYMPHOMAS: AN INTRODUCTION

Ian Magrath

Definitions and pathogenetic considerations

The non-Hodgkin's lymphomas are neoplasms of the component cells of the immune system and their precursors.[1] While, as a group, these tumours have many features in common, they also reflect the diversity of their normal counterpart cells and exhibit a wide range of immunological and biological characteristics. Particularly striking are the differences in the natural history of the *untreated* patient. Some patients with low grade lymphomas, defined according to the National Cancer Institute (NCI) Working Formulation (*see* Chapter 4), may remain well for many years with minimal or no treatment, while within the high grade group, the untreated patient may sometimes have a lifespan measured only in weeks. Morphologically, the cells of the non-Hodgkin's lymphomas bear sufficient resemblance to their normal counterpart cells that a diagnosis of malignant lymphoma does not stem from abnormal cytology *per se*. Although atypical cells may be seen, diagnosis depends more upon the finding of large numbers of cells with similar cytological characteristics – infiltrating or destroying the normal lymphoid tissue architecture, or invading other tissues which normally lack organized lymphoid tissue. The morphology of the cells is critically important, however, to the determination of the subtype of lymphoma.

There is no precise definition of malignant lymphoma which is universally accepted, and although many lymphomas meet the criteria that have been proposed as indicating a malignant tumour, others lurk in the borderland between benign lymphoproliferation and true malignant neoplasia. Lymphoproliferative processes arising in organ transplant recipients, or superimposed on chronic inflammatory diseases often provide particular difficulties in this respect. At a practical level, however, it is less important to designate a disease as a malignant neoplasm than to have a clear idea of its natural history when untreated, and the most effective available therapy. Certain clinical characteristics, such as rapid progression, may dictate the initiation of treatment approaches used for malignant lymphomas even if some criteria, normally considered as indicating neoplasia (such as monoclonality or the presence of a cytogenetic abnormality), are lacking. In such circumstances, semantic debates are out of place. Nevertheless, understanding the pathological nature of any given disease is of importance to the development of new approaches to its treatment, or even prevention. In the absence of such understanding, therapeutic advances can only be made via empirical clinical trials – a relatively inefficient process which, although it has served us well to date, will hopefully be replaced by more rationally designed, more specific treatment. Recent advances in the understanding of the biology and biochemical derangements of the lymphoid tumours provide considerable optimism that this goal will ultimately be achieved.

Escape from growth regulation – implications for clonality

While a quintessential characteristic of malignant neoplasia in contradistinction to non-neoplastic lymphoproliferation may be difficult to define, one *sine qua non* of both is the partial or complete escape from the processes which normally regulate cellular proliferation. If extreme enough, no matter what the cause, inappropriate and progressive lymphoproliferation will result in the death of the patient because of interference with the function of other organs, or physical disruption of vital structures. Escape from growth control results from either a defect in the external regulatory mechanism itself or an intrinsic defect in a cell's ability to respond to regulatory signals (or to avoid being killed by cytotoxic T-cells). These two very different types of derangement provide a convenient and logical means of defining neoplastic and non-neoplastic lymphoproliferation (Table 1.1).

Defects in the host's ability to regulate the proliferation of lymphoid cells (usually cells infected by a virus) resulting from inherited or acquired immunodeficiency, imply no intrinsic abnormality in the proliferating cells themselves. Hence the proliferating cells do not conform to our modern concept of a neoplasm. The presence of intrinsic cellular defects, which of necessity are ultimately at a genetic level, might appropriately be considered as true neoplasia. Indeed, non-random genetic abnormalities are usually detectable at a cytogenetic level in malignant lymphomas (*see* Chapter 5). Failure to detect such abnormalities may be because present cytogenetic methods are not sufficiently sensitive, or because the defect lies at a molecular rather than at a chromosomal level. The development of a genetic change able to cause neoplasia is sufficiently rare that it is likely to occur in only a small number of individuals in the population. It is not

Table 1.1 Comparison between neoplastic and non-neoplastic lymphoproliferation

Neoplastic	*Non-neoplastic*
Pathogenesis	
Somatic genetic abnormality(s)	No genetic abnormality
Host immunodeficiency not essential	Host immunodeficiency essential
May evolve from non-neoplastic lymphoproliferation	
Histology	
Variety of histologies	Usually immunoblastic. Polymorphic
Immunophenotype	
B- or T-cell	Predominantly B-cell
Clonality	
Monoclonal	Polyclonal or oligoclonal
Virus infection	
May have a role in some neoplasms	Often has an essential role
Prognosis and treatment	
Fatal if untreated	May be fatal if untreated
Requires chemotherapy and may benefit from surgery and/or radiotherapy	May respond to reversal of immunosuppression
	Treatment would logically involve biological agents
	Antiviral agents may be of value. Chemotherapy or radiotherapy may be necessary

surprising, therefore, that 'true' lymphomas are essentially always monoclonal, i.e. they arise from a single cell in which an appropriate genetic change occurred. It is worth stressing that the monoclonality itself is not an essential aspect of neoplasia, only a reflection of the rarity of the events which cause it.

Lymphoproliferations in which there is no somatic genetic change may still result in the death of a patient, if extreme (witness fatal infectious mononucleosis), but because the proximate cause is a defect in the regulation of proliferation of a whole subgroup of lymphoid cells, these processes are almost always polyclonal. Frequently, however, as happens to polyclonal cell populations *in vitro*, a small number of clones will eventually predominate in the population, so that such processes may be described as oligoclonal. These predominant clones, however, may comprise only a small fraction of the population, while the remainder of the cells consist of thousands, or even millions of clones. In patients with human immunodeficiency virus (HIV) infection, oligoclonality of B-cells has been described in lymph nodes both before and after the induction of small non-cleaved lymphomas. The latter have monoclonal rearrangements of the oncogene c-*myc*, and appear to have arisen from one of the few dominant clones in the population.[2] This observation emphasizes the value of using the rearrangement of a non-lineage specific gene to measure tumour clonality wherever possible, and is also an example of a second phenomenon – the emergence of a true lymphoma from a lymphoproliferative process.

Frequent involvement of antigen receptor genes in chromosomal translocations in lymphoid neoplasia – relevance to epidemiology

In lymphoid cells in which rearrangement of T-cell receptor genes and immunoglobulin genes (involving the breaking and rejoining of a DNA strand) is a part of the normal process of lymphocyte differentiation, chromosomal translocations frequently occur within or close to these lineage specific genes, and may sometimes be a consequence of 'mistakes' in the process of physiological gene rearrangement (*see* Chapter 6). Because of this, it is not difficult to imagine a number of factors which could influence the likelihood of the occurrence of a genetic abnormality. An increase in the size of the cell population from which a particular subtype of lymphoma can evolve, for example, will increase the chances of a genetic error arising, *particularly* if the generation of this cell population implies an increased frequency of physiological gene rearrangements. This explains the development of true lymphomas superimposed upon pre-existing lymphoproliferations such as occurs in inherited or acquired immunodeficiencies and immunoblastic lymphadenopathy. Even without such an increase in a cell compartment size, situations in which DNA damage is increased, or the process of DNA repair is impaired predispose to the development of genetic abnormalities and hence the development of neoplasia, particularly lymphoid neoplasia (perhaps because of the necessity for differentiating lymphoid cells to undergo physiological genetic rearrangements). These situations include exposure to irradiation or some chemotherapeutic agents, which increase DNA damage, and certain inherited syndromes, such as ataxia telangiectasia, Bloom's syndrome and Fanconi's syndrome in which there is impaired ability to repair DNA. Clearly, in extreme situations in which the chances of a genetic error are markedly increased, more than one tumour, i.e. more than one transformational event, may develop in a single individual. We have described a patient with HIV infection, for example, who developed two clonally discrete lymphomas separated in time by about 3 years.[3] Thus clonality, although often helpful, is not an absolute means of distinguishing true neoplasia from non-neoplastic lymphoproliferation.

The role of virus infections

Virus infections of lymphoid cells may induce lymphoproliferation via either of the two primary mechanisms discussed above. The expression of viral genes may influence the expression of cellular genes involved in proliferation as is the case with Epstein–Barr virus (EBV), human B-cell lymphotrophic virus

(HBLV or HHV-6) and human T-cell lympho-trophic virus-I (HTLV-I). Such virus–induced lymphoproliferation, e.g. infectious mononucleosis, is normally readily controlled by the host's regulatory mechanisms and as such provides no continuing threat to health. However, in the presence of immunodeficiency, which could be the consequence of an inherited defect, a virus infection (e.g. HIV infection) or drug treatment, the lymphoproliferation may itself be fatal, or it may predispose to the development of a genetic change, thus evolving into a true lymphoma. It also remains possible, as is the case in animal lymphomas and leukaemias, that virus infection itself may be sufficient to induce neoplasia, either because of the introduction of a viral oncogene, or because of insertion of the proviral genome, with its accompanying transcriptional enhancing elements, in the vicinity of a cellular proto-oncogene, resulting in enhanced transcription of the oncogene. This mechanism of oncogene activation is known as insertional mutagenesis. It is of interest to note that if virus infection can cause neoplasia without the need for other genetic events (as with the acutely transforming retroviruses, which carry oncogenes and cause rapidly developing tumours in animals) such tumours, because of the large number of virus–infected cells, will be polyclonal. To date, such a phenomenon has not been described in humans.

These considerations provide a conceptual basis for understanding the epidemiology of the non-Hodgkin's lymphomas. It would appear that there is likely to be a 'basal rate' of lymphoma occurrence – a reflection of the rate at which random genetic errors occurring in lymphoid cells may happen to be of such a nature as to result in abnormal lymphoproliferation. This 'basal rate' will be much higher in kindreds where inherited defects in DNA repair are present, in patients exposed to drugs or radiation therapy which increase DNA damage and in individuals in whom the size of potential 'target' cell populations is increased as a consequence of inherited or acquired immunodeficiency[4,5] (*see* Chapter 9).

Children presumably encounter new antigens more frequently, and must generate an immunological repertoire of specific responses. Thus, the lymphoid cell mass in a child contains a higher proportion of precursor cells (manifested as relatively larger thymus size and larger bone marrow volume). It is not surprising, therefore, that lymphomas in children usually originate from genetic changes occurring in precursor cells. Age-specific incidence may also vary as a consequence of the duration of exposure to an environmental agent which significantly elevates the risk of lymphoid neoplasia.

Finally, the spectrum of environmental antigens and mitogens, including microorganisms and chemical exposure will influence the size of individual subpopulations of lymphoid cells and alter the risk of the development of particular subtypes of lymphoma. Examples of this include the predisposition to B-cell lymphomas, particularly small non-cleaved lymphomas in patients infected by HIV, the increased incidence of lymphomas in individuals exposed to organic solvents, e.g. phenoxy acids, chlorophenols and hydantoins,[4,5] the high incidence of small non-cleaved lymphomas in Africa, and the high incidence of follicular lymphomas in Europe and the USA.

Characterization and classification of non-Hodgkin's lymphomas

The major advances in the understanding of the surface and functional characteristics of normal lymphocytes have led to similar progress in our ability to characterize the neoplasms of lymphoid cells. Lymphomas retain the characteristics of their normal counterpart cells to a greater or lesser extent and can be classified on this basis, e.g. their ability to reproduce the same cytoarchitectonics (follicular versus diffuse), cell size (small or large), nuclear characteristics (cleaved or non-cleaved, convoluted or cerebriform) and their immunological characteristics (T- or B-cell) (*see* Chapter 4). In addition, the presence of cytogenetic abnormalities and, at another level, molecular genetic abnormalities, may be a particularly valuable method of classifying lymphomas, since the genetic changes are critical to pathogenesis (*see* Chapter 6). An additional characteristic which should be sought is the presence of viral genomes in the tumour cells, although at the present time it is not known whether viral genes are directly relevant to malignant transformation or to the maintenance of the transformed state (*see* Chapter 11). The most accurate definition of lymphoma type is one which includes all of these characteristics. In the case of molecular abnormalities, which are unique to the malignant clone, methods of detection have become sufficiently sensitive that the presence of neoplastic cells in some tissues can be detected in the absence of morphological (microscopic) evidence. The value of this in patient follow-up is discussed in Chapter 7.

Incidence and mortality

The non-Hodgkin's lymphomas account for approximately 3–5 per cent of the deaths from all malignant neoplasms in the more developed countries (and a similar proportion of estimated new cases), but a more variable percentage in other world regions.[6,7,8] In the USA, non-Hodgkin's lymphoma was estimated to be the eighth cancer in order of incidence in 1987 and the sixth in order of mortality. Incidence rates of non-Hodgkin's lymphoma adjusted to a world standardized population (International Classification of Diseases categories 200 plus 202) for selected registries reporting to the International Agency for Research on Cancer during sequential time periods are shown in Table 1.2. Comparison of these figures with more recent data clearly show the increase in incidence and rank order that has occurred in the USA (*see* Table 1.3). Similar increases have occurred in other Western countries, but the lower incidence in some East European countries (such as the DDR and Czechoslovakia[7]) is interesting and, at this moment in time, is unexplained. The proportion of all deaths due to non-Hodgkin's lymphoma, and the mortality rates in selected countries derived from World Health Organization figures for 1984 and 1985 are shown in Fig. 1.1. Reasons for the variation in the mortality rates include differences in incidence of subtypes of lymphoma, as well as

differences in treatment in different parts of the world. It is well recognized, for example, that the frequency of follicular lymphomas is much lower in most of the less developed countries and Japan.

Because of the many available classification schemes for the non-Hodgkin's lymphomas there is a great deal of difficulty in comparing the incidence or frequency of the histological subtypes of lymphoma in different parts of the world. The differences in overall incidence in various countries may well be caused by differences in only one or two subtypes, rather than a general increase or decrease in all subtypes. To investigate these differences further, it will be important to standardize the classification schemes used by registries. Information is available from the Surveillance Epidemiology and End Results (SEER) programme (which includes data collected from cancer registries covering 10 per cent of the population of the USA) and from the International Agency for Research on Cancer for overall incidence in some other world regions. For most of the world, however, apart from information derived from individual institutes, the relative proportions and incidence of different lymphoma subtypes in various populations is unknown. The incidence of lymphoma subtypes according to the Working Formulation is shown for the SEER data of the USA in Table 1.3. The percentage (i.e. based on actual numbers of cases rather than incidence) of each histological type of non-Hodgkin's lymphoma in centres in several countries participating in an international study organized by the International Agency for Research on Cancer is shown in Table 1.4.

Some caution should be applied to the interpretation of these figures, because information is largely derived from institutions rather than registries, and is not, except in the case of Hungary, population based. However, these data were reviewed by the same panel of histopathologists, so that the problem of reproducibility of the histological diagnoses is lessened. However, similarity of histological classification can be misleading since phenotypically different tumours may have the same histological features. Moreover, the relative

Table 1.2 Average annual incidence per 100 000 of non-Hodgkin's lymphomas in sequential time periods; data from selected registries[1]

	Incidence[2] 1973–1977		Incidence[2] 1978–1982	
	Male	*Female*	*Male*	*Female*
Brazil (Sao Paolo)	6.0	4.4	7.1	5.8
Canada (Ontario)	7.1	5.0	10.3	7.7
Jamaica (Kingston)	5.4	2.5	–	–
Netherlands (Antilles)	2.7	2.8	–	–
Puerto Rico	5.3	3.8	5.3	4.1
USA (San Francisco Bay Whites)	10.0	6.8	11.3	8.7
USA (San Francisco Bay Blacks)	8.1	4.1	7.7	5.0
USA (San Francisco Bay Chinese)	7.8	4.1	7.9	7.4
USA (Connecticut) White	8.0	6.7	10.5	7.5
USA (Atlanta Whites)	9.9	6.0	9.9	7.3
USA (Atlanta Blacks)	4.2	2.5	6.8	2.8
Czechoslovakia (Western Slovakia)	2.7	1.4	5.5	2.6
England (Birmingham and region)	4.8	3.5	5.3	3.2
England (South Thames region)	3.8	2.5	3.7	2.7
England (Trent region)	4.9	3.6	6.5	3.9
Finland	4.4	2.7	7.6	4.8
Federal Republic Germany (Hamburg)	3.1	2.2	3.5	2.3
France (Bas-Rhin)	5.3	3.3	7.5	5.5
German Democratic Republic	4.3	2.8	5.0	3.1
Sweden	6.3	4.3	7.4	4.9
Dakar (Senegal)	3.5	1.2	–	–
China (Shanghai)	3.6	2.1	3.5	2.1
India (Bombay)	3.2	1.7	3.6	2.0
Israel, Jews born in USA or Europe	8.3	5.5	10.5	7.8
Japan (Fukuoka Prefecture)	4.3	2.2	–	–
Japan (Nagasaki City)	12.1	7.5	8.5	5.4
Japan (Osaka Prefecture)	3.8	1.9	5.0	2.5
Singapore (Chinese)	4.1	2.4	5.1	2.9
Singapore (Malay)	2.8	2.6	5.4	3.2
New Zealand (non-Maori)	6.8	5.0	7.2	5.1

[1]Data from[7,8]. Listings under 'lymphosarcoma etc.', ICD-8th 200 and 'other reticuloses', ICD-8th 202 have been combined.
[2]Most data is from within this time period. In some cases the data is for a shorter time period or extends outside this period.

proportions of the subtypes differ markedly with age, particularly in children versus adults, so that some of the differences in the frequency of subtypes in different populations are due to the age structure of the population rather than true differences in incidence. High grade lymphomas, for example, account for 28 per cent of non-Hodgkin's lymphoma in US patients less than 35 years old at diagnosis, and only 6–7 per cent of tumours in patients over 35. Low grade lymphomas, on the other hand, account for 37 per cent of non-Hodgkin's lymphoma in patients between the ages of 35 and 64 at diagnosis, but only 16 per cent of patients below the age of 35.[9] Low grade lymphomas are extremely rare in children. The proportions of subtypes of non-Hodgkin's lymphomas (actual numbers of cases registered at all ages) for the USA are shown in

NON-LEUKAEMIC LYMPHOID/HAEMOPOIETIC NEOPLASMS

PERCENTAGE OF ALL DEATHS

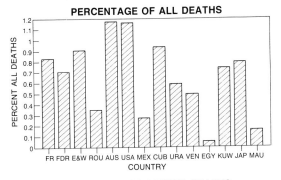

PERCENTAGE OF CANCER DEATHS

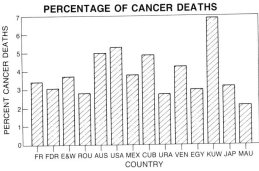

DEATHS PER 100 000 OF THE POPULATION

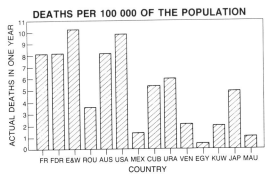

Fig. 1.1 Upper histogram: proportion of total annual deaths from non-Hodgkin's lymphoma in various countries in a single year. Middle histogram: percentage of cancer deaths in the same year. Lower histogram: mortality rate per 100 000 of the population from non-Hodgkin's lymphomas in the same year.

Percentages and mortality rates were calculated from figures available in *World Health Statistics, 1986* for the years 1984 or 1985 for the disease category, 'lymphoid and haemopoietic malignancies other than Hodgkin's

disease and leukaemias'. Available population estimates from the same source were made within 2 years of the mortality statistics. Countries include France (FR), the Federal Republic of Germany (FDR), England and Wales (E & W), Romania (ROU), Australia (AUS), the USA, Mexico (MEX), Cuba (CUB), Uruguay (URA), Venezuela (VEN), Egypt (EGY), Kuwait (KUW), Japan (JAP) and Mauritius (MAU).

Table 1.5. Of interest is the relatively lower proportion of small cleaved-cell follicular lymphomas in Blacks.

In the USA, the age-adjusted incidence of non-Hodgkin's lymphoma in White males and females combined increased from 5.9 per 100 000 in 1950, to 13.1 per 100 000 in 1985 – an increase of 123 per cent. In this same time period the mortality increased from 2.9 per 100 000 to 5.9 per 100 000 – an increase of 100 per cent.[9] The increases in incidence (and mortality) occurred predominantly in persons aged 65 and over, perhaps due in part to improvements in diagnosis. Lesser increases in incidence occurred in those aged 35–64, but there has been little change in incidence among children and young adults.

During this same period the male:female ratio decreased from 1.4:1 to 1:1, indicating a slightly greater increase in incidence in females than in males. The lesser increase in mortality compared with incidence is the result of an improvement in the five-year relative survival rate (i.e. observed survival compared with the expected survival of persons in the US population similar to the patient group with respect to age, sex, race, and calendar year). The relative survival rate increased from 28 per cent between 1950 and 1954 to 49 per cent between 1979 and 1985.[9] These improvements in survival occurred mainly in young adults and children. Relative five-year survival rates by histology for patients diagnosed in 1979–80 are shown in Table 1.3.

The age-specific incidence and mortality rates of non-Hodgkin's lymphoma in the USA are shown in Fig. 1.2. The progressive increase in the incidence of non-Hodgkin's lymphoma throughout life, which is readily apparent from these graphs, is seen in all world regions (Fig. 1.3), but the age at which the greatest number of cases occurs depends in part upon the age structure of the population. In the less developed countries, where there is a much higher proportion of young people, the peak age for the occurrence of non-Hodgkin's lymphoma is much lower than in the more developed countries. However, there are clearly differences in the age-specific incidence of non-Hodgkin's lymphoma in different parts of the world as the few selected graphs (see Fig. 1.3) show. In the USA, the highest number of cases among five-year age-groups occurred in 60–64 year-old males and 70–74 year-old females. In France, the Federal Republic of Germany, England and Wales, the USA and Japan, the greatest numbers of cases occurred above the age of 75 years; in

Australia and Japan the five-year periods 65–69 and 70–74 were approximately equal with regard to case numbers; in Mexico and Cuba peak numbers occurred between the ages of 65 and 74; in Romania, Uruguay, Venezuela, Mauritius and Kuwait peak numbers occurred between 55 and 64; while in Egypt the peak occurred between 45 and 54 years.[6]

Of interest is the difference in average annual incidence between Blacks and Whites in the USA. This is predominantly due to a relatively greater incidence in White males. In women, although the incidence in Blacks and Whites is very similar up to the age of 70 years, it is higher in Black women in the younger age groups. In men, on the other hand, the incidence is

Table 1.3 Incidence and relative survival rates at five years by the NCI working formulation (SEER data, Blacks and Whites, both sexes)

	Incidence				Survival (%)
	1977[1]	%[2]	1985[1]	%[2]	1979–80
Total	8.97		11.94		49.6
Low grade	2.31	25.75	3.14	26.30	63.7
Small lymphocytic	0.81	9.03	1.21	10.13	54.0
Follicular, small cleaved	1.17	13.04	1.30	10.89	68.6
Follicular, mixed small cleaved and large cell	0.32	3.57	0.63	5.28	68.5
Intermediate grade	4.87	54.29	5.81	48.66	41.9
Follicular, large cell	0.16	1.78	0.36	3.02	67.4
Diffuse, small cleaved	1.79	19.96	1.04	8.71	42.1
Diffuse, mixed small and large cell	0.63	7.02	0.99	8.29	44.7
Diffuse, large cell	2.29	25.53	3.42	28.64	39.1
High grade	0.37	4.12	1.14	9.55	34.9
Large cell, immunoblastic	0.10	1.11	0.58	4.86	35.2
Lymphoblastic	0.07	0.78	0.15	1.26	33.6[3]
Small non-cleaved; Burkitt's	0.19	2.12	0.41	3.43	36.0
Unclassified	1.42	15.83	1.85	15.49	–

NCI, National Cancer Institute, Bethesda, Maryland; SEER, Surveillance, Epidemiology and End Results programme
[1]Year of diagnosis.
[2]Percentage of total incidence per 100 000 for each diagnostic category. This indicates the relative incidence rather than the actual proportion of cases of each subtype.
[3]Figure is for the period between 1977 and 1984. There were insufficient numbers in 1979–1980 to make an accurate estimate.

Table 1.4 Relative proportions of different histological subtypes of NHL in various countries

	Percentage			
	H	*J*	*P*	*Pa*
Low grade				
Small lymphocytic	39	3	7	18
Follicular, small cleaved	4	3	4	8
Follicular, mixed small cleaved and large cell	2	3	2	6
Intermediate grade				
Follicular, large cell	4	9	2	6
Diffuse, small cleaved	5	1.5	2	4
Diffuse, mixed small and large cell	10	25	21	12
Diffuse, large cell	12	11	16	14
High grade				
Large cell, immunoblastic	6	20	15	6
Lymphoblastic	4	1.5	6	6
Small non-cleaved; Burkitt's	2	6	4	10
Unclassified	8	17	18	12
Other	5	0	6	0

NHL, Non-Hodgkin's lymphoma
Data for this table were assembled by Dr O'Conor. All material except that from the USA was part of an international study organized by the International Agency for Research on Cancer. All material was reviewed by a panel of experienced haematopathologists, headed by Dr O'Conor, at the International Agency's Research Centre in Lyon, France.
H, Hungarian National Lymphoma Registry, University of Pecs and National Oncological Institute, Semmelweise Institute, Budapest (330 patients); J, Aichi Cancer Centre Nagoya and Kyoto University Hospital Kyoto, Japan (65 patients); P, Instituto Nacional de Enfermedades Neoplasticas, Peru (165 patients); Pa, Armed Forces Institute of Pathology, Rawalpindi, Pakistan (51 patients).

uniformly higher at all ages in Whites than in Blacks, the difference being particularly noticeable above the age of 70. The greater differences between Blacks and Whites above the age of 70 may be explained by the possibility that underdiagnosis in the elderly occurs more often in Blacks, but this does not explain the differences at younger ages. It is interesting that the incidence in Black males and females between 1981 and 1985 is similar to that in White males and females between 1947 and 1950. These data suggest that environmental factors are mainly responsible for the differences in Blacks and Whites, and it seems likely that a continuing increase in the incidence of non-Hodgkin's lymphoma in Blacks will be seen, as differences in lifestyle are lessened. These data also suggest that differences in the incidence of non-Hodgkin's lymphoma would be found in different socioeconomic strata of the population. Further epidemiological investigations are clearly warranted.

Clinical features and treatment

Just as malignant lymphomas resemble their normal counterpart cells morphologically, they retain, to a degree, their functional attributes. In practice this means that there is a tendency for subtypes of lymphomas to have characteristic clinical features, i.e. sites of presentation, and

Table 1.5 Frequency (percentage) of different histological subtypes of NHL in the USA (SEER data)

| | Whites[1] | | Blacks[2] | |
| | Time period | | | |
	1977–81	1982–85	1977–81	1982–85
Low grade	26.6	26.2	20.5	18.0
Small lymphocytic	9.3	9.5	11.8	10.9
Follicular, small cleaved	12.9	11.6	5.7	5.1
Follicular, mixed small cleaved and large cell	4.4	5.1	3.0	2.0
Intermediate	50.7	47.2	48.5	45.1
Follicular, large cell	1.9	2.5	1.3	2.0
Diffuse, small cleaved	16.4	9.9	18.5	10.0
Diffuse, mixed small and large cell	6.3	7.5	6.5	7.3
Diffuse, large cell	26.1	27.3	22.2	25.8
High grade	4.5	9.1	5.4	10.8
Large cell, immunoblastic	1.6	4.7	2.3	6.0
Lymphoblastic	0.7	1.4	0.9	2.5
Small non-cleaved; Burkitt's	2.2	3.0	2.2	2.3
Unclassified	18.2	17.4	25.1	26.0

[1]Based on the 11 089 White males and females included in the SEER data between 1977 and 1981 and the 11 045 White males and females included between 1982 and 1985.
[2]Based on the 541 Black males included in the SEER data between 1977 and 1981 and the 604 Black males included in the data between 1982 and 1985.

complications produced by involvement or compression of surrounding structures. In some cases there are marked differences in clinical presentations, e.g. lymphoblastic lymphomas frequently present with an anterior superior mediastinal (thymic) mass whereas follicular lymphomas usually present with peripheral lymph node involvement. However, there is much overlap, since ultimately all lymphomas arise from lymphoid tissue, including the primary and secondary lymphoid organs, i.e. thymus, bone marrow, central and peripheral lymph nodes, spleen and mucosal-associated lymphoid tissue (primarily that of the alimentary canal). Involvement of the bone marrow (and consequently the peripheral blood) sometimes creates semantic problems, and uncertainty as to whether the disease is a leukaemia or lymphoma. Such a distinction is in many ways artificial. Diseases which arise in haematopoietic precursor cells predominantly present as leukaemias, but both precursors of T- and B-cells arise in the marrow, and mature lymphoid cells also circulate through the marrow. Thus, the most important considerations with respect to diagnosis and the determination of optimal treatment are the cell type and tumour burden. The terms leukaemia and lymphoma do not precisely define subsets of lymphoid neoplasms, and while it is unlikely that they will fall into disuse, their failings as taxonomic nomenclature should be recognized.

Since normal lymphocytes migrate through the body as part of their surveillance function, the vast majority of lymphomas rapidly become widely disseminated. By the time sufficient neoplastic cells have accumulated to produce symptoms, it is probable that more than 90 per cent of non-Hodgkin's lymphomas are disseminated (i.e. have more than a single

AVERAGE ANNUAL INCIDENCE AND MORTALITY RATES OF NHL
PER 100 000 POPULATION, USA, 1981-85

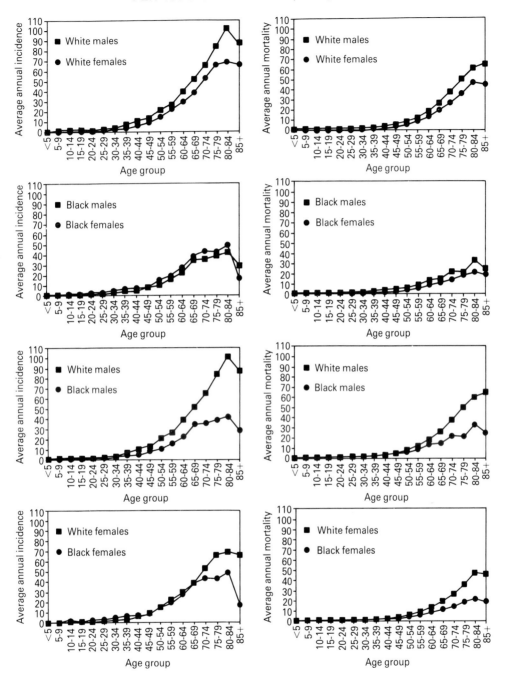

Fig. 1.2 Age-specific incidence and mortality rates for non-Hodgkin's lymphoma in the USA during the period 1981–85. (Data obtained from[9].) Average annual incidence rates are shown for White males and females on the curves on the left side of the figure, and average annual mortality rates for corresponding populations on the right.

AVERAGE ANNUAL INCIDENCE RATES OF NHL
PER 100 000 POPULATION

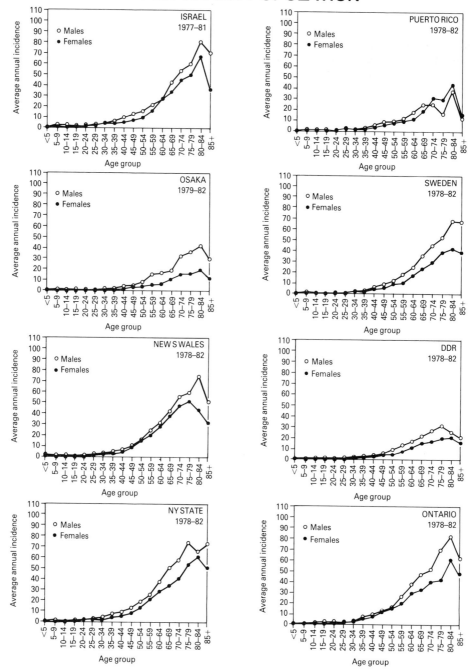

Fig. 1.3 Age-specific average annual incidence rates for Israel (all Jews) Puerto Rico, Osaka, Japan, Sweden, New South Wales, Australia, the German Democratic Republic (DDR), New York State (less New York city) and the province of Ontario. (Data obtained from the relatively low incidences in Osaka, Puerto Rico and the DDR are apparent).

tumour mass). This, of course, has implications for treatment, since radiation or surgery, directed only at known sites of disease, almost never results in cure, except in a proportion of the small group of patients with stage I disease, or an even smaller proportion of patients with stage II disease. Thus, systemic treatment, i.e. chemotherapy, must be considered the primary treatment modality, although surgery and radiation may have adjunctive roles.

Treatment must take into account the lymphoma subtype, since chemotherapy is, at present, largely palliative in the low grade lymphomas but is given with curative intent in the intermediate and high grade lymphomas. Drug regimens and schedules employed may thus differ markedly. Moreover, patients with intermediate and high grade lymphomas with a large tumour burden are very likely to develop the biochemical complications resulting from rapid tumour lysis, described in Chapter 15, which require appropriate management. Such patients may also require more intensive therapy than patients with a small tumour burden. Thus the steps involved in the management of patients with lymphoma include: the establishment, by biopsy, of as definitive a diagnosis as possible (including morphological characterization, and wherever feasible, immunophenotyping, cytogenetics and molecular studies); the determination of the extent of disease by a series of 'staging' investigations, (including history and clinical examinations, haematological and biochemical tests, radiological, radionuclide scintigraphic and sometimes magnetic resonance imaging, and additional endoscopic or biopsy procedures as indicated); the establishment of a plan for overall management, (including dealing with complications – sometimes necessary on an emergency basis prior to complete evaluation of the extent of disease); the selection of a treatment protocol; and the initiation of chemotherapy. Detailed explanations to the patient as to the nature of the disease and the therapeutic options, and the obtaining of consent for procedures and treatment according to a research protocol, are standard practice in most Western countries.

Future goals

An enormous amount has been learnt about the non-Hodgkin's lymphomas in the last 20 years, such that today we are able to ask more sophisticated questions. It now seems possible that a reasonably detailed understanding of the pathogenic events which lead to the development of each type of lymphoid neoplasm will eventually be obtained. Moreover, it is highly probable that this information will lead to the development of totally novel approaches to treatment, and possibly to prevention. In the meantime, efforts must continue to improve our use of available therapeutic modalities in order that the proportion of patients cured (predominantly patients with intermediate and high grade lymphomas) is increased. Although the treatment of patients who relapse is rather unsatisfactory, since the aim is to use optimal therapy *per primum*, research protocols for the treatment of patients with recurrent disease serve a useful purpose in that the efficacy of new drugs or new drug combinations, as well as different dosages and schedules of widely used drugs can be explored. Such patients also represent the primary patient population for the evaluation of approaches entailing the use of autologous or allogeneic bone marrow transplantation and biological response modifiers such as cytokines and monoclonal antibodies.

Relatively little progress has been made in the treatment of the low grade lymphomas, but several new approaches are being explored, including bone marrow transplantation, and the use of biological response modifiers. Ultimately, it is to be hoped that truly tumour-specific treatment can be developed, with minimal effect on normal tissues and organs. For this to become feasible, it is necessary to detect and exploit the biochemically unique aspects of lymphoma cells. This will require continued efforts to understand the genetic and consequent biochemical derangements of the lymphoid tumours. In some lymphomas such unique characteristics have already been identified (*see* Chapter 6) and hopefully, in the ensuing years, we shall witness the development of treatment approaches directed towards the root cause of the neoplastic behaviour. While it is not possible to predict with any accuracy whether and when such novel treatments will become a reality, it is indeed a mark of progress that approaches of this kind can be discussed in pragmatic terms (*see* Chapter 27) and pre-clinical experiments initiated.

References

1. Magrath IT. *Journal of the National Cancer Institute*. 1981; **67**, 501–14.
2. Pelicci P-G, Knowles DM, Arlin ZA, *et al. Journal of Experimental Medicine*. 1986; **164**, 2049–60.
3. Barriga F, Lee E, Whang-Pheng J, *et al. Blood*. 1988; **72**, 792–5.
4. Miller RW. In: Magrath IT, O'Conor GT, Ramot B eds. *Pathogenesis of Leukemias and Lymphomas.*
Environmental Influences. New York: Raven Press, 1984: 201–5.
5. Finch S. In: Magrath IT, O'Conor GT, Ramot B eds. *Pathogenesis of Leukemias and Lymphomas. Environmental Influences.* New York: Raven Press, 1984: 207–23.
6. World Health Organization. *World Health Statistics*, Geneva: 1986.
7. Waterhouse J, Muir C, Shanmugaratnam K, Powell J eds. *Cancer Incidence in Five Continents.* Vol. IV. Lyon, IARC Scientific Publications, 1982.
8. Muir C, Waterhouse J, Mack T, Powell J, Whelan S eds. *Cancer Incidence in Five Continents.* Vol V. Lyon, IARC Scientific Publications, 1987.
9. National Cancer Institute, Division of Cancer Prevention and Control, US Department of Health and Human Services, Public Health Service, National Institutes of Health. *1987 Annual Cancer Statistics Review*, Bethesda, 1988.

CHAPTER 2

HISTORICAL PERSPECTIVE: THE ORIGINS OF MODERN CONCEPTS OF BIOLOGY AND MANAGEMENT

Ian Magrath

Origins of modern concepts of malignant lymphomas

The foundations of modern pathology rest firmly upon the shoulders of Giovanni Morgagni (1682–1771), Marie Francois Xavier Bichat (1771–1802), Johannes Müller (1801–1858) and Rudolph Virchow (1821–1905). Morgagni initiated the science of the study of gross morbid anatomy, Bichat established the importance of tissues rather than organs as the matrix for disease processes, while Müller, utilizing the microscope extensively (which Bichat never did), began to base the classification of tumours on their histological appearance and made a number of seminal observations on the nature of cancer. But it is perhaps more to Virchow, a student of Müller, than to any other single individual that we owe the origins of our modern concepts of neoplastic disease.

As a young man, Virchow lived in an era when disease was generally considered to have a separate existence from the body, into which it could enter and live as a parasite. This idea was to change radically during the intellectual and political ferment of the mid-nineteenth century. Virchow himself espoused careful observation and experiment as the fundamental tools of pathology rather than the then prevalent tendency, particularly in Germany, to formulate unsupportable (and therefore frequently replaced) hypotheses. His emphasis on the value of the experimental approach followed the earlier examples of John Hunter (1728–1793) and

Claude Bernard (1813–1878). Perhaps Virchow's major contribution was to develop the concept of cellular pathology, based on the observations of Schleiden and Schwann (the latter also a student of Müller), who respectively demonstrated that the fundamental structural unit of plants, and animals, is the nucleated cell. Virchow's concept, whereby diseases are recognized as disorders in the functioning of cells, was expounded in a series of lectures in Berlin in the spring of 1858, which were subsequently assembled in a single volume entitled 'Cellular pathology'. Virchow also made important observations on the anatomy and function of the spleen and lymphoid tissues, and originated the terms *leukaemia* and *lymphoma*. His Berlin lecture series on malignant tumours, given during the winter of 1862 was published as 'Die krankhaften Geschwülste'.[1] Virchow's most distinguished pupil, Julius Cohnheim (1839–1884), was responsible for the first modern book on pathology, which emphasized the pathophysiology and experimental study of disease.

Hodgkin's disease and pseudoleukaemia

In the middle of the last century international communication was remarkably slow by modern standards and it is therefore not surprising that a number of separate concepts of lymphomas flourished in different parts of the world. Sporadic descriptions of generalized lymph node swelling of unknown cause, often associated with splenic enlargement, occur in the literature in the latter part of the eighteenth century and the first half of the nineteenth century, including those of Cruickshank, Hodgkin, Wunderlich, Wilkes and Trousseau.[2-6] Not surprisingly, several descriptive terms were used for this clinically or pathologically defined disease – in England, Hodgkin's disease (an eponym first used by Wilkes); in France, l'adenie; in Germany, Pseudoleukämie. The latter term, initiated by Cohnheim,[7] emphasized the lack of a high white blood cell count which had been observed in a clinically similar disease described by Virchow in 1845 as 'Weisses Blut'[8] and subsequently renamed 'Leukämie'. Craigie and Bennett had also observed the pathological state characterized by a very high white cell count, but had misinterpreted this as a form of suppuration of the blood.[9,10]

Each of these designations included the whole range of malignant lymphomas (both Hodgkin's and non-Hodgkin's lymphomas) as we know them today, and doubtless some non-neoplastic lymphadenopathies as well as acute leukaemias with low white blood cell counts. Initially they were clinical or gross pathological entities; histological subdivision had not been attempted. For example, in Osler's classic textbook of medicine, published in 1898, all lymphomas are included under the general term 'Hodgkin's disease', and Dreschfeld, in describing these syndromes in 1892, provided clinical subdivisions such as acute and chronic Hodgkin's disease, rather than an attempt to subdivide them on a morphological or histological basis.[11]

Lymphosarcoma

Localized lymph node swellings unrelated to a recognized disease entity such as tuberculosis, or to obvious pathology in the drainage area of a nodal group had also been recognized for some time. In Germany, such a disease usually fell under the rubric of 'Lymphosarkoma', a term with its origins in antiquity, for the word sarcoma was used in the second century by Galen to refer to any fleshy, superficial tumour. Kundrat classified Lymphosarkoma with the other sarcomas, i.e. cellular growths arising in

connective tissue, and separated it from 'lymphatic growths', a term he presumed applied to generalized lymphatic swelling.[12] In Kundrat's experience, Lymphosarkoma was confined to lymph nodes or lymphatic tissue in mucous membranes, although it tended to invade neighbouring tissues and could spread from its local origin to other lymph node groups. He referred to this progressive form as 'Lymphosarkomatosis', which he still considered, on clinical grounds (i.e. the evolution of the disease from a single site and the lack of truly widespread disease involving the liver and spleen), to be distinct from Pseudoleukämia, although his categories would clearly not correspond to any modern subdivisions (except perhaps clinical stages!).

Clearly, Lymphosarkomatosis as defined by Kundrat, like Cohnheim's Pseudoleukämia, included patients that would today be diagnosed as having Hodgkin's disease. In fact, his description of progressive anatomical involvement of other lymph node areas is more reminiscent of Hodgkin's disease than non-Hodgkin's lymphomas (which were later encompassed by the term lymphosarcoma). Moreover, some of Kundrat's major distinctions, such as invasion of the lymph node capsule and surrounding tissues, were subsequently shown to be present in both diseases when histology provided the basis for separation.

Not everybody agreed with Kundrat's views. Dreschfeld, for example, disagreed with Kundrat's opinion that Pseudolekämia and Lymphosarkoma were different diseases. He appeared to view all lymph node swellings as part of the same disease process, namely Hodgkin's disease, and did not even accept a subdivision into benign (lymphadenoma) and malignant (lymphosarcoma) forms. He did, however, recognize a more acute form of Hodgkin's disease, which he considered encompassed Kundrat's Lymphosarkoma and Lymphosarkomatosis, and a chronic form, which was more closely related to leukaemia, and therefore better called pseudoleukaemia.[11] The former was sometimes disseminated from the outset, the latter always.

This clinical era in the classification of malignant lymphomas was beset by similar problems to those encountered in the later descriptive histological period, prior to the concept of lymphomas as tumours of the immune system. The names applied to various 'diseases' had originated in several different countries, and could not be defined with precision because of the overlap in clinical features among what we now recognize as individual pathological entities. There is no doubt that these early attempts at classification bear little or no relationship to our current concepts of disease entities. But then, we should be scarcely better equipped today to produce a classification of lymphomas on clinical grounds alone.

Evolution of histological classification

Although Bichat is often considered to be the father of histology he made little or no use of the microscope, in spite of the clear indication of its potential value to the study of disease shown by the host of discoveries already made by its use. These included Malpighi's identification, in the seventeenth century, of kidney glomeruli and the splenic corpuscles that bear his name. It is probable that the prevailing concepts of disease, which were based on theories dating from the preclassical era rather than methodical observation and experiment, diverted the leading pathologists from recognizing the enormous gains to be realized from the microscopic study of diseased tissue, even after the onset of the era of pathological anatomy. It is worthy of note that Galen continued to exert sway until well into the eighteenth century. As late as 1842, Rokitansky's great *Handbuch der pathologischen Anatomie* made no use of histology.

However, after the discovery of the achromatic lens in the nineteenth century and the development of the concept of cells as the ultimate pathological unit, the stage was set for rapid progress. Virchow devoted a third of his book '*Cellular Pathology*' to normal histology, while his student Cohnheim was one of the pioneers of modern experimental pathology. The histopathological classification of diseases owes much to Jacob Henle (1809–1885), one of Müller's protégés who wrote the first text on microscopic histology, *Allgemeine Anatomie*, published in Leipzig in 1841. By this time, greatly improved techniques in the hardening, sectioning and staining of tissues had been developed.

The distinction between Hodgkin's disease and lymphosarcoma

The value of histological examination of lymphomas was not widely recognized until the twentieth century although many reports of histological appearances were published earlier than this; in 1858 Wunderlich described the histological appearance of some cases of Pseudoleukämia and mentioned the presence of giant cells.[4] However, it was the later reports of Sternberg, who described giant cells in what he considered to be 'a peculiar type of tuberculosis with the appearance of Pseudoleukämie',[13] and Dorothy Reed,[14] who refuted Sternberg's contention that the tubercle bacillus was causally involved in Hodgkin's disease, which led to the first histological separation of the lymphomas into Hodgkin's disease and non-Hodgkin's lymphomas (referred to as lymphosarcoma). The histological findings seemed to confirm previous suggestions, based on clinical and gross pathological grounds, that Hodgkin's disease (Pseudoleukämie) differed from Lymphosarkoma. Moreover, the variety of cell types in Hodgkin's disease and the apparent lack of effacement of the normal architecture of the lymph node, led to the conclusion that it was not a true malignancy but rather an inflammatory granulomatous lesion. Hence 'lymphosarcoma' became the common term for true neoplasms arising in lymphoid tissue, i.e. all tumours that we would now identify as non-Hodgkin's lymphomas.

This apparent confirmation of Kundrat's clinical impressions of a separation between Hodgkin's disease and lymphosarcoma was misleading since, as is apparent in retrospect, histology and clinical features did not separate the same groups of patients. In any event, the diagnosis of Pseudoleukämia gradually fell into disuse as the eponymous 'Hodgkin's disease' gained in popularity, perhaps because of the increasing influence of British medicine. Other terms used to describe lymph node swelling such as 'lymphadenoma' and 'lymphogranuloma' did persist, however, as synonyms for Hodgkin's disease[15], reflecting the view, stemming from Reed's paper, that Hodgkin's disease was not a neoplastic process at all.

Not all pathologists accepted this concept. Observing the same type of invasion of the lymph node capsule and surrounding tissue, the same degree of obliteration of the normal architecture, evidence of invasion and apparent spread by blood vessels as well as lymphatics, others considered that Hodgkin's disease, too, was a malignant condition.[16–18] In other words, they felt that Hodgkin's disease was merely a variety of lymphosarcoma, a view supported by the gradual merging of the histological features of the diseases at the end of the spectrum subsequently referred to by Jackson and Parker as Hodgkin's sarcoma.[19] At least some of the dissension doubtless resulted from the very small numbers of cases studied in these earlier descriptions. Gibbons concluded from a study of nine cases of Hodgkin's disease that malignant proliferation could occur from the cells of the germinal centres, the endothelium lining the sinuses and the reticulum cells of the connective tissue capsule and blood vessels.[18] He proposed that proliferation of all these tissues gave rise to the picture of Hodgkin's disease, but predominance of one or other would be more readily recognized as a sarcomatous process. The debate as to the nature of Hodgkin's disease and, therefore, its relationship to lymphosarcoma, continued until quite recently. Although few today would content that it is not a neoplastic condition, the origin of Reed-Sternberg cells has still not been completely resolved.

Reticulum cell sarcoma

By the early part of the twentieth century, histopathology was firmly established and in the ensuing years led to the recognition of new entities which fell under the rubric of lymphosarcoma. The different histological appearances were presumed to signify origins from different cellular components of lymph nodes, as proposed by Gibbons. Although no formal classification had been proposed, many pathologists had recognized that lymphosarcoma, i.e. what was left after the exclusion of lymphogranuloma (Hodgkin's disease), was probably a group of diseases, based on the variety of cell types that could be discerned. As expressed by Ewing in 1939, amidst the confusion, there was at least recognition of small cells and large cells.[20] In fact the terms 'lymphocytoma' and 'lymphoblastoma' were sometimes used to indicate the predominant cell size. Endothelial sarcoma or 'endothelioma of lymph nodes' was a term used by other pathologists to denote a tumour of larger cell type believed to arise from the endothelial lining cells of the lymph node sinuses.[21] Oberling, in France, used the terms 'reticulosarcoma' and 'reticuloendotheliosarcoma' in the context of a subset of bone tumours, described shortly before by Ewing, and which, he believed, arose in the reticuloendothelial tissue of bone marrow and had the same histogenesis as similar tumours arising in lymph nodes.[22] Roulet, in Germany, set out to characterize more precisely the third type of lymphosarcoma of lymph nodes, which he distinguished from the lymphocytic and lymphoblastic types and referred to as 'Retothelsarkom'.[23] He believed that this entity arose from the cells associated with the fibrous scaffolding of lymph nodes rather than from the endothelial lining of the lymph node sinuses, hence his preference for the elimination of the term 'reticuloendothelial sarcoma'.

The designation of a group of large cell tumours led some pathologists to limit use of the term 'lymphosarcoma' to the smaller cell varieties, but others continued to use the term to indicate all lymphomas other than Hodgkin's disease.

Giant follicular lymphoma

The occurrence of lymphomas with a follicular or nodular architecture had been recognized at least as early as 1912,[24] but came under serious consideration after the independent descriptions by Brill *et al.* and Symmers[25,26] of patients with lymphadenopathy and splenomegaly in which histological studies revealed enlarged lymphoid follicles. This disease, because of its generally protracted clinical course, also generated considerable controversy as to whether it was simply a chronic hyperplastic state, as originally believed to be the case by Brill *et al.* and Symmers, or a truly neoplastic condition. That it could evolve into a rapidly progressive malignant lymphoma was, however, accepted by all. Varying descriptions of the histology and clinical course of follicular lymphomas appear to reflect the range of tumours which fall under this rubric, and this, coupled to its relative rarity, made it difficult for any one individual to acquire a large experience. In fact, reports of series collected in the first half of this century suggest that follicular lymphoma comprised a considerably lower proportion of lymphoma cases than today, namely 4 per cent and 13 per cent of patients with non-Hodgkin's lymphoma in two large series reported in the USA.[27,28] Although this may reflect a truly lower incidence in the early part of this century, differences in diagnostic criteria or lack of referral to specialized centres could also account for the relatively low frequency in these series. Gall *et al.*[29] described four main histological forms of the disease which were quite close to present categories, types I, II and III being composed of follicles containing small cells, mixed small and large cells, and large cells respectively. Type IV referred to a variety in which there was a degree of confluence or rupture of follicles such that a diagnosis of follicular lymphoma was sometimes difficult. Such cases may have been in transition to diffuse lymphoma. It is interesting that the average duration of disease was roughly similar in all subtypes, but the duration after biopsy varied from almost 6 years in type I to about 2 years in types II and III (Table 2.1). These patients were treated almost exclusively with local kilovoltage radiation to 600 roentgens (R). Doses as high as 1800 R were occasionally used.

Histological classification schemes

The recognition of these additional histological subtypes of lymphoma paved the way for the classification scheme published by Gall and

Table 2.1 Survival (years) in patients with various histological types of follicular lymphoma, as reported in 1940[1]

Type	Duration prior to biopsy	Duration after biopsy	Total duration
I	2.0	5.7	7.7
II	3.6	3.2	6.8
III	4.1	1.8	5.9
IV	4.1	2.3	6.4

[1]From Gall *et al.*[29]

Mallory in 1942,[30] one of the first to be based on histology alone (Table 2.2). Since that time, and until very recently, histology has been the primary basis for classification, although the clinical features of the more recently recognized pathological entities such as Burkitt's lymphoma, lymphoblastic lymphoma (using the term in the sense of Nathwani and Rappaport,[31]) and adult T-cell leukaemia/lymphoma have been important in leading to their acceptance as separate tumours. Not surprisingly, a purely morphological schema untempered by any real knowledge of the functional nature of the cells which had become neoplastic was less than satisfactory, as indicated by the subsequent proliferation of alternative classification schemes. The lack of effective treatment (except radiation therapy for the relatively uncommon localized tumours) also hampered division into different prognostic groups based upon response to therapy and curability. Thus, until the development of an understanding of the compartments of the immune system at both functional and anatomical levels, and the development of effective therapy for some types of lymphoma, there was general agreement on only three major subdivisions of the non-Hodgkin's lymphomas or lymphosarcomas and some pathologists preferred a simple classification of this type:[32]

1. a group of tumours with a follicular architecture, resembling enlarged secondary lymphoid follicles. Patients with tumours in this category survived considerably longer than most other patients

Table 2.2 Evolution of histological classification systems

Custer and Bernhard	Gall and Mallory	Gall and Rappaport*	Rappaport*
	Lymphocytic	Lymphocytic, WD	Lymphocytic, WD
Lymphosarcoma	Lymphoblastic	Lymphocytic, PD	Lymphocytic, PD
		Histiocytic/lymphocytic	Histiocytic/lymphocytic, mixed
Reticulum cell sarcoma	Stem cell Clasmatocytic	Stem cell Histiocytic } RCS	Histiocytic
Follicular	Follicular	All of the above	All of the above

*In these classification schemes each cytological type of lymphoma occurs in a diffuse or nodular form. The term 'nodular' was used in preference to 'follicular' by Rappaport, because of a belief that this cytoarchitectural appearance was a consequence of a tendency of lymphoma cells to aggregate, rather than depicting an origin from germinal follicles. There was also a tendency for all lymphomas to evolve from the nodular to the diffuse form.
WD, well differentiated; PD, poorly differentiated; RCS, Reticulum cell sarcoma.

2. a group of tumours with large cells (compared to the normal lymphocyte) of disputed origin, but most commonly referred to as reticulum cell sarcoma
3. the remaining tumours, usually designated simply as lymphosarcoma or lymphocytic lymphosarcoma.

There was not an abrupt transition between these main groups and each, by dint of the efforts of numerous pathologists, were divided into equally numerous subdivisions, particularly groups 2 and 3. Such subdivisions had little practical value, in view of the limited significance either to clinical features or to duration of survival. Unfortunately, the plethora of classification schemes led to more confusion than clarification, since series of patients from different centres, and certainly from different countries, could not be compared. Moreover, as pointed out by Stout, there was clearly enormous variation in the usage of these terms.[33] In 1940 in the USA, for example, the term reticulum cell sarcoma was applied to 94 per cent of all the lymphomas in one series and 3.6 per cent of those in another. Gall also drew attention to the extremely wide variation in descriptions of tumours classified as reticulum cell sarcoma,[34] and decided to abandon this term in favour of words indicating an origin from

phagocytic cells, initially 'clasmatocyte'[30] and subsequently 'histiocyte'.[35] Not surprisingly, most clinicians found the complicated schemes confusing, and of little relevance to clinical practice.

One of the most widely used classification systems prior to the growth of immunology was that published by Rappaport[36] (see Table 2.2), which was developed from the classification of Gall and Mallory and the subsequent modification by Gall and Rappaport.[35] Rappaport's classification scheme encompassed the basic morphological elements still used today (see Chapter 3), although it has become clear that the individual categories, no matter how homogeneous morphologically, are heterogeneous at the level of phenotype, cytogenetics and molecular biology. Rappaport divided lymphomas into nodular (the same category as follicular, but renamed nodular in view of doubt as to whether the nodules were truly the neoplastic counterparts of germinal follicles[37]) and diffuse. Each category was then further subdivided on the basis of the size of the predominant cell population (small, intermediate and large, or a mixture). Small cells were referred to as well differentiated, intermediate as poorly differentiated, and large (mistakenly, as was also true of the clasmatocytic category of Gall and Mallory) as histiocytic. This system was subsequently modified to take into account the new tumours described in children,[38] but little real progress was made beyond this, in spite of continued efforts,[39–41] until the advent of a functional understanding of the cell types of the immune system, when an attempt was made to incorporate this new information into histological classification schemes.[42,43] Rappaport's classification scheme, however, devised before the development of effective chemotherapy, did prove to have prognostic relevance in the era of combination chemotherapy and has therefore continued to be used alongside the more recent classifications, although the NCI Working Formulation,[44] devised in 1982 in an attempt to allay confusion created by multiple different nomenclatures, has become the dominant classification system.

Recognition of lymphomas occurring predominantly in childhood

While the occurrence of lymphomas in childhood had been reported upon since the nineteenth century it was only quite recently that the difference in their histological spectrum from that of the adult lymphomas was recognized. In 1958 (the year in which Burkitt published his first description of the tumour named after him) Rosenberg *et al.* reported 69 cases of lymphosarcoma (non-Hodgkin's lymphoma) in children aged 15 years and younger. Data were collected over a 30-year period at the Memorial Center for Cancer and Allied Diseases in New York. During this period a total of 1269 patients with lymphosarcoma were seen at the institution.[28] Relatively small differences in the frequency of the three major subdivisions of lymphosarcoma between children and adults were reported, although the incidence of giant follicular lymphoma in childhood was rare (2.9 per cent compared with 13.2 per cent in adults) and lymphosarcoma was more common (60 per cent compared with 41.9 per cent in adults). The difficulty of distinguishing between patients with leukaemia and lymphoma was apparent, and patients with

bone marrow involvement at onset or a high peripheral white blood cell count were excluded. Lymphosarcoma was considered to be more generalized in adults than in children, doubtless in part a reflection of the investigations performed to detect occult, and particularly extranodal, sites of disease, but it was also considered to be more locally aggressive. Only 11 of the 69 cases, all with limited disease, except one patient with stage II and one with stage III disease, became long-term survivors.

In the Rappaport classification, both of the major types of childhood lymphoma, Burkitt's lymphoma and lymphoblastic lymphoma were initially classified as diffuse, poorly differentiated lymphocytic lymphomas.

Burkitt's lymphoma

The high frequency of jaw tumours in African children appears to have been first recognized by Sir Albert Cook who, with his brother, established a mission hospital in Uganda in 1897.[45,46] The high frequency of jaw tumours in West Africa was noted later in pathological reviews. Edington, in the Gold Coast, commented on the high frequency of maxillary lymphosarcoma in children[47] and Thijs, working in the Belgian Congo (Zaire), reported 74 of 145 children with malignant tumours as having lymphosarcoma.[48] De Smet, also in the Belgian Congo (Zaire), reported the frequent involvement of multiple organ sites, including the maxilla and orbit, in children with lymphosarcoma.[49] In East Africa, Burkitt recognized the high frequency of a clinical syndrome in which tumours could occur in the jaw as well as in multiple organ sites,[50] and subsequently delineated the high frequency areas as approximately 15° north and south of the equator with a southern prolongation to the east.[51,52] O'Conor described the basic pathological features of the disease in 1960,[53] and soon after this the occurrence of a tumour which was histologically indistinguishable was also reported in children in the USA and Europe.[54–57] Epstein–Barr virus (EBV) was discovered in 1964 in a cell line derived from a Burkitt's lymphoma,[58] a finding which led to the recognition of the association of African Burkitt's lymphoma with EBV.

Lymphoblastic lymphoma

The occurrence of mediastinal 'hyperplasia' in pseudoleukaemia was mentioned in Virchow's great work *Die krankhaften Geschwülste*,[1] and Ortner, somewhat later, had described the association of thymic tumours with leukaemia.[59] Sternberg described several patients with thymic sarcoma in 1905, although he thought they were of myeloid origin.[60] Our modern concept of lymphoblastic lymphoma stems from the observations of Barcos and Lukes[43,61] and Nathwani and Rappaport in 1976.[31] They described a discrete histological entity with a high frequency of mediastinal involvement occurring predominantly in children and young adults. Initially the presence of nuclear convolutions was believed to be a characteristic feature (hence Lukes and Collins term, convoluted T-cell lymphoma) but, although some lymphoblastic lymphomas have prominent convolutions, this is a variable feature and is not essential to the diagnosis.

Recognition of lymphomas as tumours of the immune system

The recent recognition that lymphomas possess many of the functional attributes of their normal counterpart cells in the immune system has led to a revolution in our understanding of these neoplasms, and provided a much more precise means of classification than the erstwhile 'image recognition'. This new perspective on lymphomas has been made possible by the burgeoning growth of immunology in the last 15 years. However, lymphoid neoplasia has not been merely a passive recipient of the fruits of immunological research but has contributed greatly to progress in the understanding of the functional attributes and interactions of the various lymphoid cell populations. This is a consequence of the monoclonality of lymphoid neoplasia, which results in the availability of large numbers of cells of a single subpopulation, permitting their detailed study, and characterization of their products. The determination of the structure of immunoglobulins and numerous cell mediators, as well as the recognition of the necessity for genetic recombinations of immunoglobulin and T-cell antigen receptor genes has been accomplished largely through the use of clonal, usually neoplastic, cell populations, including continuous cell lines derived from lymphoid tumours of mice and humans.

One of the most important immunological concepts from the perspective of lymphoma classification has been the division of the immune system into cellular (T-cell mediated) and humoral (B-cell mediated) compartments. The application of techniques to distinguish T- and B-cells to lymphoid neoplasia has led to major insights into the origins of individual lymphomas and has often confirmed the relevance of, or led to, histological distinctions. For example, the cutaneous lymphomas, i.e. mycosis fungoides/Sézary syndrome, although described as early as 1806 by Alibert,[62] were only clearly understood when recognized as neoplasms of helper T-cells. Likewise the T-cell adult lymphoma, which was first described in Japan on the basis of its pleomorphic morphology. This tumour was difficult to classify according to the recognized classification schemes,[63] and it was clearly identified as a separate entity, closely related or identical to adult T-cell leukaemia (which had been described previously[64,65]) when shown to have a T-cell phenotype.[66]

The value of an objective means of corroborating subjective diagnosis cannot be underestimated, and is of use both in confirming the true lymphoid nature of a tumour (something which is not always apparent merely by histological examination) and sub-categorizing the tumour further. Immunological phenotyping has led to the recognition that almost all the diagnostic categories in histological classification schemes are heterogeneous, being composed of both T-cell derived and B-cell derived tumours. Moreover, the construction of hybridoma monoclonal antibodies provided a means to identify lineage-specific or lineage-associated antigens, and to define the antigenic characteristics of B- and T-precursor cells as well as different functional subpopulations of lymphocytes. This has permitted the characterization of lymphomas in terms of an origin from immature lymphoid cells (e.g. lymphoblastic lymphoma) or from a specific subpopulation of lymphoid cells such as helper T-cells (e.g. adult T-cell leukaemia/lymphoma, ATLL). While some investigators have bewailed the lack of prognostic significance to characterization as of B-cell or T-cell origin, such a crude delineation, taking no account of the heterogeneity within these major immunological groups, is unlikely to be of value. Nor should prognostic value be the major criterion by which any given approach to characterization is judged. Immunological phenotyping is essential to the elucidation of the cellular origins of malignant lymphomas and provides a primary step towards resolving these tumours into individual pathological entities. Whether or not discrete tumours will respond differently to any given therapeutic approach can only be resolved, at the present time, by empirical testing.

Recognition of the pathogenetic significance of genetic abnormalities

A non-random chromosomal translocation in a lymphoid neoplasm was first detected in Burkitt's lymphoma by Zech in 1976[67] after the description of the 14q$^+$ abnormality by Manolov and Manolova.[68] Subsequently the identification of the 14;18 translocation in the majority of follicular lymphomas and the 11;14 translocation in small cell lymphomas have not only strongly supported the concept that malignant neoplasia is a consequence of genetic abnormalities occurring in lymphoid cells, but also led to the cloning of genes situated at the breakpoints on chromosomes 18 and 11[69–71] (*see* Chapter 6). The frequent occurrence of translocations involving the location of the immunoglobulin heavy chain genes on chromosome 14q32 in B-cell lymphomas and the T-cell antigen receptor genes on chromosome 14q11 in T-cell lymphomas suggests that the genetic errors may occur during the process of cell differentiation, which requires rearrangement of these loci (*see* Chapter 6). It seems likely that the translocations, or other genetic changes, lead to abnormalities of gene expression which result in neoplastic behaviour. This is almost certainly the case in Burkitt's lymphoma, in which the translocations have been shown to lead to abnormal expression of the c-*myc* oncogene (*see* Chapter 6), but much less is known of the consequences of the other chromosomal aberrations. Moreover, consistent chromosomal abnormalities have not been detected in all lymphomas (*see* Chapter 6). This may reflect limitations in available techniques, or heterogeneity at the genetic level, or both.

The present state of knowledge regarding the nature of the malignant non-Hodgkin's lymphomas contrasts dramatically with the information available even 30 years ago. Although there remains a great deal to be learnt, it seems realistic to think that we shall soon develop a reasonably complete concept of the biochemical abnormalities which occur in specific cell types and lead to malignant neoplasia.

The evolution of modern approaches to treatment

Active therapy for the malignant lymphomas has been available only during this century and it is only in the last 20 years that curative therapy for any patients, except those with localized disease, could be contemplated. Prior to radiation, arsenic, usually in the form of Fowler's solution, was frequently used, alongside various other medications which were often given as 'tonics'. Surgery as the sole modality of treatment has a very limited role, but a very small number of patients have achieved long-term survival or cure by excision of localized disease[28,72] and surgery may be beneficial in some circumstances when used prior to chemotherapy.[73] The primary modality for most of this century has been radiation, curative only for some patients with localized disease, and although responses were obtained with single agent chemotherapy, this made little impact upon survival.[28,33,74,75] It is thus only in the modern era of drug combination therapy that a significant number of patients have achieved long-term disease-free survival. In patients with diffuse intermediate or high grade lymphomas, classified according to the National Cancer Institute (NCI) Working Formulation, more than half of all patients may achieve cure when treated with effective drug combinations, even in the presence of disseminated disease, which represents the majority of cases. However, although patients with low grade lymphomas can survive for several years, they appear, with some possible exceptions, ultimately to die from their disease.

Radiation therapy

The first report of the successful treatment of cancer by X-rays was published in 1899 by Sjögren,[76] just 3 years after Roentgen had discovered X-rays. In 1902, Pusey described the use of X-rays in a 24-year-old patient with a small round cell sarcoma involving cervical lymph nodes, and two cases of Hodgkin's disease.[77] All three patients had good responses, which must have been most impressive in an era during which no therapy other than surgery had produced a significant response. The results in the early decades of radiation therapy, however, were usually temporary in so far that recurrence in the treated field or another region of the body was the rule. In addition, there was frequently severe skin and soft tissue injury and radiotherapy was further hindered by the unreliability of the early equipment. It was not until the invention of the Coolidge tube, in 1920, that 180 kilovolt (kV), and shortly thereafter, 200 and 250 kV machines became available for radiation therapy. The 250 kV machine became a standard that lasted until the era of megavoltage equipment (primarily cobalt-60 units and linear accelerators) which began in the 1950s.

Some success was obtained with radiotherapy in Hodgkin's disease in the 1930s and 1940s, largely by the irradiation of all known sites of disease followed by irradiation of adjacent healthy sites where recurrence, from experience, was likely. In 1950, Peters reported an overall survival rate of 51 per cent with rates of 88 per cent for stage I and 72 per cent for stage II Hodgkin's disease,[78] but the results in the non-Hodgkin's lymphomas were much less promising, largely because of the less predictable pattern of spread. It was noted by Gall *et al.* in 1941 that follicular lymphomas appeared to be more sensitive to radiation than lymphosarcomas or reticulum cell sarcomas, as many as 65 per cent having complete regression of lymphadenopathy with long intervals between recurrences.[29] Less than 10 per cent of patients with the more aggressive lymphomas had such a response and about 35 per cent had no response at all. Even in the megavoltage era, a high proportion of patients with localized diffuse aggressive lymphomas fail to achieve long-term disease-free survival and radiation alone can be considered only as palliative therapy in patients with more extensive disease.[79]

Chemotherapy

The modern era of chemotherapy could be said to have had its beginnings in the Second World War, when the rapid lytic effect of the β-chloroethyl amines (nitrogen mustard) on lymphoid tissue, as well as their toxic side-effects were observed.[80] In 1947 Wintrobe reported a good effect (freedom from symptoms such that the patient could return to work) of intravenous nitrogen mustard in four of 11 patients with lymphosarcoma, but a poor effect in seven.[74] By the late 1960s the results of single agent therapy, even with the much larger armamentarium available, were still limited to temporary amelioration, although occasional dramatic results were obtained.[81]

More encouraging results were obtained in childhood lymphomas. Burkitt's and others' reports of long-term remissions in patients treated with only one or two doses of cyclophosphamide[82–84] must have given the pioneer chemotherapists a tremendous boost, since it provided an indication that chemotherapy could, at least in some circumstances, eradicate disease. In childhood leukaemia, too, encouragement to pursue chemotherapy was to be found. Although prior to 1948 there were no survivors, in that year Farber *et al.* had shown that temporary remissions could be induced with aminopterin.[85] The value of other drugs such as 6-mercaptopurine and corticosteroids was demonstrated soon after,[84,86] and by 1963 occasional long-term survivors were reported (although they represented less than 1 per cent of sufferers, according to Burchenal's estimate).[84]

It was not until combinations of drugs began to be used in the 1960s, that prospects for curative chemotherapy began to improve. Notable in the development of drug combinations were workers at the National Cancer Institute in Maryland, where a number of drug combinations were evaluated in the leukaemias and lymphomas.[87–89] The MOPP regimen (nitrogen mustard, vincristine (Oncovin) procarbazine and prednisone) developed for Hodgkin's disease[90] clearly had a considerable influence on the drug combinations subsequently designed for the treatment of the non-Hodgkin's lymphomas in adults, particularly the diffuse large cell (intermediate grade) lymphomas. The substitution of cyclophosphamide for nitrogen mustard led to the combination called C-MOPP, which demonstrated for the first time that the diffuse large cell lymphomas were potentially curable.[91] The introduction of doxorubicin (Adriamycin) and bleomycin in the latter half of the 1970s permitted the successive development of the CHOP regimen (cyclophosphamide, doxorubicin, vincristine (Oncovin) and prednisone),[92] BACOP,[93] and CHOP-Bleo.[94] Both of the latter are basically CHOP regimens to which bleomycin has been added, although in spite of its activity as a single agent, it is not clear that bleomycin adds significantly to the therapeutic efficacy of CHOP.[95] In a more recent extension of these regimens (COP-BLAM) both bleomycin and procabazine were added to the drugs of the basic CHOP programme.[96] The demonstration of the activity of high dose methotrexate coupled to leucovorin rescue of normal tissues in the diffuse lymphomas[97] led to its incorporation into several regimens, including M-BACOD, ProMACE-MOPP, proMACE-CYTOBOM, COMLA, MACOB-B and CHOP-MTX, which are discussed in Chapters 13 and 21. Although initially thought to provide a significant advantage over CHOP, the relative merits of these various drug combinations remain uncertain – an issue which is currently being examined by means of randomized clinical trials.

In the very aggressive (high grade) lymphomas of childhood, the greatest influence came from the improving results in acute lymphoblastic leukaemia and Burkitt's lymphoma.[88,98–100] The high frequency of bone marrow recurrence in the childhood lymphomas supported the concept that these diseases might respond well to the same therapies used in acute lymphoblastic leukaemia, and led, in the 1970s, to the use of the LSA$_2$L$_2$ and APO[75,101] regimens in children with non-Hodgkin's lymphomas. The conflicting approaches – short duration therapy with intermittent pulses of drug combinations which always contained an alkylating agent (usually cyclophosphamide), and long duration therapy with daily drug administration and minimal or no use of alkylating agents – prompted the design of a study to examine the relative value of lymphoma versus leukaemia therapy. In 1977, a randomized trial of these approaches was initiated by the Children's Cancer Study Group (CCG) in the USA, although the lymphoma treatment arm (COMP) deviated from the regimens used to treat Burkitt's lymphoma in that it was continued for 18 months. The COMP regimen included methotrexate with leucovorin rescue, after the demonstration by Djerassi of the efficacy of this approach in childhood lymphomas.[102] The CCG trial demonstrated a significant difference in the results achieved with these different treatment approaches for the two main histological groups of childhood lymphomas, showing superiority for the LSA$_2$L$_2$ regimen in lymphoblastic lymphomas, and better results with COMP in non-lymphoblastic lymphomas.[103] The results of this trial have been confirmed in other centres using the same regimens, although the apparently clear cut result may be slightly misleading, for reasons discussed in Chapters 16 and 17. A number of other drug combinations have been developed for the non-lymphoblastic lymphomas in children, all of which include methotrexate with leucovorin rescue (*see* Chapter 17).

It is now widely accepted that combination chemotherapy regimens represent the primary and most effective therapy for the diffuse non-Hodgkin's lymphomas. However, because of the historical reliance upon radiation and the fact that a fraction of patients with localized disease can be cured by radiation alone, there has been a reluctance to depart from its use, particularly in early stage lymphomas. There has had to be a shift in philosophy, now largely accomplished, so that the role of radiation therapy as *adjuvant*, rather than *primary* treatment is evaluated. In most clinical trials it appears to add little, except toxicity, to combination chemotherapy. Meanwhile, there has been considerable focus on defining the subgroups of patients which still have a poor response to conventional drug combinations, in order to preselect them for even more aggressive regimens, sometimes involving bone marrow transplantation (*see* Chapter 25).

Treatment of the low grade, predominantly follicular, lymphomas is much more controversial, since it has been widely accepted, until recently, that such patients are incurable with currently available therapy. Here, there are still a variety of approaches, the two main schools being minimal treatment or treatment only in specific circumstances – the object being to maintain the highest possible quality of life for as long as possible for a presumptively incurable disease – versus strategies aimed towards the development of curative therapy. Clearly, the evaluation of toxic, potentially life-threatening regimens in patients who could enjoy several years of high quality life poses an ethical dilemma, but the possibility of cure with intensive chemotherapy regimens, possibly supported by bone marrow transplantation, has led to the early, tentative exploration of much more aggressive approaches. Other approaches involving a variety of modalities, including biological response modifiers, are also being studied, inspired by the very different biology of these tumours (in some senses at least, the small cleaved cell variety can still be considered a 'benign' process with the potential for malignant conversion, as originally conceived).

The benefits and disadvantages of these widely different approaches to treatment can only be determined by empirical clinical trials. It is to be hoped, however, that as more is learnt of the biology of the malignant lymphomas, quite new approaches, derived from a knowledge of the biochemical changes specific to each tumour type, which have led to neoplastic behaviour, may be developed. Such possibilities are discussed in Chapter 27.

References

1. Virchow R. In: *Die krankhaften Geschwülste. Dreissig Vorlesungen gehalten während des Winter-semesters 1862–1863 an der Universitat zu Berlin.* Berlin: Hirschwald, 1864–1865: 564–620.
2. Cruickshank W. *The Anatomy of the Absorbing Vessels of the Human Body.* London: G Nichol, 1768.
3. Hodgkin T. *Transactions of the Medical and Chirurgical Society of London.* 1832; **xvii**, 68–114.
4. Wunderlich CA. *Archiv für Physiologische Heilkunde* 1858; **12**, 122–31.
5. Wilkes S. *Guy's Hospital Report.* 1856; **17**, 102–32.
6. Trousseau A. *Clinique Médicale de l'Hôtel-Dieu de Paris.* 1865; **3**, 555–81.
7. Cohnheim J. *Virchows Archiv.* 1862; **33**, 451–4.
8. Virchow R. *Neue Notizen aus dem Gebiet der Natur und Heilkunde (Froriep's Neue Notizen).* 1845; **36**, 151–6.
9. Craigie D. *Edinburgh Medical and Surgical Journal.* 1845; **64**, 400–13.
10. Bennett JH. *Edinburgh Medical and Surgical Journal.* 1845; **64**, 413–23.
11. Dreschfeld J. *British Medical Journal.* 1892; **1**, 893–6.
12. Kundrat H. *Wien klinische Wochenschrift.* 1893; **6**, 211–13 and 234–9.
13. Sternberg C. *Zeitschrift für Heilkunde.* 1898; **xix**, 21–90.
14. Reed DM. *Johns Hopkins Hospital Report.* 1902; **x**, 133–96.
15. Ghon A, Roman B. *Frankfurter Zeitschrift für Pathologie.* 1916; **xix**, 1.
16. Beda C. *Verhandlung der Deutsche Pathologische Gesellschaft.* 1904; **vii**, 123–31.
17. Yamasaki M. *Zeitschrift fuÿ Heilkunde.* 1904; **xxv**, 269–313.
18. Gibbons HW. *American Journal of Medical Science.* 1906, **cxxxii**, 692–704.
19. Jackson H Jr, Parker F Jr. *New England Journal of Medicine.* 1944; **231**, 35–44.
20. Ewing J. *Bulletin of the New York Academy of Medicine.* 1939; **15**, 92–103.
21. Oliver J. *Journal of Medical Research.* 1913; **xxix**, 191–207.
22. Oberling C. *Bulletin de l'Association Francais pour l'Etude du Cancer.* 1928; **17**, 256–9.
23. Roulet F. *Virchows Archiv für Pathologische Anatomie.* 1930; **277**, 15–47.
24. Foix C, Roemmele A. *Archives de Medicine Experimentale et d'Anatomie Pathologique.* 1912; **24**, 111.
25. Brill NE, Baehr G, Rosenthal N. *Journal of the American Medical Association.* 1925; **84**, 668–71.

26. Symmers D. *Archives of Pathology*. 1938; **26**, 603–47.
27. Evans TS, Doan CA. In: *Annals of Internal Medicine*. 1954; **40**, 851–80.
28. Rosenberg SA, Diamond HD, Dargeon HW, *et al. New England Journal of Medicine*. 1958; **259**, 505–12.
29. Gall EA, Morrison HR, Scott AT. *Annals of Internal Medicine*. 1941; **14**, 2073–90.
30. Gall EA, Mallory TB. *American Journal of Pathology*. 1942; **18**, 381–429.
31. Nathwani BW, Kim H, Rappaport H. *Cancer*. 1976; **38**, 964–83.
32. Custer RP, Bernhard WG. *American Journal of Medical Sciences*. 1948; **216**, 625.
33. Stout AP. *New York State Journal of Medicine*. 1947; **47**, 158–64.
34. Gall EA. *Minnesota Medicine*. 1955; **38**, 674.
35. Gall EA, Rappaport H. *Proceedings of 23rd Annual Seminar*. American Society of Clinical Pathology, 1958.
36. Rappaport H. In: *Atlas of Tumor Pathology, Section III, Fascicle 8*. Washington DC: Armed Forces Institute of Pathology, 1966.
37. Rappaport H, Winter WJ, Hicks EB. *Cancer*. 1956; **9**, 792.
38. Rappaport H, Braylan RC. In: Rebuck JW, Berard CW, Abell MR (eds). *The Reticuloendothelial System; International Academy of Pathology*. Baltimore: Williams & Wilkins Co., 1975; 1–19.
39. Bennett MH, Farrer-brown G, Henry K. *et al. Lancet*. 1974; **i**, 1295.
40. Dorfman RF. In: Rebuck JW, Berard CW, Abell MR (eds). *The Reticuloendothelial System; International Academy of Pathology*. Baltimore: Williams & Wilkins Co., 1975; 262.
41. Mathé G, Rappaport H, O'Connor GT, *et al. Histological and Cytological Typing of Neoplastic Diseases of Hemopoietic and Lymphoid Tissue*. World Health Organization, Geneva; 1976.
42. Lennert K, Mohri N, Stein H, *et al. British Journal of Haematology*. (supply. II), 1975; **31**, 193.
43. Lukes RJ and Collins RD. *British Journal of Cancer*. 1975; **31** (suppl. II), 1–28.
44. National Cancer Institute sponsored study of classifications of non-Hodgkin's lymphomas. Summary and description of a working formulation for clinical usage. *Cancer*. 1982; **49**, 2112–35.
45. Davies JNP, Elmes S, Hutt MSR, *et al. British Medical Journal*. 1964; **1**, 259–64.
46. Davies, JNP, Elmes S, Hutt MSR, *et al. British Medical Journal*. 1964; **1**, 336–41.
47. Edington GM. *British Journal of Cancer*. 1956; 10: 595.
48. Thjis A. *Annales de la Société Belge de la Médicine Tropicale*. 1957; **37**, 483–514.
49. De Smet MP, *Annales de la Société Belge de la Médicine Tropicale*. 1956; **36**, 53–70.
50. Burkitt D. *British Journal of Surgery*. 1958; **46**, 218–23.
51. Burkitt D. *British Medical Journal*. 1962; **2**, 1019–23.
52. Burkitt DP. In: *Burkitt's Lymphoma*. Edinburgh: Livingstone, 1970; 186–97.
53. O'Conor GT, Davies JNP. *Journal of Pediatrics*. 1960; **56**, 526–35.
54. O'Conor G. *Cancer*. 1960; **14**, 270–83.
55. O'Conor G, Rappaport H, Smith EB. *Cancer*. 1965; **18**, 411–17.
56. Dorfman RF. *Cancer*. 1965; **18**, 418–30.
57. Wright DH. *International Journal of Cancer*. 1966; **1**, 503.
58. Epstein MA, Achong BG, Barr YM. *Lancet*. 1964; **i**, 702–3.
59. Ortner N. *Wien klinische Wochenschrift*. 1890; **3**, 937–8.
60. Sternberg C. *British Journal of Pathology*. 1905; **61**, 75–100.
61. Barcos MP, Lukes RJ. In: Sinks JF, Godden JO (eds). *Conflicts in Childhood Cancer: an Evaluation of Current Management*. New York: 1975; Liss, 147–78.
62. Alibert JLM. *Description des Maladies de la Peau*. Paris: Barrois L'Ainé et Fils. 1806.
63. Suchi T, Tajima K, Namba K, *et al. Acta Pathologica Japonica*. 1979; **29**, 755–66.
64. Uchiyama T, Yodoi J, Sagawa K, *et al. Blood*. 1977; **50**, 481–92.
65. Yodoi J, Takatsuki K, Masuda T. *New England Journal of Medicine*. 1974; **290**, 572–3.
66. Shimoyama M, Tobinai K, Hirose M, *et al.* In: Hanaoaka M, Takatsuki K, Shimoyama M, (eds). *Gann Monograph on Cancer Research no. 28*. Tokyo and New York: Japan Scientific Societies Press and Plenum Press; 1982; 23–35.
67. Zech L, Hagland U, Nilsson K, *et al. International Journal of Cancer*. 1976; **17**, 47–56.
68. Manolov G, Manolova Y. *Nature*. 1972; **237**, 33–4.
69. Tsujimoto Y, Finger LR, Yunis J, *et al. Science*. 1984; **226**, 1097–9.
70. Bakhshi A, Jensen JP, Goldman P, *et al. Cell*. 1985; **41**, 899–906.
71. Tsujimoto Y, Yunis J, Onorato-Showe L, *et al. Science*. 1984; **224**, 1403–6.
72. Gall EA. *Annals of Surgery*. 1943; **118**, 1064–70.
73. Magrath I, Lwanga S, Carswell W, *et al. British Medical Journal*. 1974; **2**, 308–12.
74. Wintrobe MM, Huguley CM Jr, McLennan MR, *et al. Annals of Internal Medicine*. 1947; **27**, 529–40.

75. Wollner N, Burchenal JH, Liebermann PH, *et al. Cancer.* 1976; **37**, 123.

76. Sjögren T. *Forhandlingar vid Sammankomster Svenska Lakaresallskapets.* 1899; **0**, 208.

77. Pusey WA. *Journal of the American Medical Association.* 1902; **38**, 166–9.

78. Peters MV. *American Journal of Roentgenology.* 1950; **63**, 299–311.

79. Miller TP, Jones SE. *Cancer Chemotherapy and Pharmacology.* 1980; **4**, 67–70.

80. Goodman LS, Wintrobe MM, Dameshek W, *et al. Journal of the American Medical Association.* 1946; **132**, 126.

81. Karnovsky DA. In: Zarafonetis CJD ed. *Proceedings of the International Conference on Leukemia-lymphoma.* Philadelphia: Lea and Febiger, 1968; 409–22.

82. Burkitt D. *Cancer.* 1967; **20**, 756–9.

83. Clifford P. *Cancer Research.* 1967; **27**, 2578–615.

84. Burchenal JH. In: Zarafonetis CJD ed. *Proceedings of the International Conference on Leukemia-lymphoma.* Philadelphia: Lea and Febiger, 1967: 469–74.

85. Farber S, Diamond LK, Mercer RD, *et al. New England Journal of Medicine.* 1948; **238**, 787–97.

86. Burchenal JH, Murphy ML, Ellison RR, *et al. Blood.* 1953; **8**, 965–99.

87. Moxley JG III, DeVita VT Jr, Frei E. *Cancer Research.* 1967; **27**, 1258–63.

88. Frei E III, Freireich EJ, Karon M. *Proceedings of the American Association for Cancer Research.* 1964; **5**, 20.

89. Frei E, Freireich EJ, Gehen E, *et al. Blood.* 1961; **18**, 431.

90. De Vita VT Jr, Serpick A, Carbone PP. *Annals of Internal Medicine.* 1970; **73**, 881–95.

91. DeVita VT Jr, Canellos GP, Chabner B. *Lancet.* 1975; **i**, 248–50.

92. McKelvey EM, Gottleib JA, Wilson HE. *Cancer.* 1976; **38**, 1484–93.

93. Schein PS, DeVita VT Jr, Hubbard S. *Annals of Internal Medicine.* 1976; **85**, 417–22.

94. Rodriguez B, Cabanillas F, Burgess MA. *Blood.* 1977; **49**, 325–33.

95. Koziner B, Little C, Kurland E. *Proceedings of the American Association for Cancer Research.* 1982; **450** (abstract), 115.

96. Laurence J, Coleman M, Allen SL. *Annals of Internal Medicine.* 1982; **97**, 190–5.

97. Skarin AT, Zuckerman KS, Pitman SW. *Blood.* 1977; **50**, 1039–47.

98. George P, Hernandez K, Borella L, *et al. Cancer Research.* 1966; **7**, 23.

99. Arseneau JC, Canellos GP, Banks PM, *et al. American Journal of Medicine.* 1975; **58**, 314–21.

100. Ziegler JL. *New England Journal of Medicine.* 1977; **297**, 75–80.

101. Weinstein HJ, Cassady JR, Levey R. *Journal of Clinical Oncology.* 1983; **1**, 537.

102. Djerassi I, Kim JS. *Cancer.* 1976; **38**, 1043–51.

103. Anderson JR, Wilson JF, Jenkin RD, *et al. New England Journal of Medicine.* 1983; **308**, 559.

CHAPTER 3

LYMPHOCYTE ONTOGENY: A CONCEPTUAL BASIS FOR UNDERSTANDING NEOPLASIA OF THE IMMUNE SYSTEM

Ian Magrath

Neoplasia of the immune system

Our understanding of the homeostatic mechanisms by which the body eliminates foreign materials is relatively recent. Early attempts to classify lymphoid neoplasms – i.e. neoplasms of the cells which make up the immune system – were therefore purely descriptive in nature, being based initially upon clinical features, and subsequently upon the morphological appearance of the neoplastic tissue and its component cells (*see* Chapter 2).

Our modern understanding of malignant lymphomas began approximately 20 years ago with the subdivision of the immune system into humoral (i.e. mediated by circulating antibodies) and cellular (cell-mediated) components. These major subdivisions are currently referred to as B (bone marrow-derived) and T (thymus-derived) compartments because of the anatomical locations from which they are replenished after birth. Each of these compartments consists of precursor cells, derived from a common haemopoietic/lymphocytic stem cell, and a large number of mature cell types which subserve different functions. Mature B-cells primarily differ from each other with regard to the class of antibody they secrete, while mature T-cells subserve a variety of regulatory functions including the destruction of cells infected by micro-organisms (or foreign cells) and the control of the proliferation and differentiation of normal lymphoid and non-lymphoid cells.

With the development of methods whereby functionally different lymphocyte subpopulations could be identified, it became clear that lymphoid neoplasms could also be distinguished from each other by virtue of their possession of the attributes of specific normal lymphocyte populations. Thus, it would appear that malignant lymphomas not only arise from specific cell subpopulations within the larger B and T compartments but also retain many of the characteristics of their normal counterpart cells.[1]

A quintessential feature of cells of the immune system is their ability to recognize foreign antigens through their possession of antigen receptor genes (immunoglobulin in the case of B-cells). These genes are central to lymphocyte function and their expression defines the cell lineage. Both sets of receptor genes belong to the same supergene family, which includes the genes for histocompatibility antigens (HLA) as well as those for a number of the other surface molecules present on lymphoid cells. Because of the need to recognize and react to several million epitopes, mechanisms of generating receptor diversity have evolved. These mechanisms could only be guessed at until the development of recombinant DNA technology, which has permitted a much more detailed understanding of the structure of T- and B-cell receptor genes as well as the changes that these genes undergo during cell differentiation. Such knowledge has also led to a new ability to examine the molecular changes associated with neoplastic behaviour in lymphoid cells (*see* Chapter 6) as well as providing a broad range of tools of value in diagnosis, follow up, and potentially even treatment of patients with lymphoid malignancies (*see* Chapters 7 and 27). This is because the antigen receptor genes are frequently involved in the genetic abnormalities (usually chromosomal translocations) which are associated with lymphoid neoplasms and believed to be of pathogenetic significance.

Genetic abnormalities in lymphoid neoplasia

The cells of individual lymphomas may undergo a greater or lesser degree of differentiation, giving rise to some degree of heterogeneity within the malignant clone. However, a primary attribute of lymphoid neoplasia (indeed, perhaps of the majority of neoplasms) is a degree of autonomy such that malignant lymphoid cells fail to respond appropriately to the complex series of regulatory signals which govern the proliferation and differentiation of normal lymphoid cells. The process by which a lymphoid neoplasm is generated may thus be thought of as a series of cellular changes whereby a once normal lymphoid cell (or cell clone) becomes refractory to the regulation of its differentiation and proliferation. These changes are, of necessity, genetic, whether induced by mutation, chromosomal translocation or deletion, or the insertion of foreign genes (e.g. viral genes) into the cells. Translocations generally result in altered expression of an adjacent gene. Deletions may cause loss of genes involved in regulation of other genes, or loss of genes necessary for differentiation to occur (e.g. a differentiation factor receptor). Mutations could have any of these effects, while viruses are likely to exert their effect either on adjacent genes, via the virus promoters or enhancers, or on distant genes via one or more virus proteins able to 'transactivate' other genes. Such transactivating genes are usually involved in the control of virus production, but may also be able to influence cellular genes. In the case of virus infections, however, the infected cell normally expresses viral antigens and so can be destroyed by specific or non-specific cytotoxic cells. If virus-infected cells are to become malignant, a

mechanism for avoiding destruction by the immune system is an additional necessity e.g. suppression of the expression of certain viral antigens, or of cell surface molecules necessary for immune recognition, such as HLA class I molecules or leucocyte adhesion molecules.

It is worth noting that alterations in proliferation are not necessarily confined to increases in the rate of proliferation, or in the proportion of proliferating cells in a population. Prolongation of life span (e.g. by imposition of a block to differentiation, by preventing exit from the differentiation compartment or by a genetic change which 'immortalizes' the cell (e.g. renders it unable to respond to regulatory signals) may also give rise to the progressive accumulation of a single clone of malignant cells (Fig. 3.1). It is likely that the low grade non-Hodgkin's lymphomas fall into this category, thus accounting for their relatively long natural histories.

Antigen receptor diversity

Both B- and T-cells have developed remarkable mechanisms whereby their antigen receptors, while retaining a similar basic structure, or framework, contain variable regions which differ from one molecule to the next. Such regions confer upon each receptor molecule the capacity to react specifically with one (or a small number) of antigens among the millions to which the cell may be exposed. The mechanisms by which antigen receptor diversity is generated are of seminal importance, not only to an understanding of the whole basis of specific immunological recognition, but also to many aspects of lymphoid neoplasia. The fact that variable and constant components of antigen receptor genes are separated in the cell genome and must be assembled into complete genes by a multistep process during lymphocyte differentiation[2-5] has several repercussions.

First, the antigen receptor gene loci are particularly likely to be involved in chromosomal translocations. This is either because of mistakes occurring during the normal process of approximation of variable to constant regions, or because these sites are among the more fragile of the sites in lymphocytes because of the need to alter the chromatin structure of relatively long lengths of DNA to permit enzyme access. In either case, chromosomal translocations are more likely to occur in precursor cells when the chromatin is 'open', in order to provide access for recombinases involved in the normal process of antigen receptor gene rearrangement. A proportion of such translocations result in altered expression of genes adjacent to the breakpoints and so, when these genes are

(a) (b) (c) (d)

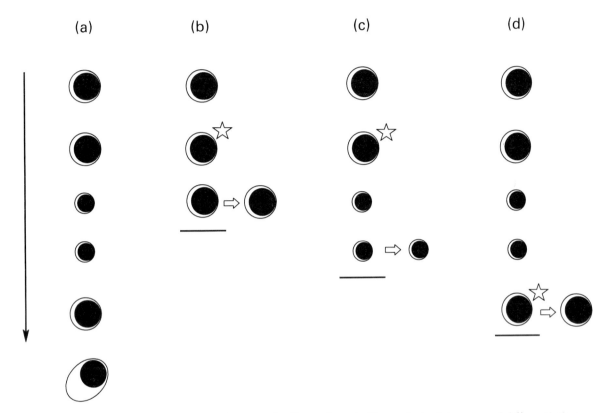

Fig. 3.1 Scheme depicting possible mechanisms leading to lymphoid neoplasia. (a), a normal differentiation sequence of lymphocytes showing progression from precursor cells to resting forms of immunocompetent cells, and after activation to immunoblasts and plasma cells. Memory cells are also represented by the small lymphocytes. The arrow indicates the direction of differentiation; (b), genetic abnormalities (shown by a star – e.g. a translocation involving lineage specific genes) in a rapidly proliferating precursor cell lead to inability to down-regulate a gene involved in proliferation and accumulation of immature cells – not necessarily at the exact point in the differentiation pathway at which the genetic abnormality occurred. There is secondary failure of differentiation resulting from the constant proliferative state. Some high grade lymphomas such as the small non-cleaved and lymphoblastic lymphomas may fall into this category; (c), a genetic change results in a primary differentiation block which leads to accumulation of the cell clone at the stage whose further differentiation, or in this case, activation, is prevented. This is the equivalent of increasing the life span of the particular cell type whose differentiation is blocked, thus preventing exit from the particular differentiation compartment. Other genetic changes which 'immortalize' the cell, however, may also be required. Note that the genetic change, although occurring in a precursor cell has no effect until a later cell stage. Some low grade lymphomas, e.g. small cell lymphomas and follicular lymphomas may fall into this category; (d), a genetic change occurring in an activated cell causes accumulation of cells at the same level of differentiation. This is similar in principle to b, although the genetic lesion may be quite different, e.g. deletion of a suppressor gene rather than translocation. Some large cell lymphomas may fall into this category.

important to differentiation or proliferation, the chromosomal translocation contributes to, or causes, neoplasia. The fact that these lineage-specific genes must be expressed throughout essentially all stages of differentiation, probably also contributes to the frequency of their involvement in pathogenetically important chromosomal translocations. Genes brought into the sphere of influence of their regulatory regions are likely to be constitutively expressed, and unable to be down-regulated. When such lineage-specific genes inappropriately regulate genes which cause proliferation, the resultant neoplasm is likely to be rapidly progressive. An excellent example of this is the small non-cleaved lymphomas (*see* Chapter 17).

Secondly, because the rearrangement of the antigen receptor genes is unique to each cell clone, a highly specific clonal marker is generated which gives information about the cell lineage (B-cell versus T-cell receptor gene rearrangements) and, in the case of precursor cells, the level of differentiation. The latter is possible because recombination of antigen receptor genes takes place in a series of steps and at different stages of differentiation (see below). In addition, in T-cells, there are two main sets of receptor genes, only one of which is rearranged in any given mature cell type, suggesting that the particular set of receptor genes employed by a cell may have functional significance.

Lymphocyte activation

Another highly relevant aspect of the differentiation of normal lymphocytes is the process of lymphocyte activation. Because of the need for a wide range of antigen specificities, and because antigen encounters are intermittent, mature lymphoid cells whether of B- or T-cell lineage, are normally maintained in a non-proliferative state (resting cells); they are activated by contact with the specific antigen with which they react. This results in the major advantage that only very small numbers of cells able to react with a specific antigen need be retained in the body. Resting cells which have already encountered their specific antigen may be retained as relatively long-lived cells, able to undergo rapid clonal expansion at the next

antigen encounter; these cells are operationally defined as memory cells. Whether memory cells differ phenotypically from resting cells which have not yet been exposed to antigen is a controversial issue. However, even the need for only a small number of cells able to react with any antigen likely to be encountered (whether a first or subsequent exposure) has obvious disadvantages. First, a large number of lymphocyte clones would need to be maintained, but many would probably never come into contact with an antigen able to activate them. Secondly, the contact of any given antigen with a potentially reactive cell (i.e. the selection of an appropriately reactive clone, according to the clonal selection theory) would become less and less likely, the fewer the number of cells present in each antigen specific clone.

Possible role of CD5 bearing B-cells

A mechanism of overcoming these shortcomings has recently been proposed, based on the characterization of a B-cell subpopulation which accounts for some 18 per cent of circulating B lymphocytes and is distinguished by the expression of the CD5 antigen also present on the majority of T-cells. Such CD5-positive B-cells make antibodies which have low affinities and which are able to bind to a relatively wide range of antigens, including some autoantigens.[6] It has been proposed that, after activation by an antigen with which they may only weakly react, these cells have a high propensity to serially modify the variable region of their immunoglobulin molecules. Such a modification may occur either by substitution of the bulk of the variable region by another (by virtue of a second recombinational event), or by a process of somatic mutation of the variable region, or both.[7] Any modified clones which have a higher antigen affinity will be selected for as long as the antigen remains present. In this way, higher and higher affinity antibodies, which are also more and more specific, are selected for in daughter generations of activated cells. This process would obviate the need for the entire antibody repertoire to be present in every individual.

One might ask, therefore, why the lymphoid

precursor compartment persists throughout life (albeit at a progressively decreasing level), since once the antigen repertoire has been fully developed the maintenance of each clone should take place at the memory cell level. However, in practice, it is suspected that clones of memory cells which are not repeatedly stimulated eventually die out. If the generation of a complete antigenic repertoire were truly a chance phenomenon, very large numbers of clones would have to be generated continuously in order to ensure that the complete repertoire is continuously available. Interestingly, if the hypothesis referred to above regarding the CD5 population of B-cells is correct, and if a homologous population of T-cells exists, antigen responses would continually deplete the population of virgin immunocompetent cells, still giving rise to a need for continual replenishment. However, this need would be less than would be required for the maintenance of a broad range of antigenic specificities by a classical clonal selection process, and could also be limited to replacement of a specific type of cell, perhaps containing only one or a few particular variable regions. These initially selected variable regions, are destined to be replaced or modified on a random basis in activated cells in the presence of antigen, permitting much more efficient clonal selection.

Activation antigens

Regardless of these considerations, strict control mechanisms must be in place so that activated cells undergo an appropriate amount of clonal expansion, followed by suppression of proliferation after the antigen with which they react has been eliminated. The process of activation is therefore associated with the generation of 'activation antigens' e.g. Ki-1, Ki-67, the transferrin receptor and interleukin-2 receptor (IL-2R).[8,9] Activation antigens are predominantly concerned with the process of proliferation and its control, i.e. many of them are growth factor receptors, which are generated upon encounter with antigen; others may be molecules with which T-cells or their chemical mediators (lymphokines) can react. Such antigens are frequently recognized on the surface of lymphoid neoplasms.

It is important to realize that lymphocyte activation also entails differentiation – some of the activation antigens are known to be receptors for differentiation factors. A resting B lymphocyte when activated, for example, becomes first a large immunoblast and then a plasma cell, which is capable of secreting large quantities of the same antibody specified by the small lymphocyte. While the immunoblast and plasma cell are in one sense more differentiated cells, the cell from which they arose is not an immature cell. Rather it is an immunocompetent cell, capable of subserving its function when stimulated by the appropriate antigen. Since the progeny of the activated cell are also capable of giving rise to additional small, resting lymphocytes (memory cells), however, this process resembles stem cell differentiation associated with self-renewal. Thus, to distinguish the processes of differentiation which result, on the one hand, in the production of immunocompetent but resting cells from immature precursor cells, and, on the other hand, cells subserving their role as part of an immune response, the terms 'antigen dependent' and 'antigen independent' differentiation are often used.

Differentiation pathways of normal B-cells

In postpartum mammals, cells committed to lymphoid differentiation arise in the bone marrow from multipotential stem cells. Whereas T-cells undergo further differentiation in a circumscribed location – the thymus – there is no similar organ that serves exclusively as a site for the early phases of B-cell differentiation (i.e. antigen independent differentiation). This is not the case in birds, where the Bursa of Fabricius serves this function. Because of this, the characteristics of immature B-cells in mammals are less well known than those of immature T-cells. Moreover, the bone marrow, the site at which primary B-cell differentiation occurs in mammals, is both a primary and secondary lymphoid organ. It contains the most mature (plasma cells) and the most immature cells of the B-cell series (committed B-cells not yet synthesizing immunoglobulins), as well as a large number of other cell lineages. Consequently, it has not proved possible to obtain pure populations of immature B-cells and investigate the stages of early differentiation, as has been done so elegantly for T-cells. Currently existing information regarding the sequence of events occurring in antigen independent differentiation in man has been derived predominantly from the analysis of acute lymphoblastic leukaemia of pre-B origin.[10] It must be borne in mind that this information is derived from neoplastic cells, and may not reflect normal processes in every respect. It remains, however, the best information available in humans at the present time.

Molecular events occurring in B-cell precursors

The molecular events occurring in B-cells during differentiation are directed towards the generation of an immunoglobulin molecule with reactivity to an antigen, or rather to a specific epitope of an antigen. The immunoglobulin genes are situated on chromosome 14 (q32) and arranged in tandem sequence, while lambda light chain genes are on chromosome 22 (q11) and kappa chain genes on chromosome 2 (p11) (Fig. 3.2). The diversity of the humoral immune response is partly brought about by the rearrangement (i.e. approximation) of the initially separate components of the immunoglobulin genes with deletion of intervening non-coding sequences, known as introns (Fig. 3.3).[2-4] The generation of a gene coding for a functional heavy chain immunoglobin molecule requires the approximation of one of the multiple variable regions with the constant region via one each of the other multiple discontinuous segments called D (diversity segment) and J (joining region). In the heavy chain locus, one of the 20 or more D segments first joins to one of the six J_H segments which lie immediately upstream of the first heavy chain constant region expressed during development, namely $C\mu$. In general, DJ joining occurs simultaneously on both chromosomes. This process is mediated through heptamer–nonamer signal sequences (consensus CACAGTG) located on the 3′ side of each D segment (where they are separated by 12 base pairs) and the 5′ side of each J_H segment (where they are separated by 23 base pairs).[11] Subsequently, one of the 50 to several 100 variable regions on one of the two chromosomes

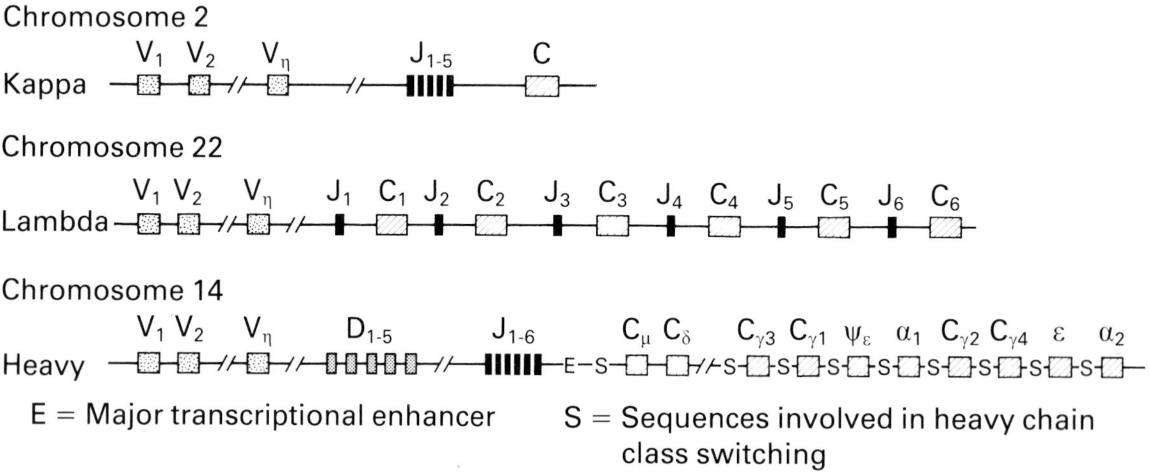

Fig. 3.2 Diagrammatic representation of the arrangement of the heavy and light chain immunoglobulin genes on chromosomes 14 (heavy), 2 (kappa) and 22 (lambda). V, variable; D, diversity; J, joining regions; S, switch regions; E, the major enhancer region in the heavy chain locus. A similar enhancer (not shown) is present in the kappa locus.

is approximated to the DJ region. Similar heptamer–nonamer signal sequences are involved in the V–D joining process, the repeat sequences 3' of V (variable segment) being separated by 23 base pairs, those 5' of D, like those 3' of D, being separated by 12 base pairs. The V region brings with it the promoter and leader regions of the immunoglobulin gene which now come under the influence of the enhancer region of the immunoglobulin locus situated 3' of the J_H region. This enhancer region is a non-transcribed DNA element which can bind regulatory proteins and which acts on the promoter of the immunoglobulin gene to initiate transcription. Other such promoter regions are probably present within the immunoglobulin heavy chain locus, and they may be important in influencing the expression of genes aberrantly brought into juxtaposition with them by a chromosomal translocation (*see* Chapter 6). Successful production of a μ gene in the cytoplasm is the hallmark of a pre-B-cell.

In the light chain loci similar events occur, although these genes lack D segments. In the kappa locus, one of the 200 or so variable regions is directly approximated to one of the five J_{kappa} regions. The heptamer–nonamer signal sequences are similarly involved, although in the kappa locus, the heptamer–nonamer separation is 12 base pairs near the V region and 23 base pairs near the J_{kappa} segment. As in the heavy chain region, a protein-binding enhancer region has been described between the J_{kappa} and C_{kappa} regions. Less information is available about the lambda locus, which is more complex, there being at least six constant regions, each with its own J region. However, the basic process of VJ joining is similar to that in the kappa locus. If a functional light chain is produced, it binds to the μ chain in the endoplasmic reticulum vesicles, displacing a retention protein from the heavy chain and permitting the whole immunoglobulin molecule to be transported via the Golgi apparatus to the cell surface. The expression of surface immunoglobulin is the hallmark of a B-cell.

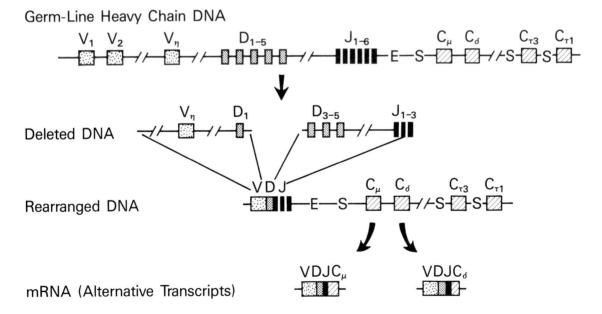

Fig. 3.3 Diagrammatic representation of rearrangement of the heavy chain immunoglobulin μ gene during B-cell differentiation in order to approximate the variable region to the constant region prior to expression and production of an immunoglobulin μ chain. V, variable; D, diversity; J, joining regions; S, switch regions; E, the major enhancer region in the heavy chain locus.

Based on studies in acute lymphoblastic leukaemia,[12] there appears to be an ordered sequence of immunoglobulin gene rearrangements, the first being VDJ joining of one of the two μ alleles. If the recombination is precise and a functional immunoglobulin gene is created (errors resulting in non-functional genes occur in as many as one third of attempts), the second μ gene on the allelic chromosome remains unrearranged so that only one antibody specificity is generated per cell – a process known as allelic exclusion. The gene product itself (i.e. a μ chain) appears to be responsible for inhibiting the joining of V to D on the allelic chromosome.[11] If a functional gene is not created, the second allele is rearranged. If the resultant gene is still not functional, the cell presumably cannot become a B-cell. It is possible, based on the occurrence of rearranged μ genes in a small proportion (approximately 10 per cent of T-cell acute lymphoblastic leukaemias, that such cells may sometimes go on to rearrange their T-cell receptor genes and become T-cells. If a functional μ gene is produced, signalled by the synthesis of μ chains, VJ joining of one kappa allele occurs. Again, only if unsuccessful does the second allele undergo VJ joining, and only if this is also unsuccessful do the lambda genes undergo sequential rearrangements in similar fashion to the kappa genes.

The generation of antibody diversity

The recombinational processes which result in the approximation of variable regions to constant regions is one of the mechanisms for generating antibody diversity. Since this process occurs in both heavy and light chain loci, and since both heavy and light chain variable regions make up the final antigen combining region of the immunoglobulin molecule, a considerable amount of diversity of immunoglobulin molecules is generated at this level alone. However, another important mechanism for generating diversity is the variability of the precise splice junctions between the various gene segments and the random replacement of nucleotides (so called N (nucleotide) regions) at the imprecise join sites between variable and D region domains and between D and J domains,

during the process of VDJ joining. This is accomplished by an enzyme expressed in immature lymphoid cells called terminal deoxyribonucleotide transferase (TdT), which inserts nucleotides into a DNA chain without the need for a DNA template.[13] Interestingly, the insertion of N regions appears not to occur at VJ junctions in light chains. Additional somatic mutations occur at random in the variable region subsequent to VDJ recombination. It is probable that these modifications are primarily responsible for the acquisition of increasing affinity of the antibodies which is produced in the course of an immune response. This process presumably depends upon competition for antigen and the selection of cells in which mutation of the variable region has led to increased affinity for the epitope in question.

Phenotypic changes during antigen independent B-cell differentiation

Although B lineage associated surface antigens have been detected on the surface of pre-B-cells, the expression of cytoplasmic μ chains heralds their commitment to antibody production. Pre-B-cells express the enzyme TdT as well as histocompatibility (HLA) class II antigens (DR), and a B-cell specific antigen known as Cluster of Differentiation antigen (CD) CD19.[2–4,14] Subsequently, other B-cell specific or associated (i.e. not confined to B-cells) antigens, including the common ALL antigen (CD10), CD24, CD20, CD22 and finally CD21 (the C3d complement component receptor) are sequentially expressed. Pre-B-cells are large, rapidly dividing cells, but shortly before the expression of surface IgM, they became small resting cells. The expression of IgM is accompanied by loss of TdT and CD10 reactivity. IgM is the first immunoglobulin to be expressed. IgD is then expressed in conjunction with IgM, and subsequently, by the process of heavy chain class switching, other heavy chain constant regions can be substituted for μ and delta in the immunoglobulin heavy chain. Recently generated virgin B-cells which have never encountered antigen leave the bone marrow and circulate for a short time through the perifollicular lymphoid tissue in lymph nodes and the marginal zone of the spleen.[15]

As mentioned above, at least a proportion of virgin B-cells belong to the CD5 positive population of B-cells.[6] Malignant lymphomas of small lymphocytic origin, as well as the mantle zone lymphomas and 'lymphomas of intermediate differentiation', express CD5 and appear to be neoplasms of this subgroup of B lymphocytes (*see* Chapter 4).

Molecular and phenotypic changes in B-cells following antigenic stimulation

B-cells express a wide range of B-cell specific and B-cell asssociated surface antigens and receptors in addition to surface immunoglobulin. Among these are CD19, CD20, CD22, CD24 and receptors for interleukin 4 (IL-4 formally known as BSF-1), and the complement fragments C3b, C4b and C3d. The C3d receptor, also known as CD21, is a molecule which also functions as a receptor for Epstein–Barr virus. CD10 is not expressed by mature B-cells, except for a proportion of the cells in germinal centres. Under normal circumstances virgin B-cells appear to be short-lived, being converted to long-lived lymphocytes only if they encounter antigen. It seems likely that circulating lymphocytes which express both IgM and IgD, a phenomenon which involves differential splicing of a long RNA transcript which reads through both μ and δ constant regions[2,4], are long-lived lymphocytes, and presumably, therefore, memory B-cells. These cells recirculate through the primary follicles of lymphoid tissue, and if antigen is encountered they are activated and enter the germinal centre of a secondary follicle (Fig. 3.4). The cells surrounding the germinal centre (i.e. the cells which make up the mantle zone) have the same characteristics as those of the primary follicles, namely surface IgM and IgD. Antigen activated B-cells may promote T-cell help in further dif-

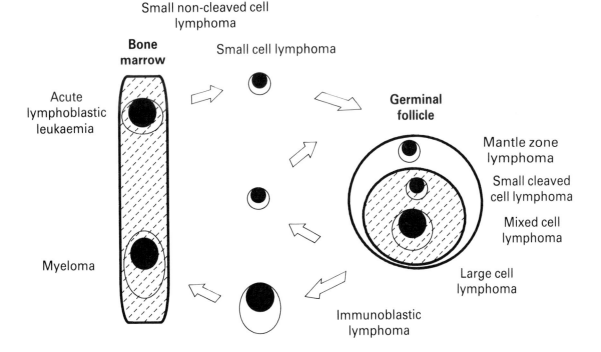

Fig. 3.4 Diagrammatic representation of the differentiation pathways and anatomical location of B-cells. Lymphoid neoplasms which correspond phenotypically to specific stages of differentiation of normal B-cells are indicated adjacent to the relevant cell types. The secondary follicle is composed of an outer mantle zone and an inner germinal centre.

ferentiation by recruiting T-cells which are specifically reactive to the antigen to which the B-cell is reacting. This antigen is processed by the B-cell and expressed on its surface in the cleft of HLA class II molecules which are expressed at a higher level by activated B-cells. Activated B-cells (normally resident in germinal centres of lymph nodes) also express additional growth factor and differentiation factor receptors,[8] including Ki-1, Ki-67, CD23 (Blast-2, an antigen expressed by circulating activated cells, but not cells in the germinal centre), interleukin-2 (IL-2), transferrin receptor, and receptors for IL-5 and 6. At least a proportion of germinal centre cells express CD10 (CALLA).[16] Although CD19 and CD20 expression persists, CD22 and CD23 expression is lost by germinal centre lymphocytes.[14]

The germinal follicle may be the predominant site for somatic mutation of V regions and of class switching (i.e. the site at which the immune response is more precisely tailored with regard to the affinity for antigen)[15], and the reapproximation of the variable region to constant regions with different functional capacities (e.g. complement fixation, the ability to bind to different F_c receptors etc.). In the latter process, the variable region is moved from its position adjacent to the μ constant region to a position adjacent to one of the other heavy chain constant regions.[2-4,17] This recombination occurs at specific sites in the immunoglobulin locus, called switch regions, which lie immediately upstream (5') of the constant regions. During heavy chain class switch recombination, the DNA sequences between two switch regions are deleted, the switch regions fuse, and a new transcript composed of the same variable sequences as before, coupled now to a new heavy chain constant region (e.g. γ or α) is synthesized (Fig. 3.5). Cells which secrete antibody also process the IgG messenger RNA differently, in that the

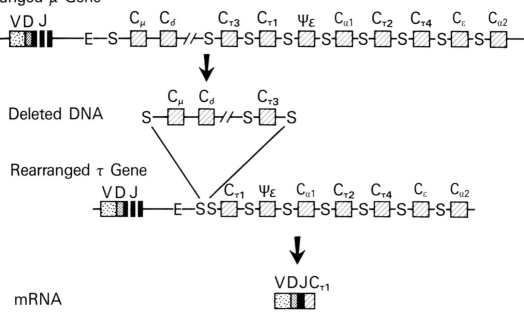

Fig. 3.5 Diagrammatic representation of heavy chain class switching. In this process, the μ gene is broken at the switch region and the segment containing the variable region is approximated to another constant region, in this case γ, via its adjacent switch region. Intervening DNA is deleted. In some cases expression of a heavy chain other than μ or δ may occur via differential splicing, without structural alteration of the gene, as occurs in simultaneous μ/δ expression. V, variable; D, diversity; J, joining regions; S, switch regions; E, the major enhancer region in the heavy chain locus.

region coding for the membrane anchoring lipophilic region at the carboxy terminal of the molecule is spliced out of the RNA.[18] The resultant molecules are not inserted into the cell membrane, but exported from the cell.

At a morphological level, activated B-cells tend to develop nuclear clefting and undergo rapid enlargement. While still small in size, they are referred to as small cleaved cells. As they enlarge within a germinal centre, they become large cleaved cells which may lose most of their surface Ig including surface IgD.[19] There is some evidence that it is during this phase of lack of expression of surface immunoglobulin that further somatic mutation occurs. After re-expression of the immunoglobulin which contains a mutated variable region, cells which express immunoglobulins with the highest affinity for antigens being presented to them by dendritic reticulum cells will be selected for further clonal expansion.[15]

Eventually the nuclear clefts are lost and the cells develop large quantities of rough endoplasmic reticulum as they begin to synthesize large quantities of immunoglobulin. Such cells are referred to as immunoblasts, and are usually found in the medullary cords of the lymph node, having left the germinal follicle. Finally, the cells take on the appearance of plasma cells. Many of them return to the bone marrow, which is the predominant site of antibody production in a secondary immune response. By now they have lost their surface immunoglobulin, as well as most of the B-cell specific and B-cell associated antigens, and they express plasma cell associated antibodies such as T10 and PCA-1.[20] They also possess large amounts of cytoplasmic immunoglobulin, containing both heavy and light chains, unlike pre-B-cells.

Differentiation pathways of normal T-cells

Because T-cell differentiation occurs predominantly in a specific anatomical location (the thymus), it has been relatively easy to explore the stages through which T-cells pass during their maturation (Fig. 3.6). Pre-T-cells arise in the marrow and migrate to the thymus during which time there is progressive rearrangement of T-cell antigen receptor genes (Ti, the i indicating that the antigen is idiotypic) and progressive alteration in the expression of surface receptors.[5,21–23]

Molecular events occurring in T-cell precursors

There are four Ti loci which code for α, β, τ and delta chains. The α locus, in which the delta locus is embedded, is on chromosome 14 (q11), while the β and τ loci are on chromosome 7 (q35-6 and 7p15 respectively).[24–27] The genomic organization of the mouse T-cell receptor genes, which is similar to that of man, is shown in Figure 3.7. A complete antigen receptor molecule is composed of two chains, either α and β, or τ and delta, which form a heterodimer similar to an immunoglobulin molecule composed of heavy and light chains. Both heterodimers are associated with another molecule, T3 (CD3), on the cell surface to form the complete antigen detection complex.[5,9] T-cells can only recognize antigen, however, when presented in the cleft of either a class I or class II HLA molecule.[5] Recent evidence also suggests that antigen recognition by T-cells is considerably enhanced in the presence of either CD4, in the case of T-cells interacting with class II molecules, or CD8, in the case of T-cells interacting with class I molecules.[5]

The rearrangement of the T-cell antigen receptor genes is very similar to that of the immunoglobulin genes. Each allele has discontinuous variable (V), joining (J) and constant (C) regions in the germline (unrearranged) state, while the β and δ loci also have D regions, thus making them the homologues of the immunoglobulin heavy chains. There are two C regions for β. A functional gene is formed when one of a small number of V regions, perhaps only 15 for this locus, joins to one of the six D regions and one of the six J regions (DJ joining precedes VD joining as in the immunoglobulin locus) which are located upstream of both the $C\beta_1$ or $C\beta_2$ regions.[28] A similar recombinational process occurs in the other T-cell receptor loci, although each varies with regard to the number of V, J

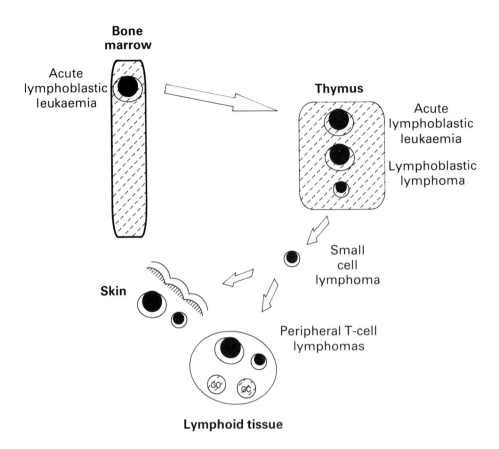

Fig. 3.6 Diagrammatic representation of the differentiation pathways and anatomical location of T-cells. Lymphoid neoplasms which correspond phenotypically to specific stages of differentiation of normal T-cells are indicated adjacent to the relevant cell type.

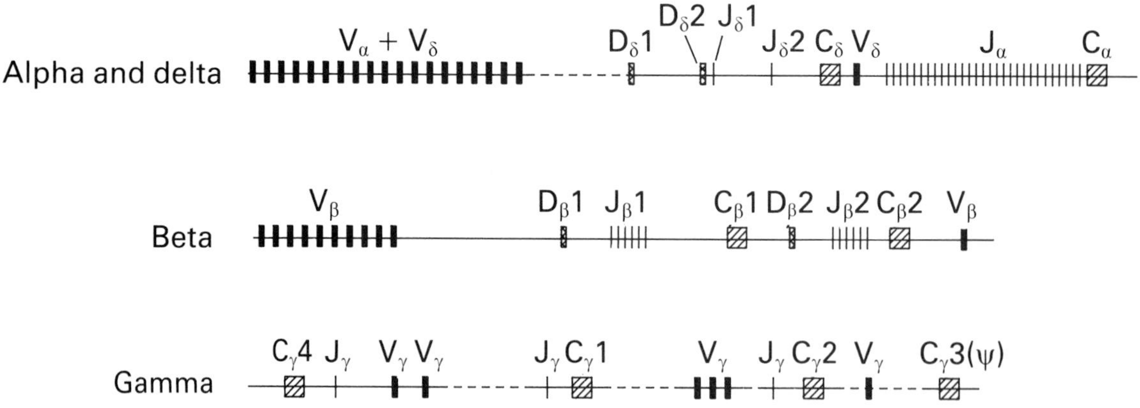

Fig. 3.7 Diagrammatic representation of the mouse T-cell antigen receptor genes. Note that the δ gene is embedded within the α gene. Variable, diversity and joining regions are designated as V, D, and J respectively. Modified from Davis HM, Bjorkman PJ. *Nature.* 1988; **334**, 395–402.

and C regions. In the mouse, for example, the α locus probably uses 75–100 V regions, while only about 10 V regions have been identified for δ. In addition, in the case of both β and δ, a single V region has been identified immediately downstream of the C locus.

During thymocyte differentiation it appears that the T_τ and T_δ are the first genes to rearrange, followed by the T_β gene and finally the T_α gene.[5,21,29] Although it has been suggested that α:β rearrangement occurs only if a functional T-cell receptor is not made as a consequence of τ:δ rearrangement, there is evidence that the two varieties of T-cell receptor are expressed in cells with functionally different capacities. γ:δ receptors have, however, also been identified in a variety of functionally different T-cell populations including helper and cytotoxic/ suppressor T-cells.[5,30] The β chain, like the immunoglobulin μ chain, is expressed in the cytoplasm prior to the expression of the complete antigen receptor complex which includes α and T3 (CD3) molecules.[31] As in B-cell tumours, the enzyme TdT has been shown to be involved in adding random nucleotides to either side of the D or J segments in all 4 of the rearranging Ti genes[5,29] although, unlike B-cells, somatic mutation does not appear to be a mechanism involved in the generation of antigen receptor diversity.[28]

Phenotypic changes during T-cell differentiation

Early thymocytes, which enter the cortex of the thymus from the bone marrow and account for some 10 per cent of thymocytes, express CD7, an antigen of unknown function which is recognized by several monoclonal antibodies, 3A1, 4H9 (leu 9) and WT1. It is expressed at all levels of thymic differentiation as well as in a proportion of mature T-cells and may be the best marker of thymic neoplasms.[32-34] The CD5 antigen, present on all mature T-cells and most thymocytes, is also frequently expressed and some, but not all, early T-cells (and the majority of all thymocytes and T-cells) express CD2 – the sheep erythrocyte receptor – which was formerly detected by the formation of rosettes with sheep erythrocytes.[22,23] T-cells (including thymocytes)

can be activated via this receptor, which is expressed on the majority of thymocyte and peripheral T-cells.[9] In addition, early thymocytes express the transferrin receptor (T9) and an antigen also present on activated T-cells and plasma cells (T10), but no other antigen which has so far been identified on more mature T-cells. T_τ, but not T_β receptor genes are rearranged at the earliest stage of intrathymic differentiation. TdT is expressed by the majority of thymocytes but tends to be lost in the most mature cells of the thymic medulla.

At an intermediate level of differentiation, a level which accounts for approximately 70 per cent of thymocytes, the antigens expressed include CD2, CD5, CD7, and both CD4 and CD8. T10 continues to be expressed, but T9 is not.[35] Intermediate thymocytes also express an antigen which occurs only in the intermediate thymic compartment (CD1). Intermediate thymocytes rearrange their T_β and/or T_δ genes and synthesize receptor proteins, but do not express Ti molecules or the associated T3 at the cell surface.[29,31] As the cells mature further and enter the late thymic compartment in the thymic medulla, before leaving the thymus, they lose CD1, T10 and eventually TdT, but continue to express CD5. They also begin to express the antigen receptor (Ti) in conjunction with CD3. Rearrangement of the T_α gene occurs at this stage of differentiation.

Mature, CD4-positive cells are helpers of other cell types, including B-cells responding to antigen and mitogen stimulation, suppressor and cytotoxic T-cells and antibody-producing cells. The CD4 molecule also functions as the receptor for the human immunodeficiency virus (HIV). CD8-positive cells include suppressor and cytotoxic cells of various kinds. Because T-cells may either help or destroy cells which express foreign antigens, the mode of antigen presentation is crucial to the outcome of the cellular interaction with T-cells. HLA class I molecules are found on essentially all normal cells, whereas class II molecules are confined to antigen-presenting cells such as dendritic macrophages, B- and activated T-cells. Thus the majority of cells can only present antigen embedded in class II antigens and thus stimulate CD4 cells and obtain T-cell help. Self HLA antigens appear to be necessary for the development of helper cells in the thymus.[22]

Events in T-cells following antigenic stimulation

Activation of T-cells is associated with the expression of a variety of 'activation' antigens including Il-2, transferrin receptor (T9), HLA class II antigens, T10, Ki-1, Ki-67 and antigens known as TA_1, TA_2 and TA_3.[9,35] As is the case for B-cells, some, at least, of these activation antigens are growth factor receptors. Others are associated with the need to bind to other cell types, including other T-cells, during immune responses. The latter are known as lymphocyte functional antigens – e.g. LFA-1, LFA-3 and ICAM-1.[36,37]

Anatomical distribution of mature T and B lymphocytes

Mature T- and B-cells differ in their anatomical locations in lymphoid tissue. T-cells primarily occupy the paracortical or interfollicular regions of lymph nodes and gut-associated lymphoid tissue, including the tonsils. In the spleen, T lymphocytes are found mainly in the periarteriolar regions of the Malphighian corpuscles. Unlike B-cells, T-cells must be activated frequently at the initial site of antigen exposure (e.g. the skin, lungs or bowel). This may account for the high frequency of extranodal sites (e.g. the skin) in T-cell neoplasia.

B lymphocytes are found predominantly in the lymphoid follicles of lymph nodes, spleen, Peyer's patches and other lymphoid tissue. Primary lymphoid follicles are homogeneous collections of small lymphocytes, while secondary follicles contain a germinal centre – an expanded area of small and large lymphoid cells surrounded by a crescentic mantle zone, with its convexity to the outer edge of the lymph node or lymphoid aggregate. In normal germinal centres (which are the site of expansion of B-cell clones reacting to antigenic stimulation) there is a polarity across the follicle, with smaller cells collecting at one pole and larger cells at the other. Infiltrating T-cells, almost all of which express CD4, are present in large numbers among the large cells but not among the small cells. Large, antigen-activated B-cells (immunoblasts) leave the germinal follicles and the lymph node via the medullary cords and migrate to the bone marrow, the major site of IgG antibody production. Thus, lymphocyte traffic is from the bone marrow to the peripheral blood, and thence, circulation through lymph nodes (primary follicles and mantle zones) and spleen. Antigen responses occur both in the parafollicular regions (T-cells and Ki-1-positive T- and B-cells) and in the secondary germinal follicles. Terminally differentiated cells return to the bone marrow, and memory cells re-enter the blood and lymphatic circulation.

The entry of lymphocytes into the lymph nodes is mediated by specific interactions between lymphocytes and specialized endothelial cells lining the postcapillary venules. Because of these specialized cells, the postcapillary venules are known as 'high endothelial venules'. Monoclonal antibodies have been derived which react with structures on the lymphocyte surface which are able to bind to the specialized endothelial cells and effect lymph node entry.[38]

Prelymphomatous states

Since lymphomas arise from the constituent cells of the immune system, it is not surprising that disorders associated with abnormal regulation of lymphocytes are associated with an increased incidence of non-Hodgkin's lymphomas. This is probably a consequence of alterations in the size and proliferative (or self-renewal) potential of selected lymphoid subpopulations. Epstein–Barr virus (EBV) also appears to be important in the pathogenesis of lymphomas in immunodeficiency states, since the majority of these lymphomas contain EBV genomes.[39,40] One possible explanation of this is that defective T-cell regulation permits the expansion of EBV-infected clones of B-cells which would normally be tightly controlled, but which, due to the influence of viral genes, have a selective growth advantage over uninfected cells. Such cell clones would then be at increased risk to develop a genetic change capable of causing neoplastic behaviour. In such patients, however, the borderline between non-neoplastic lympho-proliferation and true neoplasia is not easy to discern, and is perhaps to some extent a semantic debate.

Some families carry a sex-linked disorder known as X-linked lymphoproliferative syndrome (XLP) which is characterized by the occurrence of aplastic anaemia, fatal infectious mononucleosis and malignant non-Hodgkin's lymphomas.[40] Whether or not patients succumb to fatal infectious mononucleosis or lymphoma presumably reflects the degree to which immune reactivity against EBV infection is impaired. Individuals with essentially no ability to regulate the proliferation of EBV-infected cells die as a consequence of primary EBV infection. However, those individuals with some ability to control EBV-infected cells may simply be at increased risk for a B-cell lymphoma, the result of an enlarged pool of EBV-infected B-cells and the consequent increased risk of the development of a genetic abnormality leading to a clonal lymphoma. It is of interest that in patients with the acquired immunodeficiency syndrome (AIDS), some of the lymphomas which develop have the histology of small non-cleaved lymphomas and also carry the same chromosomal abnormalities, including break-point locations similar to those in sporadic small non-cleaved lymphomas (*see* Chapter 6).[41-43] Prior to the development of these lymphomas there is B-cell hyperplasia, in which expansion of a small number of clones occurs, but in which the genetic changes associated with small non-cleaved lymphoma are not present,[43] strongly supporting the above interpretation. HIV is not present in the tumour cells themselves, although it may be present in interspersed lymphocytes.

In children, the genetically determined immunodeficiency syndromes with the greatest risk of lymphoma development are ataxia telangiectasia, Wiskott–Aldrich syndrome, common variable immunodeficiency disease, severe combined immunodeficiency syndrome (SCID) and XLP. The estimated risk of non-Hodgkin's lymphoma in these syndromes is between 1 per cent (SCID) and 35 per cent (XLP). Some 12 to 14 per cent of patients with Wiskott–Aldrich syndrome develop non-Hodgkin's lymphomas. Other genetically determined immunodeficiency syndromes are associated with a much lower risk of lymphoma development. It is possible that in some of these syndromes the decreased ability to repair DNA and the predisposition to chromosomal abnormalities (e.g. in ataxia telangiectasia, Bloom's syndrome and xeroderma pigmentosum) also play a role in the induction of lymphomas (*see* Chapter 9).

Transplant recipients are also at risk of developing non-Hodgkin's lymphomas as a consequence of iatrogenic immunosuppression and consequent lymphoid hyperplasia (lymphomas have been described in renal, heart and bone marrow recipients). In some series as many as 25 per cent of renal or cardiac allograft recipients have developed non-Hodgkin's lymphomas after one year. Patients treated with the monoclonal antibody T3 have also developed EBV-associated lymphomas, doubtless from the consequent reduction in regulatory subsets of T lymphocytes.

Additional prelymphomatous states of adults include α heavy chain disease, which is associated with an increased incidence of B-cell (α heavy chain-expressing) immunoblastic lymphoma of the bowel[44] (*see* Chapter 23), while the angiocentric lymphoproliferative syndromes, including lymphomatoid papulomatosis, lymphomatoid granulomatosis, lethal midline granuloma and angioimmunoblastic lymphadenopathy are associated with an increased incidence of T-cell lymphomas of mature origin.[45] The pathology of these syndromes is discussed in Chapter 4.

Major phenotypic subdivisions of lymphoid neoplasms

Non-Hodgkin's lymphomas appear to arise from essentially all lymphoid cell subpopulations. This includes cells of the B and T lineages and their precursor cells. Thus, 4 major subgroups of non-Hodgkin's lymphomas are immediately apparent: lymphomas arising from B- and T-cell precursors, i.e. cells undergoing antigen independent differentiation, and lymphomas arising from mature, immunocompetent B- and T- cells undergoing antigen dependent differentiation (or, at least, appearing to do so) (Figs. 3.4 and 3.6).

This simple observation has a number of implications. For example, precursor cells are usually rapidly dividing cells, since their function is to maintain the size of the compartment containing immunocompetent cells so far unexposed to antigen. Loss from the precursor compartment, and hence limitation of its size, occurs through the production of non-dividing, virgin lymphocytes (*see* Fig. 3.1). Thus, precursor cell neoplasia results from a failure to enter a resting state – i.e. the cell remains in a state of continual renewal of proliferating cells, with no differentiation into non-proliferating cells. Such a situation could be brought about by a failure to down-regulate one or more genes involved in cell proliferation. Such genes, however, would not necessarily need to be expressed at a level greater than had been the case in the normal proliferating precursor cell. This may well be pertinent to the pathogenesis of the small non-cleaved lymphomas (*see* Chapter 6) and lymphoblastic lymphoma. In such tumours the predominant cell in the neoplasm would resemble the normal counterpart cell (i.e. precursor cell) in which malignant transformation occurred if a sharp and efficient differentiation block were induced, but a small degree of differentiation beyond the target cell stage is also possible. Because tumour cells are unable to enter a resting phase, the malignant neoplasm will become manifest at the stage of differentiation at which proliferation normally ceases.

Some genetic abnormalities in precursor cells may not result in continued proliferation, but rather in a specific differentiation block – not necessarily at the stage in which the genetic lesion occurs (*see* Fig. 3.1). Thus, the cell clone may undergo normal proliferation and differentiation for a considerable part of the differentiation pathway. Tumours resulting from such genetic lesions may eventually become clinically apparent because of a greater life span (immortalization) of one differentiation stage of the malignant clone. This results in the slow but progressive accumulation of more differentiated cells (follicular lymphomas may fall into this category) at the stage at which differentiation ceases. Perhaps because of the time required to generate a neoplasm by this mechanism, increased further if some regulation of the malignant clone is retained, such tumours are essentially unknown in children.

Neoplasms caused by genetic changes in precursor cells are more likely to occur during childhood since the precursor compartments, as judged by the relative size of the thymus and bone marrow, are higher in children. Even in tumours which are manifested in adult life, because of a slow accumulation of more differentiated cells following a genetic lesion which occurred in a precursor cell, the genetic lesion could have occurred in childhood. This possibility has interesting implications with regard to the epidemiology of these tumours.

The converse of this is that neoplasms arising in cells undergoing antigen-dependent differentiation are more likely to arise in adult life. This could be a simple consequence of the gradual increase in cumulative antigen exposure throughout life, resulting in an increasing probability, with age, that a lymphoma of this type will occur. Most diffuse lymphomas in adults fall into this category, and this may explain the increasing incidence of the non-Hodgkin's lymphomas which occur in adults with age (*see* Chapter 1).

Lymphomas of the B-cell lineage

Neoplasms of B-cell precursors

Neoplasms arising in precursor cells are frequently categorized as acute leukaemia, since precursor cells arise in the bone marrow (Fig. 3.4). Neoplasms of the B-cell lineage which have the characteristics of precursor cells account for the major fraction of acute lymphoblastic leukemias (some 80 per cent), the commonest childhood malignancy in the more developed countries. Pre-B-cell tumours presenting as solid masses in lymph nodes or bone, without bone marrow involvement are rare, but have been described.[46–48] A characteristic feature of precursor B-cell neoplasms is the expression of TdT, which is also found in neoplasms of T precursor cells, but in no other lymphomas. CD19 is almost invariably expressed, and a high percentage of such tumours (60–75 per cent) express the common acute lymphoblastic leukaemia antigen, CD10.

Presumptive pre-follicule centre cell neoplasms

B-cell neoplasms, in which the malignant cell has many of the characteristics of primary B-cells not yet exposed to antigen, include small cell lymphomas and small non-cleaved cell lymphomas. In neither case is such an origin certain, but in the case of small cell lymphomas, the expression of CD5 and IgM as well as IgD strongly suggests that this is a neoplasm of primary B-cells. Small non-cleaved cell lymphomas express surface IgM as well as CD10, and other antigens, such as CD22 and CD24, which are expressed at a higher level on mantle zone cells rather than germinal centre cells.[49] This applies particularly to small non-cleaved lymphomas which lack the presence of the EBV genome which, because of its effect on cellular genes, may induce the expression of antigens which would otherwise not be expressed at the same level of cellular differentiation. Thus, attempting to determine the degree of differentiation of EBV-positive Burkitt's lymphoma simply by examination of its expression of surface markers may be misleading.

It is important to note that there are at least two types of small non-cleaved cell lymphoma, based on cytogenetic findings (*see* Chapter 17). Those tumours with 14;18 translocations probably arise from a germinal centre cell. It has been suggested by some investigators, however, that even tumours with 8;14 translocations fall into at least two categories based on phenotypic differences: those which arise from bone marrow, and those which arise in the germinal centres of lymphoid tissue.[50]

It is possible that the normal counterpart cell of both small cell lymphomas and small non-cleaved cell lymphomas is a memory cell – or even that some of these neoplasms are the malignant counterparts of memory cells and that other primary neoplasms are the counterparts of virgin lymphocytes. The marked behavioural

and morphological differences in these neoplasms which may arise from the same, or a closely related, normal cell type, are readily explained by the fact that they have different genetic abnormalities (*see* Chapters 5 and 6). While small non-cleaved lymphomas result from a marked abnormality in the regulation of proliferation, small cell lymphomas appear to result from an abnormally prolonged life span (perhaps resulting from a differentiation block) of a specific cell type.

Follicle cell neoplasms

The majority of lymphomas in the more developed countries arise from follicle centre cells. Such tumours may have a follicular or diffuse histological pattern, and lymph node involvement is usually a prominent feature of their clinical presentation. In follicular lymphomas, dendritic reticulum cells are interspersed among the tumour cells, but such cells are not seen in diffuse lymphomas.[51] A very small fraction of lymphomas have the phenotypic characteristics of cells normally found in primary lymphoid follicles or the mantle zones of secondary lymhoid follicles (*see* Fig. 3.4). These tumours include the mantle zone lymphoma (in which the neoplastic cells have the appearance of a mantle zone in that they surround normal or atrophic germinal centres), and lymphomas of intermediated differentiation (which are identical to mantle zone lymphomas except for their completely diffuse nature). Both tumours express IgM, IgD and CD5, as well as other B-cell markers, but are usually CD10-negative.[52]

Tumours of germinal centre cells may consist of small cells (cleaved), large cells (cleaved or non-cleaved) or a mixture of small and large cells. All such tumours may be manifested as follicular or diffuse forms, and frequently undergo conversion from follicular to diffuse. None of these tumours express CD5, but most express CD10 and CD21 as well as other B-cell markers. IgD expression is very uncommon.

Lymphomas of immunoblasts

In normal lymph nodes, activated B-cells which

are beginning to secrete immunoglobulin leave the germinal centre via the medullary cords. Such cells often have so-called 'plasmacytoid' characteristics, which result from the increased amount of rough endoplasmic reticulum and well developed Golgi apparatus related to increased levels of immunoglobulin production. Tumours which have these characteristics are referred to as immunoblastic lymphomas. There are other types of large cell lymphoma which do not resemble either germinal centre cells or plasmacytoid immunoblasts. These include the Ki-1-positive lymphomas which have similar phenotypic characteristics to a subset of activated parafollicular B-cells[53,54].

Lymphomas of the T-cell lineage

Neoplasms of precursor T-cells

As might be expected from a knowledge of T-cell differentiation pathways, a high proportion of T-cell precursor neoplasms present as thymic enlargement, with or without marrow involvement and lymphadenopathy (*see* Fig. 3.6). Precursor neoplasms of the T lineage differ from their B-cell counterparts with regard to the much higher proportion of such tumours in which the bone marrow remains uninvolved – without doubt a corollary of the major extramedullary site of T-cell differentiation (i.e. the thymus). However, the ratio of precursor cell neoplasms with bone marrow involvement to those without bone marrow involvement varies throughout the world. Moreover, because of differences in the definition of leukaemia (which is based solely on cell location rather than morphology or phenotype), there is considerable variation around the world with regard to the categorization of any given neoplasm as a leukaemia rather than a lymphoma. This must be taken into account in epidemiological studies.

T-cell precursor neoplasms, like those of the B-cell lineage, express TdT. Their phenotypic characteristics conform largely to those of normal thymocytes, but apparently aberrant phenotypes may also be seen.[55,56] It is possible that such cells are present in very small numbers in the normal thymus and therefore are not readily detected. The most frequently expressed markers in precursor cells in the T-cell lineage are CD7, CD5 and CD2. However, since CD1 is expressed only by thymocytes (among lymphoid cells), whenever it is present in lymphoid cells outside the thymus, this antigen is strongly suggestive of neoplasia, particularly when coupled to TdT expression. CD10 and HLA class II antigens are occasionally expressed on precursor T-cell lineage neoplasms, their presence probably signifying more immature and more mature neoplasms respectively.

Peripheral T-cell neoplasms

The broad variety of neoplasms characterized as being of peripheral T-cell origin (i.e. post-thymic) show a lack of expression of TdT and antigens associated with immature T-cells, including CD1 and CD10. These are neoplasms which represent activated T-cells and therefore generally express interleukin 2 receptors and HLA class II antigens as well as 'pan-T' antigens. Sometimes CD5 or CD3 antigens, which might be expected to be expressed on all peripheral T-cell lymphomas, are missing.[52] These neoplasms usually express either CD4 or CD8 antigens and are often functionally active and able to help or suppress in *in vitro* systems.[1,57] They frequently secrete lymphokines, a feature which may give rise to infiltrations of other cell types (e.g. epithelioid histiocytes in Lennert's lymphoma, fibroblasts, plasma cells and normal lymphocytes, including T lymphocytes) or characteristic abnormalities such as hypercalcaemia.[57–59] These neoplasms are also often tropic for particular organs or tissues, e.g. the skin (cutaneous T-cell lymphomas) blood vessels (angiocentric neoplasms) or lung (Waldron's lymphoma)[59–61] (*see* Chapter 22). One subset of peripheral T-cell lymphomas has been associated with HTLV-1, a T-cell tropic human retrovirus (*see* Chapter 11). In general, T-cell lymphomas are more pleomorphic than B-cell lymphomas, but they may have any of the histological appearances listed in the Working Formulation (*see* Chapter 4).

It is clear that over the last two decades a much improved understanding of the nature and classification of malignant lymphoid neoplasms has been gained by relating them to the differentiation sequences of normal lymphocytes. A practical consequence of this approach has been the use of phenotyping and genotyping in the diagnosis of the non-Hodgkin's lymphomas. These topics, which are discussed in succeeding chapters, have provided a new level of diagnostic precision which has, in some cases, been instrumental in identifying hitherto unrecognized pathological entities as well as leading to the identification of previously unrecognized subsets of normal lymphocytes. It is to be hoped that continued exploration of this area, coupled to detailed evaluation of the molecular genetic changes associated with specific neoplasms, will lead to an improved understanding of pathogenesis, and ultimately, to novel treatment techniques.

References

1. Magrath IT. *Journal of the National Cancer Institute.* 1981; **67**, 501–14.
2. Calvert JE, Maruyama S, Tedder TF, Webb CF, Cooper M. *Seminars in Hematology.* 1984; **21**, 226–43.
3. Vogler LB, Lawton AR. *Clinical Immunology and Allergy.* 1985; **5**, 235–52.
4. Cooper MD. *New England Journal of Medicine.* 1987; **317**, 1452–6.
5. Davis MM, Bjorkman PJ. *Nature.* 1988; **334**, 395.
6. Casali P, Burastero SE, Nakamura M, Inghirami G, Notkins AI. *Science.* 1987; **236**, 77–81.
7. Nakamura M, Burastero SE, Notkins AL, Casali P. *Journal of Immunology.* 1988; **140**, 4180–5.
8. Gordon J, Guy G. In: Bird G, Calvert JE (eds). *B Lymphocytes in Human Disease.* Oxford: Oxford University Press, 1988; 148–73.
9. Alcover A, Ramarli D, Richardson NE, Chang H–S, Reinherz EL. *Immunological Reviews.* 1987; **95**, 5–36.
10. Nadler LM, Korsmeyer SJ, Anderson KC, *et al. Journal of Clinical Investigation.* 1984; **74**, 332.
11. Alt FW, Blackwell TK, Depinho RA, Reith MG, Yancopoulos. *Immunological Reviews.* 1986; **89**, 5–30.
12. Korsmeyer SJ, Hieter PA, Ravetch JV *et al. Proceedings of the National Academy of Sciences USA.* 1981; **78**, 7096–7100.
13. Desiderio SV, Yancopoulos GD, Paskind M, *et al. Nature.* 1984; **311**, 752.
14. Nadler LM. In: Reinherz EL, Haynes BF, Nadler LM, Bernstein IO, (eds). *Leukocyte Typing II.* New York: Springer Verlag, 1986; 3–43.
15. Maclennon ICM, Gray D. *Immunological Reviews.* 1986; **91**, 61–84.
16. Hoffman-Fezer G, Knapp W, Thierfelder S. *Leukemia Research.* 1982; **6**, 761–767.
17. Radbruch A, Burger C, Klein S, Muller W. *Immunological Reviews.* 1986; **89**, 69–83.
18. Alt FW, Bothwell AKM, Knapp ALM, *et al. Cell.* 1980; **20**, 293.
19. Bhan AK, Nadler LM, Stashenko P, McCluskey RT, Schlossman SF. *Journal of Experimental Medicine.* 1981; **154**, 737–49.
20. Anderson KC, Bates MP, Slaughenhoupt B, *et al. Journal of Immunology.* 1984; **132**, 3172–9.
21. Royer HD, Ramarli D, Acuto O, *et al. Proceedings of the National Academy of Sciences USA.* 1985; **82**, 5510–4.
22. Blue ML, Schlossman SF. (1986) Serono Symposium Publications. Raven Press 28, 3–11.
23. MacDonald HR, Howe RC, Pedrazzine R, Lees RK *et al. Immunological Reviews.* 1988; **104**, 157–82.
24. Croce CM, Isobe M, Palumbo A, *et al. Science.* 1985; **227**, 1044–7.
25. Le Beau MM, Diaz MO, Rowley JD, *et al. Cell.* 1985, **41**, 335.
26. Murre C, Waldmann RA, Morton CC, *et al. Nature.* 1985, **316**, 549–52.
27. Isobe M, Russo G, Haluska FG, Croce CM. *Proceedings of the National Academy of Sciences USA.* 1988; **85**, 3933–7.
28. Hood L, Kronenberg M, Hunkapillar T. *Cell.* 1985; **40**, 225–9.
29. Haars R, Kronenberg M, Gallatin WM, Weissman IL, Owen FL, Hood L. *Journal of Experimental Medicine.* 1986; **164**, 1–24.
30. Lefranc M–P, Rabbitts TH. *Nature.* 1985; **316**, 464–6.
31. Royer HD, Acuto O, Fabbi M, *et al. Cell.* 1984; **39**, 261–6.
32. Haynes BF. *Immunobiology.* 1981; **159**, 14.
33. Vodinelich L, Tax W, Bai Y, Pegram S, Capel P, Greaves MF. *Blood.* 1983; **62**, 1108–13.
34. Link M, Warnke R, Finlay J, *et al. Blood.* 1983; **62**, 722.
35. Reinherz EL, Schlossman SF. In: Murphy SB, Gilbert JR (eds). *Leukemia Research, Advances in Cell Biology and Treatment.* New York: Elsevier Science Publishing Company Inc., 1983; 85–95.
36. Shaw S, Ginther Luce GE. *Journal of Immunology.* 1987; **139**, 1037–45.
37. Makgoba MW, Sanders ME, Ghinther Luce GE, *et al. Nature.* 1988; **331**, 86–8.
38. Streeter PR, Berg EL, Rouse BTN, Bargatze RF, Butcher EC. *Nature.* 1988; **331**, 41.

39. Saemundsen AK, Purtilo D, Sakamoto K *et al*. *Cancer Research*. 1981; **41**, 4237–42.
40. Purtilo D. In: Magrath IT, O'Conor G, Ramot B (eds). *Pathogenesis of Leukemias and Lymphomas: Environmental Influences*. New York: Raven Press, 1984; 235–57.
41. Whang-Peng J, Lee EC, Sieverts H, Magrath IT. *Blood*. 1984; **63**, 818–22.
42. Chaganti RSK, Jhanwar S, Kozinar B, *et al*. *Blood*. 1983; **61**, 1269–1272.
43. Pelicci PG, Knowles DM, Arlin ZA *et al*. *Journal of Experimental Medicine*. 1986; **164**, 2049–60.
44. Salem P, El-Hashimi L, Anaissi E, *et al*. *Developmental Oncology*. 1985; **32**, 269–77.
45. Watanabe S, Sato Y, Shimoyama M, *et al*. *Cancer*. 1986; **58**, 2224–32.
46. Cossman J, Chused TM, Fisher RI, *et al*. *Cancer Research*. 1983; **43**, 4486.
47. Link MP, Hoper M, Dorfman RF, *et al*. *Blood*. 1983; **61**, 838.
48. Grogan T, Spier C, Wirt DP, *et al*. *Diagnostic Immunology*. 1986; **4**, 81–8.
49. Sandlund JT, Kiwanuka J, Marti GE, Goldschmidts G, Magrath IT. In: Reinherz EL, Hayes BF, Nadler LM, Bernstein ID (eds). *Leukocyte Typing II*. New York: Springer Verlag, 1986; 403–10.
50. Favrot MC, Philip I, Philip T, *et al*. *Journal of the National Cancer Institute*. 1944;, **73**, 841–78.
51. Grogan TM, Spier CM, Richter LC, Rangel CS. In: Bennett JM, Foon DA (eds). *Immunological approaches to the Classification and Management of Lymphomas and Leukemias*. Boston: Kluwer Academic Publishers, 1988; 31–148.
52. Caligaris-Cappio F. In: Bird G and Calvert JE (eds). *B Lymphocytes in Human Disease*. Oxford: Oxford University Press, 1988; 323–353.
53. Stein H, Gerdes J, Tippelmann G, *et al*. In: Cavalli F, Bonnadonna G, Rosencweig M (eds). *Lymphoma: Experimental and Clinical Findings*. (Abstract published in meeting proceedings).
54. Kadin M, Sako K, Berliner N, *et al*. *Blood*. 1986; **68**, 1042–9.
55. Bernard A, Boumsell L, Reinherz EL, *et al*. *Blood*. 1981; **57**, 1105.
56. Roper M, Crist WM, Metzger R, *et al*. *Blood*. 1983; **61**, 830.
57. Wright DH. *Histopathology*. 1986; **10**, 321–6.
58. Kim H, Jacobs C, Warnke RA, Dorfman RR. *Cancer*. 1978; **41**, 620–35.
59. Greer JP, York JC, Cousar JB, Mitchell RT, *et al*. *Journal of Clinical Oncology*. 1984; 788–98.
60. Waldron JA, Leech JH, Click AD, Flexner JM *et al*. *Cancer*. 1977; **40**, 1604–17.
61. Jaffe ES. *Cancer Investigations*. 1984; **2**, 413–26.

CHAPTER 4

HISTOPATHOLOGY AND IMMUNOPHENOTYPING

Paul J Cohen and Elaine S Jaffe

The advances in the understanding of the basic biology of the immune system have been rapidly applied to the diagnosis and classsification of the malignant lymphomas. The concept of the lymphomas as tumours of the immune system continues to be confirmed and extended (*see* Chapter 2). While traditional morphological methods have been fairly successful in predicting the clinical behaviour of these diverse entities, and therefore remain the cornerstone of the pathologist's approach to tissue diagnosis, there has been an explosion of new techniques available to study lymphoid neoplasia. Some of these have been refined to the point where they can be utilized to study lymph node biopsies on a relatively wide scale. Methods such as immunohistochemistry, flow cytometry and cytogenetics are now in the process of dissemination from research centres to diagnostically-orientated clinical laboratories. This chapter reviews the combined use of morphological and immunological tools in the diagnosis of non-Hodgkin's lymphomas.

Immunological methods: general considerations

Normal and neoplastic cells of the immune system can be distinguished by the presence of selected surface molecules thought to represent markers of differentiation or of functional capacity. Antibodies which detect these determinants can therefore be used to characterize proliferations of lymphoid cells.[1] The use of hybridoma technology has given an enormous spur to this approach, as it provides an unlimited supply of monospecific antibodies directed at these markers.[2] For example, the E-rosette test was previously the best way to detect T lymphocytes, which have receptors for sheep erythrocytes, and the erythrocyte antibody complement (EAC) test was employed for the detection of cells that have receptors for the C3d component of complement.[3] These cumbersome methods have been replaced by antibodies to CD2 (the sheep erythrocyte receptor) and CD21 (the C3d receptor).

The cornucopia of monoclonals has also created some difficulties. Often monoclonals established in different laboratories were found to have identical specificity, or to recognize different epitopes of the same molecule, yet the names for the antibodies were those given by the various laboratories. In order to develop a standard nomenclature, international work-shops on leucocyte typing have been organized, patterned on the conferences which developed the system for naming HLA antigens.[4,5,6] Antibodies are grouped into 'clusters of differentiation' or 'CDs' when the evidence points to a common antigen. Thus, the 'CD3 molecule' refers to the complex of peptides linked to the T-cell antigen receptor, which is detected by several monoclonals of diverse origins (T3, OKT3, anti-Leu 4).

Monoclonals can be used to study lymphoid cells from clinical samples using tissue sections or cell suspensions. A cell preparation is incubated with an antibody to the molecule of interest, the non-adherent antibody is washed off and adherent antibody is detected by either a linked enzymatic reaction, which gives a coloured product, or by fluorescence. The advantage of immunohistochemical techniques is that cell morphology and the anatomical organization can be seen as well as the immunological phenotype. This is important, especially when one considers that neoplasms are rarely pure populations of neoplastic cells; there is invariably an admixture of normal and reactive cells, often lymphoid as well. For example, many B-cell lymphomas contain large numbers of infiltrating T-cells, sometimes T-cells can be the numerical majority.[7,8] Thus, if one were deciding whether a tumour was of B- or T-cell origin, it would be crucial to ascertain which markers were on the malignant cells, and which on the reactive cells.

The use of cell suspensions in a flow cytometer or fluorescence-activated cell sorter can give complementary information.[9] Cells labelled with fluorescent antibody can be sensed quantitatively by the laser-based optical system of these analysers. The amount of fluorescence on a given cell is proportional to the amount of antibody bound, and hence to the level of expression of antigen. Measurement of cell size is made at the same time. In addition, current models allow the labelling of two antigens on a single cell with molecules which fluoresce at different wavelengths. The output of the flow cytometer is an enumeration of cell size, number and fluorescent intensity which can be stored in computers as raw data and subjected to sophisticated analysis. One can look at tens of thousands of cells in seconds, which enables one to study a clinical sample with numerous antibodies. The sensitivity of the technique is such that, with a high affinity antibody, the flow cytometer can detect in the order of a few thousand molecules on the cell surface.

Since processing of tissue for paraffin embedding often significantly alters antigenic determinants, most antibodies are used on viable cell suspensions or frozen sections. However, several very useful antibodies do react with formalin fixed, paraffin embedded tissue,

e.g. antibody to leucocyte common antigen (CD45), Leu M1 (CD15), or cytoplasmic immunoglobulin. Leucocyte common antigen is present on virtually all lymphocytes and histiocytes and has never been demonstrated on non-haematopoietic cells. It is very useful in the differential diagnosis of lymphoma from poorly differentiated carcinoma.[10,11] Leu M1 has been reported to be present on the neoplastic cells of Hodgkin's disease, and may be helpful when the dilemma is between Hodgkin's and non-Hodgkin's lymphoma.[12,13] Cells with significant amounts of cytoplasm, if they are of B-cell origin, may demonstrate monoclonal cytoplasmic immunoglobulin in paraffin sections. Monoclonality is supportive evidence for a neoplastic nature (*see* below).

In the early phase of the application of hybridoma technology to diagnosis, it was thought that certain markers would be specific for a given entity. For example, CD10 (CALLA, J5) was initially felt to be diagnostic of common acute lymphoblastic leukaemia;[14] now, CD10 is known to be found on many normal and neoplastic lymphocytes.[15,16] However, malignant lymphomas often exhibit a characteristic profile with a panel of antibodies, as will be discussed below in the section on the pathology and classification of lymphomas. A selection of monoclonals in current use for the characterization of lymphoid malignancies is presented in Table 4.1.

Clonality, lineage and developmental stage

Malignant lymphomas are neoplastic expansions derived from a single clone. In B-cell tumours, because of allelic exclusion,[17] only one light chain will be expressed in such a monoclonal proliferation, whereas a polyclonal, reactive process will show expression of both κ and λ light chains. When monoclonality is demonstrated by immunophenotyping at this level, the correlation with malignancy is excellent.[18] (However, one must be cautious in the interpretation of minor clones detected by more sensitive methods such as Southern blotting, *see* Chapter 10.) Unfortunately, since the T-cell receptor does not express antigenic diversity analogous to light chain restriction in the B-cell series, there is no equivalent immunophenotypic marker for monoclonality of T-cell proliferations.[19] It is possible, however, to delineate proliferations of T-cells with aberrant phenotypes, such as the loss of CD7 which occurs on most peripheral T-cell lymphomas.[20] There is often a marked predominance of CD4-

or CD8-positive cells. (Most T-cell lymphomas are CD4-positive.[21,22]) However, these are not clonal markers, and such findings are not conclusive for malignancy; they are supportive if other evidence points to that diagnosis.

Monoclonal antibodies are used to identify the lineage of lymphoid cells, as well as their stages of differentiation. Lymphomas can generally be characterized as a neoplasm arising from a cell

Table 4.1 Selected antibodies used to characterize lymphoid cells

Antibody	CD	Molecular weight of antigen	Primary reactivity
T-cells			
Leu 1, T101, OKT1	CD5	67	Pan-T-cell
Leu 2a, OKT 8	CD8	33	Suppressor T-cell
Leu 3a, OKT 4	CD4	55	Helper T-cell
Leu 4, OKT 3	CD3	20–25	T-cell receptor linked molecule, pan-T-cell reagent
Leu 5, OKT 11, T11	CD2	45–50	E-rosette receptor, pan-T reagent
Leu 6, OKT 6, T6	CD1	49	Cortical thymocyte
Leu 9, 3A1	CD7	40	Pan-T-cell reagent
B-cells			
B1, Leu 16	CD20	35	Pan-B-cell reagent
B4, Leu 12	CD19	95	Pan-B-cell reagent
B2	CD21	145	C3d receptor
Leu 14	CD22	150	Pan-B-cell reagent
PCA 1			Plasma cell
Other, non-lineage restricted			
T200	CD45	200	Common leucocyte antigen, pan haematopoietic reagent
HLA DR		28–34	Class II histocompatibility antigens; B-cells, monocytes/macrophages, activated T-cells
Tac	CD25	55–60	Interleukin-2 receptor
CALLA, J5	CD10	100	Common ALL antigen
Hefi-1, Ki-1	CD 30	90–110	Activated T-cells, EBV infected B-cells, Reed–Sternberg (R–S) cells
Leu M1	CD15		Carbohydrate moiety of glycoprotein; monocytes, granulocytes, R–S cells
Leu M5	CD11c	150, 95	Monocytes, macrophages; hairy cell leukaemia
OKT 9		90	Transferrin receptor
Leu 7		110	T-cell and NK-cell subsets
Leu 11	CD16	50–70	Fc IgG receptor on NK-cells and neutrophils
Leu 17, T10	CD38	45	Plasma cells, immature T-cells (thymocytes), activated B-cells

Leu series, anti-CALLA, and anti HLA-DR from Becton-Dickinson; OK series from Ortho; B series, J5, T6, T10, T11, and PCA 1 from Coulter; T200, T101 from Hybritech; Ki-1 from H Stein, West Germany; Hefi-1 from RF Fisher and DL Longo, National Cancer Institute; Tac from T Waldmann, National Cancer Institute; 3A1 from B Haynes, currently Duke University.

'arrested' at a particular stage of differentiation. Thus, normal prothymocytes express CD7, but not CD4 or CD8; T-cell acute lymphoblastic leukaemias (T-ALL) often show such a phenotypic pattern.[23] CD4 and CD8 are coexpressed for a period of T-cell development, and a subset of both T-ALL and T-cell acute lymphoblastic lymphoma (T-LBL) also express both antigens[24] (Fig. 4.1). Similarly, in the B-cell

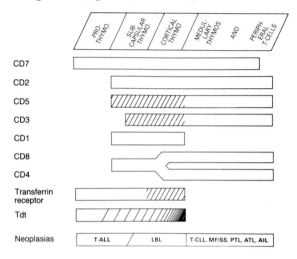

| | CD7 | CD2 | CD5 | CD3 | CD1 | CD8 | CD4 | Transferrin receptor | Tdt | Neoplasias |

Fig. 4.1 Schematic diagram demonstrating phenotypic correlates of normal T-lymphocyte differentiation. Neoplasias of T-cell origin can be related to sequential stages of T-cell differentiation. Monoclonal antibodies are identified according to CD groups established by international nomenclature panel. (Modified from Cossman J, *et al. Cancer Research.* 1983; 4486–90.

series, most B-cell lymphomas express CD19, except for those arising from cells late in the differentiation pathway such as myeloma and some plasmacytoid chronic lymphocytic leukaemias (CLLs), which lose CD19 and acquire the antigens detected by OKT10 or Leu 17 (CD 38) (Fig. 4.2).

The presumption is that as more is known about the phenotypes of the lymphomas, clinically relevant patterns will emerge. Indeed, such data are often invaluable to the pathologist when morphological features are insufficient to decide among different entities. For example, Burkitt's lymphoma and lymphoblastic lymphoma can be difficult to distinguish mor-

phologically. However, immunophenotyping will show Burkitt's lymphoma to be a B-cell neoplasm with surface immunoglobulin, whereas lymphoblastic lymphoma will have an immature phenotype, almost always T-cell, and will be terminal deoxynucleotidyl transferase (TdT)-positive.[25,26]

Phenotypic findings must be interpreted with some caution, since there is some variance from the normal in patterns found on neoplastic cells.[27] For example, CD5 is found in abundance on normal T-cells but not on most normal B-cells, yet is typically present in the cells of B-cell small lymphocytic lymphoma.[28] Some early T-cell markers such as CD7 and CD2 have been found on the blasts of acute myelogenous leukaemia (AML), though this is not the usual case. Once again it must be emphasized that no single marker should be viewed as definitive, and that the immunophenotypic profile must be considered along with morphological and clinical data.

Pathology of the non-Hodgkin's lymphomas: general comments

As with many diseases, the pathology of malignant lymphomas begins with Virchow, who recognized 'lymphosarcoma' as a tumour of the lymphoreticular system.[29] Before the turn of the century, Hodgkin's disease had been separated from the lymphomas as a disease with a different histological appearance and clinical course.[30] The term 'reticulum cell sarcoma' was introduced in the 1920s to signify a tumour presumably arising from the cells which make up the supporting structures of lymphoreticular tissue.[31] At the same time, Brill *et al.* and Symmers described 'giant follicular lymphadenopathy' (or as it became known, Brill-Symmers disease).[32,33] There was controversy at the time over the nature of this disease, whether it was benign or malignant, which is not surprising since follicular lymphoma (as we now call Brill-Symmers disease) often displays a waxing and waning course.

However, the diversity of the microscopic appearances of lymphomas failed to fit into these three categories of lymphosarcoma,

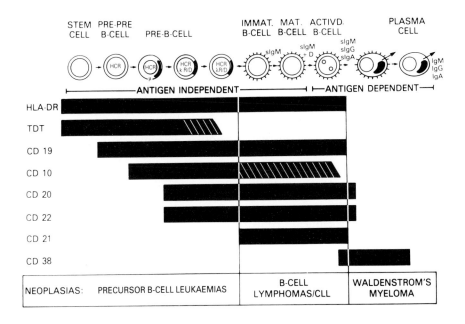

Fig. 4.2 Schematic diagram demonstrating molecular genetic and immunophenotypic correlates of normal B-cell differentiation. Monoclonal antibodies are identified according to CD groups established by international nomenclature panel. Steps of heavy and light chain immunoglobulin gene rearrangement are shown. B-cell malignancies can be related to sequential stages of B-cell differentiation. HCR, heavy chain rearrangement; κR/D, kappa light chain rearrangement or deletion; λR/D, lambda light chain rearrangement or deletion; μ, mu heavy chain synthesis.

reticulum cell sarcoma, and giant follicular lymphadenopathy. Although in present day terminology these would roughly correspond to the major categories of small lymphocytic, large cell, and follicular lymphomas, the terms were not uniformly applied. The studies of Gall and Rappaport resulted in classification schemes which were reasonably reproducible, and achieved a high degree of correlation with clinical behaviour.[34,35]

The Rappaport system[36] expanded the previous categories by combining pattern of growth with cytological characteristics of the malignant cells. Tumours were divided into nodular and diffuse patterns, and categorized as well differentiated or poorly differentiated, depending on the degree to which the cells resembled normal lymphocytes. Instead of the category of 'reticulum cell sarcoma', certain lymphomas composed of large cells with abundant cytoplasm were called 'histiocytic'

since these tumours were felt to have arisen from histiocytes, and not from the supporting cells. Lymphomas containing a mixture of the two cytological types were called 'mixed lymphocytic-histiocytic' lymphomas. 'Undifferentiated' lymphoma was a term used to define cells of intermediate size that failed to show evidence of either 'histiocytic' or 'lymphocytic' origin.

Although the Rappaport scheme enjoyed widespread use, it was formulated at a time when relatively little was known of the cells of the normal immune system. The division of lymphocytes into B- and T-cells, let alone T-cell subsets, was yet to be discovered. As the science of immunology progressed, it became clear that the conceptual underpinnings of the Rappaport system were no longer tenable. The neoplastic cells in lymphomas could not be shown to correspond to a differentiation scheme as represented in the classification system. Cells termed histiocytic were not histiocytic in origin, but actually lymphoid. Therefore, systems for classifying lymphomas were proposed which attempted to combine the clinical utility of the Rappaport approach with the newer concepts of immunology. For example, the Lukes and Collins system[37] tried to find consistent morphological correlates for immunological subtypes, but has, however, proved unreliable.[38]

Eventually, multiple different pathological schemes for the classification of malignant lymphomas were in use by different groups of pathologists throughout the world, making the comparison and analysis of clinical trials extremely problematic.[39,40,41] In an effort aimed at resolving these difficulties, the National Cancer Institute (NCI) sponsored an international study comparing the six major classification systems in use in 1982.[42] It was found that no system was significantly superior to the others. As a result, a new system of classification was developed, largely to facilitate translation from one scheme to another, although use of the new scheme for initial diagnosis is becoming increasingly widespread (Tables 4.2 and 4.3). Termed 'the Working Formulation', it is based on morphological features alone. (It has been repeatedly validated that the histological appearance of a lesion is the single most important predictor of clinical behaviour[43], and therefore the preparation of a thinly cut, properly stained slide from well-fixed tissue is essential.) The approach has its origins in the Rappaport method of dividing lymphomas on the basis of pattern and cytological appearance. For the remainder of this chapter, the Working Formulation will be employed. Entities will be related to the normal immune system if possible.

In general, a lymph node involved by a malignant lymphoma shows effacement of normal nodal architecture. Normal structures such as sinuses and follicles are replaced by neoplastic elements growing in either a nodular or diffuse pattern. Individual cells are characterized first by their size. Small cells are close to the size of a mature, non-transformed lymphocyte, whereas large cells are two to three times the diameter of a small lymphocyte, similar to the large cells seen in germinal centres.

Different entities have characteristic appearances of the nuclear contour, which may be smooth and oval, or show deep grooving or lobation such as in 'cleaved' or 'convoluted' cells. Chromatin may be finely dispersed (stippled) or coarsely clumped. Nucleoli vary in size, frequency and tinctorial properties. The neoplastic cells vary markedly in the amount of cytoplasm from one category to another. The mitotic rate can be helpful in subclassification of lymphomas. Certain features, such as the presence of numerous histiocytes containing cell debris (starry sky histiocytes) are present much more frequently in rapidly proliferative lymphomas.

The Working Formulation is organized into low, intermediate and high grade categories, which correlate with natural history and prognosis. However, many chemotherapeutic protocols make a distinction only between low grade and high grade lymphomas, and for most clinical purposes this is adequate.[44] (This division into low and high grade only will be used for the rest of this Chapter.) The low grade lymphomas usually follow an indolent course, and are associated with relatively long survival with or without chemotherapy. Clinically high grade lymphomas (which include both intermediate and high grade classes in the Working Formulation) have an aggressive natural history unless vigorously treated; many of these lymphomas are potentially curable.[45]

The cells of the low grade tumours have preserved more of the normal functions of their non-neoplastic counterparts than the cells of high grade tumours. This has clinically important consequences. The pattern of involvement of low grade lymphomas, for example, mirrors the sites where the normal cell might be found.[46] Follicular lymphomas, which are always of B-cell origin, home to the B-cell dependent areas of the lymphoid system. The cells circulate readily, and usually present as stage III or IV disease, but are rarely found in sites not normally frequented by lymphocytes, such as the central nervous system (CNS) or testis. Follicular lymphomas may be responsive to immunoregulation by other, normal components of the immune system. Host immunity has been invoked to explain the

typically waxing and w   , or by transforming into
lymphomas.[47,48,49] Deat   1a.
lymphomas usually resu   igh grade tumours are
normal haematopoietic   sive neoplasms which

Table 4.2   A Working Forn   :commendations of an expert
international panel and cor

Working formulation	

Low grade
A.   Malignant lymphoma   d lymphocytic
        Small lymphocytic
            consistent with chrc
            leukaemia
            plasmacytoid
B.   Malignant lymphoma   iated lymphocytic
        small cleaved cell
            diffuse areas
            sclerosis
C.   Malignant lymphoma   ytic histiocytic
        cleaved and large cell
            diffuse areas
            sclerosis

Intermediate
D.   Malignant lymphoma
        large cell
            diffuse areas
            sclerosis
E.   Malignant lymphoma, diffuse small cleaved cell   Diffuse, poorly differentiated lymphocytic
F.   Malignant lymphoma, diffuse mixed, small   Diffuse mixed lymphocytic-histiocytic
        and large cell
            sclerosis
            epithelioid cell component
G.   Malignant lymphoma, diffuse large cell   Diffuse histiocytic
        cleaved cell
        non-cleaved cell
        sclerosis

High grade
H.   Malignant lymphoma, large cell, immunoblastic   Diffuse histiocytic
        plasmacytoid
        clear cell
        polymorphous
        epithelioid cell component
I.   Malignant lymphoma, lymphoblastic   Diffuse lymphoblastic
        convoluted cell
        non-convoluted cell
J.   Malignant lymphoma, small non-cleaved cell   Diffuse undifferentiated
        Burkitt's
        follicular areas

Table 4.3 Comparison of commonly used classifications for the non-Hodgkin's lymphomas

Modified Rappaport classification (1966)[36]		Lukes and Collins classification (1974)[37]		Kiel classification (1974)[40]	
Nodular		Undefined cell type		**Low-grade malignancy**	
Lymphocytic, well differentiated	A*	T-cell type, small lymphocytic	A	Lymphocytic, chronic lymphocytic/leukaemia	A
Lymphocytic, poorly differentiated	B	T-cell type, Sézary—mycosis fungoides (cerebriform)	B	Lymphocytic, other	A
Mixed, lymphocytic and histiocytic	C	T-cell type, convoluted lymphocytic	I	Lymphoplasmacytoid	A
Histiocytic	D	T-cell type, immunoblastic sarcoma (T-cell)	H	Centrocytic	E
Diffuse		B-cell type, small lymphocytic	A	Centroblastic-centrocytic, follicular without sclerosis	B,C,D
Lymphocytic, well differentiated	A	B-cell type, plasmacytoid lymphocytic	A	Centroblastic-centrocytic, follicular with sclerosis	
Lymphocytic, well differentiated with plasmacytoid features		Follicular centre cell, small cleaved	B,E	Centroblastic-centrocytic, follicular and diffuse, without sclerosis	
Lymphocytic, poorly differentiated	E	Follicular centre cell, large cleaved	I	Centroblastic-centrocytic, follicular and diffuse, with sclerosis	
Lymphoblastic, convoluted	I	Follicular centre cell, small non-cleaved	D,G	Centroblastic-centrocytic, diffuse	F
Lymphoblastic, non-convoluted	I	Follicular centre cell, large non-cleaved	J	Low-grade malignant lymphoma, unclassified	
Mixed, lymphocytic and histiocytic	F	Immunoblastic sarcoma (B-cell)	D,G	**High-grade malignancy**	
Histiocytic without sclerosis	G	Subtypes of follicular centre cell lymphomas	H	Centroblastic	G
Histiocytic with sclerosis	G	1. Follicular		Lymphoblastic, Burkitt's type	J
Burkitt's tumour	J	2. Follicular and diffuse		Lymphoblastic, convoluted cell type	I
Undifferentiated	J	3. Diffuse		Lymphoblastic, other (unclassified)	
		4. Sclerotic with follicles		Immunoblastic	H
Malignant lymphoma, unclassified		5. Sclerotic without follicles		High-grade malignant lymphoma, unclassified	
Composite lymphoma		Histiocytic		Malignant lymphoma, unclassified (unable to specify 'high grade' or 'low grade')	
		Malignant lymphoma, unclassified		Composite lymphoma	

*Letters indicate equivalent or related category in the Working Formulation as shown in Table 4.2.

commonly involve extranodal and privileged sites, behaving in a fashion similar to other highly malignant, non-lymphoid tumours. Peripheral blood involvement, which is not of prognostic significance in most low grade lymphomas, is usually an ominous, preterminal event in the high grade lesions.[50] High grade lymphomas grow in a destructive pattern, and systemic symptoms are more common. Spontaneous remissions are very rare, and the course is unrelenting if untreated.

A common problem is the occurrence of divergent histologies in biopsies taken from the same patient, even when obtained at the same time. The most frequent situation is the observation of a follicular pattern in one biopsy and a diffuse infiltration in another specimen. In such cases, survival is intermediate between the two.[51] Such occurrences may represent a point in the evolution of the lymphoma, as histological progression from a low grade to a high grade category is often seen during the clinical course of an individual patient. In the experience of the National Institutes of Health, 37 per cent of patients with a follicular pattern on initial staging had progression to a diffuse pattern in specimens obtained after an interval greater than 3 months.[52]

There has been debate about whether the occurrence of two histological types of lymphomas in a single individual represents two separately occurring tumours or different manifestations of the same process. Immunophenotypic and molecular genetic data strongly favour clonal evolution as the explanation in the great majority of cases.[53,54] With modern therapy, one is seeing an increasing number of cases in which the aggressive component of a lymphoma is eradicated, but the patient relapses with an indolent histology,[55] with markers identical to the original tumour.

Malignant lymphoma, small lymphocytic

Diffuse small lymphocytic lymphoma is the Working Formulation designation corresponding to Rappaport's well differentiated lymphoma, and is the solid tumour counterpart of CLL. The cells of CLL and small lymphocytic lymphoma are both morphologically and phenotypically the same, and the two entities represent different manifestations of the same disease.[56] Even when there is no clinical leukaemia, patients with this lymphoma often have occult involvement of the bone marrow and viscera, though the usual presentation is asymptomatic lymphadenopathy. Furthermore, the natural history is commonly progression to a leukaemic phase.

The cells are closest to the resting mature lymphocyte in appearance (Fig. 4.3), and there may be some differentiation to plasma cell morphology and function. The cells may be induced to secrete immunoglobulin, which in the great majority of cases is IgM, with κ the more commonly detected light chain.[57] Secretion may occur spontaneously, which is seen in the disorder of Waldenstrom's macroglobulinaemia, accounting for up to 15 per cent of cases of small lymphocytic lymphoma. The cells of Waldenstrom's macroglobulinaemia are more plas-

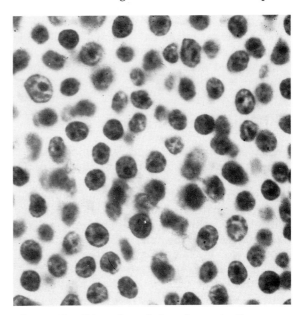

Fig. 4.3 Small lymphocytic lymphoma (well differentiated lymphocytic lymphoma of Rappaport). Lymph nodes are replaced by a monotonous diffuse proliferation of small round lymphoid cells with condensed chromatin. Occasional larger cells with prominent nucleoli (prolymphocytes) are identified.

macytoid, and tend to home to the medullary cords, which is the normal location of immunoglobulin-secreting plasma cells.[58]

Though most of the cells of small lymphocytic lymphomas are similar to mature lymphocytes, involved lymph nodes usually contain numerous aggregates of larger cells, which may be mitotically quite active. This gives rise to a 'pseudofollicular pattern' although the foci of large cells should not be mistaken for germinal centres. The larger cells are prolymphocytes, and are the proliferating component of the lymphoma. When the mitotic rate in these areas does not exceed 30 per 20 high power fields, there is not an adverse effect on prognosis. However, progression to large cell lymphoma (Richter's syndrome[59]) occurs when the larger cells emerge as a dominant, and monomorphous proliferation is no longer restricted to growth centres. Richter's syndrome occurs in approximately 1 per cent of patients.

Small lymphocytic lymphomas are B-cell tumours which are positive for the pan-B markers CD19, CD20, CD22, and CD24. These tumours also express CD5, an antigen found on normal T-cells, but not on normal B-cells; this antigen is not usually expressed on plasmacytoid cells.[60] The significance of these findings is unclear.

Follicular lymphomas

Follicular lymphomas (nodular lymphomas of Rappaport) are so-named because the neoplastic cells form aggregates resembling normal germinal centres (Fig. 4.4). The main differential diagnosis pathologically is with reactive follicular hyperplasia. A number of criteria have been developed to help in this distinction, though no one alone is definitive.[61] Normal germinal centres are composed of a heterogeneous population of cells reacting to antigenic stimulation, while nodular lymphomas are more monotonous in appearance. The mitotic rate is often lower in the neoplastic process, and the normal 'tingible body' macrophages are absent. Neoplastic nodules tend to vary less in size and shape, and overrun the normal lymph node architecture with crowding of the nodules even in the medulla. Normal germinal centres are

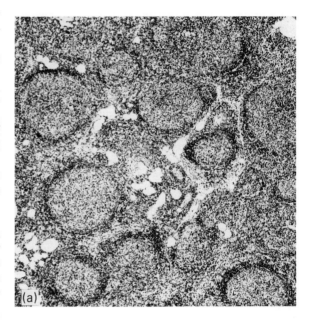

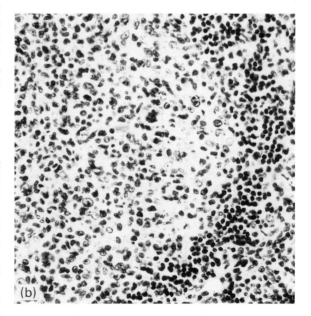

Fig. 4.4 Follicular lymphoma. (a) At low power lymph node is replaced by a monotonous nodular infiltrate. Interfollicular area is compressed. Nodules are monotonous in size and shape and have ill-defined lymphoid cuffs. (b) Cytologically nodules are composed of a mixture of follicular centre cells. In the present example there is a predominance of small cleaved cells with scattered large non-cleaved cells.

asymmetric and demonstrate a polarity orientated towards the site of antigen entry, usually the sinuses. They should also have a cuff of small lymphocytes surrounding them. These features are often lacking in lymphomatous follicles.

The Working Formulation subtypes follicular lymphomas as either predominantly small cleaved (the nodular poorly differentiated lymphomas of Rappaport), large cell, cleaved or non-cleaved (histiocytic), or mixed small cleaved and large cell (mixed lymphocytic-histiocytic). Once again it must be emphasized that the small cells and the large cells are part of the same neoplastic process, not the collision of two lymphomas. The larger cells are the more biologically aggressive, while the smaller cells exhibit more motility, but are the indolent component.

Malignant lymphoma, follicular, predominantly small cleaved cell

This is the most common form of follicular lymphoma, accounting for up to 60 per cent of cases. Follicles are composed of monotonous small lymphocytes with a characteristic indented or cleaved nucleus. There are few large cells or mitoses. The small cleaved cells may be seen in the peripheral blood, where they have been termed 'buttock' cells.

Malignant lymphoma, follicular, mixed small cleaved and large cell

This subtype is characterized by the finding of more than five large cells per high powered field in the neoplastic follicles, although an element of subjectivity in the distinction between the small cleaved and mixed cell types is probably unavoidable.[62] Mitoses are more common. This category accounts for approximately 30 per cent of the follicular lymphomas. As with the small cleaved variety, these follicular lymphomas most often present with systemic involvement. In the bone marrow, the paratrabecular location of neoplastic cells is useful in making the distinction from normal lymphoid follicles. When there is marrow or visceral involvement it is usual to find only the small cleaved cells at these sites, even when the histology is clearly

mixed in the lymph nodes; this lends support to the concept of the small cleaved cell as the circulating cell in these tumours.

Malignant lymphoma, follicular, predominantly large cell

In this variant, small cleaved cells are largely absent and the follicles contain large, mitotically active lymphoid cells. This is the least common of the follicular subtypes, accounting for about 10 per cent, perhaps because of a more rapid progression to a diffuse histology. At initial staging, there are often localized masses and until the use of aggressive systemic chemotherapy these lymphomas would frequently recur with widespread disease.[63]

As mentioned above, the finding of different histologies in multiple biopsies from the same patient is not uncommon. Often the differences are of minor clinical significance, as when both biopsies are low grade. However, they also often reflect the natural history of these lesions to progress, from a follicular to a diffuse growth pattern, and from a small cell to a large cell cytological appearance. A significant portion of tumours presenting as diffuse aggressive lymphomas probably evolved from a subclinical indolent histology. In all cases, treatment decisions should be based upon the most aggressive subtype.

All follicular lymphomas are monoclonal B-cell neoplasms, with the malignant cells usually concentrated in the follicular structures. The cells express only one light chain and one or more heavy chains, most often IgM with or without IgD, and are positive for pan-B-cell markers CD19, CD20, and CD22. They are often positive for the common ALL antigen (CD10), but in contrast to the small lymphocytic lymphomas, are negative for the T-cell antigen CD5.[15] The follicular areas contain a framework of dendritic reticulum cells, detected by antibodies such as DRC-1.[64] In the peripheral blood it is possible to detect 'clonal excess' using sophisticated flow cytometry techniques in almost all patients,[65] once again emphasizing the propensity of these malignancies to circulate and underscoring the unlikelihood that a follicular lymphoma is truly localized.

The cells in the interfollicular areas of involved

lymph nodes may be neoplastic B-cells, and as such represent a diffuse component of the tumour; or as is often the case, they may be normal, reactive T-cells. The T-cell infiltrate may be so prominent, in fact, that T-cells account for the majority of cells in samples run on the flow cytometer.[7] Numerous T-cells may also be found within the neoplastic nodules. The T-cells are phenotypically normal, with a CD4:CD8 ratio appropriate to normal lymph nodes.[8] They are functionally active, and may retain the capacity to modulate the behaviour of the neoplastic cells.[66] It is speculated that this partial responsiveness to immunoregulation may account for the typical waxing and waning of these lesions. The presence of a significant T-cell infiltrate appears to be of predictive value in identifying patients who may respond to anti-idiotype therapy.[67]

Malignant lymphoma, diffuse, small cleaved cell

This category contains within it two distinct entities. One probably represents a progression of the follicular small cleaved cell lymphoma described above, and is composed of cytologically identical cells, with the same markers. This is only a small percentage of the tumours termed diffuse small cleaved. The other entity corresponds to what Berard termed 'intermediate' differentiated lymphoma, so called because the morphology appeared in between the small cleaved cell and the small lymphocytic cell[68] (Fig. 4.5). 'Mantle zone lymphoma' is another name for this lesion, because of the phenotypic characteristics shared with the cells of the normal cuff, or mantle around germinal centres.[69,70]

In intermediate lymphoma, the cells may be a mixture of small cleaved cells and small round lymphocytes, often with a vaguely nodular growth pattern. It is common to see residual germinal centres, with the neoplastic cells encroaching upon them in the fashion of a mantle. These lymphomas, in contrast to the other B-cell tumours, are more likely to express λ light chain. They are often CD5-positive (like small lymphocytic lymphomas), but are also often CD10 positive (like follicular lymphomas), thus demonstrating consistency of im-

munophenotypic characteristics and morphological appearance.[15]

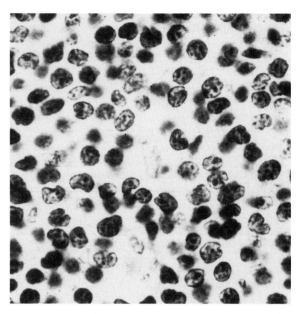

Fig. 4.5 Lymphocytic lymphoma of intermediate differentiation, so-called 'mantle zone lymphoma'. Lymph node is replaced by a monotonous proliferation of slightly irregular and angulated lymphoid cells with condensed chromatin.

Diffuse aggressive lymphomas

Several of the diffuse subtypes of lymphomas in the Working Formulation can be grouped together, as they share common clinical features. These include diffuse mixed small and large cell, diffuse large cell, and diffuse large cell immunoblastic types. They present mainly in adults, both as lymphadenopathy (65 per cent) and as extranodal disease (35 per cent). They are less selective in their homing to B- or T-cell dependent zones, and are more likely to grow as large masses, often involving privileged sites. In contrast to the low grade lymphomas, which have a continuous relapse rate over time, the aggressive lymphomas have a significant chance of cure when treated with appropriate, intensive chemotherapy.

The cells of the diffuse aggressive lymphomas may be quite aberrant immunophenotypically and often lack many of the usual cell surface markers. However, using a large battery of monoclonal antibodies (and, if necessary, Southern blotting) it is possible in almost all cases to assign the cell of origin as a B (85 per cent)- or T (15 per cent)- cell. In less than 5 per cent of cases can true histiocytic markers be demonstrated. However, while these data may have some clinical correlates with the behaviour of certain subtypes, no aspect of immunophenotyping has emerged as a consistent prognostic indicator for the diffuse aggressive lymphomas.[71]

Malignant lymphoma, diffuse, mixed small and large cell

The majority of cases of diffuse mixed lymphoma are composed of cells cytologically identical with those of the mixed cell population found in follicular lymphomas; it is only the pattern of growth which is different. These tumours have the same markers as in the follicular variants and in fact it is not infrequent that foci of nodularity are observed. Also, as in the follicular lymphomas, there is often an admixture of normal T-cells in the involved areas.

However, in a significant number of the diffuse mixed cases (approximately 35 per cent), the cells do not resemble the follicular centre cells. Instead there is a more pleomorphic range of cells, from small atypical lymphoid cells to large cells with abundant cytoplasm and prominent nucleoli, and many forms in between. There is often an infiltrate of granulocytes, plasma cells and histiocytes, similar to that seen in Hodgkin's disease (Fig. 4.6). Immunologically, the majority of cases with such an appearance will have a mature T-cell phenotype, hence the term mature, or peripheral (as opposed to thymic, or central) T-cell lymphoma.[21] Commonly, these tumours will show loss of expression of one or more normal T-cell markers (most often CD7), or a marked predominance of CD4 or CD8; once again, it must be emphasized that this is only supportive evidence, and not conclusive for malignancy.

These lesions can be confused with Hodgkin's disease – the distinction must be made with the recognition that in T-cell lymphoma the smaller lymphocytes are atypical as well as the large

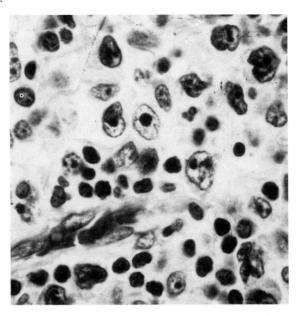

Fig. 4.6 Peripheral T-cell lymphoma subclassified in the Working Formulation as mixed small and large cell type. Atypical small lymphoid cells are admixed with large immunoblastic cells with prominent nucleoli. An inflammatory background is conspicuous.

Hodgkin's-like cells. One variant of T-cell lymphoma which has a prominent component of epithelioid histiocytes, known as 'lymphoepithelioid cell lymphomas' or 'Lennert's lymphoma'[72] was initially thought to be related to Hodgkin's disease, a concept which has not been borne out. These lymphomas should be treated as any other in the diffuse aggressive category.

Malignant lyphoma, diffuse, large cell

These lymphomas are predominantly composed of cells with nuclear diameters greater than the 'starry sky' histiocytes which are often admixed. There is usually a brisk mitotic rate. The cells may be divided into cleaved and non-cleaved variants (Fig. 4.7). The cleaved cells have a thin rim of eosinophilic cytoplasm, with somewhat less conspicuous nucleoli. Sclerosis often accompanies the cleaved cell variant, especially in extranodal sites. The large non-cleaved type has more abundant amphophilic cytoplasm, with several distinct nucleoli which are often

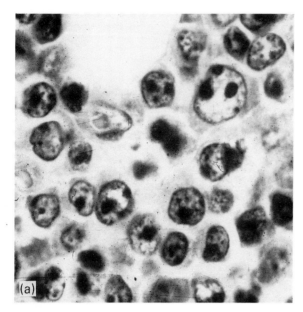

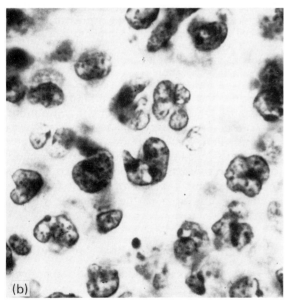

Fig. 4.7 Large cell lymphoma. (a) Tumour is composed of large non-cleaved lymphoid cells. Cells have large vesicular nuclei with multiple nucleoli, often apposed to the nuclear membrane. Cytoplasm is abundant and indistinct. (b) In large cleaved cell variant cells demonstrate marked nuclear irregularity. Chromatin is more finely distributed and nucleoli less conspicuous. Both variants of large cell lymphoma most often demonstrate B-cell markers.

adherent to the nuclear membrane. Most of the diffuse large cell lymphomas are B-cell phenotypically, in accord with their follicular centre cell morphology. In fact, many such cases carry the t(14;18) translocation that is characteristic of follicular lymphomas.[54]

Malignant lymphoma, diffuse, large cell, immunoblastic

This is the second category that is the result of the division of the Rappaport diffuse histiocytic class. It is comprised of a variety of cytological subtypes which all differ from the follicular centre cell in appearance (Fig. 4.8). While some studies have claimed a poorer prognosis for the immunoblastic category,[42] the clinical importance of the distinction from large cell non-immunoblastic is in question. These are all high grade lymphomas, with a tendency to exhibit anaplasia, and are very rapidly dividing. The plasmacytoid subtype has large pleomorphic cells with abundant amphophilic cytoplasm and eccentrically placed nuclei containing prominent nucleoli. The polymorphous subtype was included as the subtype which would best correspond to the pleomorphism seen in the T-cell large cell lymphomas (Fig. 4.9), both those associated and those not associated with human T-cell lymphotrophic virus (HTLV)-I (*see* below). The epithelioid subtype is part of the spectrum of Lennert's lymphoma, while the clear cell subtype is comprised of cells with abundant cytoplasm which is clear on routine stains.[72]

A small portion of large cell immunoblastic lymphomas will display characteristics indicating an origin from true histiocytes; these neoplasms will be discussed separately below. Another recently described variant of immunoblastic lymphoma shows a propensity to involve lymph node sinuses. The cells express an immunological marker, CD30 (Hefi-1, Ki-1) which was originally identified on a Hodgkin's disease cell line.[73] Often T-cell markers are also present, albeit inconsistently and with a markedly aberrant phenotype. Because of the sinusoidal and often focal involvement of lymph nodes, this neoplasm can easily be mistaken for metastatic carcinoma or malignant histiocytosis. It has been described as occurring in all age

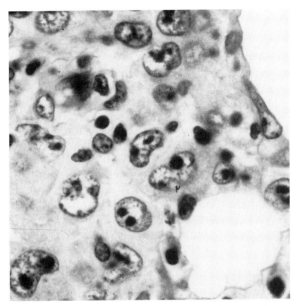

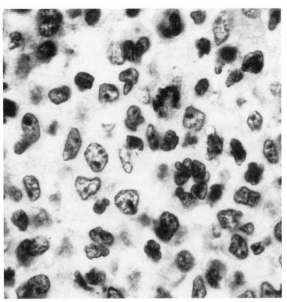

Fig. 4.8 Large cell immunoblastic lymphoma. This example expressed B-cell surface markers. Cells are large and pleomorphic with prominent nucleoli. Abundant cytoplasm is often amphophilic.

Fig. 4.9 Large cell immunoblastic lymphoma of peripheral T-cell type. Marked nuclear pleomorphism is evident. Frequent multilobated cells are seen.

groups, but appears to be unusually common in children, and has a high incidence of skin involvement.[74]

Malignant lymphoma, lymphoblastic

Morphologically, phenotypically and clinically, lymphoblastic lymphoma is related to the T-cell type of acute lymphoblastic leukaemia.[23,24,75] The cells are 'blastic', which is shorthand for cells with scant cytoplasm, have fine chromatin with small nucleoli and show an exceedingly high mitotic rate. Convoluted and non-convoluted forms are described, depending on whether the nuclei are oval-shaped with smooth contours or are markedly lobulated[76] (Fig. 4.10). Involved lymph nodes may show no remnant of normal architecture, and be replaced by a monotonous infiltrate of neoplastic cells, admixed only with a variable number of starry sky histiocytes. Alternatively, one finds preferential involvement of the paracortical, T-dependent zones, with sparing of germinal centres. The cells demonstrate a tendency to stream out into perinodal tissue, which is often termed a 'leukaemic' pattern of involvement.

Lymphoblastic lymphomas commonly present in young adults and adolescents, and show a marked male predominance. Often the initial site of disease is a mediastinal mass, though on subsequent staging a high percentage will have disseminated disease, including the CNS. Many patients progress to a frank leukaemia if treated inadequately.

Approximately 85 per cent of these tumours are T-cell in origin. Indeed, it was long postulated that this tumour arose from the thymus gland, even prior to the use of immunophenotyping.[77] These neoplasms represent proliferations of cells at an early stage of T-cell differentiation. The cells are TdT-positive. The cells of virtually all cases of both T-LBL and T-ALL express the T-cell marker CD7, and a high proportion express CD2 (the E-rosette receptor)[23,24], both of which are acquired at the prothymocyte stage of T-cell maturation in the thymus. CD5 (Leu 1) is also present in the vast majority of cases. T-cell lymphoblastic

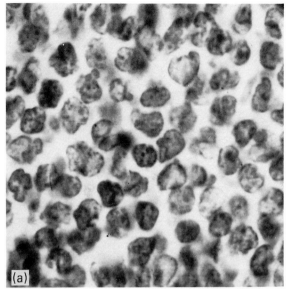

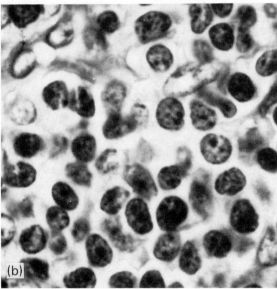

Fig. 4.10 Lymphoblastic lymphoma. (a) Convoluted subtype is most common. Cells have finely distributed chromatin and sparse cytoplasm. Nucleoli are inconspicuous. Nuclear irregularities are best appreciated when examined with an oil immersion objective. (b) Non-convoluted subtype is more difficult to distinguish from small non-cleaved cell lymphomas. Cells have finely distributed chromatin and small nucleoli. Morphological subtypes of lymphoblastic lymphoma do not correlate with phenotypic markers.

malignancies reflect normal T-cell ontogeny in the expression of the subset markers CD4 and CD8. These markers are at first absent, then co-expressed and finally expressed singly. Overall, a greater proportion of T-LBL express the more mature phenotypes, i.e. CD4+/CD8− or CD4−/CD8+ then T-ALL.[23,24,78] Many cases of T-LBL will also express the cortical thymocyte marker CD1.

The remaining 15 per cent of lymphoblastic lymphomas show an early pre-B-cell phenotype. These too are TdT-positive; hence the identification of this enzyme can be crucial in the differentiation from other high grade lymphomas. The B- and T-cell types are indistinguishable morphologically. However, patients with the B-cell type do not usually present with mediastinal masses, and lytic bone lesions have been reported in a number of cases.[24]

Malignant lymphoma, small non-cleaved cell

This category is equivalent to Rappaport's diffuse undifferentiated lymphoma, and can be further divided into Burkitt's and non-Burkitt's subtypes. The cells of Burkitt's lymphoma (Fig. 4.11) are moderately sized, approximately 15–25 μm, and show little variation from cell to cell within a tumour. They are round or oval, with coarse chromatin and several prominent basophilic nucleoli. The cells have a distinct rim of amphophilic cytoplasm, and have a diffuse growth pattern. A starry sky is characteristic, though not pathognomonic, and can be seen in all high grade lymphomas.

All cases of Burkitt's lymphoma are B-cell tumours, usually expressing μ heavy chain and a single light chain. Most are CD10-positive.[16] This neoplasm occurs in endemic[79] and non-endemic forms.[80] The endemic form is usually positive for the genome of the Epstein–Barr virus (EBV), and expresses receptors for C3d; the non-endemic cases are usually negative for both.[81] Morphologically, the endemic and non-endemic forms are indistinguishable. The endemic cases present at a median age of 7 years, most often in the face or jaw, while the non-endemic cases have a median age of 11 years, and commonly present as an abdominal mass involving the

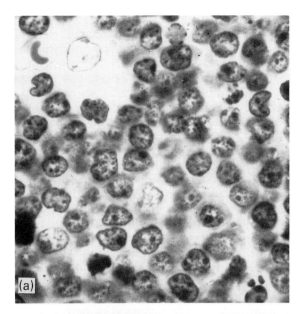

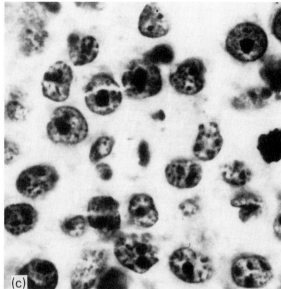

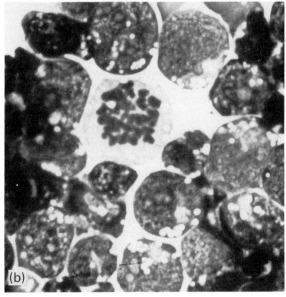

Fig. 4.11 Small non-cleaved cell lymphomas. (a) Small non-cleaved cell lymphoma, Burkitt's subtype. Cells are of uniform size and shape. Chromatin is finely clumped and multiple small basophilic nucleoli are evident. Nuclei of tumour cells approximate in size the nuclear diameter of admixed starry sky histiocytes. (b) Touch imprint of Burkitt's lymphoma stained with Wright Giemsa stain. Cells have deeply basophilic cytoplasm and prominent cytoplasmic vacuoles. (c) Small non-cleaved cell lymphoma, non-Burkitt's subtype. Nucleoli are more prominent. Most cells have single central prominent nucleolus. More variation in nuclear size and shape is typically observed.

ileocaecal region or ovaries.

Small, non-cleaved cell lymphomas of the non-Burkitt's type are distinguished from Burkitt's by a somewhat greater degree of nuclear pleomorphism (Fig. 4.11c). Occasional giant cell or bizarre forms may be seen. Usually there is a single prominent nucleolus. Small non-cleaved non-Burkitt's lymphoma most commonly occurs in adults with a median age of 34 years, most often in lymph nodes. Approximately 5 per cent of these tumours express a T-cell phenotype, suggesting that, in contrast to Burkitt's, the non-Burkitt's subtype is not a homogeneous entity. However, when this lesion occurs in children, it is probably biologically identical to classical Burkitt's lymphoma.[82,83] Moreover, both subtypes together make up the most frequent form of lymphomas that occur in the setting of the acquired immunodeficiency syndrome (AIDS). In this setting, as in the endemic cases of Burkitt's lymphoma, there is disordered T-cell regulation of B-cells due to a viral infection, and it is postulated that a common pathogenesis may be operating in both situations, involving translocations which result in juxtaposition of *myc* oncogene to an immunoglobulin locus.[84]

Mycosis fungoides/Sézary syndrome

Mycosis fungoides/Sézary syndrome (MF/SS) is a clinicopathological entity the hallmark of which is infiltration of the skin by atypical lymphoid cells displaying a marked affinity for the epidermis and superficial dermis. Some authors group MF/SS with other T-cell disorders involving the skin, including adult T-cell leukaemia/lymphoma (ATLL) and peripheral T-cell lymphoma as the 'cutaneous' T-cell lymphomas.[85] However, because of the differences in aetiology (viral in the case of ATLL – *see* Chapter 22), prognosis (MF/SS is compatible with a prolonged survival even if untreated), and histological appearances, it is preferable to maintain the nosological distinctions; hence the more specific term MF/SS is used.

Mycosis fungoides/Sézary syndrome is a neoplastic process that typically progresses from involvement of the skin, to lesions of lymph nodes, with visceral involvement occurring in advanced stages. Mycosis fungoides and Sézary syndrome are different phases of the same process, with the malignant cell expressing a T-cell phenotype, usually CD4-positive. The Sézary cell is a small, circulating lymphoid cell, while the infiltrate of mycosis fungoides is composed of a mixture of small and large lymphoid cells.[86] Both the small and large cells have a characteristic irregular infolding of the nuclei, imparting a 'cerebriform' appearance. Large multinucleated forms may occur, simulating Reed–Sternberg cells.

The earliest lesions of MF/SS in the so-called 'eczematoid' stage mimic a variety of lymphohistiocytic skin disorders such as lichen planus and Mucha-Habermann syndrome (*Pityriasis lichenoides et Varioliformis acuta*).[87] The diagnosis may be suspected, but cannot be confirmed by routine pathological methods. In the more advanced plaque, tumour, or erythrodermic skin lesions of MF/SS, the atypical lymphoid cells are more in evidence, and the histological picture is more specific. There is usually acanthosis of the epidermis, and focal parakeratosis. A requirement for the diagnosis is the presence of clusters of cells with a characteristic cerebriform appearance. Exocytosis (migration) of these cells into the epidermis, which may aggregate to form Pautrier's microabscesses (*see* Chapter 22) are highly suggestive of MF/SS, although they also occur in ATLL. In the dermis is a polymorphous infiltrate of lymphocytes, histiocytes, and the atypical cells. The infiltrate may be lichenoid or perivascular.

Patients with skin lesions of MF/SS frequently have lymphadenopathy. Most commonly these nodes show a pattern designated as dermatopathic lymphadenopathy.[88] There is paracortical hyperplasia with marked proliferation of histiocytes, lymphocytes, plasma cells and sometimes eosinophils. Often the macrophages contain lipid or melanin pigment. In addition, there is an infiltration of CD1-positive cells phenotypically identical with Langerhans cells found in normal epidermis.[89] Dermatopathic lymphadenopathy is nonspecific, and can occur in reaction to a large variety of skin disorders. In patients with MF/SS, however, nodes showing only dermatopathic changes by routine histology can be demonstrated to harbour clonal proliferations consistent with MF/SS cells by more sensitive techniques such as Southern blotting.[90] In a minority of cases, there is sufficient effacement of lymph node architecture, or large enough aggregates of atypical cells to warrant a definite diagnosis of nodal involvement.

Adult T-cell leukaemia/lymphoma (ATLL)

This is a distinct clinicopathological syndrome, originally described in southwestern Japan, which is associated with a retrovirus, HTLV-

I.[91,92] It has also been identified in other parts of the world, including the southeastern USA and the Caribbean. It may be difficult to distinguish from MF/SS in that both have a helper T-cell phenotype and involve the skin in most cases. However, patients with ATLL most commonly present with leukaemia, and leukaemia almost always develops during the course of this disease. Other clinical findings include lymphadenopathy, hepatosplenomegaly, lytic bone lesions and hypercalcaemia. The median age is 45, and in the western hemisphere it is most common among Blacks. Morphologically, the most characteristic feature is the presence of highly pleomorphic, polylobated cells in the peripheral blood[93] (Fig. 4.12). Lymph nodes may display features consistent with a diagnosis of large cell immunoblastic, or diffuse mixed lymphoma in the Working Formulation. However, evidence for infection with HTLV-I is necessary for a definitive diagnosis.

True histiocytic lymphoma

As mentioned above, a small percentage of the diffuse aggressive lymphomas will be derived from the mononuclear phagocytic cell lineage. True histiocytic lymphoma or histiocytic sarcoma represents a neoplasm of cells at a late point in the differentiation of this lineage, at the stage of the fixed tissue histiocyte. The lesion is often a localized tumour.[94] In addition to the reticuloendothelial system, the skin and bones are often involved. In lymph nodes, there is a tendency for the malignant cells preferentially to involve the sinuses. Also, the presence of phagocytic activity by the malignant cells may point to a histiocytic origin. However, no morphological criterion is diagnostic. Phagocytosis can occur in T- or B-cell lymphomas, and may be seen even in epithelial malignancies.

The cells of true histiocytic lymphomas are large, up to 50 μm, and are frankly malignant, with large nucleoli in a lobulated nucleus and abundant cytoplasm. However, the distinction from B- or T-cell malignancies relies upon cytochemical and immunochemical methods. Enzyme cytochemical studies can be performed on air-dried touch preparations or on frozen sections.[95,96] Phagocytic cells have diffuse positivity

for fluoride sensitive non-specific esterase. (Myeloid cells should be fluoride resistant.) They should be negative for alkaline phosphatase and

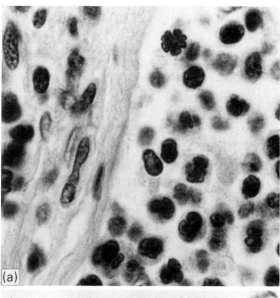

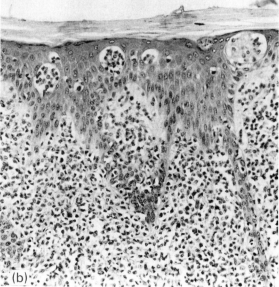

Fig. 4.12 Adult T-cell leukaemia/lymphoma. (a) Open sinus within lymph node contains markedly pleomorphic and polylobated lymphoid cells. (b) Skin demonstrating involvement of epidermis by adult T-cell leukaemia/lymphoma. Pleomorphic lymphoid cells form Pautrier abscesses within epidermis.

chloroacetate esterase activity. They should be positive for lysozyme and alpha-1 antitrypsin, which can be detected immunologically as well as cytochemically. Monoclonal antibodies raised against mononuclear phagocytes include the Mo-series,[97] and Leu M5. However, none of these tests is completely specific for true histiocytic lymphoma, and the diagnosis is made when a malignancy presents a profile which is consistent with histiocytic origin, and which lacks evidence for T- or B-cell origin.

Haemophagocytic syndromes

Florid reactive proliferations of the mononuclear phagocytic system can present difficulties in the differential diagnosis with malignant histiocytic neoplasms.[98] The disorder, formally called histiocytic medullary reticulosis (HMR)[99], was considered a variant of malignant histiocytosis. It has now been recognized as the clinical manifestations of the haemophagocytic syndromes (HPS). These syndromes were first reported as an unusual response to a viral infection in the immunocompromised host.[100] Subsequently, HPS have been reported in patients with a variety of infections, including viral, bacterial, fungal and parasitic. They usually occur in the setting of immunodeficiency, whether congenital or iatrogenic. They have also been reported in patients with lymphoid malignancies, most commonly of T-cell type.[101]

The clinical features of HPS include pancytopenia, hepatosplenomegaly, abnormal liver function tests and a coagulopathy. Histologically there is a marked proliferation of activated histiocytes throughout the reticuloendothelial system, especially the hepatic sinusoids, splenic red pulp, lymph node sinuses and bone marrow. The cells have very abundant cytoplasm which contains formed blood elements including red cells, neutrophils and platelets. Critical to the distinction with malignant histiocytosis is the lack of significant cytological atypia. Such conspicuous erythrophagocytic activity is also not a feature of true histiocytic malignancies. It is of utmost importance to distinguish HPS from malignancy, since in a patient with HPS cytotoxic therapy is contraindicated; an underlying infection should be sought, and, if possible, treated. Acyclovir has been useful in some patients with Epstein–Barr virus (EBV) infections and HPS.[102]

A provocative hypothesis is that the HPS is caused by abnormal immune regulation in the setting of an immune response to a stimulus, usually an infection. In patients with HPS secondary to EBV infection without a history of immunodeficiency, abnormal responses to T-cell dependent antigens were demonstrated.[102] A lymphokine, termed phagocytosis inducing factor (PIF), was isolated from normal T-cells, cloned T-cell lines, and mononuclear cells from patients with angiocentric immunoproliferative diseases.[103] This factor was demonstrated to be capable of stimulating the cells of the U937 histiocytic cell line to phagocytose IgG coated red blood cells, and hence could be involved in the pathogenesis of this disorder.

Lymphoid proliferations of uncertain malignant potential

In virtually every organ system in the human body lymphoid proliferations of uncertain malignant potential exist.[104] These range from clearly demonstrated reactive lymphadenopathies which are associated with an increased risk of subsequent malignant lymphoma, to atypical lymphoid proliferations that may in fact represent low grade clonal lymphoproliferative disorders.

Sjögren's syndrome and rheumatoid arthritis

A variety of autoimmune disorders are associated with an increased risk of malignant lymphoma. Individuals affected with the autoimmune complex known as Sjögren's syndrome commonly develop an atypical lymphoid hyperplasia.[105] Involved lymph nodes exhibit reactive follicular hyperplasia, marked plasmacytosis, atypical paracortical hyperplasia, and the presence of monocytoid or plasmacytoid cells in the lymphoid sinuses. Patients with this lymphadenopathy syndrome usually have a polyclonal hypergammaglobulinaemia and readily demonstrable rheumatoid factor in the serum.

Individuals with Sjögren's syndrome are also at increased risk from developing malignant lymphoma. Such lymphomas are usually, but not exclusively, of high grade B-cell types, and in the NZB mouse model for autoimmune disease, B-cell lymphomas are also seen.[106] The development of a malignant lymphoma in a patient with Sjögren's syndrome is usually accompanied by the disappearance of polyclonal hypergammaglobulinaemia and rheumatoid factor from the serum. Thus, it is likely that the reactive lymphoid proliferation disappears and is replaced by a neoplastic lymphoid proliferation no longer producing polyclonal immunoglobulins.

The lymphoid cells isolated from the salivary gland lesions are capable of secreting monoclonal immunoglobulins, and monoclonal plasma cell proliferations can also be seen in affected minor salivary glands.[107,108] It is likely that these small monoclonal proliferations represent a preneoplastic event, and that these are the cells at risk for ultimate development of malignant lymphoma. Using sensitive techniques, such as Southern blotting for detection of immunoglobulin gene rearrangements, the majority of affected salivary glands contain detectable B-cell clones.[109] As in multiple myeloma, the ultimate emergence of the malignant disease may represent a two hit phenomenon.[110] The first hit is the creation of an expanded clone of B-cells, and the second event is the oncogenic event leading to uncontrolled proliferation of the clone. Nevertheless, salivary gland involvement by lymphoma is not necessarily seen, and the lymphomas are usually both nodal and extranodal in origin.

Hashimoto's thyroiditis

Hashimoto's thyroiditis represents another autoimmune syndrome in which affected individuals are at increased risk for the development of malignant lymphoma.[111] Hashimoto's thyroiditis occurs more often in females than males. The thyroid gland is infiltrated by abundant, dense lymphoid tissue containing hyperplastic germinal centres. Plasma cells may also be present. The glandular acini are small and atrophic, and the epithelial cells exhibit acidophilic change (so-called Hürthle or Askanazy cells).

Patients with classical Hashimoto's thyroiditis, or patients with lymphocytic thyroiditis (without epithelial alterations) are both at increased risk for development of malignant lymphoma of the thyroid.[112] As one might expect, since the reactive proliferations are predominantly of B lymphocytic origin, the malignant lymphomas seen in this population are also predominantly of the B-cell type, and usually of the aggressive follicular centre cell subtypes (large non-cleaved, large cleaved, and small non-cleaved).[113]

Immunodeficiency syndromes

Patients with immunodeficiency, either congenital, acquired, or iatrogenic, have a greatly increased risk of developing malignant lymphoma. Although malignancies are seen with an increased frequency in this patient population, a simple failure of immunosurveillance cannot be invoked to explain the increased incidence of malignant lymphoma.[114,115] Malignant lymphomas are by far the most common neoplasm in patients with immunodeficiency and, in some patient populations, the incidence may approach 20 per cent. The pathogenetic mechanism that leads to development of malignant lymphoma has not been fully explained in this patient population. It is likely that abnormal immunoregulation is the underlying cause.

Immunodeficiency syndromes commonly associated with malignant lymphoma include the Wiskott-Aldrich syndrome, ataxia telangiectasia and and common variable hypogammaglobulinaemia. In this clinical setting virtually all the lymphomas seen are of high grade histological types.[116,117] Disease usually presents in extranodal sites, in particular the brain. Extensive immunological studies to document the phenotype of the malignant cells have not been performed. A similar pattern of increased incidence of malignant lymphoma is seen in association with the acquired immune deficiency syndrome (AIDS), as discussed elsewhere (*see* Chapters 10 and 11). Epstein–Barr virus may play a role in the pathogenesis of HIV-associated malignant lymphomas (*see* Chapters 7 and 8).

Angiomatous lymphoid hamartoma or giant lymph node hyperplasia (Castleman's disease)

This lymphoid proliferation has been considered either a hamartomatous or reactive process.[118] The lymphoid mass lesion may be seen in the mediastinum, retroperitoneum, or other lymph-node bearing sites. Follicles predominate in this lesion, but T-cells are present in between the proliferating follicles. The follicles are characterized by prominent central vascular tufts, often leading to a hyalinized appearance. Surrounding the follicle are circumferential rows of small normal lymphocytes, so-called 'onion-skinning'. Numerous plasma cells may be present in the interfollicular stroma and clinically the disorder may be associated with systemic symptoms and a polyclonal hypergammaglobulinaemia.

Although patients with angiomatous lymphoid hamartomas are not considered to be at risk for the subsequent development of malignant lymphoma, isolated reports have been described in which the intervening plasma cells are monoclonal.[119] At our institution, we have encountered a similar case. Thus, these limited expanded monoclonal proliferations could be considered a preneoplastic event with subsequent risk for malignant evolution. Since malignant lymphomas are not reported in this patient population either such monoclonal proliferations are exceedingly rare, or secondary malignant transformation is uncommon.

A systemic form of Castleman's disease has also been described.[120] It does not appear related to the localized form, but represents a generalized form of atypical lymphoid hyperplasia in which the lymphoid follicles demonstrate prominent central vascular tufts. An increased incidence of Kaposi's sarcoma has been described and indeed many patients appear to have the clinical and pathological findings of AIDS.[121] It is notable that even in endemic Kaposi's sarcoma involving lymph nodes, the lymphoid follicles exhibit the characteristic vascularity associated with Castleman's disease. Thus, systemic Castleman's disease may not represent a distinct disease entity, but a constellation of immune disorders which share this common morphological feature. As in AIDS, an increased incidence of malignant lymphoma has been reported, and these lymph nodes may harbour monoclonal lymphoid populations.[122]

Pseudolymphoma

The term 'pseudolymphoma' has been used to describe atypical lymphoid proliferations of tumour-like proportions. These lesions commonly occur in extranodal sites and have been described in the stomach, orbit, lung, and skin. Pseudolymphomas present clinically as mass lesions, but when examined histologically they are composed of normal lymphoid elements.[123] Sheets of relatively monotonous small lymphocytes may be seen, sometimes admixed with plasma cells. Interspersed among the small lymphoid elements are cytologically normal germinal centres. Immunoblasts or large transformed lymphoid cells may be present in variable proportions. The more polymorphous the infiltrate and the greater the number of germinal centres, the easier it is to distinguish pseudolymphoma from malignant lymphoma. Because of the preponderance of small lymphocytes in many pseudolymphomas, the principal diagnostic dilemma is usually pseudolymphoma versus a malignant lymphoma of the small lymphocytic subtype.

Definite criteria for the distinction of pseudolymphoma from malignant lymphoma are not universally agreed upon. Koss *et al.* reclassified many pulmonary lesions, which were formerly diagnosed as pseudolymphomas, as small lymphocytic lymphomas.[124] Nevertheless, many of the patients in this series continued to pursue a benign clinical course, even without systemic therapeutic intervention. Knowles *et al.* and Evans attempted to use lymphocyte surface markers to distinguish pseudolymphomas from small lymphocytic lymphomas in the orbit and skin respectively.[125,126] Their studies were not universally successful as some patients with polyclonal lesions progressed to the development of malignant lymphoma. Conversely, some patients with 'monoclonal lymphoid proliferations' continued to pursue an indolent course without systemic progression of disease. Recently Medeiros *et al.* demonstrated a close correlation between phenotypic analysis for clonality and clinical behaviour.[127]

It seems apparent that, even if many so-called pseudolymphomas are monoclonal and perhaps neoplastic, these lesions do not undergo rapid dissemination and conservative therapy is indicated. For orbital lesions localized radiotherapy is probably the treatment of choice. In other anatomical sites, such as the lung, radiotherapy may be more difficult to deliver.

In a small number of patients with pseudolymphoma, progression to a high grade malignant lymphoma, large cell lymphoma or large cell lymphoma of the immunoblastic subtype, has been documented.[128] Thus, recurrent disease should always be rebiopsied to document the presence or absence of histological progression.

In some sites it may be possible to identify the putative stimulus of the atypical lymphoid proliferation. For example, pseudolymphomas of the stomach are often associated with a chronic gastric ulcer.[129] The presence of a chronic ulcer with a granulation or fibrous tissue base is supportive evidence that the lymphoid proliferation associated with it is reactive. In contrast, in lymphomas of the stomach, although the overlying mucosa may be ulcerated the malignant lymphoid proliferation extends directly to the ulcerated tissue surface. Evidence of chronicity is not an absolute criterion for benignity, since, as noted above, pseudolymphoma may progress to lymphoma. In such cases, evidence of a chronic ulcer may be seen in the malignant lymphoid proliferation.

Angioimmunoblastic lymphadenopathy

Several disorders have been described in which the histological features may not be diagnostic of malignant lymphoma, at least at the onset of symptoms, but which commonly progress to outright malignancy. One such syndrome is angioimmunoblastic lymphadenopathy (AILD),

first described in 1975.[130,131] This most commonly occurs in older individuals, with a mean age of 68. Presenting features are generalized lymphadenopathy, constitutional symptoms and a rash. Hepatosplenomegaly, polyclonal hypergammaglobulinaemia and a positive Coombs' test are often seen. Biopsy of an involved lymph node reveals virtually complete effacement of the normal architecture, excepting the possible presence of 'burnt out' germinal centres (i.e. those with a paucity of cells and deposits of hyaline material). There is a marked proliferation of small blood vessels, and a polymorphous infiltrate of lymphocytes, immunoblasts and plasma cells. Histiocytes and eosinophils may be present, but are not essential for the diagnosis. The infiltrate is often associated with interstitial deposits of amorphous eosinophilic material, and the overall appearance is hypocellular. When lymphoma supervenes, the immunoblasts form large clusters or sheets, and the inflammatory background is partially or totally diminished.

Angioimmunoblastic lymphadenopathy is often a rapidly progressive disorder, with a mean survival of only 15 months, despite the lack of morphologically malignant cells. However, large cell immunoblastic lymphomas are found in up to 50 per cent of patients, either clinically or at autopsy.[132] The biological nature of this disease is not yet clear. Most of the immunoblastic cells are T-lymphocytes, and clonal populations of T-cells have been demonstrated in most cases. However, B-cell clones have been shown in some instances.[133,134] Such findings have been variously interpreted as arguing that AILD is neoplastic at the outset, or that it is an immunoregulatory disorder.

Angiocentric immunoproliferative lesions

Another group of disorders characterized by polymorphic proliferations of immune cells can be brought together under a common rubric of angiocentric immunoproliferative lesions (AIL). Included in this group are lymphomatoid granulomatosis (LYG), polymorphic reticulosis (PMR), and midline malignant reticulosis (MMR). These entities were described separately as occurring in different anatomical sites, LYG in the lower respiratory tract and PMR and MMR in the upper respiratory tract including the nose, nasopharynx, palate and sinuses. The latter two were associated with the clinical syndrome known as lethal midline granuloma. However, all these disorders share a similar histological picture, with an atypical lymphoid proliferation, admixed with plasma cells, eosinophils and histiocytes, displaying marked propensity to invade and destroy blood vessels (Fig. 4.13). There is often vascular destruction, and necrosis is characteristic, presumably secondary to ischaemia. The name AIL was proposed because of these similarities, under the assumption that these entities are really a single disorder.[135] Other sites which are commonly involved include the skin, the gastrointestinal tract, the kidneys and the central and peripheral nervous systems.

As with AILD, patients with AIL frequently develop overt lymphomas.[136] Survival appears to be inversely proportional to the number of large atypical cells.[137] When lymphoma does develop, it appears to have a mature T-cell phenotype.[138] A grading scheme has recently been proposed.[97] Grade I lesions lack any significant atypia. Grade II lesions display some cytological atypia whereas Grade III lesions represent clear-cut angiocentric lymphoma. It is hoped that such a grading system will aid in the decision to treat these patients with either cyclophosphamide and prednisone for the low grade lesions (grade I), or aggressive chemotherapy for the higher grades (grades II and III).

Pagetoid reticulosis, parapsoriasis *en plaque*, and alopecia mucinosa

The above lesions all represent atypical cutaneous infiltrates, which may precede the development of mycosis fungoides. Mycosis fungoides (MF) is a notoriously chronic cutaneous malignancy. Patients in whom the diagnosis of MF is ultimately made frequently give a history of cutaneous eruptions for many years. Multiple skin biopsies may be necessary over a period of years in order to document the diagnosis of mycosis fungoides. In the early stages, although atypical cerebriform

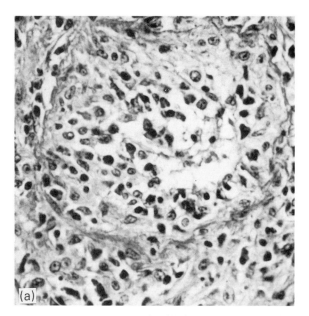

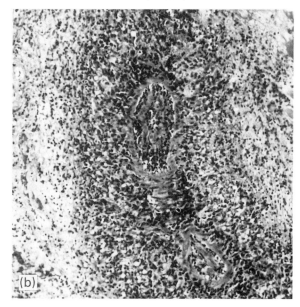

Fig. 4.13 Angiocentric immunoproliferative lesions. (a) Angiocentric immunoproliferative lesion, lung. Vessel is obliterated by angiocentric and angiodestructive lymphoid infiltrate. Infiltrate is polymorphous and composed of lymphocytes and plasma cells. (b) Buccal mucosa. Obliterated vessel is surrounded by extensive coagulative necrosis.

lymphocytes may be seen, diagnostic Pautrier abscesses are absent.

In alopecia mucinosa the atypical lymphoid cells infiltrate hair follicles, leading to destruction of the follicle and loss of hair. Pagetoid reticulosis is characterized by an atypical infiltrate of cerebriform cells throughout the epidermis.[139] In the Woringer–Kolopp variant, although histologically the lesion resembles mycosis fungoides, only single isolated keratotic plaques are present, and excision of the lesion may result in a sustained clinical remission without recurrence.[140] However, the disseminated form of pagetoid reticulosis is best considered as a morphological variant of MF and clinically it pursues an aggressive clinical course. It is likely that the isolated form of pagetoid reticulosis represents an isolated MF lesion, and that resection of this isolated lesion may lead to a prolonged disease-free survival. A recent study using molecular genetic techniques demonstrated that in one such patient the T-cells were in fact mono-clonal.[141]

Parapsoriasis *en plaque* is a disorder charac-terized by chronic recalcitrant erythematous scaling lesions.[140] The skin biopsy exhibits a high dermal infiltrate composed of atypical lymphoid cells without demonstrable Pautrier micro-abscesses. Patients with large patch lesions or exhibiting the poikiloderma variant frequently progress to MF. However, patients with only small patches may pursue a benign clinical course.

Gluten sensitive enteropathy

Gluten sensitive enteropathy is a clinico-pathological syndrome associated with villous atrophy of the small bowel, plasmacytosis of the lamina propria, diarrhoea and malabsorption, all of which can be reversed following removal of gluten from the diet. Immunological abnor-malities have also been demonstrated in these patients. As with many immune disorders, patients with gluten sensitive enteropathy or coeliac disease have an increased incidence of lymphoma.[142]

The lymphomas usually occur in the affected small bowel and may be preceded by intestinal ulcerations which are accompanied by an atypical lymphoid infiltrate.[143] Usually a history of coeliac disease has been present for many years but in some cases the two processes may present simultaneously.[144,145]

At their base the ulcerative lesions show a densely cellular infiltrate composed of lymphocytes, immunoblasts and plasma cells. The infiltrates are usually confined to the submucosa and lamina propria without involvement of the muscularis. The lymphomas seen in this setting are all of the diffuse aggressive subtypes: mixed small and large cell, large cell, and large cell immunoblastic. Although Isaacson *et al.* initially claimed that these lymphomas represented a variant of malignant histiocytosis,[146] other authors have not found evidence for a histiocytic origin of the neoplastic cells.[142–47] Recent studies employing gene rearrangement techniques have provided evidence for a monoclonal T-cell origin.[148]

Lymphomatoid papulosis (LP)

Lymphomatoid papulosis is a chronic, self-remitting atypical lymphoproliferative disorder which involves the skin.[149] Patients present with papular-nodular cutaneous lesions which spon-taneously ulcerate and heal. Histologically the lesions appear cytologically malignant but have a polymorphous cellular composition. Bizarre lymphoreticular cells are admixed with plasma cells, lymphocytes, histiocytes, and acute inflammatory cells. The bizarre cells are activated T-cells and may express the CD15 and CD30 antigens often seen in the cells of Hodgkin's disease.[150] Molecular genetic analysis using probes to the T-β antigen receptor genes have demonstrated clonal rearrangements.[151] Thus, although many of the cytological, phenotypic and genetic characteristics of this lesion would suggest malignancy, the process usually behaves in a clinically benign fashion for many years. Lymphomatoid papulosis is occasionally seen in patients with Hodgkin's disease or mycosis fungoides.[152,153] Rare patients will progress to lymph node or visceral involvement, and in such cases, the process will then pursue a malignant clinical course. Lymphomatoid papulosis is a disorder at the interface of benignancy and malignancy. It may represent a malignancy which behaves in a clinically benign fashion due to its unique microenvironment.

References

1. Jaffe ES, Cossman J. In: Rose NR, Friedman H, Fahey JL eds. *Manual of Clinical Laboratory Immunology*, 3rd edn, Washington DC: American Society for Microbiology, 1986: 779.
2. Kohler G, Milstein C. *Nature*. 1975; **256**, 495.
3. Aiuti F, Cerrottini JC, Coombs RRA, *et al. Scandinavian Journal of Immunology*. 1974; **3**, 521.
4. Bernard A, Boumsell L, Dausset J, *et al. Human Leukocyte Differentiation Antigens Detected by Monoclonal Antibodies: Specification, Classification, Nomenclature*. Berlin, Heidelberg, New York, Tokyo: Springer-Verlag, 1984.
5. Reinherz EL, Haynes BF, Nadler LM, *et al. Leukocyte Typing II: Human B Lymphocytes*. New York, Berlin, Heidelberg, Tokyo: Springer-Verlag, 1987.
6. Reinherz EL, Haynes BF, Nadler LM, *et al. Leukocyte Typing II: Human T Lymphocytes*. New York, Berlin, Heidelberg, Tokyo: Springer-Verlag, 1987.
7. Jaffe ES, Longo DL, Cossman J, *et al. Laboratory Investigation*. 1984; **50**, 27A.
8. Dvoretsky P, Wood GS, Levy R, Warnke RA. *Human Pathology*. 1982; **13**, 618.
9. Lovett EJ, Schnitzer B, Keren DF, *et al. Laboratory Investigation*. 1984; **50**, 115.
10. Battifora H, Trowbridge IS. *Cancer*. 1983; **51**, 816.
11. Warnke RA, Gatter KC, Phil D, *et al. New England Journal of Medicine*. 1983; **309**, 1275.
12. Hsu S–M, Jaffe ES. *American Journal of Clinical Pathology*. 1984; **82**, 29.
13. Dorfman RF, Gattes KC, Pulford KAF, *et al. American Journal of Pathology*. 1986; **123**, 508.
14. Greaves MF, Brown G, Rapson NT, *et al. Clinical Immunology and Immunopathology*. 1975; **4**, 67.
15. Cossman J, Neckers LM, Hsu SM, *et al. American Journal of Pathology*. 1984; **114**, 117.
16. Ritz J, Nadler LM, Bhan AK, *et al. Blood*. 1981; **48**, 648.
17. Ritchie KA, Brinster RL, Storb U. *Nature*. 1984; **312**, 517.
18. Levy R, Warnke R, Dorfman RF, *et al. Journal of Experimental Medicine*. 1977; **145**, 1014.
19. Royer HD, Reinherz EL. *New England Journal of Medicine*. 1987; **317**, 1136.
20. Weiss LM, Crabtree GS, Rouse RV, *et al. American Journal of Pathology*. 1985; **118**, 316.
21. Jaffe ES. *Cancer Investigation*. 1984; **2**, 413.
22. Haynes BF, Metzgar RS, Minna JD, *et al. New England Journal of Medicine*. 1981; **304**, 1319.
23. Reinherz EL, Nadler LM, Sallen SE, *et al. Journal of Clinical Investigation*. 1979; **64**, 392.
24. Cossman J, Chused TM, Fisher RI, *et al. Cancer Research*. 1983; **43**, 4486.
25. Braziel RM, Keneklis T, Donlon JA, *et al. American Journal of Clinical Pathology*. 1983; **80**, 655.
26. Bollum FJ. *Blood*. 1979; **54**, 1203.
27. Greaves MF, Chan LC, Furley AJW, *et al. Blood*. 1986; **67**, 1.
28. Boumsell L, Coppin H, Pham D, *et al. Journal of Experimental Medicine*. 1980; **152**, 229.
29. Virchow RLK. *Die Krankhaftern Geschwuelste*. Berlin: Hirschwald, 1983.
30. Kundrat H. *Wein klinische Wochenschrift*. 1893; **6**, 211 and 234.
31. Roulet F. *Virchows Archives*. 1930; **277**, 15.
32. Brill NE, Baehr G, Rosenthal N. *Journal of the American Medical Association*. 1925; **84**, 668.
33. Symmers D. *Archives of Pathology*. 1927; **3**, 816.
34. Gall EA, Mallory TB. *American Journal of Pathology*. 1942; **18**, 381.
35. Rappaport H, Winter WJ, Hicks EB. *Cancer*. 1956; **9**, 792.
36. Rappaport H. *Atlas of Tumor Pathology*, Section III, fascicle 8. Washington DC: Armed Forces Institute of Pathology, 1966.
37. Lukes RJ, Collins RD. *Cancer*. 1974; **34**, 1488.
38. Jaffe ES, Strauchen JA, Berard CW. *American Journal of Clinical Pathology*. 1982; **77**, 46.
39. Dorfman RF. *Lancet*. 1974; **i**, 1295.
40. Bennet MH, Farrer-Brown G, Henry K *et al. Lancet*. 1974; **ii**, 405.
41. Lennert K, Mohri N, Stein H, *et al. British Journal of Haematology*. 1975; **31**, 193.
42. Rosenberg A, Berard CW, Brown BW, *et al. Cancer*. 1982; **49**, 2112.
43. Jaffe ES. *Seminars in Oncology*. 1986; **13** (no.4, suppl. 5), 3.
44. Rosenberg SA. *New England Journal of Medicine*. 1979; **301**, 924.
45. DeVita VT, *et al. Lancet*. 1975; **i**, 243.
46. Jaffe ES. *Journal of the National Cancer Institute*. 1983; **70**, 401.
47. Foon KA, Sherwin SA, Abrams PG, *et al. New England Journal of Medicine*. 1984; **311**, 1148.
48. Cohen PJ, Lotze MT, Roberts JR, *et al. American Journal of Pathology*. 1987; **129**, 208.
49. Krikorian JG, Portlock CS, Cooney DP, *et al. Cancer Research*. 1980; **46**, 2093.
50. Come SE, Jaffe ES, Anderson JC, *et al. American*

Journal of Medicine. 1980; **69**, 667.

51. Fisher RI, Jones RB, DeVita VT Jr., *et al. Cancer.* 1981; **47**, 2022.

52. Hubbard SM, Chabner BA, DeVita VT Jr., *et al. Blood.* 1982; **59**, 258.

53. Raffeld MR, Neckers L, Longo DL, Cossman J. *New England Journal of Medicine.* 1985; **312**, 1653.

54. Raffeld MR, Wright JJ, Lipford E, *et al. Cancer Research.* 1987; **47**, 2537.

55. Head DR, Avakian J, Kjeldsberg CR, Cerezo L. *American Journal of Clinical Pathology.* 1988; **89**, 106.

56. Dick FR, Maca RD. *Cancer.* 1978; **41**, 282.

57. Cossman J, Neckers LM, Braziel RM, *et al. Journal of Clinical Investigation.* 1984; **73**, 587.

58. Harrison CV. *Journal of Clinical Pathology.* 1972; **25**, 12.

59. Richter MN. *American Journal of Pathology.* 1928; **4**, 285.

60. Royston I, Majda JA, Baird SM, *et al. Journal of Immunology.* 1980; **125**, 725.

61. Nathwani BN, Winber CD, Diamond LW, *et al. Cancer.* 1981; **48**, 1794.

62. Nathwani BN, Metter GE, Miller TP, *et al. Blood.* 1986; **68**, 837.

63. Osborne CK, Norton L, Young RC, *et al. Blood.* 1980; **56**, 98.

64. Harris NL, Nadler LM, Bhan AK. *American Journal of Pathology.* 1984; **117**, 262.

65. Ault KA. *New England Journal of Medicine.* 1979; **300**, 1401.

66. Braziel RM, Sussman E, Neckers LM, *et al. Blood.* 1985; **66**, 128.

67. Lowder JN, Meeker TC, Campbell M, *et al. Blood.* 1987; **69**, 199.

68. Berard CW, Dorfman RF. In: Roschberg SA ed. *Clinics in Hematology.* London: W.B. Saunders, Vol. 3(1), 39.

69. Weisenberger DD, Kim H, Rappaport H. *Cancer.* 1982; **49**, 1429.

70. Jaffe ES, Bookman MA, Longo DL. *Human Pathology.* 1987; **18**, 877.

71. Cossman J, Jaffe ES, Fisher RI. *Cancer.* 1984; **54**, 1310.

72. Burke JS, Butler JJ. *American Journal of Clinical Pathology.* 1976; **66**, 1.

73. Stein H, Mason DY, Gerdes J, *et al. Blood.* 1985; **66**, 848.

74. Kadin ME, Sako D, Berliner N, *et al. Blood.* 1986; **68**, 1042.

75. Nathwani BN, Kim H, Rappaport H. *Cancer.* 1976; **38**, 964.

76. Barcos MP, Lukes RJ. In: Sinks LF, Godden JO eds. *Conflicts in Childhood Cancer: An Evaluation of Current Management.* New York: Alan R Liss Inc, 1975.

77. Smith JL, Barker CR, Clein GP, *et al. Lancet.* 1973; **i**, 74.

78. Picker LJ, Weiss LM, Medeiros LJ, *et al. American Journal of Pathology.* 1987; **128**, 181.

79. Burkitt D. *British Journal of Surgery.* 1958; **46**, 218.

80. Banks PM, Arseneau JC, Gralnick HR, *et al. American Journal of Medicine.* 1975; **58**, 322.

81. Magrath IT, Freeman CB, Pizzo P, *et al. Journal of the National Cancer Institute.* 1980; **64**, 477.

82. Miliauskas JR, Berard CW, Young RC, *et al. Cancer.* 1982; **50**, 2115.

83. Grogan TM, Warnke RA, Kaplan HS. *Cancer.* 1982; **49**, 1817.

84. Croce CM, Tsujimoto Y, Erikson I, *et al. Laboratory Investigation.* 1984; **51**, 258.

85. Edelson RL. *Journal of Dermatologic Surgery and Oncology.* 1980; **6**, 358.

86. Lutzner MA, Hobbs JW, Horvath P. *Archives of Dermatology.* 1971; **103**, 375.

87. Matthews MJ. In: Jaffe ES ed. *Surgical Pathology of the Lymph Nodes and Related Organs.* Philadelphia: W B Saunders, 1985: 329.

88. Rappaport H, Thomas LB. *Cancer.* 1974; **34**, 1198.

89. Rowden G, Lewis MG. *British Journal of Dermatology.* 1976; **95**, 665.

90. Weiss LM, Hu E, Wood GS, *et al. New England Journal of Medicine.* 1985; **313**, 537.

91. Uchiyama T, Yodoi J, Sagawa K, *et al. Blood.* 1977; **50**, 481.

92. Blayney DW, Jaffe ES, Blattner WA, *et al. Blood.* 1983; **62**, 401.

93. Jaffe ES, Blattner WA, Blayney DW, *et al. American Journal of Surgical Pathology.* 1984; **8**, 263.

94. Van der Valk P, Meijer CJLM, Willemze R, *et al. Histopathology.* 1984; **8**, 105.

95. Ducatman BS, Wick MR, Morgan TW. *Human Pathology.* 1984; **15**, 368.

96. Furth RV, Raeburn JA, Van Zwet T. *Blood.* 1979; **54**, 485.

97. Todd RF, Nadler LM, Schlossman SF. *Journal of Immunology.* 1981; **126**, 1435.

98. Jaffe ES. *Seminars in Diagnostic Pathology.* 1988; in press.

99. Scott RB, Robb-Smith AHT. *Lancet.* 1939; **ii**, 194.

100. Risdall RJ, McKenna RW, Nesbitt ME, *et al. Cancer.* 1979; **44**, 993.

101. Jaffe ES, Costa J, Fauci AS, *et al. American Journal of Medicine.* 1983; **75**, 741.

102. Sullivan JL, Woda BA, Herrod HG, *et al. Blood.* 1985; **65**, 1097.

103. Simrell CR, Margolick JB, Crabtree GR, *et al. Blood.* 1985; **65**, 1469.

104. Jaffe ES. In: Henson DE, Albores-Saavedra J. eds. *Pathology of Incipient Neoplasia.* Philadelphia:

WB Saunders & Co: 1986: 87–115.

105. Anderson LB, Talal N. *Clinical and Experimental Immunology*. 1972; **10**, 199.
106. Zulman J, Jaffe R, Talal N. *New England Journal of Medicine*. 1978; **299**, 1215
107. Talal N, Asofsky R, Lightbody P. *Journal of Clinical Investigation*. 1979; **49**, 49.
108. Lane HC, Callihan TR, Jaffe ES, *et al. Clinical and Experimental Rheumatology*. 1983; **1**, 237.
109. Fishleder A, Tubbs R, Hesse B, Levine H. *New England Journal of Medicine*. 1987; **316**, 1118.
110. Salmos SE, Seligmann M. *Lancet*. 1974; **ii**, 1230.
111. Dailey ME, Lindsay S, Skahen R. *Archives of Surgery*. 1955; **70**, 291.
112. Burke JS, Butler JJ, Fuller LM. *Cancer*. 1977; **39**, 1587.
113. Maurer R, Taylor CR, Terry R, Lukes RJ. *Virchows Archives A. Pathology, Anatomy and Histology*. 1979; **383**, 293.
114. Gatti RA, Good RA. *Cancer*. 1971; **28**, 89.
115. Waldmann TA, Strober W, Blaese RM. *Annals of Internal Medicine*. 1980; **77**, 605.
116. Frizzera G, Rosai J, Dehner LP, *et al. Cancer*. 1980; **46**, 692.
117. Cotelingam JD, Witebsky FG, Hsu SM, Blaese RM, Jaffe ES. *Cancer Investigation*. 1985; **6**, 515.
118. Keller AR, Hocholzer L, Castleman B. *Cancer*. 1972; **29**, 670.
119. Schlosnagle DC, Chan WC, Hargreaves HK. Nolting SF, Brynes RK. *American Journal of Clinical Pathology*. 1982; **78**, 541.
120. Frizzera G, Banks PM, Massarelli G, Rosai J. *American Journal of Surgical Pathology*. 1983; **7**, 211.
121. Dickson D, Ben-Ezra JM, Reed J, Flax H, Janis R. *Archives of Pathology and Laboratory Medicine*. 1985; **109**, 1013.
122. Hanson CA, Kersey JH, Patton DF, Gajl-Peczalska K, Peterson BA, Frizzera G. *Laboratory Investigation*. 1988; **58**, 37A.
123. Saltzstein SL. *Pathology Annual*. 1969; **159**, 185.
124. Koss MN, Hocholzer L, Nichols PW, Wehunt WD. *Human Pathology*. 1983; **14**, 1024.
125. Knowles DM, Halper JP, Jakobiec FA. *Cancer*. 1982; **49**, 2321.
126. Evans HL. *Cancer*. 1982; **49**, 84.
127. Medeiros LJ, Harmon DC, Bhan AK, Harris NL. *Laboratory Investigation*. 1988; **58**, 62A.
128. Wolf JA, Spjut HJ. *Cancer*. 1981; **48**, 2518.
129. Brooks JJ, Enterline HT. *Cancer*. 1983; **51**, 476.
130. Lukes RJ, Tindle BH. *New England Journal of Medicine*. 1975; **292**, 1.
131. Frizzera G, Moran EM, Rappaport H. *American Journal of Medicine*. 1975; **58**, 803.
132. Nathwani BN, Rappaport H, Moran EM, *et al. Cancer*. 1978; **41**, 578.
133. Weiss LM, Strickler JG, Dorfman RF, *et al. American Journal of Pathology*. 1986; **122**, 392.
134. Lipford EH, Smith HR, Pittaluga S, *et al. Journal of Clinical Investigation*. 1987; **79**, 637.
135. Jaffe ES, Lipford EH, Margolick JB, *et al. Seminars in Respiratory Medicine*. 1988; in press.
136. Fauci AS, Haynes BF, Costa J, *et al. New England Journal of Medicine*. 1982; **306**, 68.
137. Katzenstein A, Carrington CB, Liebow AA. *Cancer*. 1979; **43**, 360.
138. Nicols PW, Koss M, Levine AM, *et al. American Journal of Medicine*. 1982; **72**, 467.
139. Braun-Falco O, Marghescu S, Wolff HH. *Hautarzt*. 1973; **24**, 11.
140. Burg G, Braun-Falco O. *Cutaneous Lymphomas, Pseudolymphomas and Related Disorders*. Berlin: Springer-Verlag, 1983.
141. Wood GS, Weiss LM, Chung-Hong H, *et al. New England Journal of Medicine*. 1980; **318**, 164.
142. Otto HF, Bettman I, Weltzien JV, Gebbers JO. *Virchows Archives A*. 1981; **391**, 9.
143. Baer AN, Bayliss TM, Yardley JH. *Gastroenterology*. 1980; **79**, 754.
144. Cooper BT, Holmes GKT, Ferguson R, Cooke WT. *Medicine*. 1980; **59**, 249.
145. Swinson CM, Slavin G, Coles EC, Booth CC. *Lancet*. 1983; **i**, 111.
146. Isaacson P, Jones DB, Sworn MJ, Wright DH. *Journal of Clinical Pathology*. 1982; **35**, 510.
147. Saraga P, Hurlimann J, Ozzello L. *Human Pathology*. 1981; **12**, 713.
148. Isaacson PG, O'Connor NT, Spencer J, Bevan DH. *Lancet*. 1985; **ii**, 688.
149. Valentino LA, Helwig EG. *Archives of Pathology*. 1973; **96**, 409.
150. Kadin M, Nasu K, Sako D, Said J, Vonderheid E. *American Journal of Pathology*. 1985; **119**, 315.
151. Weiss LM, Wood GS, Trela M, Warnke RA, Sklar J. *New England Journal of Medicine*. 1986; **315**, 475.
152. Fine RM, Meltzer HD, Rudner EJ. *South Medical Journal*. 1974; **67**, 1492.
153. Dowd PM, Munro DD, Stansfield AG. *Journal of the Royal Society of Medicine*. 1981; **74**, 68.

CHAPTER 5

CYTOGENETICS

Jacqueline Whang-Peng and Elaine C Lee

In contrast to Hodgkin's disease, the non-Hodgkin's lymphomas are composed of a wide range of tumours with histological, immunological and cytogenetic heterogeneity. The Southwest Oncology Group, in a histopathological review,[1] stated that there may be disagreement in as many as 25 per cent of the cases in diagnosis and subclassification of the lymphomas even among experienced pathologists examining fixed lymph node sections. In 6 per cent of the cases there may even be disagreement on whether or not the resected tissues show evidence of malignancy. Needle aspirations of lymph nodes may suggest a diagnosis but lack of sufficient tissue prevents accurate classification.[2] It has been demonstrated that the cellular origin of lymphoma often cannot be discerned by routine histological means. Application of newly available tools such as immunochemistry and flow cytometry still results in a certain number of undiagnosed cases. Other recently developed techniques of molecular genetics may help in diagnosis but these largely experimental methods are far from useful on a daily basis for most laboratories. Several large series of cytogenetic studies in non-Hodgkin's lymphoma have been reported.[3–7] These show that 95–100 per cent of the lymphomas exhibit cytogenetic abnormalities and that some changes can be correlated with specific histological and immunological phenotypes. Use of cytogenetics as a diagnostic aid, in predicting prognosis and as a guide to therapy may therefore be very helpful. In addition, cytogenetic abnormalities may point the way towards molecular genetic disorders which appear to be the basis of neoplastic growth.

Materials and methods

Successful cytogenetic studies of neoplastic disorders depend upon locating the tumour cells and upon the availability of dividing cells. Then it must be determined whether the anticipated chromosomal abnormalities are readily visible using standard harvesting techniques or if high resolution techniques are required to permit detection of more subtle aberrations.

The tissue of choice for study of lymphomas is the lymph node, or material from needle aspiration of the lymph node. However, other specimens can be used, including effusions such as pleural fluid or ascites. These often provide a large number of tumour cells from which cytogenetic preparations are easily obtainable. In addition, specimens from the spleen (obtained after splenectomy) may be used; splenic needle aspirations are not usually performed in the USA. In cases where there is involvement of the bone marrow, this may serve as a good source of tumour tissue. After a single cell suspension is obtained, the harvesting procedure for obtaining the cytogenetic preparations is the same for tumours, bone marrow, or peripheral blood.

Bone marrow and needle aspirations

A small amount, 0.25–0.5ml, of bone marrow or material from the needle aspiration is collected without anticoagulant. The specimen is incubated in 0.2 μg/ml colcemid in RPMI 1640 medium supplemented with penicillin, streptomycin, glutamine, and 15–20 per cent fetal bovine serum (FBS) for 30 minutes to an hour at room temperature or at 37°C. It is treated with hypotonic solution and fixed as described below. Usually, a few drops of the bone marrow are also cultured for 18–24 hours in RPMI 1640 containing FBS.

Peripheral blood

The blood sample is collected with 20 units of heparin/ml blood (preservative-free heparin is preferred). After gravity sedimentation of the erythrocytes, leucocyte-rich plasma is obtained and the cell count adjusted to a final concentration of 1–2 $\times$ 10^6 cells/ml.

Effusions

The fluids are centrifuged to collect the tumour cells, which are then washed once with culture medium containing FBS. The cell count is adjusted to 1–2 $\times$ 10^6/ml and the cells are cultured in RPMI 1640 with FBS for 1–2 days.

Lymph nodes, tumours, and spleen

Cytogenetic analyses of tumours are sometimes difficult as there is variation in the number of dividing cells. Obtaining a single-cell suspension is essential and sterile scissors or blades may be used to mince the tissue into small pieces. A single cell suspension can then be obtained by use of a stainless steel mesh, homogenizer, or repeated aspiration through a 22 gauge needle. The use of collagenase or other means of disaggregation is not necessary. In our laboratory the small pieces of tissue are forced through a 190 μm pore-sized mesh; this results in adequate numbers of viable cells. Chromosome preparations are made after 1–2 days of culture in the usual medium.

Several mitogens may be added according to the cell type found in the tumours. For T-cell malignancies, the mitogen of choice is phytohaemagglutinin (PHA) at a concentration of 0.2 ml for each 10 ml of culture. In addition, pokeweed mitogen (PWM), interleukin-2 (IL-2) or TPA (phorbol-12-myristate-12 acetate, Sigma Chemical Co., St Louis, Missouri) may be used singly or in combination. The combination, or cocktail, described by Nowell and Finan,[8] includes 1.0 ml IL-2, 0.2 ml PWM, and 0.1 ml TPA (10 μg/ml) added to a 10 ml culture. For B-cell malignancies the cocktail, PWM, LPS (lipopolysaccharide)[9] and EBV (Epstein–Barr virus) is used. The duration of the culture varies according to the mitogen used with those such as IL-2 and TPA requiring 3–4 days and LPS requiring 6–7 days.

Harvesting

Direct preparations and cultures of bone marrow, peripheral blood, lymph node, effusions, etc. are all harvested in the same way. First, the cells are arrested in metaphase, usually by incubation with colcemid at a concentration of 0.1–0.2 μg/ml for 30–90 minutes. Second, to swell the cytoplasmic membrane the cells are exposed to a hypotonic solution (1:1 mixture of 1 per cent sodium citrate and 0.75 M KCl) for 20 minutes at room temperature. After the cells have been fixed in a 3:1 mixture of absolute ethanol and glacial acetic acid for 10–15 minutes and again, in a fresh solution, for 5 minutes, air-dried preparations are made. Between steps, the cells are centrifuged at 800 r.p.m. for 5 minutes.

Staining

Metaphases are scored for modal chromosome number and frequency of chromosomal aberrations (breaks, fragments, rings and minutes that may be difficult to detect in banded preparations) using a standard Giemsa stain. In order to identify each homologue and determine the location of breakpoints, chromosomal banding analysis is mandatory and various techniques may be used to produce the banding. One of the first to be described was Q banding in which quinacrine mustard is used to stain the chromosomes which were analysed by fluorescence microscopy. The chromosomal banding pattern obtained in this way was used as the basis for all subsequent descriptions of chromosome bands. Q banding allows detection of polymorphic variants as well as the brilliantly staining region on the long arm of the Y chromosome, and the bands obtained are very similar to G-bands.[10,11] The most widely used banding analysis is the trypsin-Giemsa technique (exposure of the chromosomes to trypsin followed by staining with Giemsa stain).[12] This stain is easy, cheap, reproducible and, most importantly, does not fade. R banding, the reverse of G banding,[13] is based on thermal denaturation of DNA and is used more extensively in Europe than in the USA. C banding, resulting from alkali denaturation of DNA, reveals areas of constitutive hetero-chromatin (centromeric region, long arm of Y, etc.) and is helpful in determining whether or not abnormal chromosomes are dicentric, or if homogeneously staining regions are hetero-chromatic or euchromatic in nature.[14]

Nomenclature

The chromosomal banding nomenclature was first established at the Paris Conference in 1971,[15] was revised in 1985, and has been published as *An International System for Human Cytogenetic Nomenclature (ISCN) 1985.*[16]

Briefly, the short arm of each chromosome is known as the 'p' arm and the long arm, the 'q' arm. The designation of chromosomal location is made in the following manner: chromosome number, arm, region, band and subband. For example 1q21.2 indicates chromosome 1, q arm, region 2, band 1, and subband 2. The nomenclature for chromosomal abnormalities was also standardized at the Paris Conference. Plus (+) and minus (−) symbols in front of a chromosome indicate that there is gain or loss of a whole chromosome; when placed after the chromosome it denotes gain or loss of portions of the indicated chromosome. Many complex abnormalities are often found in neoplastic diseases and other abbreviations used to describe these include der (derivative

chromosome), dup (duplication), fra (fragile site), h (secondary constriction), i or iso (iso-chromosome), ins (insertion), inv (inversion), t (translocation), r (ring chromosome), min (minutes), and HSRs (homogenously staining regions).

Cytogenetic findings in non-Hodgkin's lymphomas

Correlation with the Working Formulation[17]

Cytogenetic studies in lymphoma patients have correlated chromosomal abnormalities with specific immunophenotypes and histology.[18–33] Tables 5.1 and 5.2 summarize the cytogenetic findings in a total of 167 of these patients. Six (3.6 per cent) had a normal karyotype with the remaining 96.4 per cent exhibiting cytogenetic abnormalities. The relationship between the classification of lymphoma and the extent of the chromosome abnormalities reveals that the diffuse, poorly differentiated lymphomas, regardless of grade, have the most changes. Specific changes reported for each type of lymphoma, according to the Working Formulation, will be described.

Ploidy and chromosome abnormalities

There are no clear-cut differences in modal chromosome number between the three main subgroups of lymphoma in the Working Formulation (low, intermediate or high grade tumours). However, when individual histologies are considered, there are differences in ploidy. Those tumours of the small cell type tend to be pseudodiploid or hyperdiploid, as do the undifferentiated and mixed-cell types, while those of the large cell type tend to be hyperdiploid or tetraploid.

Table 5.1 Chromosome abnormalities in non-Hodgkin's lymphomas

Dx: Total no. Patients	N	Ploidy				Chromosomal abnormalities						
		Hypo	Pseudo	Hyper	Tetra	N	1	2	3	4	5–9	≥10
Low grade												
A 29	1	3	14	11	0	1	14	3	3	2	5	1
B 36	0	3	14	18	1	0	1	7	5	2	17	4
C 14	3	1	3	6	1	3	1	1	0	2	3	4
Intermediate												
D 11	0	0	2	6	3	0	1	1	0	1	4	4
E 12	0	1	2	6	3	0	1	1	2	0	4	4
F 15	1	0	7	6	1	1	1	2	0	3	6	2
G 23	0	1	2	17	3	0	0	0	1	1	12	9
High grade												
H 11	0	1	2	6	2	0	2	0	0	1	5	3
I 9	1	1	5	2	0	1	2	2	2	1	1	0
J 7	0	0	6	1	0	0	0	3	3	0	1	0
167	6	11	57	79	14	6	23	20	16	13	58	31

Dx: Diagnosis according to the Working Formulation (see Table 5.2)

Table 5.2 Most frequent chromosomal abnormalities found in the non-Hodgkin's lymphomas

Low grade
A *Malignant lymphoma, small lymphocytic* (29 patients)
Numerical: +12 (7×), −9 (2×)
Structural:

14q32 (8×)	14q22 (2×)	11q (7×)	6q (5×)	12p13 (3×)
t(1;14)(p32;q32)	del(14)(q22)	dup(11)(q13;q25)	del(6)(q15) (2×)	t(12;?)(p13;?)
t(11;14)(p11;q32)	t(7;14)(p22;q22)	del(11q) (2×)	t(X;6)(q27;?)	t(12;13)(p13;q22)
t(11;14)(q22;q32)		del(11)(q21)	t(6;12)(q21;p13)	(see 6q)
t(11;14)(q13;q32)		inv ins(11)(q14.2q23)	t(6;?)(q27;?)	
t(14;?)(q32;?) (3×)		(see 14q)		
t(14;19)(q32;q13)				

B *Malignant lymphoma, follicular, predominantly small cleaved cell* (36 patients)
Numerical: +3 (4×), +2 (3×), +7 (2×), −8 (2×), −9 (3×), +12 (2×), +X (2×)
Structural:

18q (25×)	14q32 (32×)	6q (11×)	(i17q) (3×)
t(14;18)(q32;q21) (22×)	t(14;?)(q32;?) (3×)	del(6)(q)	
t(6;18)(q21;q23)	t(1;14)(q42;q32)	del(6)(q21) (3×)	
t(18;?)(q23;?)	t(11;14)(q23;q32)	del(6)(q22) (2×)	
t(4;18)(p15;q21)	t(7;14)(q34;q32)	del(6)(q23) (2×)	
	t(5;14)(q23;q32)	del(6)(q15)	
	t(6;14)(q21;q32)	t(6;17)(q15;p13)	
	t(8;14)(q22;q32)	i(6p)	
	t(3;14)(p21;q32)		
	(see 18q)		

C *Malignant lymphoma, follicular, mixed, small cleaved and large cell* (14 patients)
Numerical: +3 (4×), +7 (4×), +12 (3×), +X (3×), +2 (2×), +8 (3×), +16 (2×),
Structural:

14q32 (8×)	18q (6×)	13p13 (2×)
t(14;18)(q32;q21) (5×)	18q−	t(5;13)(q15;p13)
14q+	(see 14q32)	t(13;?)(p13;?)
t(1;14)(q42;q32)		
t(14;?)(q32;?)		

Table 5.2 continued

Intermediate
D   *Malignant lymphoma, follicular, predominantly large cell* (11 patients)
Numerical: +7 (3×), +10 (3×), +12 (3×), +21 (3×)
Structural:

14q32 (10×)	17q (4×)
t(14;18)(q32;q21) (6×)	t(1;17)(q25;q24)
t(2;14)(q23;q32)	dup 17(q22-24)
t(1;14)(q42;q32)	i(17q)
t(14;16)(q32;q21)	t(17;?)(q25;?)
t(14;17)(q32;q21)	

E   *Malignant lymphoma, diffuse cleaved cell* (12 patients)
Numerical: −9 (4×), +3 (4×), +4 (3×), +7 (3×), +10 (3×), +12 (3×), +14 (3×), +17 (3×), +20 (3×)
Structural:

14q32 (5×)	1q (5×)	6q (5×)	3q (3×)
t(14;18)(q32;q21)	del(1)(q23)(2×)	del(6)(q21)(2×)	t(3q9q)
t(14,?,14)(q32;?;q13)	inv ins(X;1)(p22;q31qter)	del(6)(q)(2×)	t(3q9p)
t(14;14)(q32;q24)	dup(1)(q21;q32)	i(6p)	del(3)(q21)
t(2;14)(q21;q24)	der(1)t(1;1)(pter->		
14q+,	q32::q21->qter)		

F   *Malignant lymphoma, diffuse mixed small and large cell* (15 patients)
Numerical: +12 (3×), +18 (3×), +1 (2×)
Structural:

14q + (8×)	1p (4×)	1q (3×)
t(8;14)(q24;q32)	t(1;2)(p11;q11)	del(1)(q32)(2×)
t(14;18)(q32;q21)(?)(2×)	t(1;6)(p22;q24)	t(1;18)(q25;q23)
t(11;14)(q23;q32)	t(1;?)(p36;?)(2×)	t(1;10)(q42;q22)
t(10;14)(q22;q32)		
t(14;19)(q32;q13)		
t(14;?)(q32;?)(2×)		

G   *Malignant lymphoma, diffuse large cell* (23 patients)
Numerical: +7 (8×), +12 (7×), +2 (5×), +3 (5×), +21 (5×), +10 (3×), +13 (3×), +19 (3×), +20 (3×)
Structural:

14q32 (15×)	6q (13×)	t(3;)(7×)	18q (8×)	1q (5×)
t(8;14)(q24;q32)(5×)	t(2;6)(q37;q21)	t(3;22)(q21;q11)(2×)	t(X;18)(p22;q12)	t(1;3)(q32;q27)
t(14;18)(q32;q21)(4×)	t(3;6)(q27;q21)	t(3;9)(p21;q34)	del(18)(q12)(3×)	dup(1)(q22-44)
t(11;14)	t(3;6)(p25;q21)	t(3;11)(p21;q23)	t(18;?)(q23;?)	dup(1)(q)
t(14;?)(q32;?)(3×)	del(6)(q21)(5×)	(see 1q)	t(2;18)(q14;q23)	t(1;3)(q23;p26)
t(1;14)(q23;q32)	del(6)(q15)(3×)		(see 14q32)	(see 14q)
t(3;14)(p21;q32)	t(5;6)(q15;q27)			

High grade
H   *Malignant lymphoma, large cell, immunoblastic* (11 patients)
Numerical: +12(3×), −6(2×), −21(2×), +11(2×)
Structural:

8q (3×)	6q21 (3× or 4×)
t(8;14)(2×)	del(6)(q21)(2× or 3×)
t(8;13)(q22;q32)	t(6;11)(q21;p14)

I   *Malignant lymphoma, lymphoblastic* (9 patients)
Structural:

14q (4×)	14q11 (3×)
t(8;14)(q11;q32)	del(14)(q11)
inv(14)(q11;q32)	t(9;14)(q34;q11)
t(14;15)(q;q)	t(11;14)(p11 or 13;q11)
14q+	

J   *Malignant lymphoma, small non-cleaved cell, Burkitt's and non-Burkitt's* (7 patients)
Structural:

t(8;14)(q24;q32)(7×)	dup(1q)(2×)

The number of patients with each abnormality is indicated in parentheses, e.g. +12 (7×) indicates seven patients with an additional chromosome 12.

Numerical and structural abnormalities

Low grade

MALIGNANT LYMPHOMA, SMALL LYMPHOCYTIC.
Eighty-six per cent of the 29 tumours examined were pseudodiploid or hyperdiploid and 21 per cent had more than five structural rearrangements.

The most frequent numerical abnormality was +12 (24 per cent of the patients), followed by loss of chromosome 9.

The most frequent structural abnormalities were translocations involving chromosome 14 with the breakpoint in the q32 region (28 per cent of the patients). Translocations with chromosome 11 were found in three cases, with chromosome 1 and with chromosome 19 in one case each, and with an unknown chromosome in three cases. In two instances a higher breakpoint on 14, at q22, was noted with t(7;14) occurring in one case and del(14)(q22) in the second. Abnormalities of 11q and 6q were the next most frequent structural abnormalities.

MALIGNANT LYMPHOMA, FOLLICULAR, PRE-DOMINANTLY SMALL CLEAVED CELL. Eighty-nine per cent of the 36 tumours were pseudo- or hyperdiploid, and 58 per cent had more than five chromosomal rearrangements.

Numerical abnormalities included +3(4×), +2(3×), −9(3×), +7(2×), −8(2×), +12(2×), and +X(2×).

Again, translocations involving chromosome 14 at band q32 were the most frequent structural abnormalities, occurring in 32 of 36 patients (89 per cent). Twenty-two of 36 patients (61 per cent) had t(14;18)(q32;q21) (Fig. 5.1), and the remainder had translocations with other chromosomes including 1, 3, 5, 6, 7, 8, 11, or, in three instances, with unidentified chromosomes. In addition to the 18q21 breakpoint associated with t(14;18), there was one patient with t(4;18) (p15;q21), and there were translocations involving 18q23 in two patients. One had a translocation with chromosome 6 and one with an unknown chromosome. Structural abnormalities of chromosome 6 were also frequent in this group (30 per cent). Many of these were deletions that

consisted of breaks at q15, q21, q23, and q33; in one instance there was absence of the entire long arm, i(6p). In one patient there was a translocation t(6;17)(q15;p13). (Fig. 5.1: NIH patient)

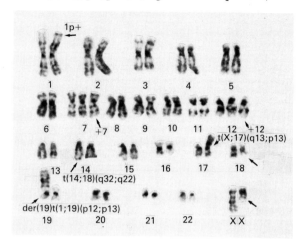

Fig. 5.1 A karyotype prepared from a one day culture of pleural fluid obtained from an NIH patient with malignant lymphoma, follicular, small cleaved cell type showing 48,X,+7,+12,1p+,t(X;17)(q13;p13), t(14;18)(q32;q22),der(19)t(1;19)(p12;p13).

MALIGNANT LYMPHOMA, FOLLICULAR, MIXED, SMALL CLEAVED AND LARGE CELL. Sixty-four per cent of these 14 tumours were either pseudo- or hyperdiploid, and 50 per cent had more than five structural abnormalities.

Numerical abnormalities included +3(4×), +7(4×), +8(3×), +12(3×), and +X(3×). Eight of the patients (57 per cent) had chromosomal rearrangements involving chromosome 14 at band q32; five had t(14;18)(q32;q21) and one each had 14q+, t(1;14)(q42;q32), or t(14;?)(q32;?). There were two cases with a rare change, involvement of 13p13.

Intermediate

MALIGNANT LYMPHOMA, FOLLICULAR, PREDOMINANTLY LARGE CELL. The majority of these 11 tumours (82 per cent) were hyperdiploid or near tetraploid and 73 per cent had five or more chromosomal abnormalities.

Numerical changes seen included +7(3×), +10(3×), +12(3×), and +21(3×).

Structural changes occurred mostly in the 14q32 region (91 per cent of the patients). Sixty per cent of these were t(14;18)(q32;q21) and the others involved translocations with chromosomes 1, 2, 16, and 17.

MALIGNANT LYMPHOMA, DIFFUSE CLEAVED CELL. Either hyperdiploidy or near tetraploidy was found in the majority of these 12 tumours (75 per cent) and 67 per cent of the patients had more than five structural abnormalities.

The most frequent changes in chromosome number were $-9(4\times)$, $+3(4\times)$, $+4(3\times)$, $+7(3\times)$, $+10(3\times)$, $+12(3\times)$, $+14(3\times)$, $+17(3\times)$, and $+20(3\times)$.

Chromosome 14 at band q32 was again the chromosome most frequently involved in structural abnormalities. There was one patient with t(14;18) (q32;q21), one with a translocation involving a second 14, one with a three-way translocation involving a second 14 and an unknown chromosome, one with a translocation involving chromosome 2 and one with a translocation involving an unknown chromosome. Abnormalities of the long arm of chromosome 1 either as a duplication or translocation and deletions of 6q also occurred frequently.

MALIGNANT LYMPHOMA, DIFFUSE MIXED SMALL AND LARGE CELL. Eighty-seven per cent of these 15 tumours were pseudo- or hyperdiploid and 53 per cent had more than five structural abnormalities.

The most frequent numerical abnormalities were $+12(3\times)$, $+18(3\times)$, and $+1(2\times)$.

Structural abnormalities of 14q32 were once again the most frequently found and occurred in 60 per cent of the patients. Two, or possibly three patients had t(14;18)(q32;q21), in two the identity of the second chromosome was not known, one had t(8;14)(q24;q32) and the remaining three had translocations with chromosome 10, 11, or 19. Involvement of 1p occurred in four tumours and of 1q in three tumours.

MALIGNANT LYMPHOMA DIFFUSE LARGE CELL. The majority of these 23 tumours were hyperdiploid (74 per cent) and 91 per cent had more than five structural abnormalities.

The most common numerical changes were associated with $+7(8\times)$, $+12(7\times)$, $+2(5\times)$, $+3(5\times)$, and $+21(5\times)$. Other changes included $+10(3\times)$, $+13(3\times)$, $+19(3\times)$, and $+20(3\times)$.

Sixty-five per cent of the patients had structural abnormalities of 14q32. In five instances, there was a translocation t(8;14)(q24;q32) and in four instances a translocation t(14;18)(q32;q21). The rest had translocations with chromosomes 1, 3, 11, or in three cases, with unidentified chromosomes. Abnormalities of 6q were also very frequently described in this group, occurring in 35 per cent of the patients. The most frequent finding was del(6)(q21) followed by deletions at q15. In 17 per cent of the cases there was a translocation involving chromosomes 2, 3, and 5. Deletion 18q12 was noted in three instances and a translocation with an unknown chromosome involving a breakpoint at 18q23 was also reported. Duplication, deletion or translocations of chromosome 1q involving bands q22, q23, q26, and q32 were found in four cases and a duplication was reported in a fifth case although the breakpoints were not identified.

High grade

MALIGNANT LYMPHOMA, LARGE CELL, IMMUNOBLASTIC. Fifty-five per cent of the 11 tumours had chromosome numbers in the hyperdiploid range and 73 per cent had more than five structural abnormalities.

Trisomy $12(3\times)$ was the most frequent numerical change; translocations involving chromosome 8q were the most frequent structural abnormality; two patients had t(8;14) and one had t(8;13)(q22;q32). Three, and possibly four, patients had abnormalities of 6q21; these occurred as deletions or translocations.

MALIGNANT LYMPHOMA, LYMPHOBLASTIC. Chromosome numbers in these tumours clustered in the pseudodiploid or hyperdiploid region (78 per cent) and most of the nine tumours had one to four structural abnormalities (78 per cent). The most frequent structural abnormalities again occurred on 14q (78 per cent) although not usually at band q32. In one case each there was t(8;14)(q11;q32) and t(14;15). there were four instances in which 14q11 was involved either as a deletion or as a translocation with chromosome 9 or 11, or was associated with inv(14)(q11;q32).

MALIGNANT LYMPHOMA, SMALL NON-CLEAVED CELL. Most of these patients have been reported as single cases; only seven are included here. Six patients were pseudodiploid and one was hyperdiploid. The majority had fewer than three structural abnormalities and only one case had five. All of these tumours had t(8;14)(q24;q32) and in two cases there was duplication of 1q.

The Burkitt's lymphomas and the non-Burkitt's lymphomas are included in this category. Many cytogenetic studies have been carried out on these patients and the findings may have important implications in the aetiology of all lymphomas.

Burkitt's lymphoma (BL), which is endemic in Africa and New Guinea, is closely associated with Epstein–Barr virus (EBV), approximately 95–98 per cent of these tumours containing the EBV genome; in contrast a much lower percentage of EBV positivity (15–20 per cent) is found in the sporadic or non-endemic tumours occurring in other areas.[34] Burkitt's lymphoma was the first neoplasm in which chromosomal aberrations were linked to a possible viral aetiology and it has been suggested that karyotypic evolution and the interaction of other risk factors, including impaired T-cell function, along with the EBV infection may be correlated with clinical and epidemiological patterns of BL.

In a review of 36 published reports of both endemic and sporadic cases, Berger and Bernheim[35] described cytogenetic findings in 121 BL patients and 65 cell lines. The most common specific translocation was t(8;14)(q24;q32) found in almost 80 per cent of the tumours. Variants included t(8;22)(q24;q11) found in about 15 per cent of the patients and t(2;8)(p12;q24) in approximately 5 per cent of the patients. In other cases there was a 14q+ or 8q−, although the presence of t(8;14) could not be determined. These abnormalities are similar to those described in B-cell acute lymphoblastic leukaemia (ALL) of the FAB L3 type (French–

American–British classification). Sporadic tumours usually have other chromosomal abnormalities such as duplication of 1q and deletion of 6q as well as abnormalities involving chromosomes 13, 3, 4, 9, X, and Y (Fig. 5.2: NIH patient).

Ziegler *et al.*[36] during an investigation of Kaposi's sarcoma in the homosexual population of the San Francisco Bay area found four cases of Burkitt-like lymphoma and suggested an outbreak of BL in this population. Several cytogenetic studies have been reported in patients with acquired immunodeficiency syndrome (AIDS)[37–39]. Of the two patients reported by Chaganti *et al.*[37] one had t(8;14)(q23;q32) and the other had t(8;22); neither had additional abnormalities. Whang-Peng *et al.*[38] also reported two patients with AIDS; one had t(8;14)(q24;q32) and the other t(8;22) (Fig. 5.3: NIH patient). Both of these had duplication of 1q with the duplicated segment either remaining on chromosome 1 (in both) or being translocated, in some cells, to chromosome 4 or 19. Cytogenetic findings in a young Haitian immigrant with AIDS and concomitant Burkitt-like lymphoma also showed t(8;14)(q24;q32) but no other abnormalities.[39]

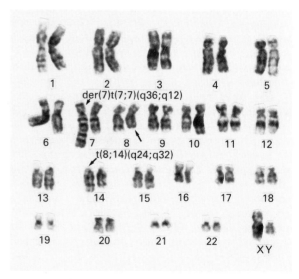

Fig. 5.2 A karyotype from a one day culture of peripheral blood of an NIH Burkitt's lymphoma patient showing
46,XY,der(7)t(7;7)(q36;q12),t(8;14)(q24;q32).

In most AIDS patients, the tumour cells have B-cell markers but a few cases with T-cell markers have been described. Berman *et al.*[40] reported partial expression of T-cell markers in a 45-year-old male who also had a 2-year history of AIDS. The karyotypes of the tumour cells were 47, XY, +12, t(8;14)(q24;q32) (70 per cent) and the same karyotype with dup 1(q22–31) (30 per cent).

Other chromosomal abnormalities have also been reported. Cytogenetic studies in a 44-year-old White male with Burkitt's lymphoma/leukaemia revealed a variant translocation t(8;22)(q24;q11), t(3;17)(q27;q12–21) and del(15)(q22).[41] The breakpoints of chromosomes 17 and 15 are similar to those found in acute promyeloctyic leukaemia (APL).

Miscellaneous lymphomas

Cutaneous T-cell lymphoma (CTCL)

The criteria for diagnosis of CTCL were established by the National CTCL workshop[42] and four clinical stages were established: IA, limited plaques; IB, generalized plaques; IIA, generalized plaques with adenopathy; IIB, cutaneous tumours with or without adenopathy; III, erythroderma; IVA, any skin involvement with histologically positive nodes; and IVB, any skin stage with visceral involvement.

In our study of 41 CTCL patients,[43] there were four patients with limited plaques, 13 with generalized plaques, eight with cutaneous tumours and 16 with generalized erythroderma. Cytogenetic abnormalities were found in many of these patients in specimens of peripheral blood and lymph nodes, although these tissues were histologically negative: 62 per cent of the peripheral blood samples were cytogenetically positive versus 49 per cent morphologically positive; 80 per cent of the lymph nodes were cytogenetically positive versus 45 per cent morphologically positive; 6 per cent of the bone marrow samples were cytogenetically positive versus 3 per cent morphologically positive. No specific chromosomal abnormalities were found in CTCL. Structural abnormalities of chromosome 1 and numerical abnormalities of

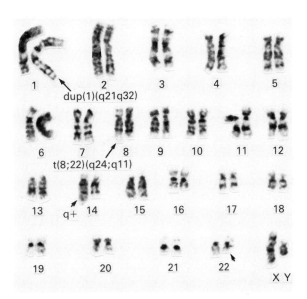

Fig. 5.3 A karyotype from an NIH patient with AIDS and Burkitt's lymphoma obtained from a one day culture of ascites fluid; it shows 46,XY,dup(1)(q21;q32), t(8;22)(9q24;q11),14q+.

chromosomes 11, 21, and 22 were the most frequent. Extensive cytogenetic abnormalities and lack of clone formation are two characteristics seen in early stages. Clone formation is seen only in advanced disease (eight patients) along with hyperdiploidy and near tetraploidy, and is associated with poor prognosis and short survival. Other investigators have confirmed that cytogenetic abnormalities parallel clinical symptoms and that there are fewer changes in the early stages. In a study of 124 patients with CTCL, Vonderheid *et al.*[44] found that a total cerebriform count above 15 per cent on a blood smear obtained at the time of cytogenetic study strongly correlated with the presence of chromosomally abnormal malignant clones, and that the appearance of polyploid cells reflected poor survival. Other reports of cytogenetic studies include a study by Gamperl[45] of a 66-year-old male in the tumour phase of mycosis fungoides who had a clone with a karyotype of 49,XY,+8,11p-,+17,int del(14)(q22q24) in PHA-stimulated peripheral blood cells, and a study by Barbieri *et al.*[46] of a 62-year-old female with mycosis fungoides (stage IIB) who had cytogenetic abnormalities including 45-46,X,-X,t(4;16)(q34;q21),inv(12)(q15;q24),+12,-18,del(21)(q11q21),±21.

Adult T-cell lymphoma/leukaemia (ATLL)

Human T-cell lymphotrophic virus (HTLV-I) was the first exogenous retrovirus to be demonstrated in a human cancer: adult T-cell lymphoma/leukaemia (ATLL).[47] Affected patients are geographically clustered in southwestern Japan, the Caribbean basin and southeastern USA. The virus is endemic in these areas, although only a small portion of those with antibodies to the virus will develop leukaemia. The clinical course includes acute onset, rapidly developing skin lesions, wide spread infiltration of lymph node and other organs, development of opportunistic infections and a syndrome of increased bone turnover that leads to bone lesions and hypercalcaemia.[48]

Cytogenetic findings in patients with ATLL suggest that more complex numerical and structural abnormalities are found in those patients with a more aggressive clinical course. Cytogenetic studies of five healthy adults who were seropositive showed that three had clonal abnormalities.[49] One had rearrangements of chromosomes 7 and 14, one had a minute chromosome of unknown origin and one had a few cells with clonal abnormalities. The determination of the significance of these findings will require careful follow-up. Cytogenetic studies may provide a means of monitoring seropositive individuals who appear to be healthy. In a review of 85 ATLL patients, Pandolfi[50] related relevant genes or oncogenes to structural rearrangements of regions of eight chromosomes. In descending order of frequency of occurrence these are: 14q11–12,q32(T-receptor α chain, c-*fos*, the putative proto oncogene *tcl*-1, IgH chain); 6q15-q21 (c-*myb*, c-*yes*-2); 2q11–24, 13q21, 1p (B-*lym*-1), 3q; 7q32 or 35 (T receptor β chain); and 10p14-15 (IL-2 receptor) (Fig. 5.4). Both HTLV-I-positive and -negative patients tend to have chromosomal breakpoints at the same band locations. Adult T-cell lymphoma/leukaemia was categorized into three clinical stages by Samada *et al.*,[51] acute, chronic, and smouldering ATLL. Eight of the nine patients with acute ATLL had trisomy 3 and/or 7, but none of these abnormalities was found in patients with chronic ATLL. Patients with smouldering ATLL were normal cytogenetically. We studied 11 patients with HTLV-I-positive ATLL, 10 of whom had numerous and complex changes involving every chromosome pair[48] (Figs. 5.5 and 5.6: NIH patients). The most common structural abnormalities were of the long arm of chromosome 6 found in six patients, and involved breakpoints at q11, q13, q16;q23, q21;q23, q22;q24, and q23;q24. Typically these patients had a characteristic clinical course with aggressive disease, high white blood cell count (WBC), hypercalcaemia with bony lesions as well as poor response to chemotherapy and short survival, while those patients without abnormalities of 6q tended to have a more indolent course.

Lymphoepithelioid cell lymphoma (Lennert's lymphoma)

In the late 1960s, a special variant of Hodgkin's disease that was characterized by clusters of epithelioid cells and only sporadic Sternberg-Reed cells was described.[52] Later it was determined that this disease was not a variant of Hodgkin's disease and it was designated lymphoepithelioid cell lymphoma (LEL) or Lennert's lymphoma. It was also determined, by immunohistochemical means, that the proliferating cells were of T-cell origin. Cytogenetic studies have been reported in a total of eight patients. Seven of these had numerical or structural abnormalities of chromosome 3; three had +3 as the sole abnormality, two had multiple abnormalities in addition to +3, and two had structural abnormalities (one had der(3)t(3;9)(q22;p13) and the other had der(3)(pter→q24::q22→pter). The remaining patient had a normal karyotype. Other structural abnormalities involved chromosomes 1, 7, 18, and 19. The structural abnormalities of chromosome 1 appeared to be random with the exception of one patient with duplication of 1q at q32 and two other patients who had breakpoints at 1q13.2 (abnormalities that occur in other lymphomas).

Angioimmunoblastic lymphadenopathy (AILD)

Angioimmunoblastic lymphadenopathy has been considered by some to be a benign proliferative process. The architecture of the lymph nodes shows loss of germinal centres as a result of infiltration by a wide spectrum of polymorphic cells, lymphocytes, immunoblasts, histiocytes, plasma cells and eosinophils.

Cytogenetic findings have been reported in 13 patients. Kaneko *et al.*[54] studied six patients and reviewed seven published cases. Although the karyotypes of the bone marrow were normal, there were chromosomal abnormalities, both numerical and structural, in the lymph nodes. Non-random abnormalities included +3 (six patients), +5 (five patients), and 14q+ (four

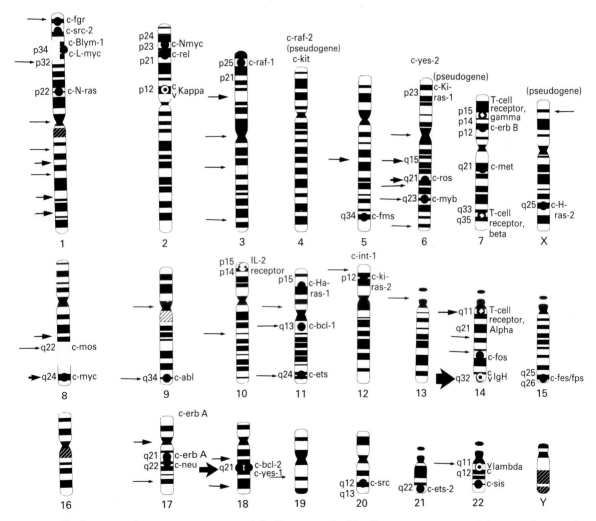

Fig. 5.4 The location of oncogenes, immunoglobulin genes, the T-cell receptor genes, and the most frequently occurring chromosomal breakpoint in patients with non-Hodgkin's lymphoma are shown. ●: Oncogenes (for those oncogenes placed on top of the chromosomes, the precise location on the chromosome has not been determined); ◉: immunoglobulin genes; ◗: T-cell receptor genes; ◓: IL-2 receptor; ▸: most frequently occurring breakpoints; ➤ ➤ ➢ : size of arrow indicates frequency of breakpoints with the largest indicating the most frequent.

patients). These findings led the authors to suggest that although this disease is not necessarily monoclonal in the early stages, one clone may become dominant in later stages.

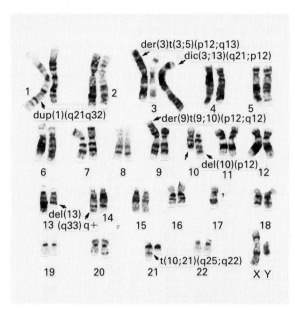

Fig. 5.5 Karyotype from NIH patient obtained from a one day culture of peripheral blood showing 46,XY,− 17,dup(1)(q21;q32),der(3)t(3;5)(p12;q13), dic(3;13)(q21;p12),der(9)t(9;10)(p12;q12),del(10) (p12),del(13)(q33),14q+,t(10;21)(q25;q22).

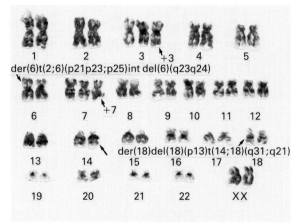

Fig. 5.6 Karyotype from a one day peripheral blood culture of a patient with ATLL showing 48,XX,+3,+7,der(6)t(2;6)(p21p23;p25),int del(6) (q23;q24),der(18)(del)(18)(p13)t(14;18)(q31;q21).

They also felt that AILD should be considered a malignant disease that requires aggressive chemotherapy.

Richter's syndrome

Richter's syndrome is a term which has been applied to a small group of patients with chronic lymphocytic leukaemia (CLL) who develop diffuse histiocytic lymphoma (DHL). Nowell *et al.*[55] performed sequential chromosome studies in a patient with untreated T-cell CLL who later developed subcutaneous and abdominal diffuse histiocytic lymphoma. In the early, indolent phase, the karyotype of the lymphocytes was pseudodiploid with 3q+ and 14q+ chromosome markers. After development of DHL, the lymphocytes became hypertriploid (70–74 chromosomes) and had the same 3q+ and 14q+ markers. This study indicates that in this patient the DHL evolved from the leukaemic T-cells.

Discussion

Although the aetiology of lymphoma is unknown, there are individuals with inherited immunological deficiencies, chromosomal instability syndromes or certain constitutional chromosomal abnormalities who have a predisposition to lymphoma. These patients have diseases such as Chediak–Higashi syndrome, ataxia telangiectasia (A-T), Wiscott–Aldrich syndrome, Swiss-type aggammaglobulinaemia, common variable immunodeficiency disease, acquired hypogammaglobulinaemia, renal transplant recipients, Sjögren's syndrome, rheumatoid arthritis, sytemic lupus erythematosus and Klinefelter's syndrome.[2,56] Patients with a newly described autosomal recessive disorder characterized by microcephaly with normal intelligence, a 'bird'-like facial appearance, cellular and humoral defects also have an increased risk for development of lymphoreticular malignancies.[57] There is also a report of a 17-year-old boy with Down's syndrome who had a poorly differentiated lymphoma in which the tumour had a karyotype of 47,XY,+21,14q+.[32] The chromosomal abnormalities associated with the lymphomas arising in these types of patients are the same as those described for all lymphomas and include rearrangements at 14q32 (t(8;14)(q24;q32), and t(14;18)(q32;q21) as well as those described in Table 5.2.

Abnormalities of 14q

Structural rearrangements of chromosome 14 at bands q11–13, q22;q24, and q32 are the most common structural abnormalities found in the lymphomas.[58–61] The breakpoint at 14q32 occurs in more than 60 per cent of all lymphomas and is found predominantly in the follicular small cleaved cell type (as t(14;18)(q32;q21) and in Burkitt's lymphoma (as t(8;14)(q24;q32) (Table 5.2). In all of the patients with the various forms of follicular lymphoma, t(14;18)(q32;q21) was found in 23 of 36 patients with the small cleaved cell type, five of 14 patients with mixed cell type and six of 11 patients with large cell type. In contrast, only five of the 97 patients with other lymphomas had t(14;18). These findings suggest that t(14;18)(q32;q21) is a specific chromosomal marker for the follicular lymphomas, particularly the small cleaved cell subtype. In a study of 71 patients with follicular lymphoma, Yunis *et al.*[62] found 85 per cent to have t(14;18) and this translocation appeared to be specific for follicular lymphoma. They noted that those patients with a single chromosome defect t(14;18) had the histological feature of the small cleaved cell type and did not usually require treatment for one to four years after diagnosis. In contrast, patients with t(14;18) and del(13)(q32) developed haematological features of leukaemia and an accelerated phase of the disease. Kaneko *et al.*[63] also reported t(14;18) in follicular small cleaved cell lymphoma while large non-cleaved cells have different abnormalities with modal chromosome numbers in the near tetraploid or tetraploid range. Those patients who were near tetraploid had the longest median survival (69 months) and those with t(14;18) as the sole abnormality had the next longest survival (48 months).

In view of the high frequency of involvement of 14q32, it has been suggested[61] that rearrangements in this region may play a role in the genesis of lymphoid malignancies and that other regions of chromosome 14 especially 14q11-13 and 14q24 may contain genes responsible for promotion of the malignant processes. Genes for the T-cell receptor chain α (TCR Cα) and the immunoglobulin heavy chain reside on 14q11 and 14q32 respectively (Fig. 5.4). Baer *et al.*,[64] in an investigation of α chain genes in a T-cell line with inv(14)(q11;q32), found a rearrangement in which the immunoglobulin heavy chain variable gene (V_H) has joined with a Jα segment, forming V_H-JαCα. This rearrangement is productive at the genomic level, and may encode for a hybrid immunoglobulin/T-cell receptor polypeptide that is important in T-cell oncogenesis. Using chromosomal *in situ* hybridization, Kennaugh *et al.*[59] showed that the 14q32 breakpoint in an ataxia telangiectasia (A–T) cell clone with t(14;14)(q11;q32) was outside the IgH locus and proximal to it with respect to the centromere. In addition, the chromosome bands 14q11→14qter containing the constant region of the TCR Cα were translocated to the q32 region of the homologous 14. The translocated TCR Cα gene may confer a growth advantage for this clone of cells, although other chromosomal changes may be required for development of a malignancy. McCaw *et al.*[60] also provide evidence that structural rearrangements of 14q especially 14q32 in A-T may be one cytogenetic step in the process leading to lymphoma. Other investigators[65,66] have determined that breakpoints of chromosome 14 are focused at the 5′ end of the joining regions of the immunoglobulin gene, and believe that this indicates that chromosomal translocation occurs at a pre-B-cell stage during attempted heavy chain joining. Ohyashiki *et al.*[31] have suggested two categories of chromosomal changes of 14q; translocations involving 14q32 that may be the primary change for development of lymphoid malignancy and rearrangement involving bands other than 14q32 in 14q+ that may constitute a secondary process in lymphoma.

Studies by Tsujimoto *et al.*[67] of the breakpoint region of chromosome 18 in patients with t(14;18), showed that rearrangements occurred in approximately 60 per cent of the cases. The breakpoint involved a small (2.1 kilobase) region localized to segment 18q21, and the gene coding for RNA transcripts (the *bcl*-2 gene) is apparently interrupted. They further found that *bcl*-2 from 18q21 is inserted into the heavy chain locus creating a unique J_H;18q21 rearrangement that most likely represents a transformation event. Lipford *et al.*[68] as well as other investigators (*see* Chapter 6) have generated DNA probes that permit the 14;18 junction on the der(14) or der(18) to be identified; these provide a molecular approach to identifying t(14;18) when an obvious reciprocal partner is lacking. They found that approximately 60 per cent of the patients with unselected follicular lymphomas, 20 per cent of those with diffuse large cell lymphoma and 50 per cent of those with adult undifferentiated non-Burkitt lymphomas had the 14;18 rearrangement within the major breakpoint region. Studies using these DNA probes on restriction fragments can thus complement routine cytogenetic studies in these patients.

Deletion 6q

Deletion of 6q is another common chromosome abnormality found in the non-Hodgkin's lymphomas. These deletions are found in a significant portion of patients with large cell lymphomas of both the diffuse (52 per cent) and the immunoblastic varieties (27 per cent), and also frequently in the small lymphocytic or small cleaved cell varieties and HTLV-I-positive ATLL patients. The most frequent breakpoints are located at q15, q21, and q27. Those ATLL patients with deletion of 6q had a clinical picture characterized by presence of a high white count, hypercalcaemia and bony lesions, poor response to chemotherapy, an aggressive course and short survival. Bloomfield *et al.*[20] found that 82 per cent of the patients with del(6)(q21) had large cell lymphoma. Yunis *et al.*[5] also found deletion 6q in five of seven patients with diffuse large cell lymphoma and in two cases of follicular mixed small and large cell lymphoma. All of these studies indicate that deletion 6q may be as specific for lymphomas that have a large cell component as the t(14;18) is for follicular lymphomas. Deletion of 6q along with either complete or partial trisomy of 7 and/or 12 is associated with the more aggressive mixed or large cell types of lymphoma.[62]

Abnormalities of chromosome 11

Abnormalities of this chromosome are very often associated with low grade, small lymphocytic lymphoma as t(11;14), but they have also been found in patients with poorly differentiated diffuse lymphocytic lymphoma.[5] Abnormalities generally affect the long arm but have also occasionally been reported for the short arm. These include deletion, inversions and insertions. Yunis *et al.*[5] have presented evidence that del(11)(q13.5) is a common abnormality in the non-Hodgkin's lymphoma of the small lymphocytic type.

It has been reported[28] that the oncogene Hu-*ets*-1 located on 11q23 was rearranged and amplified approximately 10-fold in a case of small lymphocytic cell lymphoma with inverted insertion that involved 11q23. It is suggested that Hu-*ets*-1 may be unusual in that, depending on which other chromosome locations are involved in abnormalities, different phenotypes may be expressed or Hu-*ets*-1 may be altered according to differentiation-specific pathways.

In addition, Rudd and Teshima[69] reported a constitutional deletion, 11(q14;q21), resulting from a paternal balanced deletion/insertion of chromosome 11 in a child who developed a malignant lymphoma of the thymus and suggested non-random involvement of this region, 11q13 or 14, in the occurrence or progression of certain lymphomas.

Trisomy 12

Trisomy 12 is the most commonly reported acquired numerical abnormality and occurs very frequently in B-cell CLL although it can also be found in a subtype of small cell lymphocytic lymphoma.[70] In the current review, trisomy 12 occurs in all the categories of malignant lymphoma although most frequently in the small lymphocytic type.

Abnormalities of chromosome 2, 3, 18 or 21

Trisomy of 3, 18 or 21 was found almost exclusively in the large cell lymphomas and trisomy 2 or duplication of 2p was often associated with a poor response to treatment.[62]

The presence of an extra chromosome 3 along with other chromosomal abnormalities was found most usually in the diffuse cleaved cell or the diffuse large cell lymphomas. In addition, structural changes including translocations and deletions (of both the long and short arms) was occasionally seen. Slavutsky et al.[71] reported one case of follicular small cleaved cell lymphoma, one case of immunoblastic lymphoma, and one case of secondary acute non-lymphocytic leukaemia (ANLL) (M4) all of whom had a t(2;3). They reviewed 19 published cases of t(2;3) (eight cases of non-Hodgkin's lymphoma) and suggested that chromosomal breaks between 3q26 and q29 and between 2p11 and p21 (usually at 2p21 and q11–31) may result in activation of genes related to these neoplasms.

Trisomy 7

Trisomy 7, in addition to other chromosomal abnormalities, has been reported in about 30 per cent of the intermediate grade lymphomas. Trisomy 7 has also been reported in four of 10 previously published patients with γ heavy chain disease, a rare B-cell lymphoproliferative disorder characterized by the production of a monoclonal IgG heavy chain fragment in the absence of light chain.[23] In somatic cell hybrids between murine and SV40 transformed human cells, where human chromosome 7 was known to be carrying the SV40 genome, it was responsible for the expression of malignancy.[72] The occurrence of i(7q) seems to be specific for acute lymphoblastic leukaemia and lymphoma.[32]

Abnormalities of chromosome 1

Structural abnormalities of chromosome 1, especially duplication of part or all of 1q, are found in many different malignancies and are also frequently found in the intermediate grades of non-Hodgkin's lymphoma. Fukuhara et al.[30] described duplication of 1q in a case of histiocytic lymphoma. This abnormality, dup(1)(q12q;31q), in addition to dup(1)(q21;q31), is also seen in Burkitt's lymphoma (both endemic and non-endemic types and in some patients with AIDS

in addition to BL) as a non-random marker and indicates a poor prognosis.[38,73]

Immunological markers

In 1986, Levine et al.[74] correlated immunological phenotype with karyotype in 118 patients with malignant lymphoma. Those patients with T-cell lymphomas have more normal metaphases and more frequent abnormalities such as trisomy 19 and translocations or deletions involving breakpoints at 1q21, 2q21, 3q27, 4q21, and 17q21. In patients with B-cell lymphomas certain chromosome abnormalities were associated with the expression of specific immunoglobulin heavy chains. Breakpoints at 14q22 or q24 were associated with surface δμ immunoglobulin ($P = 0.02$), trisomy 22 or breaks at 22q12 and a break at 2q32 were associated with surface γ-immunoglobulins ($P \leq 0.01$), and trisomy 12 and breaks at 2p13 with cytoplasmic γ-immunoglobulins ($P \leq 0.01$). Among B lymphomas, lack of CD24 surface antigen was associated with breaks in 2p25, 5q15-34, 6q21 while lack of CD9 occurred in those patients with del(6)(q15).

Breaks are common at 14q32, the genomic site of the immunoglobulin heavy chain, in B, non-B non-T and T lymphomas. There is no definite association between immunological phenotype and cytogenetic abnormalities involving this band in T-cell lymphomas and recurring breakpoints associated with these lymphomas are generally found at the chromosomal locations of genes coding for the various T-cell antigens.

In a study of immunological markers found in Burkitt's lymphoma, Preudhomme et al.[76] demonstrated a correlation between variant chromosomal translocations and expression of light chain immunoglobulins. In normal cells the gene for the light chain κ is located on 2p12 and λ is located on 22q11. In the variant translocations, these genes are split with the sequences encoding for the variable ($V_κ$ or $V_λ$) portion of the immunoglobulin molecule remaining on chromosome 2 and 22 respectively. However, the constant regions either Cκ (from 2) or Cλ (from 22) are translocated to 8q. In general, tumours with t(2;8) express κ, and those with t(8;22) express λ chains. If the tumour has t(8;14) the cells may express either κ or λ chains. However, Magrath *et al.*[76] and Denny *et al.*[77] have reported cases with t(8;22) in which synthesis of the κ chain was seen.

There is evidence that expression of the immunoglobulin heavy chain genes is associated with t(8;14). In hybrids derived from the fusion of two Burkitt's lymphoma cell lines, Daudi and P3HR-1, the normal chromosome 14 carries the transcribed IgH gene.[78] In contrast, in ROS-1, the 14q+ chromosome is carrying the expressed gene coding for the μIg heavy chain.[79]

Oncogene expression

In a very thorough review of the possible role of oncogenes in the aetiology of the non-Hodgkin's lymphomas, Chenevix–Trench[80] lists those oncogenes that are found at frequently occurring chromosomal breakpoints in non-Hodgkin's lymphomas; these are c-*myc*, c-*bcl*-1, c-*bcl*-2, c-*yes*-1, c-*ets*-1, and c-*abl* (Fig. 5.4). The oncogenes found by transfection assays to be activated include c-*abl*, c-N-*ras*, c-B*lym*-1, and c-T*lym*-1, while those that are expressed include c-*abl*, c-*erb* B, c-*ets*-1, c-*fos*, c-Ha-*ras*, c-Ki-*ras*, c-*myb*, and c-*myc*. At the present time the pattern of oncogene activation that has been observed is heterogeneous. Although c-*myc* rearrangement has been reported in diffuse large cell lymphomas[18] and in B and T lymphoid tumours,[81] there is no consistent relationship between specific oncogenes and specific subtypes of non-Hodgkin's lymphoma. It is likely that, with more than 30 known oncogenes, interactions between them may play a role in malignant transformation (*see* Fig. 5.4).

Chromosomal breakpoints

There is preferential involvement of some of the breakpoints associated with translocations in the aneuploid cells of the 167 lymphoma patients described here. The most frequently occurring breakpoint was at 14q32, found in 60 per cent of the patients. Breakpoints at 18q21 occurred in 28 per cent of the patients, and 6q21 and 8q24 in about 10 per cent of the patients. Breakpoints occurring four to five times are at 1q32, 5q15,

8q21, 18q23, 14q11, 1q23, 3p21, at the centromere of 17 and 8q12. The remainder of the translocation breakpoints were present in only two or three patients, these are shown in Fig. 5.4 (breakpoints occurring in only one patient are not shown). Chromosomal breakage may be the initial step for chromosomal translocation, deletion, or inversion. Many of these breakpoints are either located close to or in important constitutional genes or oncogenes (*see* Fig. 5.4). It is highly probable that the consequences of chromosomal rearrangement provide essential steps in the development of malignant transformation. More careful examination, using DNA probes, etc., of the breakpoints involved in chromosomal rearrangements in these tumours may help to identify those genes, either singly or in combination, most likely to be involved in oncogenesis.

In Burkitt's lymphoma, Berger and Bernhein[35] stated that translocation and rearrangement of the c-*myc* oncogene into the immunoglobulin region occur with breaks at different points in the nucleotide sequence of the gene, although the rearrangement of c-*myc* did not occur in all BL (it was found in eight out of 12 cases including one with t(2;8), and in five out of 15 B-cell lymphomas with t(8;14)). They also observed that there was transcriptional activation of the translocated c-*myc* even if no rearrangement had occurred; this suggested that translocation alone was sufficient for transcriptional activation. Those BL lines with a rearranged c-*myc* gene expressed c-*myc* transcripts lacking normal untranslated leader while those with a non-rearranged c-*myc* gene expressed normal c-*myc* transcripts.

Prognostic implications

There are several parameters of cytogenetic studies that have prognostic value in the non-Hodgkin's lymphomas.

Ploidy and proliferative activity

Bauer *et al.*[82] in a study of 50 patients with diffuse large cell lymphoma, noted that the single most important pretreatment adverse prognostic factor was high proliferative activity which they defined to be less than 80 per cent of the cells in G_0 or G_1 as measured by flow cytometry. However, they felt that DNA aneuploidy, detected in 62 per cent of the patients, was not of prognostic significance.

Cytogenetic findings

One hundred and six patients with non-Hodgkin's lymphoma were classified by Kristoffersson *et al.*[3] according to cytogenetic findings, comparing them in different ways to determine the prognostic significance of chromosome analysis. The authors came to the following conclusions. There was a significant difference in survival between those with abnormal metaphases (AA) or with all normal (NN) metaphases irrespective of whether the sample was taken at diagnosis or during relapse. Survival was significantly shorter for patients with 10 or more clonal aberrations than for those with no or only one to four aberrations. Further, there was no significant difference between patients with high grade lymphomas and those with low grade lymphomas. There were no differences in survival between those patients with reciprocal translocations and those with other abnormalities, but both groups had a significantly shorter survival than those who were NN. The survival was significantly shorter in patients with either completely or partially unidentified marker chromosomes. Survival was significantly shorter in patients who were hypodiploid than in those with NN karyotypes. When patients were categorized according to the chromosome involved in numerical or structural abnormalities, those with 1p+ had a significantly shorter survival. In those who had an additional chromosome 7, there was a borderline significantly decreased survival.

In a report by Bloomfield *et al.*[20] of 73 patients who were examined cytogenetically at the time of diagnosis (prior to treatment), 65 per cent of the patients achieved a complete remission, but there was no significant correlation between achieving a remission and cytogenetic findings. Survival in these patients varied according to the percentage of normal karyotypes as well as with the nodal chromosome number. Patients who had more than 20 per cent normal metaphases had a significantly longer survival and patients who had a modal number of 46 survived longer than those who were either hypo- or hyperdiploid.

In summary, clonal chromosomal abnormalities have been reported in 95–100 per cent of the patients with non-Hodgkin's lymphoma; most had multiple chromosomal abnormalities. When cytogenetic findings are related to the types of lymphoma classified according to the Working Formulation most of the structural abnormalities appear to be evenly distributed among the types. However, t(14;18)(q32;q21) is frequently found in various types of follicular lymphoma, particularly the small cleaved cell type, while deletions of 6q were frequently found in lymphomas with a large cell component. Trisomy of 3, 18, or 21 was found almost exclusively in the large cell type and trisomy 2 or duplication of 2p was often associated with a poor response to treatment.

Translocations found frequently in Burkitt's lymphoma include t(8;14), t(2;8), and t(8;22); all are associated with a breakpoint at 8q24. In all types of lymphoma, the single most commonly occurring abnormality is of 14q32; this is followed by deletion of 6q, trisomy 12, loss of 7 and structural abnormalities of chromosomes 11, 3 and 1. Patients with T-cell lymphomas have more normal metaphases, trisomy 19 and breaks at 1q21, 2q21, 3q27, 4q21, and 17q21 than other lymphomas. B-cell lymphomas with structural abnormalities at breakpoints 14q22q24, 2q32, 2p13 or + 12 were associated with the expression of specific heavy chains..

The cytogenetic findings in patients with non-Hodgkin's lymphomas appear to have prognostic implications, based on reports that survival is significantly longer in patients with more than 20 per cent normal cells, while the prognosis was poor and survival short in patients who had unidentified marker chromosomes, who were hypo- or hyperdiploid, who had 1p+ or who had multiple chromosomal markers. In addition, those patients with follicular lymphomas who have only t(14;18) usually have a more indolent course and may not require treatment for several years.

References

1. Jones SE, Butler JJ, Byrne GE Jr., *et al. Cancer.* 1977; **39**, 1071.
2. Devita VT, Hellmann S. In: DeVita VT, Hellman S, Rosenberg SA eds. *Cancer. Principles and Practice of Oncology,* Philadelphia: JB Lippincott Company, 1985; 1623.
3. Kristoffersson U, Heim S, Mandahl N, *et al. Cancer Genetics and Cytogenetics.* 1987; **25**, 55.
4. Rowley JD, Fukuhara S. *Seminars in Oncology.* 1980; **7**, 255.
5. Yunis JJ, Oken MM, Theologides A, *et al. Cancer Genetics and Cytogenetics.* 1984; **13**, 27.
6. Levine EG, Arthur DC, Frizzera G, *et al. Blood.* 1985; **66**, 1414.
7. Koduru PRK, Filippa DA, Richardson MW. *Blood.* 1987; **69**, 97.
8. Nowell P, Finan J. (Personal communication).
9. Gahrton G, Robert KH, Friberg K, *et al. Blood.* **56**, 640.
10. Caspersson T, Farber S, Foley GE, *et al. Experimental Cell Research.* 1968; **49**, 219.
11. Dutrillaux B, deGrouchy J, Finaz C, *et al. Comptes Rendues, Académie des Sciences, Paris.* 1971; **273**, 587.
12. Seabright MA. *Lancet.* 1971; **ii**, 72.
13. Dutrillaux B, Lejeune J. *Comptes Rendues, Académie des Sciences, Paris.* 1971; **272**, 2638.
14. Arighi FW, Hsu T. *Cytogenetics.* 1971; **2**, 81.
15. Paris Conference (1971). In: *Standardization in Human Cytogenetics. Birth Defects*: Original Article Series VIII. New York: The National Foundation, 1972.
16. ISCN. Harnden DG, Klinger HP eds. *An International System for Human Cytogenetic Nomenclature.* New York: March of Dimes Birth Defects Foundation, 1985.
17. The non-Hodgkin's lymphoma pathologic classification project. *Cancer.* 1982; **49**, 2112.
18. Gaunt KL, Callaghan J, Roberts DF. *Annals of Genetics.* 1986; **29**, 82.
19. Yunis JJ, Oken MM, Kaplan ME, *et al. The New England Journal of Medicine.* 1982; **307**, 1231.
20. Bloomfield CD, Arthur DC, Frizzera G, *et al. Cancer Research.* 1983; **43**, 2975.
21. Mark J, Dahlenfors R, Ekedahl C. *Cancer Genetics and Cytogenetics.* 1979; **1**, 39.
22. Takeuchi J, Ochi H, Minowada J, *et al. Cancer Genetics and Cytogenetics.* 1985; **14**, 257.
23. O'Conor GT, Wyandt HE, Innes DJ *et al. Cancer Genetics and Cytogenetics.* 1985; **15**, 1.
24. Brusamolino E, Bernasconni P, Pasquali F, *et al. Cancer Genetics and Cytogenetics.* 1984; **13**, 279.
25. Slavutsky I, de Vinuesa ML, Dupont J, *et al. Cancer Genetics and Cytogenetics.* 1981; **3**, 341.
26. Panani A, Ferti-Passantonopoulou A, Dervenoulas J. *Cancer Genetics and Cytogenetics.* 1984; **11**, 87.
27. Clare N, Boldt D, Messerschmidt G, *et al. Blood.* 1986; **67**, 704.
28. Rovigatti U, Watson DK, Yunis JJ. *Science.* 1986; **232**, 398.
29. Kaneko Y, Abe R, Sampi K, *et al. Cancer Genetics and Cytogenetics.* 1982; **5**, 120.
30. Fukuhara S, Rowley JD, Variakojis D, *et al. Blood.* 1978; **52**, 989.
31. Ohyashiki K, Yoshida MA, Ohyashiki J, *et al. Cancer Genetics and Cytogenetics.* 1985; **17**, 325.
32. Oshimura M, Ohyashiki K, Tonomura A, *et al. Cancer Genetics and Cytogenetics.* 1981; **4**, 245.
33. De Braekeleer M. *Leukemia Research.* 1985; **12**, 1571.
34. Klein G. *New England Journal of Medicine.* 1975; **293**, 1353.
35. Berger R, Bernheim A. *IARC Scientific Publications.* 1985; **60**, 65.
36. Ziegler JL, Miner RC, Rosenbaum E, *et al. Lancet.* 1982; **ii**, 631.
37. Chaganti RSK, Jhanwar SC, Koziner B, *et al. Blood.* 1983; **61**, 1269.
38. Whang-Peng J, Lee EC, Sieverts H, *et al. Blood.* 1984; **63**, 818.
39. Gyger M, Laverdiere M, Gagnon A, *et al. Cancer Genetics and Cytogenetics.* 1985; **17**, 283.
40. Berman M, Minowada J, Loew JM, *et al. Cancer Genetics and Cytogenetics.* 1985; **16**, 341.
41. Daly P, Brito-Babapulle V, Lawlor E, *et al. British Journal of Haematology.* 1986; **64**: 561.
42. Bunn PA, Lamberg SI. *Cancer Treatment Reports.* 1979; **63**, 725.
43. Whang-Peng J, Bunn PA, Knutsen T, *et al. Cancer.* 1982; **50**, 1539.
44. Vonderheid EC, Sobel EL, Nowell PC, *et al. Blood.* 1985; **66**, 358.
45. Gamperl R. *Cancer Genetics and Cytogenetics.* 1986; **19**, 341.
46. Barbieri D, Spanedda R, Castoldi GL. *Cancer Genetics and Cytogenetics.* 1986; **20**, 287.
47. Gallo RC, de-The GB, Ito Y. *Cancer Research.* 1981; **41**, 4738.
48. Whang-Peng J, Bunn PA, Knutsen T, *et al. Journal of the National Cancer Institute.* 1985; **74**, 357.
49. Fukuhara S, Inuma Y, Gotoh Y, *et al. Blood.* 1983; **61**, 205.
50. Pandolfi F. *Diagnostic Immunology.* 1986; **4**, 61.
51. Samada I, Tanaka R, Kumagai E, *et al. Blood.* 1984; **65**, 649.
52. Lennert K, Mestadagh J. *Virchows Archiv für Pathologische Anatomie und Physiologie und für*

Kleinishce Medizin. 1968; **344**, 1.

53. Godde-Salz E, Feller AC, Lennert K. *Leukemia Research*. 1986; **10**, 313.

54. Kaneko Y, Larson RA, Variakojis D, *et al. Blood*. 1982; **60**, 877.

55. Nowell P, Finan J, Glover D, *et al. Blood*. 1981; **58**, 183.

56. Becher R. *Cancer Genetics and Cytogenetics*. 1986; **21**, 271.

57. Seemanova E, Passarge E, Beneskova D, *et al. American Journal of Medical Genetics*. 1985; **20**, 639.

58. Fukuhara S, Ueshima Y, Shirakawa S, *et al. International Journal of Cancer*. 1979; **23**, 739.

59. Kennaugh AA, Butterworth SV, Hollis R, *et al. Human Genetics*. 1986; **73**, 254.

60. McCaw BK, Hecht F, Harnden DG, *et al. Proceedings of the National Academy of Sciences, USA*. 1975; **72**, 2071.

61. Ueshima Y, Rowley JD, Variakojis D, *et al. Blood*. 1984; **63**, 108.

62. Yunis JJ, Frizzera G, Oken MM, *et al. New England Journal of Medicine*. 1987; **316**, 79.

63. Keneko Y, Rowley JD, Variakojis D, *et al. International Journal of Cancer*. 1983; **32**, 683.

64. Baer R, Chen KC, Smith SD, *et al. Cell*. 1985; **34**, 705.

65. Bakhshi A, Jensen JP, Goldman P, *et al. Cell*. 1985; **41**, 899.

66. Raffeld M, Wright JJ, Lipford E, *et al. Cancer Research*. 1987; **47**, 2537.

67. Tsujimoto Y, Cossman J, Jaffe E, *et al. Science*. 1985; **228**, 1440.

68. Lipford E, Wright JJ, Urba W, *et al. Blood*. 1987; **70**, 1816.

69. Rudd NL, Teshima IE. *Human Genetics*. 1983; **63**, 323.

70. Sadamori N, Hant T, Minowada J, *et al. Hematology Oncology*. 1983; **1**, 243.

71. Slavutsky I, de Vinuesa ML, Larripa I, *et al. Cancer Genetics and Cytogenetics*. 1986; **21**, 335.

72. Croce CM. In: Crowell RL, Friedman H, Prier JE eds. *Tumor Virus Infections and Immunity*, Baltimore: University Park Press, 1976: 223.

73. Douglass EC, Magrath IT, Lee EC, *et al. Blood*. 1980; **55**, 148.

74. Levine EG, Arthur DC, Gajl-Peczalska K, *et al. Cancer Research*. 1986; **46**, 6481.

75. Preud'Homme JL, Dellagi K, Guglielmi P, *et al. IARC Scientific Publications*. 1985; **60**, 47.

76. Magrath I, Erikson J, Whang-Peng J, *et al. Science*. 1983; **222**, 1094.

77. Denny CT, Hollis GF, Magrath IT, *et al. Molecular and Cellular Biology*. 1985; **5**, 3199.

78. Erikson J, ar-Rushdi A, Drwinga HL, *et al. Proceedings of the National Academy of Sciences, USA*. 1983; **80**, 820.

79. Versnel MA, van Dongen JJM, Geurts van Kesse AHM, *et al. Cancer Genetics and Cytogenetics*. 1986; **9**, 321.

80. Chenevix-Trench G. *Cancer Genetics and Cytogenetics*. 1987; **27**, 191.

81. Adams JM, Cory S. *Proceedings of the Royal Society of London [Biol]*. 1985; **226**, 59.

82. Bauer KO, Merkel DE, Winter JE, *et al. Cancer Research*. 1986; **46**, 3173.

CHAPTER 6

THE MOLECULAR GENETICS OF NON-HODGKIN'S LYMPHOMAS

Frank G Haluska, Yoshihide Tsujimoto and Carlo M Croce

There exist several conceptual frameworks within which to understand the pathogenesis of non-Hodgkin's lymphoma (NHL). These relate the biology of lymphoid malignancy to the biology of the immune system, to histopathological morphology, or to non-random chromosome alterations. These three perspectives have been presented in preceding chapters and, taken together, they summarize in impressive fashion a body of understanding which is perhaps more extensive than for any other group of neoplasms. Yet the depth of our knowledge is best illustrated in the extent to which we have attained a molecular comprehension of lymphomagenesis for some tumours. The elucidation of the molecular biology of these lymphomas has been predicated upon a synthesis of the aforementioned biological, histopathological and cytogenetic methods of analyses.

In this chapter we discuss the molecular biology of several of the non-Hodgkin's lymphomas, including Burkitt's and undifferentiated lymphomas, follicular lymphomas and some diffuse lymphomas. Each of these groups of tumours has come to be understood on a molecular level by the dissection of the non-random chromosome translocations associated with them. This strategy has been rewarding in several respects.[1] It has led to a formulation of the general features of activation of known oncogenes, especially c-*myc*, by chromosome translocation. It has also led to the identification of novel putative oncogenes, such as *bcl*-2. It has

been extended to other malignancies, most notably the lymphoid leukaemias. Finally, it has enabled the generation of molecular diagnostic probes, tools certain to further our knowledge regarding these diseases. Our discussion will focus on each of these aspects of the molecular biology of NHL.

General principles

The lymphoid neoplasms which have been amenable to analysis share a number of consistent features. Although details regarding each of these common features vary from one class of malignancy to another, by and large a broadly applicable molecular pathogenesis can be sketched in outline form.[1] The mechanisms discussed here may not apply to all tumours of lymphoid origin, but they do constitute the basis for a model which has been employed predictively with success in several instances.

The lymphomas under consideration each carry consistent, non-random chromosome translocations. The importance of cytogenetic analyses to the characterization and diagnosis of lymphoid tumours has been discussed in detail in Chapter 5. Nonetheless, it must be stressed that chromosome translocations serve two purposes in the molecular analysis of lymphomagenesis. First, they provide evidence that tumours of diverse phenotypes carry a common genetic alteration. For instance, endemic Burkitt's lymphomas, sporadic Burkitt's lymphomas, undifferentiated lymphomas, some large cell lymphomas and acute lymphoblastic leukaemias of FAB L3 morphology all exhibit t(8;14) translocations. Thus, we infer that a similar pathway to neoplasia has been followed in each of these cases. Second, they provide clues regarding the nature of the genetic lesion. In the examples just mentioned, a rationale for examining the genetic regions involved in the translocations on chromosomes 8 and 14 is clearly evident.

An important feature of the translocations observed in various NHLs is the consistent involvement of cytogenetic loci prone to rearrangement in what one might term a lympho-specific manner. That is, the immunoglobulin loci and the T-cell receptor loci, each of which rearrange physiologically during lymphocyte ontogeny, are repeatedly involved in chromosome translocation in B- and T-cell malignancies, respectively.

The reciprocally involved chromosome region is often one known to be the cytogenetic location of a gene involved in the control of cellular proliferation, such as c-*myc*. Alternatively, the molecular analysis of the reciprocally involved chromosome reveals the presence of such a gene, e.g. *bcl*-2. The salient finding in both cases is the abnormal juxtaposition of one locus expressed in a highly lymphospecific manner to a second locus crucial to the control of cell proliferation. The consequence of this pathological arrangement is the expression of the proliferative-control gene at inappropriate levels or at inopportune times. This dysregulation contributes directly to oncogenesis.

Finally, the mechanism by which chromosome translocation occurs involves the aberrant operation of lymphocytic enzymatic machinery.[2] Recombinases, enzymes which function during physiological V-D-J recombination or during isotype switching, apparently make mistakes. Interchromosomal recombination in the lymphomas appears to take place as a consequence of the infidelity of these enzymes.

These are the central features of the molecular pathogenesis of the non-Hodgkin's lymphomas as they are presently understood. We shall now turn to an examination of the specific experimental findings for a number of individual classes of lymphoma. We begin with the best understood of the NHLs, Burkitt's lymphoma.

Chromosomal abnormalities in Burkitt's lymphoma

The first lymphoma for which a consistent cytogenetic abnormality was noted is Burkitt's lymphoma. Initial studies of chromosomal preparations obtained from samples of this malignancy led to the observation by Manolov and Manolova[3] of a 14q+ chromosome in the majority of cases. Later, refined banding techniques enabled the demonstration that the 14q+ chromosome was one product of a reciprocal translocation between chromosome 8 and chromosome 14: a t(8;14) (q24;q32) translocation.[4] More than 80 per cent of Burkitt's lymphomas carry this t(8;14) translocation. A minority of cases carry what are termed variant translocations.[5] The variant translocations comprise t(2;8) or t(8;22) translocations. These are illustrated in Fig. 6.1.

Further insight into the nature of these translocations was gained from work which resulted in the localization of the immunoglobulin genes on the human chromosome map. Using somatic cell hybrid technology or *in situ* chromosome hybridization, the immunoglobulin heavy chain (IgH) locus was mapped to chromosome band 14q32.[6] The light chain loci were also localized; κ was demonstrated to reside at 2p11,[7] and λ at 22q11.[8] Strikingly, each of these chromosome locations is a site of chromosome translocation in Burkitt's lymphoma. The first suggestion that these genes play a direct role in the pathogenesis of the Burkitt's lymphoma translocations was derived directly from cytogenetic analyses.

The other chromosome involved in the Burkitt's translocation is always chromosome 8, and the breakpoint is always at band 8q24. This was demonstrated by our laboratory and others to be the location of the human c-*myc* proto-oncogene.[9,10] It was shown by somatic cell hybrid and Southern blot analysis that the c-*myc* gene is situated on the 14q+ chromosome as a consequence of the t(8;14) translocation.[9,10] The c-*myc* gene was demonstrated to be rearranged

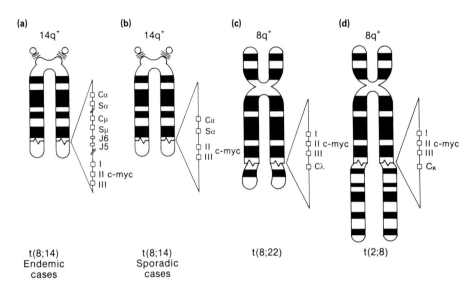

Fig. 6.1 Chromosome translocations observed in Burkitt's lymphomas. The configurations of the immunoglobulin and juxtaposed c-*myc* genes resulting from the translocations, as revealed by molecular cloning studies, are illustrated. The 14q$^+$ chromosome resulting from the t(8;14) translocation is shown in (a) and (b) for endemic and sporadic cases, respectively. (c) and (d) illustrate the variant translocations.

in approximately 50 per cent of these cases.[9–12] In several cases the rearranged c-*myc* restriction fragment also carried C_μ or C_γ sequences,[11] and the translocation was established as involving J_H[13] or switch segments. Furthermore, in the variant translocations, c-*myc* remains on the chromosome 8q$^+$, and C_κ[14] or C_λ[15] segments are juxtaposed on the 8q$^+$. Thus the common genetic feature of Burkitt's lymphoma was surmised from cytogenetic and Southern blot studies. Each case exhibits the juxtaposition of the c-*myc* proto-oncogene and one of the Ig heavy or light chain genes.

Molecular analyses of Burkitt's translocations

The juxtaposition of the well-defined c-*myc* and Ig loci, and the ready availability of molecular probes encompassing this region, allowed for the rapid molecular dissection of the Burkitt's translocations. Molecular cloning revealed a remarkable heterogeneity in genetic architecture surrounding the chromosome breakpoints.[1]

Sites of breakage on chromosome 14 (in the much more common t(8;14) translocations) are distributed throughout the heavy chain locus. Translocations were shown to occur near D_H segments,[16] J_H segments[13,17] and S_μ,[18–20] S_γ,[21,22] and S_α[23] regions (Fig. 6.2). Each of these is a region prone to physiological rearrangement during the normal sequence of V-D-J recombination or isotype switching,[24] suggesting a mechanism for chromosome translocation, a point to which we shall return.

On chromosome 8, breakpoints are similarly distributed (Fig. 6.2). The c-*myc* gene consists of three exons.[25] The first exon is non-coding, and the second and third exons encode the entire 439 amino acid c-*myc* protein.[25] The t(8;14) translocations occur far 5' of c-*myc*,[16,17] upstream of the gene[20,21] or within intron I.[18,20,23,26–28] The t(8;14) translocations thus leave the c-*myc* coding region intact. The variant translocations occur 3' of c-*myc* and also leave the gene intact.

Given the wide variance in the molecular structure underlying the Burkitt's lymphoma translocations, generation of a plausible molecular mechanism to account for

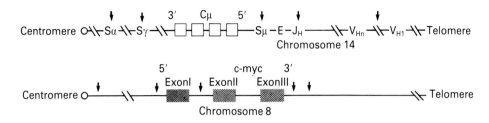

Fig. 6.2 Heterogeneity of translocation breakpoints in Burkitt's lymphoma. On chromosome 14 (top), chromosome breakage has been demonstrated in S_μ, S_γ, S_α, J_H, and D_H regions, as indicated by arrows. On chromosome 8 (bottom), breakpoints are 5' of *c-myc* or within the first intron in cases carrying t(8;14) translocations. Thus, *c-myc* may assume either an intact or truncated configuration. The variant translocations result in breakage 3' of an intact *c-myc*.

oncogenesis in this setting would seem to be a daunting task. However, several features are common to all of the translocations. First, the *c-myc* gene always remains grossly intact. Coding capacity is uniformly maintained. This strongly suggests that deregulation of *c-myc* expression, and not mutation of the *c-myc* gene product, is the operative transformation mechanism in these tumours. That changes are known to occur in *c-myc* regulatory regions following transformation (possibly as a manifestation of tumour progression) supports this contention.[29] Second, *c-myc* deregulation occurs generally as a consequence of its juxtaposition to Ig elements, regardless of the orientation of *c-myc* relative to the involved Ig locus. How this takes place is poorly understood in molecular terms, but it is likely that *cis*-acting genetic control mechanisms must be responsible. Finally, breakage of the Ig loci occurs at sites subject to B-cell ontogenetic recombination. This supports a model in which translocation occurs due to aberrant enzymatic activity.[2]

Deregulation of *c-myc*

The *c-myc* oncogene is known to play a central role in both the cellular response to proliferative stimuli and in the process of transformation.[25] It is the cellular homologue of the avian myelocytomatosis virus MC 29 transforming gene.[30] Additionally, it has been intensively studied as one of the earliest genes to be expressed following mitogenic stimulation of quiescent cells.[31,32] It encodes a phosphoprotein

which localizes to the cell nucleus,[33] and recent data indicate that this protein functions in DNA replication.[34] A more complete review of the molecular biology of *c-myc* can be obtained in several recent reviews.[25,35]

In Burkitt's lymphoma the expression of *c-myc* is clearly aberrantly regulated.[13,14,18,36] The gene is expressed constitutively at levels which approximate those seen in proliferating normal cells.[37,38] It is most important to realize, however, that this expression is inappropriate for B-cells. An extensive series of experiments utilizing somatic cell hybrids has underscored this fact. The normal *c-myc* in its germline configuration is not expressed when it is introduced into a murine B-cell background; however *c-myc* genes on tumour-associated 14q+ chromosomes are expressed when hybridized with murine B-cell lines.[39,40] This expression is lymphospecific; that is, when hybrids are constructed between Burkitt's lymphomas and fibroblast lines, the *c-myc* gene is not expressed.[41] Finally, in Burkitt's lymphomas, S1 protection experiments have demonstrated that only the translocated *c-myc* allele is expressed.[36] In sum, only the translocated *c-myc* gene is expressed inappropriately in a lymphoid background.

Although several hypotheses for this phenomenon have been put forward,[1] it appears that it is best explained by the presence of enhancers or enhancer-like elements within the Ig loci.[13,14] These are capable of acting *in cis* over long molecular distances. Additional support for this proposition comes from transfection experiments, in which a linked *c-myc* gene and

Ig enhancer are introduced into recipient cells, resulting in high levels of c-*myc* transcription.[42] Moreover, transgenic mice develop lymphomas only when the c-*myc* transgene is linked to Ig enhancers.[35] Thus the defined Ig enhancers or additional, as yet undefined, *cis*-acting elements probably play a central role in c-*myc* deregulation due to translocation.

The mechanisms of chromosome translocations in Burkitt's lymphomas

As previously stated, the distribution of chromosome breakpoints on chromosome 14 provides some clues regarding the mechanisms of chromosome translocation in t(8;14) translocations. It is immediately apparent from an examination of a map of the localization of these breakpoints that there is a non-random clustering of breakage sites (Fig. 6.2). Breakpoints localize upstream of D_H and J_H segments or within switch regions upstream of C_μ, C_γ or C_α. These sites have functional significance in the developing B-cell. Ordinarily, the immature B-cell precursor possesses an Ig configuration which is identical to that of every other somatic cell. However, unlike other somatic tissue, lymphoid cells undergo a precise programme of genetic rearrangement which allows them to diversify the ability to mount a response to antigen.[24] Early in B-cell maturation, heavy chain antibody variable region exons are constructed by the recombination of separated variable (V), diversity (D), and joining (J) segments of DNA.[24] This allows for the production of functional IgM by the transcription of the variable (V-D-J) exon and μ constant region (C_μ) exons. The V-D-J recombinase enzymes catalyse this process. Later, isotype switching occurs, so that new constant regions replace the C_μ region downstream of the utilized V-D-L segments. This, too, is an enzymatically controlled process. Thus two separate recombination mechanisms function, at different times, in the developing B cell.

The Burkitt's translocation breakpoints correspond with high fidelity to the sites of chromosome rearrangement due to the operation of one or other of the B-cell recombinases. Importantly, the distribution of breakpoints also relates to the phenotype of Burkitt's lymphoma. Burkitt's lymphomas occur with two presentations.[43,44] Endemic Burkitt's lymphoma occurs in equatorial Africa and is almost uniformly associated with Epstein–Barr virus (EBV) infection.[43] Endemic Burkitt's lymphoma tumour cells or cell lines derived from such cases usually exhibit low levels of surface Ig, predominantly IgM, and usually secrete little Ig.[45,46] In contrast, sporadic Burkitt's lymphoma occurs throughout the world. It exhibits a much lower level of association with EBV (less than 30 per cent.)[43] Sporadic Burkitt's lymphomas display higher levels of surface Ig and secrete Ig as well.[46,47] These appear to represent a more mature B-cell than endemic tumours.

On the molecular level, endemic and sporadic Burkitt's lymphomas also differ (Fig. 6.3). Endemic cases do not carry rearrangements of the c-*myc* gene detectable by conventional Southern blot.[17,48] Most breakpoints in these tumours lie far 5' of c-*myc* on chromosome 8 and involve the D_H[16] or J_H[17] segments on chromosome 14. Furthermore, cloning of translocation breakpoints from several endemic cases has revealed evidence of the operation of the V-D-J recombinase in the genesis of the translocations.[16,17] The breakpoints occur immediately 5' of D_H or J_H segments and contain N regions, thought to occur as a consequence of the operation of terminal deoxynucleotidyl transferase (TdT).[49] On the normal chromosome 8 counterpart of the translocated region, sequences homologous to the heptamer-nonamer signal sequences, recognized by the recombinase, are found.[2] These findings strongly suggest that these translocations occur due to recombination operation. Taken together with the immunophenotype data, the molecular evidence suggests that the endemic Burkitt's lymphomas arise in a pre-B-cell which is actively rearranging its Ig genes. It also implies, since the phenotype of the tumour cell is actually that of an early B cell, that to some extent differentiation of the cell carrying the translocation must occur for the full acquisition of malignant behaviour.

In contrast, sporadic Burkitt's lymphomas usually exhibit rearranged c-*myc* loci. Translocations occur immediately upstream or within the c-*myc* transcription unit on chromosome 8 and in switch regions on chromosome 14. These translocations probably occur at a later stage of B-cell differentiation when the switch recombinases are active. It has been demonstrated that the switching enzymes function in pre-B-cells. It is thus likely that in sporadic cases, as in endemic cases, some cell differentiation occurs following translocation. The molecular features of endemic and sporadic Burkitt's lymphomas are compared in Table 6.1.

The pathogenesis of endemic Burkitt's lymphomas

The sum of the molecular and biological evidence presented allows one to construct a reasonable scenario for the pathogenesis of these aggressive B-cell lymphomas.[2,43,44] Endemic Burkitt's lymphomas arise in the context of widespread hyperendemic malaria and EBV infection. Epstein–Barr virus infection *in vitro* is known to promote B-cell immortalization.[43] It is possible that EBV infection *in vivo* engenders an expansion of the B-cell compartment, which is subject to T-cell control. However, an immunosuppressed individual, including a patient who has contracted malaria, suffers from defective T-cell regulation. This may allow for unabated B-cell proliferation. The enlarged population of B-cells may provide a substrate for an increased probability of recombinase error, consequent translocation, and thus malignancy. A similar situation may occur in patients with acquired immunodeficiency syndrome (AIDS) who develop aggressive Burkitt's tumours.[50] Infection with EBV, immunosuppression, and translocation-associated malignancy are all features of this disease association.[2]

Recombinase errors are also responsible for

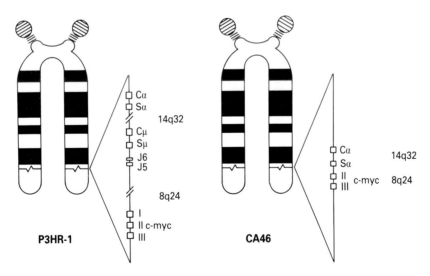

Fig. 6.3 Differences in the t(8;14) chromosome translocation between the endemic African Burkitt's lymphoma P3HR-1 and the sporadic Burkitt's lymphoma CA 46. The 14q⁺ chromosome is illustrated for each. In P3HR-1, the breakpoint lies upstream of J5 on chromosome 14, and greater than 50 kb 5′ of the intact c-*myc* on chromosome 8. The recombinase may have mediated this translocation. In contrast, the CA 46 translocation joins chromosome 14 switch sequences with the intron separating the first (I) and second (II) exons of c-*myc*. This may have occurred through the action of isotype switching enzymes. These findings typify those seen in endemic and sporadic Burkitt's lymphomas in general.

Table 6.1.   Comparison of endemic and sporadic Burkitt's lymphomas

	Endemic	*Sporadic*
Geographic location	Equatorial Africa	Europe and North America
EBV presence	+	−
IgM secretor	−	+
c-*myc* rearranged	−	+
Recombinase-mediated translocation	+	−
Isotype switch-mediated translocation	−	+

EBV: Epstein–Barr virus

the translocations consistently observed in other non-Hodgkin's lymphomas. In fact, involvement of J$_H$ segments and the presence of evidence of recombinase operation at translocation breakpoints were first described for the t(11;14) translocation found in chronic lymphocytic leukaemia (CLL) and diffuse lymphomas[51] and the t(14;18) of follicular lymphomas.[52,53] We shall now turn to a discussion of these malignancies.

The molecular biology of follicular lymphomas

The most common B-cell lymphomas display a follicular architecture (follicular small cleaved cell, follicular mixed or follicular large cell by the Working Formulation),[54] and 85 per cent of these tumours carry t(14;18) (q32;q21) translocations.[55] Using probes for the Ig J$_H$ segments, our laboratory and others have successfully cloned the breakpoints from a number of these tumours.[52,56,57] This work has led to the identification of a new gene, *bcl*-2 (for B-cell leukaemia and lymphoma-2), implicated in the pathogenesis of follicular lymphoma.[52] The *bcl*-2 gene is rearranged in up to 90 per cent of cases of follicular lymphoma, and in addition in about 28 per cent of patients with diffuse large cell lymphoma,[58,59] and thus its characterization has provided important diagnostic reagents.

The *bcl*-2 gene was first identified upstream of J$_H$ sequences at the t(14;18) breakpoint.[59] Probes from this region of chromosome 18 identified rearrangements in a majority of follicular lymphoma samples (Fig. 6.4); in addition, these

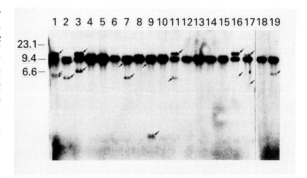

Fig. 6.4 Rearrangement of genomic DNAs from follicular lymphomas carrying t(14;18) translocation. Sst I-digested cellular DNAs probed with a DNA probe from the *bcl*-2 gene which recognizes the breakpoint cluster region. Rearranged fragments are indicated by the arrows. Such a technique is directly applicable to molecular diagnosis.

probes recognize a transcript in B-cells.[59] The *bcl*-2 transcriptional unit comprises two exons transcribed into three messages of 8, 5 and 3.5 kb. These arise by differential splicing and polyadenylation.[60,61] The transcripts encode two proteins which differ at their carboxyl termini. *bcl*-2 α is 239 amino acids long, whereas *bcl*-2 β consists of 205 amino acids[60]. The *bcl*-2 proteins function in an unknown manner; however, they are highly conserved in the mouse,[62] and their expression is modulated in response to mitogenic stimuli.[63] It seems likely that they play an important role in B-cell proliferation, and that the deregulation of their expression which occurs as a consequence of chromosome translocation results in malignant transformation.

The expression of *bcl*-2 is deregulated at the

level of transcription in cells carrying the t(14;18) translocation. Almost all translocations occur 3' of the *bcl*-2 transcription unit. In 60–70 per cent of cases, a small 100 bp region in the 3' non-coding portion of the gene, the major breakpoint cluster region (mbcr), is the site of translocation.[53] Additional translocations occur farther 3', or in one case 5',[64] of the gene. In all instances, the coding structure of *bcl*-2 is unaffected. In addition, the constancy of breakpoint anatomy which is seen in cases of follicular lymphoma (FL) leaves the *bcl*-2 gene closely linked to the Ig enhancer in most cases. Thus, the *in cis* influence of the Ig enhancer is implicated in the deregulatory process in these malignancies.

Breakpoints cluster 5' of J_H segments on chromosome 14 (Fig. 6.5). The translocation breakpoints consistently exhibit the same evidence of recombinase activity described earlier.[53] Despite the mature B-cell phenotype commonly observed in cases of follicular lymphoma, this finding suggests that these translocations must arise in pre-B-cells (Fig. 6.6). We have analysed one case of follicular lymphoma carrying a t(14;18) which progressed to an acute pre-B-cell leukaemia.[65] Initially, the patient's tumour was of mature, TdT⁻ phenotype. However, following progression, the tumour cells were TdT⁺ and carried both a t(14;18) and a t(8;14) translocation. Thus, despite

the mature phenotype of the original tumour cells, TdT⁺ cells capable of undergoing a second translocation must have been present. As has already been argued for Burkitt's lymphoma, it is clear that translocations occur early in B-cell ontogeny, and that follicular lymphomas must undergo differentiation before they manifest a malignant phenotype. Residual early B-cells which carry the translocation must be present for this type of progression to occur.

bcl-2 and molecular diagnosis

Because of the tight clustering of chromosome breakpoints on both the involved chromosomes, 14 and 18, in follicular lymphomas, these tumours are excellent candidates for the application of techniques to enable the genetic detection of malignancy. The translocation serves as a highly specific and sensitive tool for diagnosing follicular lymphomas or to a lesser extent diffuse large cell lymphoma, as noted previously, using conventional Southern blots.

One desired application for molecular diagnosis would be to employ molecular probes to detect low levels of malignant cells. This application is not well achieved by Southern blot technology, which typically detects sequences which are present in between 5 and 10 per cent of sample cells. However, the polymerase chain

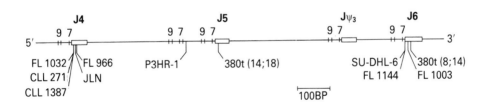

Fig. 6.5 Clustering of chromosome breakpoints 5' of J_H segments at the immunoglobulin heavy chain locus on chromosome 14. The close spacing of breakpoints at the nucleotide level strongly suggests that the recombinase is implicated in the mechanism of translocation in these various B-cell malignancies. Chromosome translocation occurs at or near the 5' end of each J_H segment, and downstream from the heptamer-nonamer signal sequences (indicated by 9 and 7). These are precisely the sites of physiological V_H-D-J_H joining. Breakpoints designated FL, JLN and SU-DHL-6 are from follicular lymphoma cases; CLL, chronic lymphocytic leukaemia; 380 is an acute pre-B-cell leukaemia carrying t(8;14) and t(14;18) translocations; P3HR-1 is an African Burkitt's lymphoma (note that while the site of translocation in this tumour is upstream of J5, a heptamer-nonamer is situated at the break, and nucleotides 3' of the breakpoint demonstrate some features of a pseudo-J_H segment). *See* reference 2 for more details.

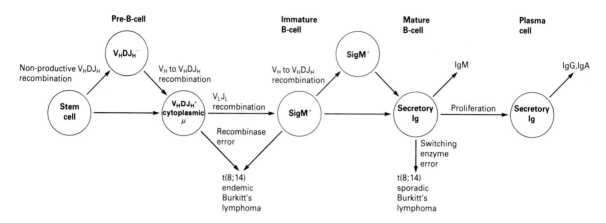

Fig. 6.6 Correlation between B-lymphocyte ontogeny and the point at which translocations leading to malignancy occur. The recombinase functions in pre-B-cells or immature B-cells. At these stages of differentiation, its physiological function is to implement V_H-D-J_H joining, V_H to V_H-D-J_H recombination, or V_L-J_L joining. Errors at these steps may give rise to translocations, as observed in follicular lymphoma, chronic lymphocytic leukaemia, acute lymphoblastic leukaemia and endemic Burkitt's lymphoma. In these cases, differentiation may occur before expression of the malignant phenotype is manifested. In more mature cells, isotype switching takes place following antigenic stimulation, and translocations of the type seen in sporadic Burkitt's lymphomas may occur.

reaction (PCR) is excellently suited for this purpose.[66] It can be utilized to detect cells carrying the specific translocation even when they only comprise 10^{-5} of the analysed cell population. It will be feasible to detect residual tumour cells in peripheral blood or bone marrow even when an exceedingly small fraction of the population is malignant. With such genetic data at hand, the clinician will be better able to tailor therapy to patients undergoing induction or being followed in remission.

The molecular biology of the t(11;14) translocation

The t(11;14) translocation is observed predominantly in cases of chronic lymphocytic leukaemia. However, it is also found in a fraction of diffuse small and large cell lymphomas. The breakpoints of t(11;14) translocations have been cloned from several cases of chronic lymphocytic leukaemia.[67] Like the endemic Burkitt's lymphomas and the follicular lymphoma cases already discussed, breakage occurs in the IgH locus 5' of J_H segments in a manner strongly

suggestive of recombinase activity.[51,68] Breakpoints also cluster on chromosome 11 at band q13, in a region we have termed *bcl*-1.[69] However, as yet no transcription unit has been identified in this region.

T-cell lymphomas and chromosome translocations

T-cell lymphomas are much less frequent than B-cell lymphomas, and thus they are not so well studied. However, there is substantial reason to believe that the fundamental elements of the molecular biology of T-cell lymphomas should differ little from that of B-cell lymphomas. Like B-cell tumours, T-cell malignancies exhibit non-random chromosome abnormalities. The most commonly involved chromosome region[1] is chromosome 14q11, the site of the T-cell receptor (TCR) α[70] and δ[71] chain loci. The TCR genes rearrange in a manner similar to the Ig loci, and in fact the same enzyme is capable of performing both recombination operations.[72] The TCR genes are active in a T-cell-specific manner and they contain genetic enhancer elements to facilitate this activation. In short, these genes function analogously to the Ig genes, both during lymphocyte ontogeny and during oncogenesis.

Some of the findings discussed below derive not from T-cell lymphomas but from T-cell chronic lymphocytic leukaemias or acute lymphoblastic leukaemias (ALL). It should be emphasized, however, that one expects to find extensive genetic similarity among lymphocytic malignancies. For example, B-cell ALL of the FAB L3 subtype has been demonstrated to be identical to Burkitt's lymphoma with regard to the organization of the t(8;14) translocation.[73] Thus some of the work detailed below will certainly eventually apply to lymphomas as well as to leukaemias.

Cytogenetics of T-cell lymphoma and leukaemia

Four chromosome abnormalities are commonly found in T-cell malignancies (Fig. 6.7). These include the t(14;14)(q11;q32) translocation, inv(14)(q11;q32) inversion, the t(8;14)(q24;q11) translocation, the t(10;14)(q24;q11) translocation, and the t(11;14)(p13;q11) translocation.[1,74]

Each of these involves chromosome 14q11. This is the site of two TCR genes, embedded one within the other. The TCR δ chain locus is situated within TCR α, with the δ constant region lying approximately 85 kb upstream of the α constant region.[71] TCR δ is expressed quite early in T-cell ontogeny, while TCR α is expressed in more mature cells. Although the precise workings of the control of TCR expression are still poorly understood it is known that the TCR genes undergo physiological recombination and that the features of V-D-J recombination are similar to V-D-J joining in B-cells.

Molecular analyses of T-cell translocations

The most completely understood T-cell lymphoma translocation is that of the cell line SUP T1 derived from a young patient with T lymphoblastic lymphoma. This cell line carries an inv(14) chromosome inversion. Molecular cloning studies have shown that this rearrangement joins an immunoglobulin variable segment

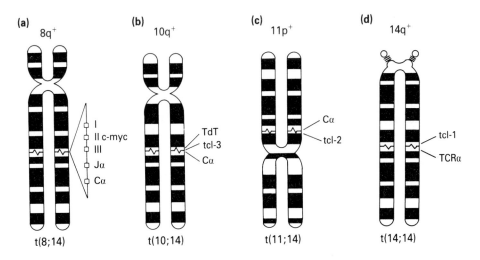

Fig. 6.7 Translocations exhibited by T-cell leukaemias and lymphomas. Cloning of the t(8;14) translocation (a) has revealed an organization similar to the variant Burkitt's lymphoma translocations, but involving the TCRα locus. Knowledge of the t(10;14) and t(11;14) translocations (b) and (c) derives from somatic cell hybrid studies; locations of putative *tcl* oncogenes and relevant chromosome markers are illustrated. In (d), the t(14;14) translocation is shown.

to a TCR α joining segment.[75,76] In effect, an intrachromosomal recombinase error engendered this inversion. However, several studies suggest that this translocation was not primary to the pathogenesis of this patient's lymphoma. Another translocation from this same line, t(7;9), has recently been cloned and demonstrated to involve the TCR β chain.[77] In addition, translocations in several T-cell malignancies carrying t(14;14) translocations have been studied. These demonstrate that the most frequent site of breakage at 14q32 is not within the IgH locus, but is instead 3' to it.[78,79] It is likely that a gene carrying transforming potential lies in this region and that oncogenic translocations result in its activation. We have named this hypothetical oncogene *tcl*-1.[70]

Several other translocations have been cloned which involve the 14q11 region. A t(8;14)(q24;q11) translocation from a T-cell leukaemia has been studied in detail.[80,81] This translocation resulted from a recombinase error which joined a TCR Jα segment to sequences 3' of c-*myc*.[81] A second case carrying a t(8;14) was employed to demonstrate that, as a consequence of the translocation, c-*myc* expression was deregulated.[80] As was the case in B-cells, somatic cell hybrid studies showed that the translocated c-*myc* allele is expressed inappropriately in hybrids between the malignant cells and murine T-cells. We have recently demonstrated that the t(8;14) translocation in this second case joins TCR Jδ and chromosome 8 sequences.[71]

The t(10;14)[82] and t(11;14)[83] translocations in T-cells have been shown by analysis of somatic cell hybrid clones, to result in the separation of Cα and Vα sequences. It is likely that these translocations involve TCR δ rearrangements as well.

Summary

A consideration of the molecular pathogenesis of non-Hodgkin's lymphomas of both B- and T-cell origin reveals several consistent features. Chromosome translocations facilitate the identification of the genetic lesion responsible for oncogenesis in most cases. The chromosome translocations consistently involve regions of the genome expressed in a lymphospecific fashion. Because they must be expressed at high levels, these loci are prone to the activation of genes pathologically placed nearby, and such genes can induce transformation when important to the control of the cellular proliferative programme. Because the loci must remain capable of developmental rearrangement, they are subject to recombination mistakes, the results of which include translocations. Finally, although translocations take place very early in lymphoid ontogeny, tumour phenotypes may be more differentiated; this suggests a limited degree of maturation is allowed or is necessary before the expression of the malignant state.

These principles are at best an incomplete foundation for the further elucidation of the genetic basis of NHL, and indeed of malignancy in general. In the future we can hope for an extension in the diagnostic utility of these studies and look forward to the rational molecular design of therapy for the non-Hodgkin's lymphomas.

Acknowledgements

We thank Ms Charlotte Long and Mrs Kathy Reinersmann for preparing and editing the manuscript. Frank G. Haluska is a trainee of the Medical Scientist Training Program at the University of Pennsylvania School of Medicine (NIH T32 GM 07170). This work was supported by grants from the National Institutes of Health Outstanding Investigator's Award CA 39860 (CMC) and the NIH Training Program in Basic Cancer Research CA 09171 (FGH).

References

1. Haluska FG, Tsujimoto Y, Croce CM. *Annual Review of Genetics.* 1987; **21**, 321.
2. Haluska FG, Tsujimoto Y, Croce CM. *Trends in Genetics.* 1987; **3**, 11.
3. Manolov G, Manolova Y. *Nature.* 1972; **237**, 33.
4. Zech L, Haglund U, Nilsson K, Klein G. *International Journal of Cancer.* 1976; **17**, 47.

5. Croce CM, Nowell PC. *Advances in Immunology.* 1986; **38**, 245.
6. Croce CM, Shander M, Martinis J, *et al. Proceedings of the National Academy of Sciences USA.* 1979; **76**, 3416.
7. Malcolm S, Barton P, Murphy C, Ferguson-Smith MA, Bentley DL, Rabbitts TH. *Proceedings of the National Academy of Sciences USA.* 1982; **74**, 4957.
8. Erikson J, Martinis J, Croce CM. *Nature.* 1981; **294**, 173.
9. Dalla-Favera R, Bregni M, Erikson J, Patterson D, Gallo RC, Croce CM. *Proceedings of the National Academy of Sciences USA.* 1982; **79**, 7824.
10. Taub R, Kirsch I, Morton C, *et al. Proceedings of the National Academy of Sciences USA.* 1982; **79**, 7837.
11. Bernard O, Cory S, Gerondakis S, Webb E, Adams JM. *EMBO Journal.* 1983; **2**, 2375.
12. Dalla-Favera R, Martinotti S, Gallo RC, Erikson J, Croce CM. *Science.* 1983; **216**, 963.
13. Erikson J, ar-Rushdi A, Drwinga H, Nowell PC, Croce CM. *Proceedings of the National Academy of Sciences USA.* 1983; **80**, 820.
14. Erikson J, Nishikura K, ar-Rushdi A, *et al. Proceedings of the National Academy of Sciences USA.* 1983; **80**, 7581.
15. Croce CM, Thierfelder W, Erikson J, *et al. Proceedings of the National Academy of Sciences USA.* 1983; **80**, 6922.
16. Haluska FG, Tsujimoto Y, Croce CM. *Proceedings of the National Academy of Sciences USA.* 1987; **84**, 6835.
17. Haluska FG, Finver S, Tsujimoto Y, Croce CM. *Nature.* 1986; **324**, 158.
18. Hayday AC, Gillies SD, Saito H, *et al. Nature.* 1984; **307**, 334.
19. Saito H, Hayday AC, Wiman K, Hayward WS, Tonegawa, S. *Proceedings of the National Academy of Sciences USA.* 1983; **80**, 7476.
20. Wiman KG, Clarkson B, Hayday AC, Saito H, Tonegawa S, Hayward WS. *Proceedings of the National Academy of Sciences USA.* 1984; **81**, 6798.
21. Hamlyn PH, Rabbitts TH. *Nature.* 1983; **304**, 135.
22. Rabbitts TH, Forster A, Baer R, Hamlyn PH. *Nature.* 1983; **306**, 806.
23. Showe LC, Ballantine M, Nishikura K, Erikson J, Kaji H, Croce CM. *Molecular and Cellular Biochemistry.* 1985; **5**, 501.
24. Tonegawa S. *Nature.* 1983; **302**, 575.
25. Cole MD. *Annual Review of Genetics.* 1986; **20**, 361.
26. Gelman EP, Psallidopoulos MC, Papas T, Dalla-Favera R. *Nature.* 1983; **306**, 799.
27. Murphy W, Sarid J, Taub R, *et al. Proceedings of the National Academy of Sciences USA.* 1986; **83**, 2939.
28. Saito H, Hayday AC, Wiman K, Hayward WS, Tonegawa S. *Proceedings of the National Academy of Sciences USA.* 1983; **80**, 7476.
29. Cesarman E, Dalla-Favera R, Bentley D, Groudine M. *Science.* 1987; **238**, 1272.
30. Graf T, Stehelin D. *Biochemistry Biophysics Acta Reviews Cancer.* 1982; **651**, 245.
31. Greenberg ME, Ziff EB. *Nature.* 1984; **311**, 433.
32. Kelly K, Cochran B, Stiles CD, Leder P. *Cell.* 1983; **35**, 603.
33. Cole MD. *Annual Review of Genetics.* 1986; **20**, 361.
34. Studzinski GP, Brelvi ZS, Feldman SC, Watt RA. *Science.* 1986; **234**, 467.
35. Adams JM, Harris AW, Pinkert CA, *et al. Nature.* 1985; **318**, 533.
36. ar-Rushdi A, Nishikura K, Erikson J, Watt R, Rovera G, Croce CM. *Science.* 1983; **222**, 390.
37. Campisi J, Gray HE, Pardee AB, Dean M, Sonnenshein GE. *Cell.* 1984; **36**, 241.
38. Keath EJ, Kelekar A, Cole MD. *Cell.* 1984; **37**, 521.
39. Croce CM, Erikson J, ar-Rushdi A, Aden D, Nishikura K. *Proceedings of the National Academy of Sciences USA.* 1984; **81**, 3170.
40. Nishikura K, Erikson J, ar-Rushdi A, Huebner K, Croce CM. *Proceedings of the National Academy of Sciences USA.* 1985; **82**; 2900.
41. Nishkura K, ar-Rushdi A, Erikson J, DeJesus E, Dugan D, Croce, CM. *Science.* 1984; **224**, 399.
42. Feo S, Harvey R, Showe L, Croce CM. *Proceedings of the National Academy of Sciences USA.* 1986; **83**, 706.
43. Klein G, Klein E. *Nature.* 1985; **315**, 190.
44. Ziegler JL. *New England Journal of Medicine.* 1981; **305**, 735.
45. Gunven P, Klein G, Klein E, Norin T, Singh S. *International Journal of Cancer.* 1980; **25**, 711.
46. Benjamin D, Magrath IT, Maguire R, Janus C, Todd HD, Parsons RG. *Journal of Immunology.* 1982; **129**, 1336.
47. McKeithan TW, Shima EA, LeBeau MM, Minowada J, Rowley JD, Diaz MO. *Proceedings of the National Academy of Sciences USA.* 1986; **83**, 6636.
48. Pelicci P-G, Knowles DM II, Magrath I, Dalla-Favera R. *Proceedings of the National Academy of Sciences USA.* 1986; **83**, 2984.
49. Desiderio SV, Yancopoulos GD, Paskind M, *et al. Nature.* 1984; **311**, 752.
50. Ziegler JL, Miner RC, Rosenbaum E, *et al. Lancet.* 1982; **ii**, 631.
51. Tsujimoto Y, Jaffe E, Cossman J, Gorham J, Nowell PC, Croce CM. *Nature.* 1985; **315**, 340.
52. Tsujimoto Y, Finger LR, Yunis J, Nowell PC, Croce CM. *Science.* 1984; **226**, 1097.
53. Tsujimoto Y, Gorham J, Cossman J, Jaffe E, Croce

CM. *Science.* 1985; **229**, 1390.

54. Report of the Non-Hodgkin's Lymphoma Pathologic Classification Project Writing Committee. *Cancer.* 1982; **49**; 2112.

55. Yunis JJ, Frizzera G, Oken MM, McKenna J, Theologides A, Arnesen M. *New England Journal of Medicine.* 1987; **316**; 79.

56. Bakhshi A, Jensen JP, Goldman P, *et al. Cell.* 1985; **41**, 899.

57. Cleary ML, Sklar J. *Proceedings of the National Academy of Sciences USA.* 1985; **82**; 7439.

58. Weiss LM, Warnke RA, Sklar J, Cleary ML. *New England Journal of Medicine.* 1987; **317**, 1185.

59. Tsujimoto Y, Cossman J, Jaffe E, Croce CM. *Science.* 1985; **228**, 1440.

60. Tsujimoto Y, Croce CM. *Proceedings of the National Academy of Sciences USA.* 1986; **83**, 5214.

61. Cleary ML, Smith SD, Sklar J. *Cell.* 1986; **47**; 19.

62. Negrini M, Silini E, Kozak C, Tsujimoto Y, Croce CM. *Cell.* 1987; **49**, 455.

63. Reed JC, Tsujimoto Y, Alpers JD, Croce CM, Nowell PC. *Science.* 1987; **236**, 1295.

64. Tsujimoto Y, Bashir MM, Givol I, Cossman J, Jaffe E, Croce CM. *Proceedings of the National Academy of Sciences USA.* 1987; **84**, 1329.

65. Gauwerky C, Haluska FG, Tsujimoto Y, Croce CM. *Proceedings of the National Academy of Sciences USA.* 1988; **85**, 8548.

66. Lee M-S, Chang K-S, Cabanillas F, Freireich EJ, Trujillo JM, Stass SA. *Science.* 1987; **237**, 175.

67. Van Den Berghe H, Vermaelen K, Louwagie A, Criel A, Mecucci C, Vaerman JP. *Cancer Genetics and Cytogenetics.* 1984; **11**, 381.

68. Tsujimoto Y, Yunis J, Onorato-Showe L, Erikson J, Nowell PC, Croce CM. *Science.* 1984; **224**, 1403.

69. Erikson J, Finan J, Tsujimoto Y, Nowell PC, Croce CM. *Proceedings of the National Academy of Sciences USA.* 1984; **81**, 4144.

70. Croce CM, Isobe M, Palumbo A, *et al. Science.* 1985; **227**, 1044.

71. Isobe M, Haluska FG, Russo G, Croce CM. *Proceedings of the National Academy of Sciences USA.* 1987; **85**, 3933.

72. Yancopoulos GD, Blackwell TK, Suh H, Hood L, Alt FW. *Cell.* 1986; **44**, 251.

73. Care A, Cianetti L, Giampolo A, *et al. EMBO Journal.* 1986; **5**, 905.

74. Hecht F, Morgan R, Hecht BK-M, Smith SD. *Science.* 1984; **226**, 1445.

75. Baer R, Chen K-C, Smith SD, Rabbitts TH. *Cell.* 1985; **43**, 705.

76. Denny CT, Yoshikai Y, Mak TW, Smith SD, Hollis GF, Kirsch IR. *Nature.* 1986; **320**, 549.

77. Reynolds TC, Smith SD, Sklar J. *Cell.* 1987; **50**, 107.

78. Russo G, Isobe M, Pegoraro C, Finan J, Nowell PC, Croce CM. *Cell.* 1988; **53**, 137.

79. Mengle-Gaw L, Williard HF, Smith CE, *et al. EMBO Journal.* 1987; **6**, 2273.

80. Erikson J, Finger L, Sun L, *et al. Science.* 1986; **232**, 884.

81. Finger LR, Harvey RC, Moore RCA, Showe LC, Croce CM. *Science.* 1986; **234**, 982

82. Kagan J, Finan J, Letofsky J, Besa EC, Nowell PC, Croce CM. *Proceedings of the National Academy of Sciences USA.* 1987; **84**, 4543.

83. Erikson J, Williams DL, Finan J, Nowell PC, Croce CM. *Science.* 1985; **299**, 784.

CHAPTER 7

MOLECULAR GENETIC MARKERS IN THE DIAGNOSIS AND CLASSIFICATION OF NON-HODGKIN'S LYMPHOMAS

Riccardo Dalla-Favera, Antonino Neri and Daniel M Knowles

In the last decade, molecular genetic techniques have been increasingly applied to resolve critical issues of human pathology. Perhaps for no human cancer is the impact of this technology more evident than for lymphoid neoplasms, where molecular genetic approaches have led to impressive advances both in understanding their pathogenesis and in improving diagnosis and classification.

Most of this progress has followed the elucidation of the structure and mechanism of expression of antigen receptor genes, i.e. immunoglobulin genes and T-cell receptor genes.[1-3] As part of the normal mechanism that produces antibody diversity these genes undergo somatic rearrangements which are unique and specific for each lymphoid cell and therefore can be used as irreversible genetic markers of their lineage and clonality.[4] The analysis of rearranged immunoglobulin and T-cell receptor genes has been instrumental in:

1. defining the lineage of neoplasms which are of controversial origin
2. determining the clonality, oligoclonality or polyclonality of various lymphoproliferative disorders
3. determining the stage of differentiation of normal and malignant B- and T-cell precursors
4. diagnosing and monitoring the clinical behaviour of lymphoid malignancies.

In addition, the identification of pathological recombinations between antigen receptor genes and various oncogenes in the context of tumour-specific chromosomal translocations has led to major advances in understanding the pathogenesis of lymphoid neoplasms. Molecular assays capable of recognizing these tumour-specific recombinations are currently being developed and may lead to significant improvements in the differential diagnosis and classification of these tumours.

In this chapter we review these different molecular markers and discuss their usage as diagnostic tools.

Antigen receptor gene rearrangements as markers of lymphoid lineage, clonality and differentiation

Molecular genetic approaches to the study of lymphoid neoplasia have been developed by exploiting a unique feature of lymphocytes: their ability to somatically rearrange and mutate their genome in order to be able to code for a virtually unlimited repertoire of antigen receptor molecules. Starting from a concise set of genes – immunoglobulin (Ig) genes active in B-cells and T-cell receptor genes (TCR) active in T-cells – more than 10^9 different molecules can be generated by the immune system using a comparably large number of newly assembled coding units.[1-3] Understanding the mechanisms involved in the diversification of Ig and TCR genes represents the basis for understanding the molecular genetic assays of lineage, clonality and differentiation of lymphoid cells.[4]

The germ line genome contains three known Ig genes – the heavy chain gene (Ig_H) and the two light chain (Ig_{Lk} and $Ig_{L\lambda}$) genes, and four known TCR genes (TCR α, β, γ, δ chain).[4–6]. Each gene is comprised of several coding domains which are discontinuously arranged in clusters along their respective chromosomes and which are then sequentially brought together by DNA rearrangements in order to produce functional genes in lymphocytes. These domains have analogous structural and functional features in both Ig and TCR genes, encoding variable (V), diversity (D) (only in Ig_H, TCR_β and TCR_δ), joining (J) and constant (C) regions. The first recombination step necessary to produce a functional Ig or TCR gene joins a V region to the adjacent D or J coding domains. In most cases a V region is directly joined to J region (V-J joining); for other genes (Ig_H, TCR_β), the J region is first joined to a D region and the resulting D-J segment is then joined to a V region (V-D-J joining). Since each V-J or V-D-J joining event involves the selection of one of many V regions (one thousand in the case of Ig_H genes) and one of several D and J regions, these rearrangements provide a first level of geometric expansion of the repertoire of functional Ig or TCR genes. A second level of expansion is provided by imprecision in the point of joining between V-D, D-J and V-J. Here a few nucleotides may be deleted or a few new nucleotides, known as N-regions, may be added. A third level of expansion occurs when Ig genes undergo point-mutations after rearrangement. These mutations, which mainly involve V region sequences, are thought to allow the selection during the immune response of genes coding for molecules displaying increased affinity for the antigen.

A consequence of these rearrangements and mutations is the appearance of novel DNA fragments that can be specifically recognized by molecular genetic techniques. These novel DNA sequences can be considered as markers of:

1. *Lineage:* antigen receptor gene rearrangement and expression is restricted to lymphoid lineages where, with some exceptions to be described below, Ig gene rearrangements occur in B-cells and TCR genes in T-cells. Therefore, the presence of these rearrangements distinguishes lymphoid elements from other haematopoietic and non-haematopoietic cells.

2. *Clonality:* a critical feature predicted by the genetic rearrangements is that any developing lymphocyte will possess a unique rearrangement, and that the progeny of a particular B- or T-cell will carry the same rearrangement as the parent cell. Therefore, if the cells in a given population all display the same rearrangement the population is a clonal expansion of a single lymphoid cell.

3. *Differentiation:* rearrangement and expression of different Ig and TCR genes occur at discrete stages of B- and T-cell development and follow a hierarchical order that correlates with discrete stages of lymphoid differentiation (Figs. 7.1 and 7.2). Therefore, Ig or TCR rearrangements can be used as markers of differentiation which in combination with immunophenotypic markers can be used in the diagnosis and classification of non-Hodgkin's lymphoma (NHL).

These concepts have been extensively applied to the analysis of malignant lymphoid

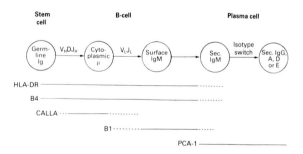

Fig. 7.1 Coordinate sequence of Ig gene rearrangements and parallel expression of cell-surface markers during B-cell development. Ig_H gene rearrangements ($V_H D J_H$) are followed by Ig_L gene requirements ($V_L J_L$), then expression of surface and secretory IgM molecules and eventually antibody isotype switch. These stages in Ig gene rearrangement and expression are paralleled by the acquisition of various cell surface marker antigens. Continuous lines indicate the presence of the marker and dashed lines indicate variable time of onset or disappearance.

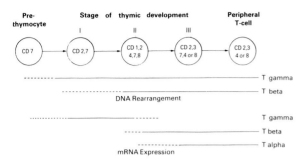

Fig. 7.2 Coordinate sequence of TCR rearrangements and expression and parallel expression of cell-surface markers during T-cell development. Stages of pre-thymic, thymic and post-thymic (peripheral T-cell) development have been identified based on the onset or disappearance of specific cell surface markers (CD). These maturation stages correlate with rearrangements and expression (mRNA) of various TCR genes. Continuous lines indicate the presence of TCR rearrangements or TCR mRNA, while dashed lines indicate variable times of occurrence of these events.

populations using the Southern blot hybridization technique.[7] A Southern blot is performed by first digesting cellular DNA with a restriction endonuclease – an enzyme which cuts the DNA molecules into fragments of specific lengths determined by the location of the sequence motif recognized by each enzyme. The various fragments are separated according to their size by gel electrophoresis, transferred to a nitrocellulose or nylon filter, and hybridized with labelled probes consisting of cloned segments of relevant genes. The hybridized fragments are visualized by autoradiography and their sizes compared to control DNA samples containing unrearranged (germ-line) genes. Examples of the use of these assays in the analysis of Ig_H, Ig_{Lk} and TCR_β gene rearrangements in non-lymphoid cells, in normal polyclonal lymphocytes and in biopsies from B- and T-cell malignancies are seen in Figs. 7.3 and 7.4, respectively.

Diagnostic applications of antigen receptor gene rearrangement analysis

Determination of the lineage of neoplastic cells

Extensive surveys of the frequency and patterns of Ig and TCR gene rearrangements have been performed on a wide array of human malignancies.[4] A summary of the results relative to the types of malignancies where clonal rearrangements have been found is reported in Table 7.1. This summary includes data on Ig_H, Ig_L, TCR_β and TCR_γ genes. Comprehensive data on the frequency of TCR_α and TCR_δ gene rearrangements are not available, due to the difficulty of analysis of the large TCR_α locus and to the only recent availability of TCR_δ probes.[6] Note that all the main types of lymphoid malignancies carry Ig or TCR gene rearrangement, and that for most tumour types the presence of *either* Ig *or* TCR gene rearrangements is consistent with the B- or T-lineage assignment determined by immunophenotypic analysis. For instance, a pattern involving rearrangement of Ig genes without rearrangement of TCR genes strongly supports a diagnosis of B lineage since it is found in the majority of tumours displaying B-cell specific markers.[8,9] On the other hand, a pattern involving rearrangements of TCR_β and/or TCR^γ is diagnostic of T lineage since it is consistently found in T-cell chronic lymphocytic leukaemia (T-CLL), T-NHL, adult T-cell leukaemia (ATL) and in the vast majority of T-cell adult lymphoblastic leukaemias (T-ALL).[10–12] In most cases, therefore, gene rearrangement analysis correctly predicts the B or T lineage of a given lymphoid malignancy.

In a sizeable number of cases, however, both Ig_H and TCR rearrangements are found in the same malignant population[13–17] and a fraction of immature myeloid and undifferentiated leukaemias also display clonal rearrangements of Ig_H or TCR genes.[18–22] It has been shown that TCR_γ gene arrangements and incomplete (D-J) Ig_H and TCR_β gene rearrangements are not entirely lineage restricted,[23,24] due most probably, to the presence of common

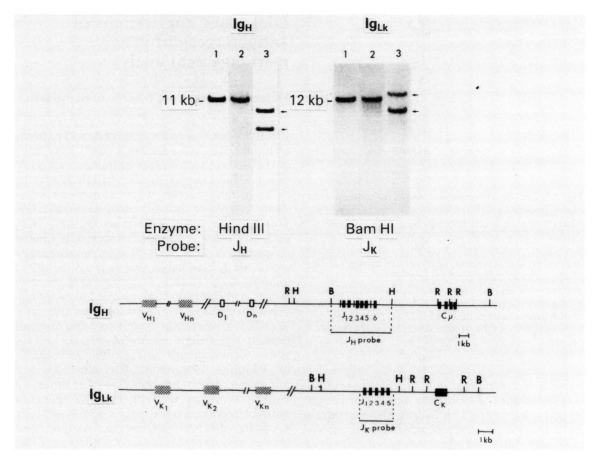

Fig. 7.3 Example of Ig gene rearrangement analysis by Southern blot hybridization. DNAs fron non-lymphoid cells (human fibroblasts, lanes 1) peripheral blood lymphocytes (lanes 2) and a B-NHL biopsy (lanes 3) are analysed using the indicated Ig probes and restriction endonucleases. Schematic representations of the Ig_H and Ig_{Lk} genes and the probes used are shown below. Restriction endonuclease sites are indicated as: R: EcoRI; BamHI; H: Hind III. Note that the germ-line configuration of both Ig_H and Ig_{Lk} genes is conserved in the non-lymphoid DNA (lanes 1) and in DNA derived from normal peripheral blood lymphocytes containing a small percentage of polyclonal Ig_{Lk} B-cells (lanes 2). Two rearrangement bands corresponding to clonal rearrangement of both the Ig_H and Ig_{Lk} alleles are present in DNA derived from the NHL biopsy (lanes 3). No germ-line Ig_H fragment is visible in this case indicating that the percentage of contaminating normal cells is below 5–10%.

recombinases capable of recognizing similar signal sequences within some Ig and TCR genes.[25] While this certainly complicates the use of these rearrangements as markers of lineage, it should be noted that, if IgL chain gene rearrangements are taken as markers of B-lineage commitment (without regard to the presence of TCR gene rearrangements) and TCR_δ and β (without regard to Ig_H) gene rearrangements are taken as marker of T-lineage commitment, there

is a high level of concordance between immuno-phenotypic and immunogenotypic lineage designation. Tumour types which cannot be un-equivocally assigned to either lineage by these criteria display a very immature (non-B non-T ALL) and/or a mixed (Ki-1[+]-NHL,AUL,TdT[+]-AML, *see* Table 7.1) phenotype which may reflect the accumulation of promiscuous rearrangements in cells frozen at an early stage of differentiation. Regardless of the mechanism

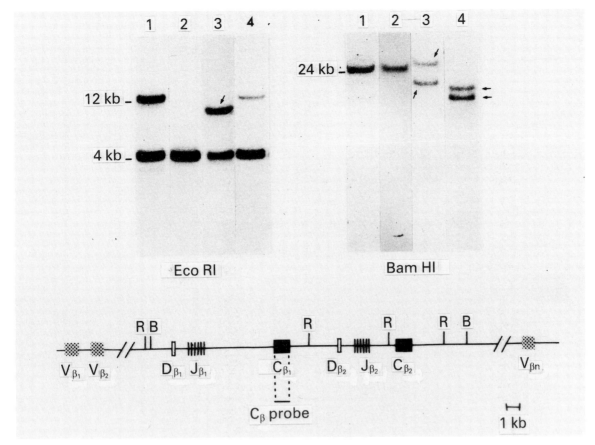

Fig. 7.4 Examples of TCR_β gene rearrangement analysis by Southern blot hybridization. DNAs from non-lymphoid cells (human fibroblasts, lanes 1), purified normal human T-lymphocytes (lanes 2), and biopsies from two T-NHL cases (lanes 3 and 4) were analysed using the indicated restriction endonucleases and a probe homologous to the constant region of TCR_β gene. This probe is highly homologous to the $C_{\beta 2}$ region and therefore recognizes two fragments (12kb: $C_{\beta 1}$; 4kb: $CB_{\beta 2}$) in EcoRI digested DNA. Note that in T lymphocytes both $D_{\beta 1}J_{\beta 1}$ and $D_{\beta 2}J_{\beta 2}$ rearrangements lead to the loss of the germ-line 12Kb $C_{\beta 1}$ fragment. Therefore, the absence or decreased intensity of this 12kB $C_{\beta 1}$ hybridization band indicates either a monoclonal or a polyclonal T-cell population. Note also that only clonal rearrangements involving $D_{\beta 1}J_{\beta 1}$ (case 3), but not those involving $D_{\beta 2}J_{\beta 2}$ (case 4), are detectable by EcoRI digestion, since the cross-hybridizing $C_{\beta 2}$ EcoRI fragment is not directly involved in the rearrangement. Therefore both EcoRI and BamHI digestion are necessary for a complete analysis. In lane 4 EcoRI, a faint band corresponding to the 12kb germ-line fragment indicates the presence of non-T cells contaminating the samples. Symbols for restriction endonucleases are as in Fig. 7.3.

involved, these observations clearly point toward the need for a combined immunophenotypic and immunogenotypic approach in order to determine the lineage of lymphoproliferative disorders.

For non-Hodgkin's lymphomas, however, the lineage specific pattern of rearrangements appear relatively well-conserved and, with the exception of Ki-1 positive NHL and possibly of a small minority of peripheral T-cell NHL,[26] the presence of either Ig_H and Ig_L or TCR_γ and TCR_β rearrangements correctly identifies the lineage of B- and T-NHL cases, respectively. This immunogenotypic analysis represents a useful complement to the lineage determination by classic immunophenotypic methods during

Table 7.1. Frequency of clonal Ig and TCR gene rearrangements in lymphoproliferative disorders*

Ig / TCR	– / –	H,L / –	H,L / γ and/or β	H / –	H / γ and/or β	– / γ	– / γ,β
NHL							
B-NHL	–	60	40	–	–	–	–
T-NHL	–	–	–	–	–	–	100
Ki-1+NHL	–	–	–	–	80	–	20
*MM**	–	100	–	–	–	–	–
*ALL**							
B-ALL	–	70	20	–	10	–	–
T-ALL	5	–	–	–	20	–	75
Non-B-non-T-ALL	5	–	–	30	65	–	–
*ATL**	–	–	–	–	–	–	100
*CLL**							
B-CLL	–	75	25	–	–	–	–
T-CLL	–	–	–	–	–	–	100
Tγ-LPD	10	–	–	–	–	5	90
*AML**	70	–	–	5	15	5	5
*AUL**	–	–	–	–	100	–	–
*HD**	100‡	–	–	–	–	–	–
Suggested Lineage	–	B	B	pre-B?	pre-B? pre-T?	Pre-T?	T

* The distribution of patterns of antigen receptor (Ig$_H$, Ig$_L$, TCR$_\beta$, TCR$_\gamma$) rearrangements within major types of lymphoproliferative diseases identified by immunophenotypic analysis is expressed as per cent (approximate) of the total number of cases examined.

** NHL: B-cell (B-NHL), T-cell (NHL) non-Hodgkin's lymphoma.
MM: multiple myeloma.
ALL: B-cell (B-ALL), T-cell (T-ALL), null and common (non-B-non-T-ALL) acute lymphoblastic leukaemia.
ATL: adult T-cell leukaemia.
CLL: B-cell (B-CLL), T-cell (T-CLL) chronic lymphocytic leukaemia; TγLPD: Tγ-lymphoproliferative disorder.
AML: acute myeloblastic leukaemia.
AUL: acute undifferentiated leukaemia.
HD: Hodgkin's disease.

‡ This percentage refers to the absence of rearrangements representing major (>50%) clonal lymphoid population in the biopsy (*see* text).

routine diagnostic procedures. In addition, this method has been instrumental in clearly establishing the lineage derivation of T-cell lymphoma cases with peculiar immunocytochemical and morphological characteristics such as Lennert's lymphoma.[27]

Determination of clonality

Perhaps the most important application of the analysis of antigen receptor gene rearrangements involves the distinction among polyclonal, oligoclonal and monoclonal lymphoproliferative disorders. Since clonality appears to be a critical feature of malignancy, the possibility of unequivocally determining the clonality of a given lymphoid population has several important diagnostic and pathogenetic implications. At least three assays of clonality have been traditionally available, but all of them have significant drawbacks. The demonstration of specific chromosomal abnormalities[28] represents a laborious assay which requires specialized technical skill and cannot be applied to those cases that appear to be karyotypically normal. A second method, based on the identification of single glucose-6-phosphate dehydrogenase alleles in tumour cells,[29] can be applied only to heterozygous females. Finally, a more widely applicable determination of clonality, based on unbalanced IgLκ or Lλ chain expression[30] also has serious limitations because it is difficult to apply to tumour cases containing mixed lymphoid populations with a minority of tumour cells and, most notably, because it is not applicable to B-cell tumours which do not express surface Ig, or T-cell tumours.

Compared to these approaches, the analysis of Ig and TRC gene rearrangements by means of Southern blot hybridization has the advantages of:

1. relative technical ease
2. applicability to all individuals
3. applicability to both B- and T-cell tumours regardless of the expression of Ig or TCR genes
4. applicability to pathological biopsies containing clonal populations as small as 1–5 per cent of the total cell sample (*see* below).

This method of analysis is now part of 'state of the art' diagnostic procedures and has also been instrumental in resolving controversies on the clonality of a number of diseases including chronic lymphocytic leukaemia,[31,32] angioimmunoblastic lymphoadenopathy,[33] mycosis fungoides,[34] dermatopathic lymphadenopathy,[34] and lymphomatoid papulosis.[35]

With respect to malignant lymphoma, the analysis of Ig and TCR gene rearrangements has a critical role in several diagnostic contexts. Although in the majority of cases the diagnosis of non-Hodgkin's lymphomas is unambiguous, a significant proportion of cases presents serious diagnostic challenges because the differential diagnosis encompasses disease entities requiring dramatically different therapeutic interventions. In the diagnostic examination of *nodal* biopsies the immunogenotypic analysis of clonality represents a critical complement to morphological and immunophenotypic examination in all those cases in which the differential diagnosis between lymphoma and reactive lymphoid hyperplasia is problematic. Perhaps even more crucial is the role of antigen receptor gene rearrangement analysis in the diagnosis of extranodal biopsies containing lymphoid infiltrates. In such cases the differential diagnosis between clonal, malignant, well-differentiated lymphocytic lymphoma and polyclonal, presumably benign, pseudolymphoma is traditionally difficult. This is particularly true for small lymphocytic infiltrates of the ocular adnexae, and lung, and, to a lesser extent, gastrointestinal tract, skin, and salivary glands.[36] In all these cases the detection of a clonal population by Ig or TCR gene rearrangement represents a highly objective diagnostic criterion which helps in substantiating a diagnosis based on more subjective morphological criteria.[37]

Immunogenotypic determination of clonality can be applied not only for diagnostic purposes but also for the clinical monitoring of disease. As shown in Fig. 7.5 Southern blot hybridization analysis using DNA probes radiolabelled at high specific activity allows the detection of a clonal lymphoid population representing as little as 1–5 per cent of the pathological specimen. Although

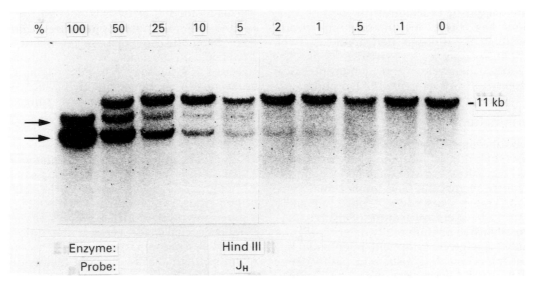

Fig. 7.5 Sensitivity of clonality assay based on Ig_H gene rearrangement analysis. DNA from a B-NHL cell line was serially diluted with DNA from non-lymphoid cells to mimic the presence of various amounts of contaminating non-malignant cells in a tumour biopsy. DNAs were then analysed as in Fig. 7.3. The two hybridization bands corresponding to clonally rearranged Ig_H alleles in B-NHL DNA can still be detected when tumour DNA constitutes as little as 1–5% of the sample.

this level of sensitivity is not significantly higher than that obtained by standard morphological or immunophenotype analysis, the specificity of the molecular assay is definitely higher. In fact, this approach has already been proven of some utility in the diagnosis of bone marrow infiltration and in the detection of minimal residual disease, both for monitoring the effects of therapy and for the early detection of relapse.[37–41] It is, however, likely that the widespread application of these assays to the clinical monitoring of lymphoma awaits the development of new technologies allowing a level of sensitivity substantially higher than that currently obtainable.

While in most cases the presence of a major clonal lymphoid population reflects a malignant lymphoma, two alternative situations which can be encountered deserve discussion because of their important clinical and biological implications. First, gene rearrangement patterns suggesting the presence of more than one clonal population may be detectable. These cases require careful analysis since only in a limited number of them have biclonal tumours been de-

monstrated. In most instances, mutations occurring during tumour development are responsible for either the multiple concurrent or temporally distinct patterns of rearrangements.[42–45] Second, a clonal lymphoid population does not necessarily imply the presence of a malignant lymphoma since clonality is a necessary but not sufficient feature of malignancy. In fact, the presence of monoclonal or oligoclonal lymphoid populations has been demonstrated in the absence of malignancy in a number of clinicopathological situations including post-transplant immunosuppression, acquired immunodeficiency syndrome (AIDS) and angioimmunoblastic lymphadenopathy.[46–49] In these situations the expansion of 'benign' clonal B-cell populations in the absence of clinically evident malignancy may reflect escape from impaired immunosurveillance mechanisms, which allow the growth of cells altered by chronic antigenic stimulation and/or by viruses, most often Epstein–Barr virus.[46–49] Despite their apparent benign character these clonal populations may nevertheless represent potential substrates for additional genetic alterations that can lead to malignancy, since all the above-mentioned diseases are accompanied by a significantly increased frequency of lymphoma.[46–49]

AIDS presents a particularly intriguing example of the presence of oligoclonality in the absence of malignancy and of the use of antigen receptor gene rearrangement analysis for monitoring these phenomena. As shown in Fig. 7.6, oligoclonal B-cell expansions are detectable by Ig gene rearrangement analysis in nodal biopsies from AIDS-associated lymphadenopathy syndrome (LAS) cases as well as in AIDS-associated non-Hodgkin's lymphoma (AIDS-NHL) biopsies in which a major clonal population is also detectable. These multiple B-cell clones do not represent malignant clones, yet they may represent a compartment at increased risk for the occurrence of the genetic alteration which is characteristic of AIDS-NHL, i.e. the chromosomal translocation and resultant rearrangement of the c-*myc* oncogene locus.[49,50] In fact, this alteration is not detectable in LAS biopsies while it is detectable in a single major B-cell clone in AIDS-NHL biopsies (*see* Fig. 7.6).

Antigen receptor gene rearrangement analysis has also been applied to investigate the clonality and the possible lymphoid lineage of Reed-Sternberg (RS) cells in Hodgkin's disease (HD). The results of these investigations have been quite controversial since evidence of sizeable clonal populations identified by rearrangements of Ig or TCR genes has been reported by some groups in a significant percentage of cases,[51–53] while no clonal lymphoid populations or only minor ones (< 5 per cent) have been found by others.[54–56] Possible explanations for these discrepancies may include differences in (i) diagnostic criteria for HD; (ii) sensitivity of hybridization techniques; (iii) interpretation of percentage of clonal cells. Representative results of our screening are shown in Fig. 7.7 where the comparative analysis of typical panels of NHL and HD biopsies are shown. It can be seen that, while a major (> 70 per cent) clonal B-cell population is clearly identified by a relatively intense hybridization signal detectable in all NHL biopsies, HD biopsies representative of different HD subtypes are consistently characterized by the absence of any clonal rearrange-

ments or, in a minority of cases, by faint hybridization signals reflecting the presence of minor (< 10 per cent) clonal B-cell populations. These

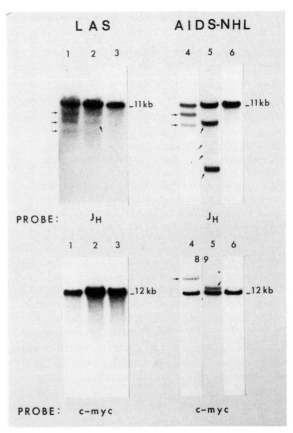

Fig. 7.6 Identification of oligoclonal, monoclonal and malignant populations by Ig and oncogene rearrangement analysis. DNAs extracted from nodal biopsies of two patients with AIDS-related lymphadenopathy syndrome (lanes 1,2), from control non-lymphoid DNA (LAS, lanes 3,6) and from nodal biopsies of two patients with AIDS-NHL (lane 4,5) were analysed for Ig_H (top panels Ig_H probe) and c-*myc* oncogene (bottom panels, c-*myc* probe) rearrangements. *Minor* oligoclonal populations are detectable by Ig_H gene rearrangement analysis in both LAS and AIDS-NHL biopsies (lane 5). In AIDS-NHL biopsies at least one major clonal population is also identifiable. In AIDS-NHL, but not in LAS, c-*myc* oncogene rearrangement analysis identifies a clonal population carrying a c-*myc* allele rearranged as a consequence of a tumour-specific chromosomal translocation event.

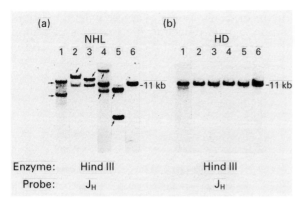

Fig. 7.7 Immunoglobulin gene rearrangement analysis in Hodgkin's disease (HD). DNAs from several NHL and HD biopsies were analysed for Ig_H gene rearrangement. Note the consistent presence of rearrangement bands representing abundant (>70%) clonal B-cell populations in NHL biopsies. In HD biopsies, such bands are either entirely absent or occasionally present (lane 1, HD) as faint bands representing 10% or less of the biopsy population.

clonal cells do not appear to be RS cells since no clonal lymphoid population was detectable in a set of exceptional HD biopsies containing more than 30 per cent RS cells.[54] Based on these results we have suggested that antigen receptor gene rearrangement analysis may be helpful for the sometimes difficult differential diagnosis between NHL and HD. This should be considered as a working hypothesis for additional extensive studies investigating the presence, relative abundance and the potential clinicopathological and prognostic correlations of clonal lymphoid populations in HD. In the meantime, a practical and conservative integration of all the available results would suggest that the absence of clonal Ig or TCR gene rearrangements in a biopsy considered for differential diagnosis between NHL and HD indicates a diagnosis of HD, whereas the presence of clonal Ig or TCR rearrangements under the same circumstances, although suggestive of NHL, cannot be considered as an unequivocal diagnostic marker.

Oncogene rearrangements as genetic markers of malignancy

As described in detail elsewhere in this book malignant lymphomas are associated with non-random chromosomal abnormalities.[57] It has been repeatedly predicted that these chromosomal abnormalities play a pathogenetic role in lymphomagenesis and that the association of NHL with different types of abnormalities could serve as a diagnostic criterion based on pathogenetic mechanisms rather than on phenotypic characteristics.[58] A continuously increasing body of experimental evidence based on the molecular analysis of some of these chromosomal aberrations is beginning to confirm these predictions. Oncogenes have been found adjacent to chromosomal breakpoints in a number of well-characterized cases and the structural and functional alterations caused by chromosomal breakages are consistent with their role in tumour development. These findings, which are discussed in detail in Chapter 5, are contributing significantly to our understanding of the pathogenesis of NHL. In addition, these studies have led to the identification of molecular probes capable of specifically recognizing novel DNA sequences generated by the chromosomal breakpoints. These novel sequences can be considered as a second generation of molecular genetic markers potentially capable of identifying not only lineage and clonality, but also malignancy and the type of lesion involved in malignancy. Although currently in development and still applicable only to a limited set of NHL cases, molecular assays based on these markers deserve discussion because of their potential usefulness as diagnostic and prognostic tools.

At least two NHL-specific chromosomal aberrations have been extensively characterized at the molecular level (*see* Chapter 5) and represent classic examples of this approach. In the endemic and sporadic forms of Burkitt's lymphoma (BL), in AIDS-associated NHL and in L3-type acute lymphoblastic leukaemia, reciprocal chromosomal translocations (t(8;14), t(2;8) and t(8;22)) involving the c-*myc* oncogene locus on chromosome 8 and Ig loci on chromosomes 14 (IgH), 2(IgLκ) or 22 (IgLλ) are consistently found.[59–61] In the sporadic form of BL and in AIDS-NHL the (8;14) translocation joins the c-*myc* locus to Ig_H switch sequences[62–64] generating a novel DNA fragment which can be recognized by Southern blot hybridization using c-*myc* specific probes (*see* Fig. 7.6). In NHL of follicle centre origin, both of diffuse and follicular growth pattern, pathological recombinations between J sequences within the Ig_H locus and the *bcl*-2 locus on chromosome 14 are frequently found.[64–66] Using probes specific for different breakpoint clusters around the *bcl*-2 gene these recombinations can be detected as rearrangements of the *bcl*-2 locus.[67,68] A number of other chromosomal translocations involving pathological recombinations between Ig or TCR gene and different oncogenes are currently under investigation and it is conceivable that molecular probes capable of detecting most tumour-associated aberrations, and thus most NHL types, will become available.

The use of these probes in the diagnosis and classification of NHL would, in many respects, represent significant progress compared to presently available Ig- or TCR-based assays. First, unlike physiological Ig or TCR gene rearrangements, oncogene translocations/rearrangements represent tumour-specific markers which have never been found in normal or pre-malignant cells. The data shown in Fig. 7.6 exemplify how oncogene rearrangements can identify the presence of a malignant clone among other clonally expanded yet non-malignant lymphoid cells. Second, oncogene rearrangements not only identify the malignant clone but also the genetic lesion which is involved in tumour development. Diagnostic classification based on pathogenetic mechanisms rather than on phenotypic characteristics may provide more biologically meaningful prognostic and therapeutic criteria. Third, because these cytogenetic aberrations create interchromosomal junctions which are presumably unique to tumour cells, they can be detected by the recently developed polymerase chain reaction method.[69] This method can detect a given chromosomal translocation even when present in only one part per 10^5–10^6 of the analysed cell population.[70] Comparing the sensitivity of this approach with that obtained using Southern blot hybridization (1 per cent) and considering its specificity for the malignant clone, it is reasonable to expect that the use of the polymerase chain reaction will substantially influence present biological and clinical concepts of minimal residual disease.

Summary and perspectives

The elucidation of the structure and mechanism of expression of various antigen receptor genes has allowed rapid progress in the development of molecular genetic assays for the diagnosis and classification of lymphoid malignancies. The use of rearrangements of immunoglobulin and T-cell receptor genes as markers of clonality represents substantial progress compared to previously available methods and allows a number of well-established applications, mostly in the diagnosis of non-Hodgkin's lymphomas. However, the application of these assays to the clinical monitoring of these malignancies, i.e. to the detection of minimal residual disease after treatment and/or during remission, is still limited because their sensitivity is only marginally higher than that obtained using currently available pathological methods. Antigen receptor gene rearrangements can also be helpful for the determination of B- or T-cell lineage derivation but, due to the lineage promiscuity of some rearrangement mechanisms, correct lineage determination requires a combined immunophenotypic and immunogenotypic evaluation.

A second generation of molecular genetic markers derived from the analysis of specific human chromosomal translocations involving antigen receptor genes and several oncogenes is in rapid development. These markers will allow the development of molecular assays for the determination of clonality as well as malignancy and type of pathogenetic alteration. These assays are expected to be significantly more specific and sensitive than any currently available morphological, immunphenotypic, or immunogenotypic method.

Acknowledgements

We are grateful to several collaborators, namely Pier-Giuseppe Pelicci, Milayna Subar and Frances Flug, for contributing some of the experimental work on which this chapter is based. This work was supported by grants from the National Institute of Health (CA44029 to RD-F, EYO6337 and CA49236 to DMK) and by a Scholarship of the Leukemia Society of America (to RD-F).

References

1. Tonegawa S. *Nature.* 1983; **301**, 575.
2. Leder P. *Scientific American.* 1982; **246**, 72.
3. Hood L, Kronenberg M, Hunkapiller T. *Cell.* 1985; **40**, 225.
4. Waldmann TA. In: Dixon EJ, ed. *Advances in Immunology*, vol. 40, New York, Academic Press, 1987; 247.
5. Toyonaga B, Mak TW. *Annual Review of Immunology.* 1987; **5**, 585.
6. Takihara Y, Champagne E, Griesser H, et al. *European Journal of Immunology.* 1988; **18**, 283.
7. Southern EM. *Journal of Molecular Biology.* 1975; **98**, 503.
8. Arnold A, Cossman J, Bakhshi A, et al. *New England Journal of Medicine.* 1983; **309**, 1593.
9. Cleary ML, Chao J, Warnke R, Sklar J. *Proceedings of the National Academy of Sciences USA.* 1984; **81**, 539.
10. Flug F, Pelicci P-G, Bonetti F, et al. *Proceedings of the National Academy of Sciences USA.* 1985; **82**, 3460.
11. Waldman TW, Davis MM, Bongionvanni KF, et al. *New England Journal of Medicine.* 1985; **313**, 776.
12. Minden MD, Toyonaga B, Ha K, et al. *Proceedings of the National Academy of Sciences.* 1985; **82**, 1224.
13. Kitchingman GR, Rovigatti U, Maner AM, et al. *Blood.* 1985; **65**, 725.
14. Pelicci P-G, Knowles DM II, Dalla-Favera R. *Journal of Experimental Medicine.* 1985; **162**, 1015.
15. Tawa A, Hozumi N, Minden M, et al. *New England Journal of Medicine.* 1985; **312**, 1033.
16. Chen Z, Le Paslier D, Dausset J. *Journal of Experimental Medicine.* 1987; **165**, 1000.
17. Subar M, Pelicci P-G, Neri A, et al. *Leukemia.* 1988; **2**, 19.
18. Rovigatti U, Mirro J, Kitchingham G, et al. *Blood.* 1984; **63**, 1023.
19. Ha K, Minden M, Hozumi N, et al. *Cancer Research.* 1984; **44**, 4658.
20. Seremetis SV, Pelicci P-G, Tabilio A, et al. *Journal of Experimental Medicine.* 1987; **165**, 1703.
21. Foa R, Casorati G, Giubellino ML, et al. *Journal of Experimental Medicine.* 1987; **165**, 879.
22. Cheng G, Minden MD, Mak TW, et al. *Journal of Experimental Medicine.* 1986; **163**, 414.
23. Yancopoulos GD, Alt F. *Annual Review of Immunology.* 1986; **4**, 339.
24. Tawa A, Hozumi N, Minden M, Mak TW, Gelfand EW. *New England Journal of Medicine.* 1985; **313**, 1033.
25. Yancopoulos GD, Blackwell KT, Sah H, et al. *Cell.* 1986; **44**, 251.
26. Weiss LM, Picker LJ, Grogan TM, et al. *American Journal of Pathology.* 1988; **130**, 436.
27. Feller AC, Griesser H, Mak TW, Lennert K. *Blood.* 1986; **86**, 663.
28. Rowley JD, Fukuharas S. *Seminars in Oncology.* 1980; **7**, 255.
29. Fialkow PJ, Klein E, Klein G, et al. *Journal of Experimental Medicine.* 1973; **138**, 89.
30. Levy R, Warnke R, Dorfman RF, Haimovich J. *Journal of Experimental Medicine.* 1977; **45**, **1014**.
31. Foa R, Pellici PG, Migone N, et al. *Blood.* 1986; **67**, 247.
32. Aisenberg AC, Krontiris TG, Mak TW, Wilkes BM. *New England Journal of Medicine.* 1985; **313**, 529.
33. Lipford EH, Smith HR, Pittaluga S, et al. *Journal of Clinical Investigation.* 1987; **79**, 637.
34. Weiss LM, Hu E, Wood GS, et al. *New England Journal of Medicine.* 1985; **313**, 539.
35. Weiss LM, Wood GS, Trela M, et al. *New England Journal of Medicine.* 1986; 315, **475**.
36. Knowles DM. *Seminars in Diagnostic Pathology.* 1985; **2**, 14.
37. Neri A, Jakobiec FA, Pelicci P-G, et al. *Blood.* 1987; **70**, 1519.
38. Swanson G, Hu E, Sklar J, Levitt LJ. *Blood.* 1985; **66**, 246a.
39. Zehnbauer BA, Pardoll DM, Burke PJ, Graham ML, Vogelstein B. *Blood.* 1986; **67**, 835.
40. Wright JJ, Poplack DG, Bakhski A, et al. *Journal of Clinical Oncology.* 1987; **5**, 735.
41. Bregni M, Siena S, Dalla-Favera R, Gianni AM. *Annals of the New York Academy of Sciences.* 1987; 473.
42. Sklar J, Cleary ML, Thielmans K, et al. *New England Journal of Medicine.* 1984; **311**, 20.
43. Siegelman MH, Cleary ML, Warnke R, et al. *Journal of Experimental Medicine.* 1985; **161**, 850.
44. Raffeld M, Neckers LM, Longo DL, et al. *New England Journal of Medicine.* 1985; **312**, 1653.
45. Meeker T, Lowder J, Cleary ML, et al. *New England Journal of Medicine.* 1985; **312**, 1658.

46. Shearer WT, Ritz J, Fibegold M, *et al. New England Journal of Medicine.* 1985; **312**, 1151.
47. Fizzera G, Hanto DW, Gaji-Peczalska KJ, *et al. Cancer Research.* 1981; **41**, 4262.
48. Starzl TE, Porter KA, Iwatsuki S, *et al. Lancet.* 1984; i, 583.
49. Pelicci P-G, Knowles DM, Arlin ZA, *et al. Journal of Experimental Medicine.* 1986; **164**, 2049.
50. Subar M, Neri A, Inghirami G, *et al. Blood.* 1988; **72**, 667.
51. Weiss LM, Strickler JG, Hu E, *et al. Human Pathology.* 1986; **17**, 1009.
52. Sundeen J, Lipford E, Uppenkamp M, *et al. Blood.* 1987; **70**, 96.
53. Griesser H, Feller AC, Mak TW, Lennert K. *International Journal of Cancer.* 1987; **40**; 157.
54. Knowles DM, Neri A, Pelicci P-G, *et al. Proceedings of the National Academy of Sciences.* 1986; **83**, 7942.
55. Roth MS, Schnitzer B, Bingham EL, *et al. American Journal of Pathology.* 1988; **131**, 331.
56. Raghavachar A, Binder T, Bertram CR. *Cancer Research.* 1988; **48**, 3591.
57. Junis JJ, Oken MM, Kaplan ME, *et al. New England Journal of Medicine.* 1982; **307**, 1231.
58. Klein G, Klein E. *Nature.* 1985; **315**, 190.
59. Dalla-Favera R, Bregni M, Erikson J, *et al. Proceedings of the National Academy of Sciences, USA.* 1982; **79**, 7824.
60. Taub R, Kirsch I, Morton C, *et al. Proceedings of the National Academy of Sciences, USA.* 1982; **79**, 7837.
61. Dalla-Favera R, Neri A, Cesarman E, Lombardi L. In: Gale RP, Golde DW eds. *Recent Advances in Leukemia and Lymphoma.* New York: Alan R Liss, 1987; 165.
62. Pelicci PG, Magrath I, Knowles DM, Dalla-Favera R. *Proceedings of the National Academy of Sciences USA.* 1986; **83**, 2984.
63. Neri A, Bariiga F, Knowles DM, Magrath I, Dalla-Favera R. *Proceedings of the National Academy of Sciences USA.* 1988; **85**, 9268.
64. Tsujimoto Y, Finger LR, Yunis J, *et al. Science.* 1984; **226**, 1097.
65. Bakshi A, Jensen JP, Goldman P, *et al. Cell.* 1985; **41**, 899.
66. Cleary ML, Smith SD, Sklar J. *Cell.* **47**, 19.
67. Tsujimoto Y, Cossman J, Jaffe E. *et al. Science.* 1985; **228**, 1440.
68. Lee MS, Blink MB, Pathak S, *et al. Blood.* 1987; **70**, 90.
69. Saiki R, Sahrf S, Faloona F, *et al. Science.* 1985; **230**, 1350.
70. Lee MS, Chang KS, Cabanillas F, *et al. Science.* 1987; **237**, 175.

CHAPTER 8

PATHOGENESIS OF NON-HODGKIN'S LYMPHOMAS: CLUES FROM GEOGRAPHY

Dennis H Wright

The geographical distribution of neoplasms may provide clues to their aetiology and many of the more common carcinomas show major variations in incidence throughout the world. Changes in incidence in migrant populations suggest that these variations are usually due to environmental, rather than genetic factors. In comparing cancer incidence in different communities, allowance must be made for the availability and quality of diagnostic services and the age structure of the population at risk. Studies of the epidemiology of malignant lymphomas have been handicapped by variations in the terminology and classification systems used and by the very high incidence of histological inaccuracy in diagnosing these neoplasms. The ICDO classification which, until the ninth revision, divided non-Hodgkin's lymphomas into only two categories (lymphosarcoma and reticulum cell sarcoma) makes geographical comparisons based on these data almost meaningless. Consequently, much of the epidemiology of non-Hodgkin's lymphomas is derived from the study of tumour syndromes that have unique features, causing them to stand out from the background of lymphoreticular tumours.

Burkitt's lymphoma (BL)

The delineation of the tumour syndrome, now known as BL, was the result of pioneering observations made by Denis Burkitt while working as a government surgeon in Uganda.[1] Examples of this tumour were recorded in the medical records of Mengo Mission Hospital at the turn of the century[2] and sporadic cases were recorded in the medical literature from Africa before Burkitt's first publication in 1958. Burkitt was the first to note that the jaw tumours and abdominal lymphomas seen in African children were part of the same tumour syndrome and to note the restricted geographical distribution of the tumour in Africa.

Jaw tumours are age dependent, occurring most frequently at 3 years of age and falling progressively in incidence thereafter, to a frequency of about 10 per cent at age 15.[3] In Uganda the mean age of diagnosis of BL is 7 years and the overall incidence of jaw tumours is 50 per cent. The low incidence of jaw tumours recorded in some reports of BL might be related to the older age of the patients in these studies. The jaw tumours form a highly characteristic feature of the tumour on which the epidemiological studies could be based. Solitary jaw tumours may be superficially mimicked by other tumours but the more characteristic multiple tumours, with loosening and shedding of the teeth, are almost pathognomonic of BL.

Other features of the tumour, such as thyroid involvement and bilateral renal (95 per cent), ovarian (75 per cent) and testicular involvement, in children of the appropriate age, are almost as pathognomonic. Combinations of these tumours are frequently seen, increasing yet further the certainty of clinical diagnosis. It was on these features that Burkitt was able to map the distribution of the tumour in Africa and to show its dependence on temperature and humidity with restriction to the wet tropics. This restriction was the feature that led to the proposition that BL is due to an infectious agent and that set in train the search for an aetiological virus.

Burkitt's lymphoma has a characteristic cytology and histology.[4] Essentially it is composed of rounded blast cells with intensely basophilic cytoplasm (rich in polyribosomes), often containing lipid droplets. Typically the histology shows sheets of these blast cells, exhibiting a high mitotic rate and a corresponding high rate of cell death with many apoptotic nuclei. The tumour cells are usually interpersed with prominent, vacuolated, phagocytic macrophages giving a characteristic 'starry-sky' pattern to the tumour. Cell kinetic studies have shown that almost 100 per cent of BL cells are in cycle and that they have a doubling time of 24–48 hours. This phenomenal growth rate is consistent with the rapid clinical progression of the tumour and the high mitotic rate seen in histological sections.

Immunological studies have shown that BL cells have membrane immunoglobulin,[5] placing them in the B-cell lineage, further along the differentiation pathway than B-lymphoblastic lymphomas which either express no immunoglobulin or contain cytoplasmic μ chains only. Burkitt's lymphoma cells show rearrangement of immunoglobulin genes consistent with their B-cell lineage. The majority also show a characteristic chromosomal translocation between chromosome 8, at the site of the *myc* proto-oncogene, and chromosome 14, at the site of the immunoglobulin heavy chain genes. Less commonly, translocations are seen between chromosome 8 and chromosome 2 (site of kappa light chain gene) or chromosome 22 (site of lambda light chain gene).[6]

Soon after BL was reported from tropical Africa a search was made for similar tumours elsewhere in the world. The tumour was found to occur in Papua, New Guinea, at a similar frequency to that seen in Africa.[7] In Papua, New Guinea, the tumour appeared to be restricted by similar parameters of temperature and humidity, as seen in Africa, with few tumours occurring in the relatively arid region around Port Morsby and in the cool mountainous highlands. Apart from Africa and Papua, New Guinea, the tumour was described sporadically from many countries throughout the world. Table 8.1 shows the incidence of BL in various countries. The incidence rate appears to be of the order of 100 times greater in tropical Africa than the USA.

Most of the non-African cases were identified as BL on the basis of histology and some showed very similar features to the African cases with jaw tumours and extensive visceral involvement in the absence of peripheral lymphadenopathy.[15] The establishment of the American Burkitt Lymphoma Registry, however, allowed the comparison of a carefully evaluated series of non-African cases with the African disease. When this was undertaken, it became apparent that, although some American cases showed similarities to the African cases, as a group they showed a number of significant differences. In particular, they had a lower incidence of jaw tumours and a higher incidence of tumours in the nasopharynx and terminal ileum.[13,16] Similarly, in the Middle East, histologically identified patients with BL have a high incidence of abdominal tumours with a predilection for the ileocaecal region,[17] a site rarely involved in African cases.[18] Is this a different tumour in terms of histogenesis, or are the different anatomical sites of predilection a result of different aetiological factors?

These differences in the clinical features of BL in African and non-African cases raise the problem of how BL should be defined. As stated above, the clinical features alone were characteristic enough to permit the delineation of the tumour distribution in tropical Africa, but they would not be precise enough to identify borderline cases or to allow for possible variations due to environmental factors. Since most neoplasms are categorized according to their histogenesis it might be worth trying to define BL on this basis.

Burkitt's lymphoma is a B-cell lymphoma with blastic morphology and a high replication rate. The unusual anatomical distribution of the tumour has led to the suggestion that it is

Table 8.1. Incidence of Burkitt's lymphoma in children

Country and years	Rate per 10^5 defined population per year	Reference
Uganda (1964–1968)	0–6.0	8
Ibadan, Nigeria (1960–1966)	7.6 (11.2 males, 4.0 females)	9
North Mara, Tanzania (1964–1971)	5.7 (6.2 males, 5.1 females)	10
Papua, New Guinea (1962–1971)		7
Lowlands	0.5–1.8	
Highlands	0.07–0.17	
Islands	0.1–1.1	
Israel (1967–1968)	0.43 (0.62 males, 0.22 females)	11
USA		
TNCS* 1969–1971	0.06	12
SEER** 1973–1977	0.10	13

* TNCS, Third National Cancer Survey
** SEER, Surveillance, Epidemiology and End Results Study
Table reprinted from Parkin DM, Sohier R, O'Conor GT.[14]

derived from the mucosa-associated lymphoid tissue, rather than nodal or follicle centre cell lymphocytes.[19] One piece of evidence in favour of this hypothesis is the massive involvement of the breasts, analogous to the migration of mucosa-associated lymphocytes to the breasts, in females who develop BL during pregnancy or lactation.[20] It is proposed that a similar migration of mucosa-associated lymphocytes occurs to the jaws at the time of active tooth development and that this accounts for the age-related involvement of the jaws by BL.

Unfortunately, no subset markers exist to identify the putative lineage of cells that give rise to BL. Morphology alone, even on the best quality preparations, will not reliably identify all cases of BL. It is apparent that, although pathologists can differentiate between lympho-blastic lymphoma and BL, they cannot reliably differentiate between BL and similar blastic tumours (undifferentiated non-Burkitt's).[21] The characteristic chromosomal translocations found in BL may occur in other B-cell lymphomas and

cannot be used as the diagnostic hallmark for BL. The cases recorded in the American Burkitt Lymphoma Registry[13] probably consist of at least two groups of blastic tumours with similar light microscopic morphology, but different clinical behaviour. One of these groups may be equivalent to African BL.

The apparent temperature and humidity dependence of African BL led to the hypothesis that it might be caused by an insect-vectored virus.[22] However, all attempts to implicate known arboviruses were in vain. Eventually a previously unknown herpes virus, the Epstein–Barr virus (EBV), was identified in cultured tumour cells from Ugandan cases of BL.[23] It is a paradox that the search for the cause of a geographically localized tumour had led to the discovery of the most widespread virus known. Epstein–Barr virus exhibits many features that suggest it is an oncogenic virus. It immortalizes B lymphocytes in culture, enabling them to grow continuously without the addition of growth factors. It causes intense lymphoproliferation in some patients[24] and in sub-human primates.[25,26]

Virtually all African children with Burkitt's lymphoma have high antibody titres to EBV. The virus genome can be identified in the tumour cells by DNA hybridization and virus particles can be identified in the tumour cells under suitable culture conditions. How then can a virus that causes lifelong infection, in almost the whole of the human population, be responsible for a climate-dependent African tumour? Epstein–Barr virus isolates from African cases of BL have not shown significant differences from isolates made elsewhere in the world. The pattern of EBV infection does, however, appear to differ in Africa from that in other parts of the world in that it is acquired at a very young age.[27] In the West Nile district of Uganda, an area of high prevalence, most children have antibodies to EBV by the age of one year. It is not clear why this should be so. Possible explanations include transmission via breast milk, saliva in pre-chewed food (60 per cent of African mothers have transforming EBV in their saliva)[28] or biting insects, but these factors must exist in other communities. Indeed, the same pattern of acquisition of antibodies seen in the lowlands of West Nile is also seen in highland areas where BL does not occur.[29] One study, unfortunately curtailed by civil unrest in West Nile, suggested that children with high antibody levels to EBV were at greater risk of subsequently developing BL than those with average levels.[30]

If EBV is an aetiological agent for BL then presumably one or more co-factors must exist to account for the localization of the disease in Africa. Anyone working in tropical Africa cannot fail to be impressed by the impact of falciparum malaria on children in that region. Dalldorf, in 1962, suggested that holoendemic falciparum malaria might be the co-factor accounting for the geographical distribution of BL.[31]

The evidence in favour of this has been reviewed by Morrow[32] and can be summarized as follows:

1. The high degree of geographical correlation between the incidence rate of BL and the intensity of *Plasmodium falciparum* transmission, both at a global level and within individual countries.

2. The close correlation between the age incidence of BL and the age of acquiring maximum levels of antimalarial immunoglobulin.

3. The relative protection from BL by residence in urban areas where levels of malaria transmission are lower compared with rural areas.

4. The decline in BL incidence in areas where death rates, due to malaria, have declined and, within such areas, a differential decline in BL incidence in people making better use of health facilities.

5. The older age of onset in patients who have migrated from low intensity to high intensity malaria areas, as compared with patients born in the high intensity areas.

6. The inverse geographical correlation between the average age of onset of BL and the intensity of falciparum malaria infection. An inverse association of BL with sickle-cell trait (AS haemoglobin) would provide strong evidence for the role of intense falciparum malaria, but most studies to date have not achieved statistical significance. Time, space clustering and reports of seasonal variation in BL incidence would indicate that a precipitating factor operates over a relatively short time span, at least in some areas.

Klein[33] put forward a multi-step hypothesis for the induction of BL. The first step involved EBV-induced immortalization of B lymphocytes. A feature of the children who develop BL would be the early and intense infection with EBV. The second step is stimulation of the proliferation of EBV-carrying B-cells. This step is facilitated in the presence of malaria through B-cell stimulation and suppression of T-cells involved in the control of proliferating EBV infected B-cells.[21] The third and final step is the reciprocal translocation that leads to *myc* deregulation and to the development of a malignant clone.

Lenoir and Bornkamm[34] argued against this sequence on the grounds that the characteristic chromosomal translocations of BL are most likely to occur when B-cells are rearranging their immunoglobulin genes. This would seem to be the only reasonable explanation for the constant involvement of one of the immunoglobulin gene loci. Epstein–Barr virus infects B lymphocytes which will, presumably, already have rearranged their immunoglobulin genes. Lenoir and Bornkamm, therefore, proposed an alternative model for the development of Burkitt's lymphoma. The first step is the generation of lymphoid cells at high risk of developing translocations involving the immunoglobulin loci. This is most likely to be caused by the intense immunological stimulation of holoendemic malaria. The second step is the appearance of the translocation involving c-*myc* and one of the immunoglobulin loci. The third step is infection by EBV of a B-cell carrying the specific translocation. This would immortalize the infected cell and allow further neoplastic progression. It may be that the young age at primary infection with EB virus, together with the suppression of immune reactivity against the virus, induced by malarial infection, increases the risk of tumour progression.

Adult T-cell leukaemia/lymphoma

It has long been apparent that the incidence and pattern of malignant lymphomas in Japan differs from that in Europe and North America. In particular, chronic lymphocytic leukaemia and Hodgkin's disease have a low prevalence in Japan. Uchiyama *et al.* first drew attention to a characteristic form of peripheral T-cell leukaemia/lymphoma in 1977 that appeared to have a high prevalence in south-western Japan, notably in Kyushu, the most southern of Japan's four main islands.[35] This tumour has been called adult T-cell leukaemia/lymphoma (ATLL), although some cases are non-leukaemic (NLATL).

Adult T-cell leukaemia/lymphoma occurs predominantly in the sixth decade, has a male to female ratio of 1.4:1 and has a characteristic clinical profile with lymphadenopathy, hepatomegaly, splenomegaly, frequent skin rashes and hypercalcaemia (probably due to the production of an osteoclast-stimulating factor by the neoplastic cells). The skin rashes take the form of erythematous patches, papules or nodules. Histologically, these lesions resemble mycosis fungoides with epidermotropism and Pautrier's microabscesses. It is an aggressive disease with an actuarial 50 per cent survival rate of only 9 months.[36] Many patients exhibit evidence of immunodeficiency and have a high incidence of opportunistic infection at autopsy. Less aggressive forms of ATLL have been described in which patients usually do not show leukaemia or hypercalcaemia.

The histopathological features of ATLL are highly characteristic and to a large extent pathognomonic of the disease. The neoplastic cells vary in size but are characterized by the extreme pleomorphism of their nuclei, variously described as gyriform, cerebriform, walnut-shaped, maple leaf and flower cells. Cells with multilobated nuclei (flower cells) are seen in tissue sections and haematological preparations. Cerebriform giant cells are said to be characteristic of human T-cell lymphotrophic virus (HTLV-I)-positive tumours and to be a fairly reliable indicator of virus positivity (*see* below).[37] The tumour cells are usually CD4-positive and CD8-negative (helper phenotype) although in experiments *in vitro* they appear to function as suppressor cells.

Catovsky *et al.*[38] reported six Black patients, living in London, five born in the West Indies and one in Guyana, with a disease similar to ATLL in its clinical, haematological and histopathological features. Five of the patients had hypercalcaemia. They ranged in age from 21 to 55 years (generally younger than the Japanese cases of ATLL and also differed from the Japanese cases in having a male to female ratio of 1:2). In 1983, Bunn *et al.*[39] reported 11 cases (seven males and four females) of ATLL from the USA. It was from one of these patients that HTLV-I was first isolated. In four of the patients the presence of antibodies to HTLV-I was retrospectively confirmed in stored serum. The patients were generally young, with a mean age of 33 years (range 24–62 years), seven had been born in the south-eastern USA, two in Jamaica and one each in Israel and Equador. The latter two patients were White, all the others being Black. Skin lesions and hypercalcaemia were prominent features of most cases. Eight of the 11 suffered from opportunistic infections before therapy. These reports established the

Caribbean and south-eastern USA as a second endemic area for ATLL, the disease in these areas being similar to that seen in Japan except for a younger age incidence and a higher frequency of hypercalcaemia.

Hinuma *et al.*[40] reported the finding of C-type virus particles in cultured tumour cells from an ATLL patient. This virus was designated ATLV. All patients with ATLL were found to have serum antibodies to an antigen (ATLA) present in the cultured cell line. Antibodies to ATLA were found in the sera of more than 20 per cent of healthy adults living in the endemic area for ATLL, but only rarely in the sera of non-endemic areas. In 1980, workers at the National Cancer Institute isolated a retrovirus from cultured T-cells of a patient initially thought to have mycosis fungoides, but subsequently recategorized as ATLL.[41] This virus, designated human T-lymphotrophic virus type I,[42] was the prototype of over 100 isolates from various parts of the world. Few patients in the USA had antibodies to HTLV-I but when coded sera from Japanese cases of ATLL were tested they were found to be 100 per cent positive. Subsequent studies established that the Japanese virus, ATLV, and HTLV-I are identical.[43]

Human T-cell lymphotrophic virus type I particles are not seen in biopsies of ATLL but appear in cultured tumour cells. Similarly, virus can be isolated from the cultured peripheral white blood cells of otherwise healthy persons seropositive for HTLV-I, indicating a persistent latent infection.[44] All ATLL cells contain HTLV-I provirus DNA integrated in a clonal or oligoclonal manner, indicating that the virus was present in the cell before neoplastic transformation and that it is not simply a passenger virus.[43] The site of integration of HTLV-I, although the same in any one tumour, varies from one patient to another. The inconsistency of the integration site suggests that the virus does not induce neoplasia by being inserted close to an oncogene but that it operates through a transactivating mechanism. In this respect it resembles bovine leukaemia virus. The risk of developing ATLL amongst HTLV-I positive Japanese is reported to be 2.2 per 1000 males and 0.8 per 1000 females, per annum. Human T-cell lymphotrophic virus shows 95 per cent homology with the simian T-lymphotrophic virus (STLV-I), a retrovirus prevalent in Old-World monkeys especially African green monkeys.[43]

In a similar way to which the seroepidemiology of EBV became of importance in the study of the epidemiology of Burkitt's lymphoma, studies of the epidemiology of ATLL focused on the seroepidemiology of HTLV-I. The seropositivity of HTLV-I among Japanese patients with ATLL is 100 per cent.[45] All 122 cases studied by Yoshida and Seiki[45] also had provirus DNA detected in the neoplastic cells, but this was not found in other lymphoreticular neoplasms arising in Japanese patients, although a minority of these had antibodies to the virus. In Jamaica only 19 of 24 patients with ATLL had antibodies to HTLV-I.[46] It is not clear how many of these had provirus DNA in their tumour cells. Assuming that these seronegative cases were truly cases of ATLL it is still possible that they were infected with the virus.

Nakano *et al.*[47] showed that 13 of 16 infants, born to HTLV-I-positive mothers, were infected with the virus but that only four developed antibodies. Several studies in Japan have shown a relationship between the prevalence of antibodies to HTLV-I and the geographic distribution of ATLL. The rate of seropositivity, however, varies widely. Thus, in a study on Tsushima Island, within the area of Kyushu where ATLL is endemic, the seropositivity for HTLV-I varied among 58 villages between 2 and 50 per cent.[48] The incidence of antibodies to HTLV-I in the endemic areas of Japan increases with age.[49,50] This could reflect continued exposure to the virus throughout life, although it has been suggested that it may be a cohort effect. This age effect is also seen in the Caribbean and the USA with rates of HTLV-I seropositivity of 1–2 per cent in persons below and 6 per cent in persons above the age of 50.[51]

In Hawaii, Japanese migrants from Okinawa showed a seropositivity rate for HTLV-I of 20 per cent. Okinawa is an area endemic for ATLL with a seropositivity rate for HTLV-I of 40 per cent. The incidence of antibodies shows a proportional increase with the age of the migrant when he left Okinawa. Seropositivity of HTLV-I rises with age until 50 when it levels off, both in residents of Okinawa and in migrants. Migrants to Hawaii from Niigata, a low endemnicity area for ATLL, show a low rate of seropositivity for HTLV-I that does not increase with age. Seropositive cases of ATLL have been recorded in Hawaii among second generation migrants in their sixth decade of life, indicating that the virus is transmitted in this area. These data suggest that HTLV-I is transmitted in Hawaii but that transmission is within the family and not in the wider community. Blattner *et al.*[52] suggest that the increase in seropositivity seen with age may be due to continued transmission of the virus but could also be due to activation of the virus in patients latently infected in childhood. This hypothesis is supported by the observation of Nakano *et al.*[47] that only a minority of children of seropositive mothers infected at birth developed antibodies to HTLV-I as neonates. In a further study in Okinawa of 65 seropositive mothers only 10 had seropositive children, followed to the age of 18 years.[53] It would have been of interest to know whether the 55 seronegative children were latently infected.

In a study of 462 healthy Chinese men, mostly from eastern China, 5 per cent were found to have antibodies to HTLV-I.[54] Two recent studies of over 12 000 cases of malignant lymphomas detected an excess of T-cell non-Hodgkin's lymphoma in eastern China, where the histological distribution of non-Hodgkin's lymphomas is said to resemble that seen in Japan, whereas in central and western China the distribution is similar to that seen in western countries.[54,55] These observations suggest that ATLL may be endemic in eastern China, but more detailed immunological and virological studies are needed to confirm this.

Outside the areas endemic for ATLL a high prevalence of antibodies to HTLV-I has been reported from Africa, although, as in the ATLL endemic areas, the incidence in different communities varies widely. A high prevalence of HTLV-I antibodies was found among the Black Jews or Falashas who migrated from Ethiopia to Israel.[56] Hunsmann *et al.*[57] found only two of 231 Kenyan students to be seropositive. Bigger *et al.*[58] also found a relatively low incidence of seropositivity in the Nairobi

area, but a high incidence, rising to 70 per cent seropositivity, among the pastoralist Turkana tribe living in northern Kenya. It may be of significance that the Turkana have an almost 100 per cent positivity for hepatitis B virus infection.

Bartholomew *et al.*[59] found a higher prevalence of seropositivity to HTLV-I in Tobago than in Trinidad and noted that this appears to be correlated with poorer socioeconomic conditions and is associated with hepatitis A and B antibodies. Infection with HTLV-I, like hepatitis B virus, is transmitted by blood transfusion and has an increased prevalence in intravenous drug abusers, although, unlike hepatitis B virus, it cannot be transmitted by cell-free blood products.

Human T-cell lymphotrophic virus has been found in breast milk and has been shown to be transmitted orally in non-human primates. The virus is present in semen and it is suggested that sexual transmission accounts for the higher rates of seropositivity found in older females than males.[60] In addition to non-human primates,[61] HTLV-I is capable of infecting mice, rats and rabbits.[62]

It is difficult, at the present time, to relate the rather fragmentary information on the sero-epidemiology of HTLV-I to the known geographical distribution of ATLL. Approximately 1 per cent of those infected with the virus in childhood develop ATLL, often in late adult life, suggesting that other co-factors may be implicated. The virus is also associated with a neurological disease known as tropical spastic paraparesis or HTLV-I associated myelopathy.[63]

The available data on the seroepidemiology of HTLV-I suggest that transmission occurs mainly as a result of close family contact, presumably by the transmission in blood or body fluids of latently infected lymphocytes. The suggestion that the virus is present in rodents in the endemic areas of Japan and that this is the source of the human infection can probably be discounted. Gallo *et al.* have suggested that HTLV-I, which is closely related to STLV-I originated in Africa and was taken to Japan and the West Indies by Portugese traders in the sixteenth century.[43,64] This hypothesis links the two areas endemic for ATLL, but leaves unanswered the question why the virus became endemic in these areas and not in others, such as Portugal itself and why ATLL is not endemic in Africa. To answer these questions more data are needed on the epidemiology of ATLL and the seroepidemiology of HTLV-I.

Human T-cell lymphotrophic virus type II (HTLV-II)

The virus designated HTLV-II was first isolated from an unusual case of hairy cell leukaemia of the T-cell phenotype.[65] Type-II shares only 60 per cent DNA homology with HTLV-I but, like HTLV-I, can infect and transform normal T cells *in vitro* producing immortalized T-cell lines. Few subjects with antibodies to HTLV-II have been identified, although serological evidence of infection has been reported in intravenous drug abusers in Great Britain.[66] The report of a second isolate of HTLV-II from a case of atypical hairy cell leukaemia of the T-cell phenotype suggests that the association of this virus with this unusual neoplasm is more than fortuitous.[67] The HTLV-II provirus DNA, in this case, was oligoclonally integrated into DNA isolated from the leukaemic cells. Further studies of the T-cell variants of hairy cell leukaemia are clearly indicated.

Human immunodeficiency virus (HIV) – associated lymphomas

A dramatic rise in the incidence of mainly high-grade malignant lymphomas in young adults has been seen in the USA in the past decade.[68] These tumours occur in patients with HIV-infection, with AIDS or pre-AIDS.[69,70,71] There appears to be a particularly high incidence of malignant lymphomas in male homosexuals and intravenous drug abusers. The Centers for Disease Control includes lymphoma as one of its diagnostic criteria for AIDS. The lymphomas in HIV-infected patients are usually extranodal in their distribution with involvement of the gastrointestinal tract, including intraoral and anorectal lymphomas as the second most frequent site after the central nervous system.

The majority of the lymphomas would be categorized as diffuse large cell in the terminology of the Working Formulation, although some have been categorized as Burkitt's lymphomas. The latter contain one of the chromosomal translocations characteristic of Burkitt's lymphoma and some have been shown to contain EBV DNA.[72] There appears to be defective control of EBV regulation in patients with HIV infection, presumably related to their T-cell deficiency.[73] On this basis, it has been suggested that at least some of the lymphomas evolve in the context of EBV-driven B-cell proliferation. However, many infective agents become opportunistic pathogens in patients with AIDS and EBV may not be central to the induction of the lymphomas.

The recently isolated human B-cell lymphotrophic herpes virus (HBLV)[74] is a possible candidate for the role of an oncogenic virus in patients with AIDS. It was isolated from HIV-positive patients with lymphoproliferative disease but not from 12 patients with AIDS without associated lymphoma. The virus has also been isolated from the peripheral blood lymphocytes of HIV-negative patients with lymphoproliferative disease. Only four of 220 randomly selected healthy donors were found to have antibodies to the virus. Clearly, further studies of HBLV are indicated, particularly in patients with HIV-associated lymphoma.

Middle East lymphoma

The relative incidence of malignant lymphoma is high in the Middle East, accounting for approximately 10 per cent of all neoplasms in this region. Data are not available to indicate how this relates to age-adjusted incidence rates. A high proportion of the lymphomas are extranodal and of these the majority involve the gastrointestinal tract. Among the gastrointestinal tract lymphomas is a clinicopathological entity that has been designated 'Middle East lymphoma', 'Mediterranean lymphoma' or 'alpha-chain disease'.[75] The tumour affects mainly young adults and has a mean age of onset of 25 years. It has a male:female ratio of 2.2:1. The major clinical features of Middle East lymphoma are abdominal pain, diarrhoea, weight loss and clubbing of the fingers and toes. Malabsorption with diarrhoea may be present for months or years before diagnosis.

At laparotomy the patients are frequently found to have diffuse thickening of much of the small intestine without tumour masses.[76] This thickening is due to a lymphoplasmacytic infiltrate involving large segments of the small intestinal mucosa and it is in the setting of this infiltrate, that has been called 'immunoproliferative small intestinal disease' (IPSID), that frank tumour masses may develop. Some patients with IPSID are found to have an incomplete IgA heavy chain molecules in the circulation (alpha heavy chain disease).[75] Alpha heavy chains can be detected with greater frequency in duodenal secretions from patients with IPSID than from serum.

The relationship between Middle East lymphoma and IPSID has been a matter for debate. Some authors have regarded IPSID as an inflammatory/reactive process in which lymphomas develop with increased frequency. Evidence in favour of this hypothesis includes the observation that some patients with IPSID respond to broad-spectrum antibiotic therapy.[75] However, the length and permanence of that response has not been documented. It has been argued that IPSID is a form of mucosa-associated lymphoma which, like other mucosal lymphomas, may remain localized for many years until neoplastic progression results in the emergence of a more aggressive, frankly malignant clone of cells.[77] Alpha heavy chain can be detected in the plasma cells that infiltrate the lamina propria of the gut in IPSID.[78] However, since the abnormal alpha chain product does not join with light chains to form a whole immunoglobulin molecule, it is rarely possible to use light chain restriction to determine whether the infiltrate is monotypic (presumed neoplastic) or polytypic (reactive).[79,80] Recent studies on DNA from patients with IPSID have shown monoclonal heavy and light chain gene rearrangements,[81] supporting the concept that IPSID, itself, is a neoplastic process.

Middle East lymphoma has been recorded with greatest frequency in those countries bordering the Eastern Mediterranean and the Arabian Gulf. A small number of cases have been reported from South Africa. Apart from rare, single case reports, the disease does not occur in the rest of the world. In Israel the disease is found with much greater frequency in Jews who have migrated from North Africa and countries bordering the Arabian Gulf than in those from Europe. This division correlates with socioeconomic standards and it has been suggested that poor standards of hygiene may be causally related to IPSID.[75] If this were so, it would have to be due to a specific agent associated with poor hygiene, since Middle East lymphoma does not occur in much of the world where socioeconomic standards are probably worse than in the Middle East.

Since patients with alpha chain disease are unable to form secretory IgA, their vulnerability to gastrointestinal tract pathogens is increased and in studying these patients it is important to discriminate between cause and effect. The restricted geography of the disease suggests that a genetic defect or, less likely, a localized specific environmental agent leads to the development of a neoplastic clone of mucosal-associated lymphocytes that form an abnormal alpha heavy chain. The failure of this heavy chain to join with light chains, together with the absence of idiotypic determinants, may result in escape from network control which is mediated by idiotype recognition. Colonization of the mucosa of the small intestine by these cells would lead to IPSID and further mutations in the neoplastic clone to solid tumour masses. Intestinal antigens, possibly specific for the Middle East, might drive this process. The absence of strong familial clustering would suggest that the genetic defect, alone, if it exists, is not sufficient for development of IPSID.

Further studies of this disease should include cytogenetics and molecular biology of biopsy tissue and peripheral blood lymphocytes from patients with IPSID and their relatives, with particular attention to the alpha chain locus on chromosome 14.

Malignant lymphoma associated with coeliac disease

Patients with coeliac disease have a 200-fold increased risk of developing lymphoma.[82] These are high-grade tumours, usually involving the small intestine. Although originally thought to be of monocyte/macrophage origin and designated malignant histiocytosis of the intestine,[83] recent immunohistochemical and gene rearrangement studies have shown them to be derived from T-cells and they are now called enteropathy associated T-cell lymphoma.[84] Initial reports suggest that this tumour is much more frequent in Great Britain and Ireland than in the USA. Coeliac disease is particularly prevalent in the west of Ireland and is associated with HLA DR3[85], suggesting a genetic influence in its pathogenesis. It is surprising that enteropathy associated T-cell lymphoma has not been reported more frequently from the USA with its large Irish immigrant population. This might point to specific environmental features in the genesis of the lymphoma.

Follicular lymphomas

Follicle centre cell lymphomas with a follicular growth pattern are the commonest non-Hodgkin's lymphomas seen in North America and Europe. Thus, in the National Cancer Institute sponsored study of the classification of non-Hodgkin's lymphomas, 34 per cent had a follicular growth pattern.[86] In contrast, non-Hodgkin's lymphomas with a follicular growth pattern are uncommon in Africa, China, Japan and the Middle East.[87,88] Differences in the age structure of the populations being studied may account for part of this observation but, even allowing for this, follicular tumours are clearly uncommon in these areas. The natural progression of follicle centre cell lymphomas is from tumours composed predominantly of small cells with a follicular growth pattern to large cell tumours with a diffuse growth pattern. An argument advanced to explain the low frequency of follicular lymphomas in the underdeveloped world is that patients frequently present late,

particularly with diseases that do not have severe systemic symptoms and that by the time they present their disease has become diffuse and large cell. This explanation is unlikely to be correct, since small cell follicular lymphomas almost always present with stage III or IV disease and, in particular, often have bone marrow involvement, whereas diffuse large cell lymphomas frequently present with stage I or II disease.

A characteristic chromosomal translocation is seen in follicle centre cell lymphomas between chromosomes 14 and 18.[89] The breakpoint on chromosome 14 is in the region of the immunoglobulin heavy chain locus and that on chromosome 18 in the region of the *bcl*-2 proto-oncogene. The constancy of this translocation in follicle centre cell lymphomas suggests that it occurs during B-cell differentiation at the time of immunoglobulin gene rearrangements. Yunis *et al.*[89] found that low-grade follicle centre cell lymphomas showed the 14;18 translocation but that the more aggressive tumours, including some with a diffuse growth pattern, had, in addition, other chromosomal abnormalities. They suggested that the 14;18 translocation was the primary defect in follicle centre cell lymphoma and that multiple, recurrent genomic defects accounted for the progression from an indolent tumour to the more aggressive forms. Weiss *et al.*[90] used a number of chromosome 18 DNA probes to detect the 14;18 translocation in a series of malignant lymphomas. The translocation is found in virtually all follicular neoplasms and in about 28 per cent of diffuse large cell lymphomas. The advantage of this technique is that it is more easily applied to solid tumours than standard cytogenetic methods and, thus, may facilitate epidemiological studies of the 14;18 translocation. If the 14;18 translocation is found to be present in non-Hodgkin's lymphomas in areas in which follicular lymphomas are uncommon it might suggest that environmental factors result in rapid tumour progression before clinical presentation. If this is so, it would be expected that the tumours would exhibit other cytogenetic abnormalities in addition to the 14;18 translocation.

Occupational risks of non-Hodgkin's lymphomas

An excess of malignant lymphomas, particularly of the aggressive subtypes has been reported to occur in farming communities.[87] This has raised the possibility that exposure to herbicides and pesticides may be involved in the aetiology of these neoplasms. However, a recent case control study in the USA indicates that the excess mortality from non-Hodgkin's lymphomas is associated only with those workers who handle meat.[91] This raises the possibility of the transmission of oncogenic viruses from animals to man, although no evidence for this has yet been deduced.

Conclusions

The study of the geography of non-Hodgkin's lymphomas has uncovered two tumour syndromes, Burkitt's lymphoma and ATLL, which have both had a major impact on the investigation of the virological and molecular biological aspects of neoplasia. These tumours have clinical and pathological features that set them apart from other non-Hodgkin's lymphomas. Middle East lymphoma has attracted less attention than the former, perhaps because of the difficulty of studying the disease in its endemic setting. As a neoplastic disorder of the mucosal immune system it would undoubtedly repay deeper study. The starting point for the study of the epidemiology of non-Hodgkin's lymphomas is careful clinical observation. This, in turn, must be supported by critical histopathological evaluation backed up with good immunology and immunohistochemistry. As observed in this chapter, the study of the geography of Burkitt's lymphoma and ATLL had then to be related to studies of the seroepidemiology of EBV and HTLV-I.

A number of non-Hodgkin's lymphomas have been shown to exhibit characteristic cytogenetic abnormalities, often involving the locus of proto-oncogenes and the immunoglobulin, or T-cell receptor gene loci. It is likely that these abnormalities occur during gene rearrangement associated with B- and T-cell differentiation. Is this a random event and does immunostimulation increase its frequency? If so, it is likely that populations with a larger burden of infective and parasitic disease will show an increase in such abnormalities. What further factors are required to promote tumour progression with the development of frank neoplasia? The answers to these questions may well come from the molecular biologists. However, the epidemiological study of lymphomas may in the future, as in the past, provide vital clues.

References

1. Burkitt D. *British Journal of Surgery*. 1958; **46**, 218.
2. Davies JNP, Elmes J, Hutt MSR, *et al. British Medical Journal*. 1964; **1**, 336.
3. Burkitt DP. In: Burkitt DP, Wright DH eds. *General Features and Facial Tumours in Burkitt's Lymphoma*. Edinburgh: E & S Livingstone, 1970; 6.
4. Berard C, O'Conor GT, Thomas LB, Torloni H. *Bulletin of the World Health Organization*. 1969; **40**, 601.
5. Gunven P, Klein G, Klein E, Norin T, Singh S. *International Journal of Cancer*. 1980; **25**, 711.
6. Lenoir GM, Preud'Homme JL, Bernheim A, Berger R. *Nature*. 1982; **298**, 474.
7. Wiley IS. *Journal of the National Cancer Institute*. 1973; **50**, 1703.
8. MacCrae AWR, Pike MC. In: Hall SA, Langlands BE eds. *Uganda Atlas of Disease Distribution*. Nairobi: East Africa Publishing House, 1975.
9. Edington GM, Hendrikse M. *Journal of the National Cancer Institute*. 1973; **50**, 1623.
10. Brubaker G, Geser A, Pike MC. *British Journal of Cancer*. 1973; **28**, 472.
11. Sacks MI, Hulu N, Selzer G, Steinitz R. *Journal of the National Cancer Institute*. 1973; **50**, 1669.
12. Young JL, Miller RW. *Journal of Pediatrics*. 1975; **86**, 254.
13. Levine PH, Kamaraju LS, Connelly RR, *et al. Cancer*. 1982; **49**, 1016.
14. Parkin DM, Sohier R, O'Conor GT. In: Lenoir GM, O'Conor GT, Olweny CLM eds. *Burkitt's Lymphoma: A Human Cancer Model*. Lyon: IARC Scientific Publications, 1985.
15. Wright DH. *International Journal of Cancer*. 1966; 1, **503.**
16. Banks PM, Arseneau JC, Gralnick HR, *et al. American Journal of Medicine*. 1975; **58**, 322.
17. Al-Attar A, Al-Mondhiry H, Al-Bahrani Z, Al-

Saleem T. *International Journal of Cancer*. 1979; **23**, 14.

18. Burkitt DP. In: Burkitt DP, Wright DH eds. *Burkitt's Lymphoma*. Edinburgh: E & S Livingstone, 1970.

19. Wright DH. In: Lenoir G, O'Conor GT, Olweny CLM eds. *Burkitt's Lymphoma: A Human Cancer Model*. Lyon, IARC Scientific Publications, 1985.

20. Shepherd JJ, Wright DH. *British Journal of Surgery*. 1967; **54**, 776.

21. Wilson JF, Kjeldsberg CR, Sposto R, *et al. Human Pathology*. 1987; **18**, 1008.

22. Haddow AJ. *East African Medical Journal*. 1963; **40**, 429.

23. Epstein MA, Achong BG, Barr YM. *Lancet*. 1964; i, 702.

24. Purtilo D. *Lancet*. 1980; i, 200.

25. Miller G, Shope T, Coope D, *et al. Journal of Experimental Medicine*. 1977; **145**, 948.

26. Sundar SK, Levine PH, Ablashi DV, *et al. International Journal of Cancer*. 1981; **27**, 107.

27. de Thé G. *Lancet*. 1977; **i**, 335.

28. Gerber P, Nkrumah FK, Pritchett R, Kieff E. *International Journal of Cancer*. 1976; **17**, 71.

29. Geser A, de Thé G, Lenoir G, Day NE, Williams EH. *International Journal of Cancer*. 1982; **29**, 397.

30. de Thé G, Geser A, Day NE, *et al. Nature*. 1978; **274**, 756.

31. Dalldorf G. *Journal of the American Medical Association*. 1962; **181**, 1026.

32. Morrow RH. In: Lenoir GM, O'Conor GT, Olweny CLM eds. *Burkitt's Lymphoma: A Human Cancer Model*. Lyon: IARC Scientific Publications, 1985.

33. Klein G. *Proceedings of the National Academy of Sciences USA*. 1979; **76**, 2442.

34. Lenoir RM, Bornkamm GW. *Advances in Viral Oncology*. 1986; **7**, 173.

35. Uchiyama T, Yodoi J, Sagawa K, Tatasuki K, Uchino H. *Blood*. 1977; **50**, 481.

36. Kikuchi M, Mitsui T, Takeshita M, *et al. Hematological Oncology*. 1986; **4**, 67.

37. Suchi T, Lennert K, Tu L-Y, *et al. Journal of Clinical Pathology*. 1987; **40**, 995.

38. Catovsky D, Greaves MF, Rose M, *et al. Lancet*. 1982; i, 639.

39. Bunn PA, Schechter GP, Jaffe E, *et al. New England Journal of Medicine*. 1983; **309**, 257.

40. Hinuma Y, Nagata K, Hanaoka M, *et al. Proceedings of the National Academy of Sciences USA*. 1981; **78**, 6476.

41. Poiesz BJ, Ruscetti FW, Gazdar AF, *et al. Proceedings of the National Academy of Sciences USA*. 1980; **77**, 7415.

42. Poiesz BJ, Ruscetti FW, Reitz MS, Kalyan Araman VS, Gallo RC. *Nature*. 1981; **294**, 268.

43. Wong-Staal F, Gallo RC. *Nature*. 1985; **317**, 395.

44. Matutes E, Dalgleish AG, Weiss RA, Joseph AP, Catovsky D. *International Journal of Cancer*. 1986; **38**, 41.

45. Yoshida M, Seiki M. *Hematological Oncology*. 1986; **4**, 13.

46. Gibbs WN, Murphy EL. *American Journal of Epidemiology*. 1986; **124**, 501.

47. Nakano S, Ando Y, Saito K, *et al. Journal of Infection*. 1986; **12**, 205.

48. Tajima K, Kamura S, Ito S, *et al. International Journal of Cancer*. 1987; **40**, 741.

49. Hinuma Y, Komoda H, Chosa T, *et al. International Journal of Cancer*. 1982; **29**, 631.

50. Maeda Y, Fukuhara M, Takehara Y, *et al. International Journal of Cancer*. 1984; **33**, 717.

51. Blayney DW, Blattner WA, Jaffe ES, Gallo RC. *Hematological Oncology*. 1983; **1**, 193.

52. Blattner WA, Nomura A, Clark JW, *et al. Proceedings of the National Academy of Sciences USA*. 1986; **83**, 4895.

53. Kusuhara K, Sonada S, Takahashi K, *et al. International Journal of Cancer*. 1987; **40**, 755.

54. Yang K, Li YW, Li JW, *et al. National Cancer Institute Monograph*. 1985; **69**, 35.

55. The Nationwide Lymphoma Pathology Cooperative Group (NLPCG). *Japanese Journal of Clinical Oncology*. 1985; **15**, 645.

56. Ben-Ishai Z, Haas M, Triglia D, *et al. Nature*. 1985; **315**, 665.

57. Hunsmann G, Schneider J, Schmitt J, Yamamoto N. *International Journal of Cancer*. 1983; **32**, 329.

58. Bigger RJ, Johnson BK, Oster C, *et al. International Journal of Cancer*. 1985; **35**, 763.

59. Bartholomew C, Saxinger C, Cleghorn F, *et al. American Journal of Epidemiology*. 1987; **126**, 756.

60. Tajima K, Tominaga S, Suchi T, *et al. International Journal of Cancer*. 1986; **37**, 383.

61. Miyoshi I, Fujishita M, Taguchi H, *et al. International Journal of Cancer*. 1983; **32**, 333.

62. Kotani S, Yoshimoto S, Yamato K, *et al. International Journal of Cancer*. 1986; **37**, 843.

63. Weiss RA. *Journal of Clinical Pathology*. 1987; **40**, 1064.

64. Gallo RC, Sliski A, Wong-Staal F. *Lancet*. 1983; ii, 962.

65. Kalyanaraman VS, Sarngadharan MG. Robert-Guroff M, *et al. Science*. 1982; **218**, 571.

66. Tedder RS, Shanson DC, Jeffries DJ, *et al. Lancet*. 1984; ii, 125.

67. Rosenblatt JD, Golde DW, Wachsman W, *et al. New England Journal of Medicine*. 1986; **315**, 372.

68. Chase-Boring C, Brynes RK, Chan WC, *et al. Lancet*. 1985; i, 857.

69. Ahmed T, Wormser GP, Stahl RE, *et al. Cancer.* 1987; **60**, 719.
70. Biggar RJ, Horm J, Goedert JJ, Melbye M. *American Journal of Epidemiology.* 1987; **126**, 578.
71. Ziegler JL, Beckstead JA, Volberding PA, *et al. New England Journal of Medicine.* 1984; **311**, 565.
72. Chaganti RSK, Jhanwar SC, Koziner B, *et al. Blood.* 1983; **61**, 1269.
73. Birx DL, Redfirld RR, Tosato R. *New England Journal of Medicine.* 1986; **314**, 874.
74. Salahuddin SZ, Ablashi DV, Markham PD, *et al. Science.* 1986; **234**, 596.
75. *Bulletin of the World Health Organization.* 1976; **54**, 615.
76. Salem P, El-Hashimi L, Anaisse E, *et al. Cancer.* 1987; **59**, 1670.
77. Isaacson P, Wright DH. *Cancer.* 1983; **52**, 1410.
78. Isaacson P. *American Journal of Surgical Pathology.* 1979; **3**, 431.
79. Asselah F, Slavin G, Sowter G, Asselah H. *Cancer.* 1983; **52**, 227.
80. Isaacson PG, Price SK. *Journal of Clinical Pathology.* 1985; **38**, 601.
81. Smith WJ, Price SK, Isaacson PG. *Journal of Clinical Pathology.* 1987; **40**, 1291.
82. Swinson CM, Slavin G, Coles EC, Booth CC. *Lancet.* 1983; **i**, 111.
83. Isaacson P, Wright DH. *Lancet.* 1978; **i**, 67.
84. Isaacson PG, O'Connor NTJ, Spencer J, *et al. Lancet.* 1986; **ii**, 688.
85. O'Driscoll BRC, Stevens FM, O'Gorman TA, *et al. Gut.* 1982; **23**, 662.
86. The non-Hodgkin's lymphoma pathologic classification project. *Cancer.* 1982; **49**, 2112.
87. Harrington DS, Yuling YE, Weisenberger DD, *et al. Human Pathology.* 1987; **18**, 924.
88. Dorfman RF. In: Roulet FC ed. *Symposium on Lymphoreticular Tumours in Africa.* Basel: S Karger, 1963; 211.
89. Yunis JJ, Frizzera G, Oken MM, *et al. New England Journal of Medicine.* 1987; **316**, 79.
90. Weiss LM, Warnke RA, Sklar J, Cleary ML. *New England Journal of Medicine.* 1987; **317**; 1185.
91. Pearle NE, Sheppard RA, Smith AH, Teague CA. *International Journal of Cancer.* 1987; **39**, 155.

CHAPTER 9

LYMPHOPROLIFERATIVE DISORDERS ASSOCIATED WITH IMMUNODEFICIENCY

AH Filipovich, R Shapiro, L Robison, A Mertens and G Frizzera

Cancer, and lymphoid tumours in particular, represent a common and often fatal complication of genetically determined (primary) immunodeficiency disorders. Recent publications of estimated cancer incidence figures for certain primary immunodeficiency disorders[1-4] confirm earlier suspicions that the inheritance of genetic defects associated with clinical immunodeficiency ranks among the highest known risk factors for tumour development in humans.[5,6] Acquired immunodeficiency, secondary to immunosuppressive therapy for allografting, or following infection with human immunodeficiency virus (HIV), also increases susceptibility to lymphoproliferative disorders.[7-9]

Earlier analyses of lymphoproliferative disorders or 'lymphomas' in patients with primary, as well as, secondary immunodeficiencies stressed the predominance of B lymphocyte proliferation. During the past few years, newer diagnostic techniques have been applied to tumours from immunodeficient patients, including immunophenotyping with monoclonal antibodies and DNA probing for clonal rearrangement of immunoglobulin (Ig) or T-cell receptor (TCR) genes. Such genetic studies have confirmed previous impressions, based on histopathological examination, that these lymphoproliferative disorders represent a full spectrum of lymphocyte activation, ranging from polyclonal reactive lesions, to oligoclonal foci of lymphocyte proliferation, and finally, to malignant tumours with identifiable cytogenetic abnormalities, and that these findings can be observed in a single immunodeficient patient. In addition to the frequent finding of B-cell lymphoproliferative disorders in immunodeficient hosts, aberrant expansion and/or malignant transformation of other cells in the immune network, e.g. T-cells and large granular lymphocytes can also complicate underlying immunodeficiency.

In some cases, viruses, especially Epstein–Barr virus and HIV (both discussed elsewhere in this book), have been identified as important co-factors in the development of fatal lymphoproliferative lesions in immunodeficient hosts. This observation implies that effective antiviral therapy, when it becomes available, may play a critical role in the prevention or control of some lymphoproliferative disorders. Historically, conventional combination chemotherapy and/or radiation therapy protocols, if used, rarely benefited immunodeficient patients with lymphoproliferative disorders. While tumour responses were occasionally observed, immunodeficient patients often died during cancer treatment from either opportunistic infections, or unusually severe secondary effects of the therapies. More recent experience indicates that moderation of immunosuppression following allografting, or correction of underlying primary immunodeficiency (as with successful marrow transplantation) may significantly reduce the risk of fatal lymphoproliferative disorders in susceptible individuals. Furthermore, augmentation of existing immunological capacities through the *in vivo* administration of recombinant lymphokines (e.g. interferon, interleukin-2 IL-2) to patients with partial defects of immunity offers additional hope for the elimination of lymphoproliferative complications in the near future.

Lymphoproliferative disorders and Hodgkin's disease associated with primary immunodeficiencies

Primary, genetically determined, immunodeficiency diseases are a heterogeneous group of syndromes sharing in common inherent abnormalities in the development or maintenance of specific immune responses. The clinical presentation of primary immunodeficiency occurs variably from birth until the fifth or sixth decades of life. The genetic bases for the majority of primary immunodeficiency syndromes identified by the WHO Scientific Group on Immunodeficiency[10] are currently unknown. Premature lethality is most often attributed to overwhelming infections or the sequelae of recurrent and chronic infections, such as pulmonary insufficiency.[3] Tumours, particularly lymphoproliferative disorders, appear to be the second leading cause of death in persons with primary immunodeficiency syndromes. The incidence of tumours for three major primary immunodeficiency syndromes: Wiskott–Aldrich syndrome (WAS),[2] ataxia-telangiectasia (A-T)[3] and common variable immunodeficiency (CVID)[4] have been estimated between 15 and 25 per cent, supporting and updating the evidence from several national cancer surveys of immunodeficient patients published in the 1970s and early 1980s.[11–13] Furthermore, in certain immunodeficiency syndromes the risk of developing cancer appears to increase with age.[2]

Because primary immunodeficiencies are rare, few cases of cancer in patients with primary immunodeficiency will be diagnosed at any given medical institution. Therefore, the idea of an international registry of these cases was conceived by Dr Robert Good and his colleagues at the University of Minnesota in the early 1970s. The concept was realized in 1973 with the support of the National Cancer Institute, and the Immunodeficiency Cancer Registry (ICR) was maintained for a number of years through the efforts of Dr John Kersey and Ms B.D. Spector, registrar. Immunodeficiency Cancer Registry cases have been identified through literature review and voluntary case reports.[14]

Since 1983, the ICR has attempted to develop and maintain a detailed and validated database of cases of immunodeficiency and cancer. This information is made accessible to interested investigators for derivative studies into the clinical epidemiology and biology of cancers associated with immunodeficiency, and cancer in general. Over the past three years more than 90 per cent of new cases registered have entered the ICR through voluntary reports. More than 350 physician-investigators have generously contributed case material to the ICR. Table 9.1 shows the distribution of reported tumour types and immunodeficiencies for 500 cases in the ICR files.

Non-Hodgkin's lymphoma in the ICR

Proportionally, non-Hodgkin's lymphomas (NHL), cancers of the immune system, comprise 50 per cent of ICR cases. An excess of NHL is observed in all the immunodeficiency categories. The largest numbers of NHL cases have been reported in association with ataxia-telangiectasia (69 of 150), Wiskott–Aldrich syndrome (59 of 78), common variable immunodeficiency (55 of 120), and severe combined immunodeficiency (SCID) (31 of 42).

Characteristics of 240 cases reported as NHL in the ICR are described in Table 9.2. Approximately 20 per cent of these cases, (representing primarily more recent reports), have undergone independent pathological review by the ICR. Most, but not all, have met the histological criteria for lymphoid malignancy. For purposes of this summary of ICR data we will continue to refer to the ICR cases as NHL, although a few would be more accurately described as lymphoproliferative disorders.

The median age at diagnosis for all NHL cases was 7 years. Tumours diagnosed prior to one year of age have been reported in all but one immunodeficiency category. A male

Table 9.1 Immunodeficiency cancer registry cases: distribution of tumours and immunodeficiencies

	Adenocarcinoma	Lymphoma	Hodgkin's disease	Leukaemia	Other tumour	Total tumours
Hypogamma-globulinaemia	3(14.3)	7(33.3)	3(14.3)	7(33.3)	1(4.8)	21(4.2)
Severe combined immunodeficiency	1(2.4)	31(73.8)	4.(9.5)	5(11.9)	1(2.4)	42(8.4)
Wiskott–Aldrich syndrome	0(0)	59(75.6)	3(3.8)	7(9.0)	9(11.5)	78(15.6)
Ataxia telangiectasia	13(8.7)	69(46.0)	16(10.7)	32(21.3)	20(13.3)	150(30.0)
Common variable immunodeficiency	20(16.7)	55(45.8)	8(6.7)	8(6.7)	29(24.2)	120(24.0)
Selective IgA deficiency	8(21.1)	6(15.8)	3(7.9)	0(0)	21(55.3)	38(7.6)
Other immunoglobulin disorders	0(0)	4(40.0)	1(10.0)	0(0)	5(50.0)	10(2.0)
Hyper IgM syndrome	0(0)	9(56.3)	4(25.0)	0(0)	3(18.8)	16(3.2)
Other immunodeficiency	1(4.0)	12(48.0)	1(4.0)	4(16.0)	7(28.0)	25(5.0)
Total immunodeficiency categories	46(9.2)	252(50.4)	43(8.6)	63(12.6)	96(19.2)	500(100)

Number in parentheses is percentage

predominance is observed in all categories of immunodeficiency including ataxia-telangiectasia and CVID which have autosomal recessive inheritance.[3,15] The ICR cases illustrate important differences in the distribution of primary tumour sites and the clinical presentation of NHL (or lymphoproliferative disorders) in immunodeficient patients compared with non-immunodeficient children and adults. The development of NHL in lymph nodes is relatively uncommon in immunodeficient patients even in immunodeficiency syndromes such as WAS, where chronic massive lymphadenopathy[16,17] is a characteristic physical finding. In contrast, the brain and gastrointestinal tract are frequent presenting sites for NHL, along with the lungs and soft tissues of the head and neck. Wide anatomical dissemination of lymphoproliferative lesions at the time of diagnosis, frequently involving the central nervous system, is another common feature of NHL in immunodeficient patients, especially among patients with the most severe T-cell defects (SCID, CVID, WAS).

Because of the recent emphasis on independent histopathological review of NHL cases submitted to the ICR, we are beginning to characterize the spectrum of lymphoproliferative disorders which behave in a clinically malignant manner. The results of one such independent review of NHL cases in WAS are shown in Table 9.3. These findings complement and extend the observations from a series of nine patients reported by Cotelingam *et al.*[17] Seventeen of 22 cases reviewed were found primarily to involve B-cells. Twelve of the 17 cases expressed features consistent with pleomorphic immunocytoma (PI),[18] although four cases showed predominant characteristics of immunoblastic sarcoma of B-cells (a high grade large cell malignancy), or polymorphic B-cell lymphoma (PBCL). In addition to B-cell lymphoproliferative disorders, three cases were identified as T-cell tumours (immunoblastic sarcoma of T-cells) and two diagnoses of Hodgkin's disease were verified.

Non-Hodgkin's lymphoma cases reported to the ICR from the 1950s and 1960s reflected a high proportion of post-mortem diagnoses; greater than 30 per cent in some immunodeficiency categories. With growing awareness of the high risk of lymphoproliferative disorders associated with immunodeficiency, more diagnoses are

Table 9.2 Characteristics of non-Hodgkin's lymphomas in the Immunodeficiency Cancer Registry*

Immunodeficiency	N	Sex** M:F	Median age at diagnosis	Range (Years)	Primary tumour sites (%)				
					Brain CNS	Gastrointestinal tract	Lymph node	Multiple	Other unknown
Hypogammaglobulinaemia	7	7:0	1.2	<1–9.8	0	14.3	14.3	14.3	57.1
Severe combined immunodeficiency	31	23:7	1.6	<1–12.4	6.5	3.2	9.7	48.4	32.3
Wiskott–Aldrich syndrome	59	59:0	6.2	<1–21.6	23.7	6.8	8.5	20.3	40.7
Ataxia telangiectasia	69	40:24	8.5	<1–22.0	0	8.7	10.1	14.5	66.7
Common variable immunodeficiency	55	30:23	23.0	<1–75.0	1.8	12.7	12.7	25.5	47.3
Selective IgA deficiency	6	4:1	9.4	<1–46.0	16.7	0	0	0	83.3
Other immunoglobulin disorders	4	4:0	4.0	2.5–48.0	0	0	0	0	100.0
Hyper IgM syndrome	9	7:2	7.8	<1–46.0	11.1	22.2	22.2	0	44.4
Column total	240	174:57	7.1	<1–75.0	7.9	8.8	10.4	21.7	51.3

*This table excludes cases of non-Hodgkin's lymphoma in immunodeficiency categories with fewer than 2 cases reported
**Sex reported where known

Table 9.3 Clinical and pathological features of 22 cases of lymphoproliferative disorders in WAS reviewed by the Immunodeficiency Cancer Registry

ICR histology	ICR no.	Contributors	Reported histology	Age at diagnosis	Survival (years) post-diagnosis	Sites
Pleomorphic immunocytoma (PI)	3001	J Montgomery	RES* hyperplasia	2.3	0	Liver
	3002	R Buckley E Green	Myeloid metaplasia	1.7	0	Multiple
	3007	W Krivit	RCS**	6.6	0	Multiple (CNS)
	3012	V Marinkovich	RCS	3.1	0	Multiple (CNS)
	3036	R Schwartz Z Tomkiewicz	Astrocytoma	3.5	0.1	CNS
	3044	C Huntley	RCS	2.3	0	Multiple
	3045	J Whisnant	Malignant lymphoma NOS	7.3	Alive	GI
	3063	S Murphy	Malignant lymphoma NOS	20.1	0	LN
Immunoblastic sarcoma of B-cells	3019	D McKeell	Histiocytic lymphoma	20.1	0	LN
	3035	M Tamar	RCS	3.8	0	Multiple (CNS)
	3018	R Holland K Heidelberger L Skendzel	Histiocytic lymphoma	18.8	0.4	CNS
Lymphoplasmacytoid tumour	3003	G Guin	RCS	1.7	0	Multiple (CNS)
	3031	W London	Microglioma	8.2	0.9	CNS
	3046	J Corrigan P Johnson	Malignant lymphoma, poorly differentiated	3.1	1.6	CNS
Follicular centre cell/polymorphic B-cell lymphoma	3009	J Miller	Histiocytic lymphoma	6.2	0.1	Multiple (CNS)
PI, polymorphic B-cell lymphoma	3017	M Schulkind R Weber	Hodgkin's disease	7.5	1.3	Multiple (CNS)
	3081	A Filipovich	Polymorphic B-cell lymphoma	8.9	0.2	CNS, pericardium
Hodgkin's disease	3020	P Periman	Hodgkin's disease	16.9	1.5	LN, spleen, liver
	3050	G Schechter	Hodgkin's disease	32	Alive	LN, spleen
Immunoblastic sarcoma of T cells	3027	R Freeman	Histiocytic lymphoma	17.5	1.1	Skin
	3037	R Heyn	Histiocytic lymphoma	22.3	3.7	LN
	3043	S Leiken	Histiocytic lymphoma	2.9	0.5	CNS

*Reticuloendothelial system;
**Reticulum Cell Sarcoma
Nos, not otherwise specified;
GI, gastrointestinal tract;
LN, lymph node

Table 9.4 University of Minnesota Immunodeficiency Cancer Registry. Response to therapy of non-Hodgkin's lymphoma in Immunodeficiency Cancer Registry

ICR No.	Age at diagnosis	Sex	Immunodeficiency	NHL diagnosis	Therapy Chem	Rad	Tumour Response	Survival post-diagnosis (months)	Cause of death
2002	2	M	SCID	ML	+	–	?	6.7	Pneumocystis carinii pneumonia (PCP)
2025	4	M	SCID	Waldenstrom's macro-globulinaemia	+	–	No R	3.0	Pneumonia
2032	1	F	SCID	IS*	+	–	No R	10.0	Candida albicans brain abscess
2033	2	M	SCID	NHL	+	–	PR	0.9	Interstitial pneumonitis, secondary to VAHS
2048	4	F	SCID	BLPD	+	–	No R	0.6	Interstitial pneumonitis
3008	8	M	Wiskott–Aldrich	ML	+	+	CR	8.0	–
3009	6	M	Wiskott–Aldrich	ML*	+	+	?	0.9	Sepsis
3017	7	M	Wiskott–Aldrich	ML*	+	+	?	6.9	GI haemorrhage
3018	19	M	Wiskott–Aldrich	IS T-cells	+	+	?	4.2	IS T-cells, pneumonia
3027	18	M	Wiskott–Aldrich	HL	+	–	?	11.4	Sepsis
3028	3	M	Wiskott–Aldrich	RCS	+	+	?	5.0	–
3031	8	M	Wiskott–Aldrich	RCS*	–	+	?	11.2	RCS (brain)
3032	6	M	Wiskott–Aldrich	RCS	+	+	?	7.1	Acute hydrocephalus
3033	11	M	Wiskott–Aldrich	ML	+	–	?	2.5	Haemorrhage
3035	4	M	Wiskott–Aldrich	RCS	+	+	?	3.9	PCP
3043	3	M	Wiskott–Aldrich	IS T-cells*	+	+	?	5.2	Pneumonia
3045	7	M	Wiskott–Aldrich	PI*	+	+	?	63.9	–
3046	3	M	Wiskott–Aldrich	Immunocytoma lymphoplasmacytic*	+	+	?	19.4	–
3052	7	M	Wiskott–Aldrich	ML	+	+	?	6.9	Sepsis
3055	9	M	Wiskott–Aldrich	ML*	+	+	?	4.3	–
3063	12	M	Wiskott–Aldrich	PI*	+	+	?	5.0	–
3072	22	M	Wiskott–Aldrich	ML*	–	+	?	4.1	Encephalitis
3073	19	M	Wiskott–Aldrich	T-cell lymphoma, large cell	–	+	?	12.2	Pneumonia
3082	21	M	Wiskott–Aldrich	ML immunoblastic	+	+	?	4.7	(Alive)
3083	4	M	Wiskott–Aldrich	ML*	–	+	?	1.7	–
4021	16	M	Ataxia telangiectasia	RCS	+	+	No R	4.0	RCS
4022	2	F	Ataxia telangiectasia	RCS	+	+	No R	1.3	–
4023	11	M	Ataxia telangiectasia	Lymphosarcoma	–	+	?	8.7	–
4026	5	F	Ataxia telangiectasia	B-cell lymphoma	+	–	No R	2.6	–
4056	11	M	Ataxia telangiectasia	HL	–	+	No R	4.6	HL
4062	9	M	Ataxia telangiectasia	Lymphosarcoma			?	25.0	–
4063	7	M	Ataxia telangiectasia	ML*	–	–	No R	24.0	'Therapeutic complications'
4067	7	M	Ataxia telangiectasia	Lymphosarcoma	+	–	PR	14.8	–

ID	Age	Sex	Immunodeficiency	Lymphoma type			Response	Time	Outcome
4089	9	M	Ataxia telangiectasia	ML	+	–	NoR	82.3	–
4098	11	M	Ataxia telangiectasia	Lymphoblastic lymphosarcoma	+	–	NoR	9.4	Pneumonia
4103	8	M	Ataxia telangiectasia	NHL	+	+	?	2.9	PCP
4106	18	M	Ataxia telangiectasia	ML, undifferentiated	+	+	?	4.9	Pneumonia
4120	11	M	Ataxia telangiectasia	ML	+	+	PR	6.3	ML
4133	17	M	Ataxia telangiectasia	HL	+	–	CR	20.9	(Alive)
4134	13	F	Ataxia telangiectasia	HL	+	–	PR	21.7	–
4137	21	M	Ataxia telangiectasia	T–cell lymphoma	+	–	NoR	5.2	Pneumonia
4144	9	M	Ataxia telangiectasia	ML	+	+	CR	106.8	(Alive)
4146	12	F	Ataxia telangiectasia	B-cell lymphoma	+	–	CR, relapse	15.9	Pneumonia
4147	11	M	Ataxia telangiectasia	Burkitt's lymphoma	+	–	PR	6.1	–
4151	15	M	Ataxia telangiectasia	Burkitt's lymphoma	+	–	CR	24.7	(Alive)
4157	6	M	Ataxia telangiectasia	B-cell lymphoma	+	–	CR	19.6	Recurrent lymphoma, sepsis
4162	18	M	Ataxia telangiectasia	ML*	+	+	NoR	2.5	Pneumonia
4165	5	F	Ataxia telangiectasia	Burkitt's lymphoma	+	–	CR	5.7	(Alive)
4168	7	M	Ataxia telangiectasia	NHL, T-cell	+	–	CR	1.5	(Alive)
4169	9	M	Ataxia telangiectasia	Lymphocytic lymphoma	+	–	NoR	1.0	Sepsis
4174	10	M	Ataxia telangiectasia	Burkitt's lymphoma	+	–	NoR	?	–
5016	70	F	CVID	Lymphocytic lymphoma	+	+	CR, relapse	?	(Alive)
5027	19	F	CVID	RCS	+	–	?	11.0	RCS
5032	57	F	CVID	Lymphoblastic lymphoma	+	+	PR	0.8	GI haemorrhage
5034	5	M	CVID	Lymphosarcoma	+	+	?	1.5	–
5036	44	F	CVID	ML	+	+	PR	48.1	(Alive)
5060	49	M	CVID	ML	+	+	?	66.3	(Alive
5105	14	F	CVID	IPSID	+	+	CR	43.4	(Alive)
5107	29	M	CVID	Diffuse mixed lymphoma	+	+	CR	?	Interstitial pneumonitis
5118	53	M	CVID	T-cell lymphoma	+	–	?	19.5	Lymphoma
5122	22	F	CVID	T-cell lymphoma*	+	+	PR	3.2	Pneumonia
5127	34	M	CVID	T-cell lymphoma*	+	–	?	2.3	Lymphoma
5134	9	M	CVID	T-cell lymphoma	+	–	CR	0.6	–
6011	46	F	Selective IgA deficiency	HL	+	–	NoR	4.3	–
8017	2	M	Hyper IgM	Lymphoblastic lymphoma	+	–	CR	54.3	–

*ICR Pathology review

Chem, chemotherapy; Rad, radiotherapy; SCID, Severe combined immunodeficiency; CVID, Common variable immunodeficiency; ML, Malignant lymphoma; HL, Histiocytic lymphoma; IS, Immunoblastic sarcoma; RCS, Reticulum cell sarcoma; NHL, Non-Hodgkin's lymphoma; PI, Plasmacytic immunocytoma; IPSID, Immunoproliferative small intestine disease; PR, partial response; CR, complete response; No R, no response; GI, gastrointestinal; PCP, *Pneumocystis carinii* pneumonia being made pre-mortem and cancer therapy is more frequently recommended. Table 9.4 lists the ICR NHL cases for which information regarding therapy and outcome are available. The overall survival for this series is discouraging: 10 of 65 patients alive (six tumour-free) at the latest ICR follow-up. Only 12 of 36 patients, for whom tumour response data are known, achieved complete remission (two later relapsed). New or progressive infections accounted for the overwhelming proportion of immediate causes of death, and median actuarial survival after diagnosis was only 5.9 months. However, occasional durable remissions have been achieved in WAS, CVID, and A-T, especially among the patients who have been recently diagnosed.

Hodgkin's disease (HD) in the ICR

Forty-three cases of HD have been recorded by the ICR for an overall proportion of 8.6 per cent. Hodgkin's disease accounts for approximately 10 per cent of tumours in many primary immunodeficiency syndromes. Characteristics of the HD cases are presented in Table 9.5. The overall median age at tumour diagnosis is 10.9 years, which reflects the contribution of four cases of HD identified in very young children with SCID (median age at tumour diagnosis: 4

months). In contrast to the male predominance observed for NHL cases, the male to female distribution of HD for immunodeficiencies with autosomal recessive inheritance is approximately equal.

Table 9.6 summarizes available information regarding the 25 patients with HD who underwent cancer therapy. Five patients are currently alive, three of them in remission. Overall, eight patients achieved complete remission and seven patients partial remission. The median survival after diagnosis was 13.6 months for treated patients. Infection was identified as the predominant cause of death, followed in frequency by progressive or recurrent tumour.

In 1986 the ICR performed a case/control study[19] designed to investigate the hypothesis that HD occurring in paediatric patients with immunodeficiency is similar to that in patients without a known immunodeficiency disorder. The objective of this study was to determine whether differences exist in demographic and clinical parameters, including outcome, of ICR cases versus non-immunodeficient patients (controls) with HD. Paediatric cases from the ICR were compared with 'controls' ascertained by the Late Effects Study Group (LESG). This group is an international consortium of investigators established to study long-term survivors

Table 9.5 Characteristics of Hodgkin's disease cases in the Immunodeficiency Cancer Registry

Immunodeficiency	No.	Sex* M:F	Age at diagnosis (years) Median	Range
Hypogammaglobulinaemia	3	2:0	10.5	<1–10.9
Severe combined immunodeficiency	4	4:0	0.3	<1–4.3
Wiskott–Aldrich syndrome	3	3:0	22.3	16.9–32.9
Ataxia telangiectasia	16	9:6	10.4	<1–25.9
Common variable immunodeficiency	8	4:4	47.0	<1–73.0
Selective IgA deficiency	3	2:1	2.8	<1–7.3
Other immunoglobulin disorders	1	0:1	38.0	–
Hyper IgM syndrome	4	2:2	12.0	3.1–18.7
Chediak–Higashi syndrome	1	0:1	9.0	–
Column total	43	26:15	10.9	<1–73.0

*Sex reported where known

Table 9.6 University of Minnesota Immunodeficiency Cancer Registry. Outcome of therapy for Hodgkin's disease in Immunodeficiency Cancer Registry

No.	Age at diagnosis	Sex	Immunodeficiency	HD stage	Therapy Chem	Rad	Tumour response	Survival post diagnosis (months)	ICR Cause of death
1009	11	M	Hypogammaglobulinaemia		+	+	PR	139.6	HD, sepsis
2041	4	M	SCID	IVB	+	-	CR	7.2	Sepsis
3020	17	M	Wiskott–Aldrich	IIIA	+	+	CR	18.2	GI haemorrhage
3037	22	M	Wiskott–Aldrich		+	+	PR	44.3	Pneumonia
3050	33	M	Wiskott–Aldrich		+	+	CR	64.3	(Alive)
4027	9	M	Ataxia telangiectasia		-	+	No R	3.4	Pneumonia
4028	9	F	Ataxia telangiectasia	IIIB	+	-	CR	10.1	-
4037	4	M	Ataxia telangiectasia		+	+	No R	0.9	Sepsis
4086	11	M	Ataxia telangiectasia	IVB	+	+	?	1.4	-
4105	14	M	Ataxia telangiectasia		+	+	PR	2.9	-
4109	4	F	Ataxia telangiectasia	IA		+	?	10.8	'Therapy complications'
4136	26	F	Ataxia telangiectasia	IIIB	+	-	?	0.8	Pneumonia
4166	21	M	Ataxia telangiectasia	IV	+	-	?	14.0	(Alive)
5015	32	M	CVID	IV	+	-	?	0.6	-
5026	63	F	CVID	IV	+	-	PR	13.6	Pneumonia
5030	49	M	CVID			+	PR	5.7	HD
5042	52	M	CVID		+	+	PR	9.0	Pneumonia
5097	73	M	CVID	IV	+	+	CR	23.1	(Alive)
5106	46	F	CVID	IIB	+	+	CR	101.0	(Alive)
5110	14	F	CVID	IVB	+	-	CR	20.8	Sepsis (pneumococcal)
6013	3	F	Selective IgA deficiency	I	+	+	?	9.7	Sepsis (pneumococcal)
6029	7	M	Selective IgA deficiency	IIB	+	+	PR	29.8	-
8001	11	M	Hyper IgM		+	+	?	136.9	Congestive heart failure
8012	3	F	Hyper IgM		+	+	?	50.0	(Alive)
16004	9	F	Chediak–Higashi	IIIB	+	+	CR	79.8	-

CR, complete response; PR, partial response; No R, no response; HD, Hodgkin's disease; GI, gastrointestinal; SCID, severe combined immunodeficiency; CVID, common variable immunodeficiency of childhood cancer. Both subject groups (LESG and ICR) were similar with regard to the proportion of males to females and the distribution of stage of disease at diagnosis. Cases reported to ICR were significantly younger ($P = 0.03$) at the time of diagnosis of HD (mean 7.8 years) compared with LESG controls (mean 11.5 years). Patients with immunodeficiency were significantly less likely to achieve an initial remission ($P = 0.001$). Survival from the time of diagnosis of HD was significantly poorer ($P = 0.001$) with 5-year actuarially estimated survival rates of 18 per cent for ICR cases and 84 per cent for LESG controls. The small group of immunodeficient patients who achieved a complete remission demonstrated a 5-year survival rate of 53 per cent compared with 86 per cent in LESG controls ($P = 0.001$).

Pathology material from 12 of the ICR cases was reviewed and demonstrated an unusual distribution of histological subtypes, as classified according to the Lukes and Butler nomenclature. In comparison to literature case series of paediatric HD patients ICR cases demonstrated a large proportion of patients with the histology of mixed cellularity (42 per cent) or lymphocyte depletion (33 per cent).

Based on these findings the following comments can be made relative to the hypothesis posed for this analysis. The finding that ICR cases were younger at diagnosis is not inconsistent with a common aetiology of HD relating to an immune defect. It is reasonable to speculate that patients with the most severe immunological defects are more likely to manifest their HD at an earlier age. Also, predominance of histological subtypes observed in ICR cases (i.e. mixed cellularity and lymphocyte depletion) may be indicative of common aetiological factors in select subgroups of HD patients without a known immunodeficiency disorder. It is not known, and will be difficult to determine, to what extent differences observed in clinical outcome are affected by the primary immunodeficiency.

Unusual lymphoproliferative disorders in patients with primary immunodeficiency

Many clinical problems associated with abnormal lymphoproliferation have been described in children and adults with primary immunodeficiency. These include intestinal nodular lymphoid hyperplasia[20], 'pseudolymphoma' or lymphoid aggregates associated with hepatomegaly,[21] immunoproliferative small intestinal disease,[22] lymphocytic interstitial pneumonitis,[23] Castlemann's disease[24] and large granular lymphocytosis associated with pancytopenia (Filipovich *et al.*, personal observations). Immunophenotyping and DNA probing for Ig gene and TCR rearrangements have identified monoclonal patterns in a proportion of these lesions concordant with the histologically monotonous appearance. In our experience at the University of Minnesota, such lesions have uniformly (four out of four cases) been eradicated by cytoreductive chemotherapy and radiation combined with allogeneic marrow transplantation for the underlying immunodeficiency.[22,23] In other cases lymphoproliferative lesions with similar clinical presentations have demonstrated polyclonal features by one or more techniques and have occasionally resolved spontaneously or with immunomodulating therapy.[21]

Lymphoproliferative disorders in secondary (acquired) immunodeficiencies

During the past 10 years, attention has been drawn to the significant number of *de novo* lymphoproliferative disorders occurring in organ allograft recipients, and in patients who have received chronic immunosuppressive treatment for non-malignant disorders. The continuing requirement for immunosuppressive therapy in growing numbers of organ transplant recipients (kidney, liver, heart, lung, pancreas, marrow) has created a numerically significant population of patients at increased risk for developing lymphoproliferative disorders. Recent information regarding the evolution of immunodeficiency in retroviral diseases (e.g. HIV infection) has led to the recognition of 'new' and even larger populations of individuals who also appear to be at increased risk of malignancy (*see* Chapter 10).

Solid organ allograft transplantation

The development of cancers, and particularly lymphoma, following allografting was first highlighted by Hoover and Fraumeni in 1973.[7] The impact of this complication has subsequently been substantiated, quantified and characterized by the Tumour Transplant Registry under Penn[8], and by Kinlen *et al*.[25] Based on analyses performed in the early 1980s lymphomas accounted for approximately one-third of post-transplant tumours, excluding non-melanomatous tumours of the skin and lips. More than half of the reported histologies of post-transplant lymphomas were consistent with B-cell lymphomas (e.g. B-cell immunoblastic sarcoma). Approximately 30 per cent of reported lymphomas were restricted to the brain or central nervous system. An approximate 2:1 male to female ratio was observed.

In a recent review Penn has compared the features of post-transplant tumours in allograft recipients treated with immunosuppressive regimens including cyclosporin A (CsA) (142 tumours in 141 patients) with the historical group (2598 tumours in 2422 patients) treated with so-called 'conventional' immunosuppressive therapy consisting of prednisone, azathioprine +/− antilymphocyte globulin.[26] Twenty-five per cent of the cancer cases following CsA immunosuppression were reported from recipients of extrarenal organs (e.g. heart, pancreas) compared with 2 per cent of post-transplant cancer cases historically. Fifty per cent of cancers in the CsA-treated group were lymphomas compared with 12 per cent of the non-CsA treated cases. Non-Hodgkin's lymphomas after CsA were diagnosed at a mean of 11 months (versus 42 months) post-grafting; more frequently involved lymph nodes and gastrointestinal sites (versus CNS); and were more likely to regress following reduction in immunosuppressive therapy.[26]

Cardiac allograft recipients have been identified as a group with unusually high susceptibility to post-transplant lymphoma.[27] This risk has been attributed to high doses of CsA administered during the early years of cardiac transplantation, and/or suspected underlying immune dysfunction associated with 'idiopathic cardiomyopathy' in certain organ recipients.[28]

The current approach to moderation of CsA dosage in cardiac, as well as other allograft, transplantation has apparently resulted in a decreased incidence of post-transplant 'lymphomas'. Post-transplant lymphoproliferative disorders in recipients of both renal[29] and cardiac[30] allografts have presented with simultaneous oligoclonal lymphoproliferative foci and have frequently been associated with either primary or reactivated Epstein–Barr virus (EBV) infection.

Bone marrow transplantation

In the early 1980s, a number of bone marrow transplant centres worldwide began to use T-cell depleted haploidentical (or otherwise partially histoincompatible) bone marrow for transplantation of patients with immunodeficiencies and haematological malignancies who did not have histocompatible sibling donors. B-cell lymphoproliferative disease (BLPD) has now become recognized as a frequent (estimated incidence 10–25 per cent) and almost universally lethal complication of mismatched T-cell depleted bone marrow grafting for primary immunodeficiency. Nine such cases of post-marrow transplant 'lymphoma' have been registered with the ICR (two cases with WAS, seven cases with SCID) and two with the Tumor Transplant Registry of Penn *et al*.

At the University of Minnesota we identified post-transplant B-cell lymphoproliferative disorders in eight patients between 1984 and 1986. Three had underlying immunodeficiency and five haematological malignancies. B-cell lymphoproliferative disorders developed between 2 and 49 months post-grafting in patients with and without T-cell depletion, and EBV was implicated as an important associated factor in all cases (Table 9.7).

From our experience with more than 500

Table 9.7 Characteristics of bone marrow transplantation and EBV exposure for eight patients who developed B-cell lymphoproliferative disease

UPN	Age at BMT/sex	Pre-BMT diagnosis	Mismatched donor	T-depleted donor marrow	Pre-transplant EBV serology** Recipient	Donor	Tumour origin	EBV genome copies/cell
588	12y/M	CML	+	+	640	320	Donor	5–50
469	14m/F	ANLL	+	+	<10	320	Donor	5–20
309	8m/M	SCID	+	+	<10	320	ND	ND
600	48y/M	CML	+*	−	320	320	Donor	20
596	30y/F	CML	−	−	320	160	Donor	15–20
541	36y/M	CML	+	+	320	<10	Donor	25
332	7.5y/M	WAS	+	+	640	ND	Host	5–20
190	13m/F	SCID	+	+	<10	<10	Host	20/50

UPN, unique patient number; BMT, bone marrow transplantation; CML, chronic myelogenous leukaemia; ANLL, acute non-lymphocytic leukaemia; SCID, severe combined immunodeficiency; WAS, Wiskott–Aldrich syndrome; EBV, Epstein–Barr virus; *, unrelated matched; **, IgG (VCA); ND, not detectable allogeneic bone marrow transplants at the University of Minnesota it appeared that donor–recipient mismatching was the most significant risk factor for BLPD which was diagnosed in six of 25 (24 per cent) recipients of mismatched T-depleted marrow, one of 10 (10 per cent) recipients of unrelated marrow, none of 60 matched T-depleted transplants and one of 24 matched non-manipulated bone marrow transplants.

The most common presenting clinical features included fever (8/8), anorexia (8/8), hepatitis (7/8), and abdominal pain (7/8). Other commonly associated findings included lethargy (6/8), lymphadenopathy (5/8), central nervous system symptoms (4/8) and pharyngitis (3/8).

Serological data regarding prior exposure of donors and recipients to EBV are shown in Table 9.7. Five patients had positive IgG antibody titres to EBV capsid antigen (VCA) prior to bone marrow transplantation, indicative of past infection. One patient was seropositive before transplantation and received marrow from a seronegative donor. Three patients had negative titres before bone marrow transplantation and two of these (UPN 469 and 309) received marrow from donors who were seropositive. At the onset of BLPD both were found to have elevated IgG titres to VCA without IgM antibodies or antibodies to Epstein–Barr nuclear antigen (EBNA). The third seronegative patient (UPN 190) received marrow from a seronegative donor. This patient developed symptoms of acute infectious mononucleosis 3.7 years after bone marrow transplantation and had a rise of both IgG and IgM titres to EBV VCA indicative of a newly acquired primary infection. DNA hybridization studies demonstrating 5–50 copies of EBV genome/cell in involved tissues in seven of seven cases studied confirms the association of EBV with BLPD in this setting and supports the contention that this virus plays a major aetiological role.

Seven of the eight patients were diagnosed as having an atypical lymphoproliferative disorder by pre-mortem biopsy. One patient (UPN 600) was diagnosed post-mortem from autopsy specimens (Table 9.8). Classification of the lymphoproliferative lesions was based on the criteria developed by Frizzera *et al.* for the polymorphic B-cell processes which develop following renal transplantation.[18] Polymorphic diffuse B-cell hyperplasia (PBCH) and polymorphic diffuse B-cell lymphomas (PBCL) were both characterized by extensive invasion of blood vessels and other organ structures as well as by obliteration of the nodal architecture in lymph nodes. Both contained a mixture of B-cells with plasmacytic differentiation and small cleaved follicular centre cells. However, lesions termed PBCH showed no atypia in the large cells and no necrosis, while PBCL was characterized by frequent atypical and multinucleated large cells, and extensive coagulative necrosis.

Atypical lymphoid hyperplasia (ALH), was characterized by involvement of the paracortex of lymph nodes or interstitial tissue of extranodal organs by collections of small lymphocytes, without morphological features of invasiveness or obliteration of normal structures. The term, atypical PBCH (APBCH), was used to describe a few lesions that had features intermediate between PBCH and PBCL. Finally, some lesions were consistent with B-immunoblastic sarcoma.

Six of seven patients with adequate tissue available for study were found to have monoclonal proliferations by *in situ* immuno-fluorescence (6/7), and/or immunoglobulin gene rearrangement (4/6). Cytogenetic analysis of involved tissues from four patients showed a normal karyotype, whereas two had multiple clonal chromosomal abnormalities (Table 9.8).

Seven patients died despite aggressive attempts at therapy with combinations of antiviral, immunological and chemotherapeutic agents. Alpha interferon may have been beneficial in the two patients treated with this agent (as discussed in greater detail below).

The biological basis of increased susceptibility to lymphoproliferative disorders in patients with immunodeficiency

Similar immunological abnormalities which may predispose to lymphomas exist among patients with either genetically determined or acquired

Table 9.8 Characteristics of B-cell lymphoproliferative processes occurring after bone marrow transplantation

UPN	Post-BMT day	Site	ALH	PBCH	APBCH	PBCL	ISB	Immunophenotype	Ig gene rearrangement analysis	Cytogenetic analysis
588	36	Liver	X					Polytypic		
	36	Cervical LN		X				Polytypic		46,XX
	43	Hilar LN				X		Monotypic	Clonal	46,XX
469	79	Liver	X					Monotypic	Clonal	
	86	Liver+		X				Monotypic	Clonal	46,XY
	86	Peripheral blood+							Clonal	46,XY
309	86	Spleen+		X				Polytypic		
	89	Appendix	X					Polytypic		
	89	Liver	X					Polytypic		
600	78	LN+			X			Monotypic	Clonal	No metaphases
	78	LN+				X			Clonal	No metaphases
	78	LN+				X				No metaphases
596	77	Axillary LN				X		Polytypic	Germ line	46,XX
541	104	Pulmonary LN				X		Monotypic	Germ line	46,XY
	104	Cervical LN					X	Monotypic		46,XY
332	549	Brain				X		Monotypic		Abnormal clone*
	593	Brain					X		Clonal	Abnormal clone*
	593	Pericardial LN					X	Monotypic	Clonal	No metaphases
190	1501	Lung nodule				X		Monotypic		
	1526	Cervical LN				X		Monotypic		Abnormal clones**
	1562	Spleen+				X		Monotypic		Abnormal clones***
	1562	LN+		X						
	1562	Kidney+			X					No metaphases

UPN, unique patient number; LN, lymph node; ALH, atypical lymphoid hyperplasia; APBCH, polymorphic B-cell hyperplasia with atypia but no necrosis; PBCH, polymorphic B-cell hyperplasia; PBCL, polymorphic B-cell lymphoma; ISB, immunoblastic sarcoma; BMT, bone marrow transplantation; +, autopsy specimen

* 46,XY,del(7)(q22),t(3;6)(q25;q23),t(13;18)(q14;q23),t,(14;21)(q24;q22)
** 46,XX/49,XX,+9,+10,+11/50,XX,+9,+9,+10,+11/92,XXXX
*** 46,XX/47,XX,+9/47,XX,+11/47,XX,+15/48,XX,+9,+15

immunodeficiencies. These are imbalances in immunoregulation, and defective ability to eradicate or control certain viral infections.

Immunoregulation, is a term used to describe internal modulation of constituent populations of the immune system during periods of homeostasis, as well as perturbation. Activation of the immune system sets in motion a series of promoting and inhibiting events. Promoting signals are generally mediated by T-helper/inducer lymphocytes and inhibiting signals by T-suppressor/cytotoxic cells. In the immunocompromised host, either excess of, or decrease in promoting signals or suppressor signals can result in failure to control activated B- and/or T-cell subpopulations, resulting in an excessive proliferation of these cells. Tumours of macroscopic proportions can develop, and result in death from organ failure secondary to imposition on vital organs (such as the brain and liver). Rapid, unchecked lymphocyte proliferation may also set the stage for chance mutational events leading to irreversible cytogenetic changes and outgrowth of one or more malignant clones.

Immunocompromised patients also frequently demonstrate defects in containment of infections caused by DNA viruses such as EBV and cytomegalovirus. Such viruses, and also the human immunodeficiency (HIV) retroviruses, are themselves polyclonal activators of immune cells and/or capable of lymphocyte transformation and stimulation of lymphokine production. Because these viruses alter the immunoregulatory balance, they often have profound and catastrophic consequences.

It is also apparent that chromosome rearrangements, which may arise as a result of errors during the normal genetic developmental programme for T or B lymphocyte differentiation are more likely to arise in certain patients with chromosomal instability, and can underlie either immunodeficiency, or lymphoid cancer, or both.

Immunoregulatory dysfunction

A number of primary immunodeficiencies[31,32] and later-onset immunoregulatory disorders[33] have been associated with decreased suppressor T-cell activity as measured by one or more methods: direct quantitation of phenotypic suppressor/cytotoxic cells (e.g. $CD3^+$, $CD8^+$ lymphocytes); qualitative assays of suppressor cell activity *in vitro*;[34] or the appearance of autoimmune phenomena, implying suppressor cell dysfunction. The functional capacity of T-suppressor cells, as well as other immune effector cells, can vary over time, particularly in association with intercurrent infections or alterations in immunosuppressive therapy. Transient decreases in suppressor cell activity may be temporally associated with periods of heightened susceptibility to lymphoproliferative disorders.

Epstein–Barr virus

Epstein–Barr virus is the prototype herpes group virus, which has been closely associated with the development of lymphoproliferative disorders in patients with compromised immunological function. It infects and immortalizes B lymphocytes *in vitro* and *in vivo*, resulting in polyclonal activation and proliferation (*see* Chapter 11). In the normal host, EBV-driven lymphoproliferation is primarily controlled by EBV-specific autologous cytotoxic T-cells (which are major histocompatibility complex (MHC) restricted),[35] with a lesser role being played by humoral responses, antibody-dependent cellular cytotoxicity, natural killer cell activity, and possibly endogenous interferons. This complex of EBV-specific immunological controls is delicately balanced to maintain the EBV in latency following primary infection.

In the immunodeficient host, suppressor and cytotoxic functions (both antigen specific and MHC restricted, as well as non-specific) are often defective, and the proliferation of EBV-infected B-cells can proceed relatively unchecked. This may result in death from organ failure secondary to infiltration and destruction of tissue by lymphoid cells, as in the fatal infectious mononucleosis (IM) of X-linked lymphoproliferative syndrome (XLP).[36] Alternatively, proliferating B- (and/or T-) cells may undergo evolution from a polyclonal reactive process to a monoclonal malignant lymphoma. In both fatal IM[37] and BLPD[38] multiple distinct clones (some involving c-*myc* oncogene rearrangement) of B-cells, and occasionally T-cells, have been detected within a matter of days following EBV infection. Epstein–Barr virus associated lymphoproliferative disorders have been documented in both primary immunodeficiency: SCID,[39,40] A–T,[41] WAS,[42] X-linked lymphoproliferative syndrome[36] and as a consequence of secondary immunodeficiency, as in solid organ or bone marrow transplant recipients.[29,38]

Chromosomal translocation

It has now been proved that irreversible DNA rearrangements involving genes which are critical for specific immunological function occur during normal human lymphocyte differentiation. These rearrangements involve breakpoints on segments of chromosomes 2, 7, 14 and 22 encoding sequences which contribute to the construction of immunoglobulin and T-cell receptor molecules. When DNA is cut as a necessary prerequisite for productive splicing of a template for immunoglobulin or T-cell receptor protein, opportunities arise for the cut segments (e.g. 7q34, beta chain locus of TCR) to reattach erroneously to a mismatched gene sequence from another chromosome that is simultaneously attempting productive gene rearrangement (e.g. 14q11, alpha chain locus of TCR). The formation of such 'non-random' translocations is thought to be catalysed by the enzymatic systems normally involved in rearrangement of the Ig or TCR genes,[43] and can be found in 1/200–1/500 peripheral blood T-cells in normal individuals.[44] Recently, it has been shown in lymphoid tumours from normal individuals that genes of the joining (J) regions of both Ig heavy chain and the alpha chain of the TCR exist in translocation with the oncogene c-*myc* (chromosome 8) suggesting a general mechanism of oncogene deregulation in B- and T-cell malignancies.[43] A number of inherited syndromes linking chromosomal instability with immunodeficiency and an apparent increased incidence of cancer have been recognized. These include ataxia telangiectasia,[3] Bloom's syndrome[45] and xeroderma pigmentosum.[46] Ataxia telangictasia provides a natural model for

the association between chromosomal rearrangement and lymphoid malignancy. Extensive chromosome analyses comparing lymphocytes from A-T and normal patients[44,47] reveal that the incidence of non-random acquired rearrangements involving the Ig supergene family in *non*-malignant lymphocytes is increased nearly 25-fold in A-T patients. In addition to translocations, inversions, duplications, and deletions involving the same set of genetic loci are very common in A-T.[44] These findings suggest that A-T patients have a functional defect in accurate splicing of Ig and TCR genes, which may contribute in large part to the variable resultant immunodeficiency. Furthermore, study of translocations observed in B- and T-cell malignancies from A-T patients suggests that two mechanisms are commonly associated with malignant transformation: translocations of 14q32, the Ig heavy chain (and less often: 2p12 and 22q11, immunoglobulin light chains) with 8q24 (c-*myc*) (as in non-immunodeficient patients);[43] and translocations between members of the pair of number 14 chromosomes followed by clonal deletion of one of the two translocation partners.[44] Thus, the A-T defect appears to magnify a common mechanism of lymphomagenesis.

Approaches to prevention and therapy of lymphoproliferative disorders associated with immunodeficiency

Prevention

Several distinct approaches can be used in combination to prevent lymphoproliferative disorders associated with immunodeficiency. One general approach is to attempt full immunoreconstitution in patients with primary immunodeficiency. Failing that, various methods of boosting immune competence have been used in patients with both primary and secondary (e.g. AIDS) immunodeficiencies. A related, often secondary approach is to avoid exposure to the viral co-factor(s) most critical to the development of uncontrolled lymphoproliferation, through prophylaxis against primary or reactivated infections with EBV in susceptible patients.

Histocompatible bone marrow transplantation is the accepted method for immunoreconstitution of patients with prematurely lethal primary immunodeficiencies. Although no reliable incidence figures for cancer in SCID exist, follow-up of 48 children with SCID successfully transplanted from histocompatible siblings[48] has recorded *no* cases of cancer developing following transplantation (note: median age at diagnosis of lymphoma in the 31 ICR cases = 1.6 years, while median post-transplant follow-up is 4.6 years). The longest follow-up is now 20 years.[49] Similarly, successfully matched marrow transplantation in WAS appears significantly to decrease the risk of subsequent fatal lymphoproliferative disorders.[48]

In contrast, partial or transient immunoreconstitution in SCID with thymic epithelial transplant[48] or haploidentical T-depleted marrow grafts[50,51] does not necessarily confer resistance to subsequent lymphoproliferative complications. It has been demonstrated that both donor marrow (most adult donors are EBV seropositive) and thymic epithelial grafts are capable of introducing EBV to an immunodeficient host. Histoincompatibility between the afferent and efferent limbs of immunity has been shown in chimeras resulting from engraftment of T-depleted parental marrow (e.g. host monocytes and B-cells with donor T-cells).[52] This chimerism can lead to chronic immunodeficiency and failure to develop efficient MHC-restricted cytotoxic responses despite the post-transplant appearance of phenotypically immunocompetent T lymphocytes. In WAS, immunomodulating therapy short of bone marrow transplantation (e.g. administration of transfer factor), has not resulted in any apparent decrease in lymphomas.[53]

Two therapies alone or in combination have been proposed for the prevention of primary EBV infection and to reduce the likelihood of reactivation of latent virus: chronic intravenous immunoglobulin transfusions; and acyclovir. Intravenous IgG prophylaxis has been recommended for patients affected with XLP and Chediak–Higashi syndrome before they encounter EBV, in hopes of preventing primary infection. No information regarding the efficacy of this approach has yet been published. Intravenous IgG has been used in combination with acyclovir (or acyclovir alone) in marrow transplant recipients considered to be at high risk of post-transplant BLPD secondary to mismatching and known donor/recipient seropositivity for EBV. Although there were early hopes for this prophylactic approach, the updated experience still indicates a very high rate of post-transplant BLPD in high risk patient groups despite such prophylaxis.

Therapy

Results with conventional combination chemotherapy and/or radiation therapy protocols have been generally disappointing in patients with primary immunodeficiencies or post-marrow transplant BLPD. Poor outcomes have been attributed to fewer tumour responses,[19] excess toxicity from the cancer therapy[54] and the exceptionally high risk of fatal infections in persons with pre-existing immune dysfunction.[54] It is important to restate that although complete and sustained remissions have been achieved in patients with primary immunodeficiency, the morbidity associated with cancer therapy is higher.

In contrast, for allograft recipients, and especially those receiving CsA, reduction or removal of immunosuppressive therapy frequently results in the elimination of abnormal lymphoproliferation. Allograft recipients are inherently immunocompetent and capable of prompt immunological recovery (days to weeks) after cessation of immunosuppressive drugs.

Recently, four patients with partial immunodeficiency have been treated to determine the efficacy of *in vivo* interferon (IFN) for therapy of lymphoproliferative disease associated with EBV (Shapiro and Filipovich, unpublished observations). Two patients (previously mentioned) developed BLPD post-marrow transplant, and two were children with CVID. Three of the four patients demonstrated dramatic and complete clinical resolution of BLPD while receiving α-interferon (2 million u/

m² every day) as the primary therapeutic agent, in conjunction with weekly infusions of intravenous IgG. The two patients with post-marrow transplant BLPD (UPNs 596 and 541) developed symptoms in the third post-transplant month. Both had disease in several organs documented by computed tomography and biopsy, UPN 541 experienced stabilization of the lymphoproliferative process and temporary symptomatic improvement, but unfortunately died of superimposed cytomegalovirus pneumonitis. In UPN 596 and the other two cases, response to alpha interferon was more dramatic with resolution of life-threatening symptoms including tracheal obstruction due to circumferential tumour, and disseminated intravascular coagulation within a week of onset of therapy. UPN 596 is alive and well and has been off interferon therapy for more than 14 months. The two children with CVID are completing a scheduled 6-month treatment course; they are at home and pursuing their normal activities. Although the mechanism of action of α-interferon is unknown, it may act by: direct antiviral effect; direct antiproliferative effect on EBV-infected B-cells; and/or modulation of the host immune responses such as natural killer function or antibody dependent cellular cytotoxicity. While these four cases represent anecdotal information, the rapid and reproducible reversal of life-threatening lymphoproliferative disease in these patients is sufficiently provoking to invite a larger pilot trial of this therapy.

diagnosis; frequent association with primary or reactivated EBV infection. Lymphoproliferative disorders often arise in patients with primary and secondary immunodeficiencies who have defective suppressor T-cell function, and when associated with EBV infection typically involve B lymphocytes in the terminal stages of differentiation. However, T-cell lymphomas have been recorded in association with EBV,[54,55] and both T-cell and non-B, non-T-lymphoid malignancies are also seen, particularly in patients with chromosomal instability syndromes.[54] While probably less common than B-cell lymphoproliferative disorders, proliferative disorders of large granular lymphocytes, or expansion of T lymphocytes along with histiocytes, as in virus associated haemophagocytic syndrome (VAHS)[56] also may arise in the context of primary or acquired immunodeficiency. In these disorders, excess or unbalanced lymphokine and monokine production may be primarily responsible for the potentially life-threatening complications such as neutropenia, pancytopenia,[57] cachexia, and interstitial pneumonitis.[56]

The recent and increasing availability of recombinant lymphokines and monokines, and well-characterized probes for specific viral and human genes, may help to unravel the mechanisms underlying increased susceptibility to fatal lymphoproliferative disorders in immunodeficient hosts during the next few years, and may offer the best hope for therapeutic intervention.

Summary

This chapter brings together descriptive information regarding the incidence, proportional distribution, and therapeutic outcome of serious lymphoproliferative disorders in patients with primary and secondary immunodeficiency disease. Features of lymphoproliferative disorders common to immunodeficient hosts include: diffuse and often highly malignant morphologies at the time of diagnosis; frequent extranodal primary sites; young age at diagnosis or short latency period (following onset of immunosuppression) to

References

1. Filipovich AH, Heinitz KJ, Robison L, Frizzera G. *American Journal of Pediatric Hematology and Oncology*. 1987; **92**, 183.
2. Perry GS III, Spector BD, Schuman LM, et al. *Journal of Pediatrics*. 1980; **97**, 72.
3. Morrell D, Cromatie E, Swift M. *Journal of the National Cancer Institute*. 1986; **77**, 89.
4. Cunningham-Rundles C, Siegal FP, Cunningham-Rundles S, Lieberman P. *Journal of Clinical Immunology*. 1987; **7**, 294.
5. Good RA. *Cancer*. 1971; **21**, 89.
6. Kersey JH, Spector BD, Good RA. In: Klein G, Weinhouse S, Haddow A (eds). *Advances in*

Cancer Research. New York: Academic Press, 1973; 211.

7. Hoover R, Fraumeni JF, Jr. *Lancet* ii. 1973; **3**, 55.

8. Penn I, First MR. *Transplantation Proceedings*. 1986; **18**, 210.

9. Ziegler J, Beckstead J, Volberding P, *et al. New England Journal of Medicine*. 1984; **311**, 565.

10. WHO Scientific Group on Immunodeficiency. *Clinical Immunology and Immunopathology*. 1983; **28**, 450.

11. Hayakawa H, Iizuba N, Yata J, Vamada K, Kobayashi N. In: Japan Medical Research Foundation ed. *Immunodeficiency, Its Nature and Etiological Significance in Human Disease*. Tokyo: University of Tokyo Press, 1978: 271.

12. Fasth A. *Journal of Clinical Immunology*. 1982; **1**, 31.

13. Aiuti F, Giunchi G, Bardare M, *et al. Immunologica Clinica*. 1978; **25**, 7.

14. Spector BD, Perry GS, III, Kersey JH. *Clinical Immunology and Immunopathology*. 1978; **11**, 12.

15. Morrell D, Chase CL, Swift M. *Genetic Epidemiology*. 1986; **3**, 17.

16. Snover DC, Frizzera G, Spector BD, Perry GS, III, Kersey JH. *Human Pathology*. 1981; **12**, 821.

17. Cotelingam JD, Witebsky FG, Hsu SM, Blaese RM, Jaffe ES. *Cancer Investigation*. 1985; **3**, 515.

18. Frizzera G, Hanto DW, Gajl-Peczalska KJ, *et al. Cancer Research*. 1981; **41**, 4262.

19. Robison L, Stoker V, Frizzera G, Heinitz KJ, Meadows AT, Filipovich AH. *American Journal of Pediatric Hematology and Oncology*. 1987; **92**, 189.

20. Hermans PE, Diaz-Buxo JA, Stobo JD. *American Journal of Medicine*. 1976; **61**, 221.

21. Snover D, Filipovich AH, Dehner L, Krivit W. *Archives of Pathology*. 1980; **105**, 46.

22. Neudorf SML, Snover S, Filipovich AH. *New England Journal of Medicine*. 1983; **309**, 1126.

23. Blazar BR, Ramsay NKC, Kersey JH, Krivit W, Arthur DC, Filipovich AH. *Transplantation*. 1985; **39**, 597.

24. Perentesis JP, Ramsay NKC, Filipovich AH. *Proceedings of the Northwest Pediatric Society*. 1985.

25. Kinlen LJ, Sheil AGR, Peto J, Doll R. *British Medical Journal*. 1979; **2**, 1461.

26. Penn I. *Transplantation*. 1987; **43**, 32.

27. Penn I. *Transplantation Proceedings*. 1979. **11**, 1047.

28. Anderson JL, Bieber CP, Fowles RE, Stinson EB. *Lancet*. 1978; ii, 1174.

29. Hanto DW, Frizzera G, Gajl-Peczalska KJ, *et al. New England Journal of Medicine*. 1982; **306**, 913.

30. Brumbaugh J, Baldwin JC, Stinson EB, *et al. Heart Transplantation*. 1985; **4**, 307.

31. Filipovich AH, Spector BD, Frizzera G, Kersey JH. In: Giraldo G, Beth E (eds). *The Role of Viruses in Human Cancer*. New York: Elsevier North

Holland, 1980: 237.

32. Graze RR, Gale RP. *American Journal of Medicine*. 1979; **66**, 611.

33. Horowitz S, Borcherding W, Molorthy A, *et al. Science*. 1977; **197**, 999.

34. Hallgren HM, Yunis EJ. *Journal of Immunology*. 1977; **118**, 2004.

35. Tsoukas CD, Fox RI, Slavin SF, *et al. Journal of Immunology*. 1981; **126**, 1742–46.

36. Sullivan JL. *Advances in Pediatrics*. 1984; **30**, 365.

37. Brichacek B, Davis J, Purtilo DT. In: Levine PH, Ablashi DV, Nonoyama M, Pearson GR, Glaser R (eds). *Epstein–Barr Virus and Human Disease*. Clifton: Humana Press Inc., 1987: 53.

38. Shapiro RS, McClain K, Blazar B, *et al.* In: Levine PH, Ablashi DV, Nonoyama M, Pearson GR, Glaser R (eds). *Epstein – Barr Virus and Human Disease*. Clifton: Humana Press Inc., 1987; 91.

39. Reece ER, Gartner JG, Seemayer TA, Joncas JH, Pagano JS. *Cancer Research*. 1981; **41**, 4243.

40. Borzy MS, Hong R, Horowitz SD, *et al. New England Journal of Medicine*. 1979; **301**, 565.

41. Saemundsen AK, Berkel AI, Henle W, *et al. British Medical Journal*. 1981; **282**, 425.

42. Model LM. *Archives of Neurology*. 1977; **34**, 633.

43. Finger LR, Harvey RC, Moore RCA, Showe LC, Croce CM. *Science*. 1986; **234**, 982.

44. Hecht F, Hecht BKM. *American Journal of Pediatric Hematology and Oncology*. 1987; **9**, 185.

45. Willis AE, Lindahl T. *Nature*. 1987; **325**, 355.

46. Hecht F, McCaw BK. In: Mulvihill JJ, Miller RW, Fraumeni JF (eds). *Genetics of Human Cancer*. New York: Raven Press, 1977: 105.

47. Aurias A, Dutrillaux B. *Human Genetics*. 1986; **72**, 210.

48. Neudorf SML, Filipovich AH, Kersey JH. In: Purtilo DT (ed). *Immune Deficiency and Cancer: Epstein–Barr Virus and Lymphoproliferative Malignancies*. New York: Plenum Press, 1984: 471.

49. Gatti RA, Allen HD, Meuwissen HF, *et al. Lancet*. 1968; ii, 1366.

50. Shearer WT, Ritz J, Finegold MJ, *et al. New England Journal of Medicine*. 1985; **312**, 1151.

51. Kapoor N, Jung LKL, Engelhard D, *et al. Journal of Pediatrics*. 1986; **108**, 435.

52. Reinherz EL, Geha R, Rappaport JM, *et al. Proceedings of the National Academy of Sciences. USA*. 1982; **79**, 6047.

53. Spitler LE, Levin AS, Fudenberg HH. *Birth Defects*. 1975; **XI**, 449.

54. Spector BD, Filipovich AH, Perry GS, III, Kersey JH. In: Bridges BA, Harnden DG (eds). *Ataxia-Telangiectasia*. Chichester: John Wiley and Sons, Ltd., 1982; 103.

55. Jones JF, Shurin S, Abramowsky C, Katz B,

Sklar J. In: Levine PH, Ablashi DB, Nonoyama M, Pearson GR, Glaser R (eds). *Epstein–Barr Virus and Human Disease*. Clifton: Humana Press, 1987; 97.

56. Reynolds CW, Foon KA. *Blood*. 1984; **64**, 1146.

57. McClain K, Gehrz R, Grierson H, Purtilo D, Filipovich AH. *American Journal of Pediatric Hematology and Oncology*. 1988; **10**: 196.

CHAPTER 10

LYMPHOMAS IN HIV-POSITIVE INDIVIDUALS

John L Ziegler and Michael S McGrath

In this chapter we consider the clinical and biological aspects of the non-Hodgkin's lymphomas in association with the acquired immunodeficiency syndrome (AIDS). We describe first the clinical features and management, followed by a discussion of pathogenesis.

Historically, patients with immune deficiencies and autoimmune disorders have an excess incidence of non-Hodgkin's lymphomas. As pointed out in Chapters 1 and 7, these tumours tend to be of intermediate or high-grade histology and appear frequently in extranodal sites. The clinical management of these patients is made difficult by the underlying immune disorder. Although the tumours respond to radiation therapy and cytotoxic drugs, the clinical outcome is determined largely by the degree and reversibility of the immunodeficiency.

In the early years of the AIDS epidemic, we encountered in San Francisco four homosexual men who inexplicably developed high grade lymphomas.[1] Their tumours were widespread and responded only temporarily to treatment; they all died ultimately of uncontrolled tumour growth and opportunistic infections. We subsequently collected a series of 90 homosexual men from five major medical centres who exhibited similar clinical features, and a clear link between lymphomas and AIDS was established.[2] Among the AIDS risk groups, homosexual men are most susceptible to development of lymphoma, followed by intravenous drug abusers, haemophiliacs and heterosexual/childhood cases. It is apparent from personal clinical experience that the incidence of AIDS-related lymphoma is rising as the AIDS epidemic matures, but precise national or international demographic estimates are not yet available. At San Francisco General Hospital, the proportion of AIDS patients with non-Hodgkin's lymphoma has nearly tripled between 1985 and 1987, from 2.5 to 7 per cent. Virtually all patients are homosexual men.

Clinical features

Since the publication of the original 90 cases of AIDS-associated lymphomas in 1984, numerous case reports and small series have appeared in the literature. Table 10.1 summarizes the largest of these series.[3–12]

The majority of histological diagnoses fall into the high grade (immunoblastic, small non-cleaved cell) or intermediate grade (large cell) categories. these histological patterns are largely consistent with B-cell origin.[13] It should be noted that while diffuse large cell lymphoma by the Rappaport classification was ranked as intermediate grade because of recent therapeutic success with this histological subtype,[14] the prognosis of patients with AIDS-associated large cell lymphomas is similar to that of high grade.[2,6]

All reports of AIDS-associated lymphomas have emphasized several atypical features:

1. there is a 5- and 20-fold increase in expected frequency of bone marrow and central

Table 10.1 Clinical features of AIDS-associated non-Hodgkin's lymphomas

			Reporting centre				
	Multi centre[2]	USF[6]	Memorial SKI[7]	UCSF[4]	NYU[10]	Pac Med Center[11]	Total (%)
Number of patients	90	63	52	40	20	18	281(100)
Pathological classification[14]							
High grade	56	56	33	21	20	8	194 (69)
Intermediate	26	7	16	19		10	78 (28)
Low grade	6		3				9 (3)
Chemotherapy response							
Complete	35/66	10/19	17/30	15/35	7/16	4/11	88/177 (50)
Partial/none	31/66	9/19	13/30	20/35	9/16	7/11	89/177 (50)
Survival of CRs							
% NED after 6 months	11/66	6/10	9/17	7/15	6/7	4/4	43/119 (36)

CR, Complete response; NED, No evidence of disease; USF, University of San Francisco; SKI, Sloane–Kettering Institute; UCSF, University of California in San Francisco; NYU, New York University; Pac Med Center, Pacific Medical Center

nervous system involvement, respectively

2. at least one-third of patients present with tumours in atypical, extranodal sites such as rectum, parotid gland, mouth, heart, orbit and lung
3. the majority (about 75 per cent in one series) have 'B' symptoms of unexplained fever, night sweats and/or weight loss, although these symptoms may be attributable to underlying human immunodeficiency virus (HIV) infection
4. approximately one-third of patients present with lymphoma as their first manifestation of HIV infection, one-third have pre-existing generalized lymphadenopathy, and one-third have AIDS at the time their lymphoma is diagnosed.

Patients with AIDS-associated lymphoma present a therapeutic dilemma because of the risk of further myelo- and immunosuppression from cytotoxic therapy. Most experts agree that management should be individualized, according to the following guidelines:

Stage I: if tumour is truly localized after extensive staging work-up, radiotherapy may be considered as the sole treatment modality, particularly in the presence of concomitant infections

Stages II–IV: combination chemotherapy regimens, tailored in intensity and composition to the patient's clinical status (e.g. avoid bleomycin in pulmonary compromise, avoid prednisone in active mycobacterial infection).

All reports emphasize the high rate of meningeal involvement and recommend intrathecal chemoprophylaxis. Finally, *Pneumocystis carinii* pneumonia is the commonest opportunistic infection in these patients, and prophylaxis with trimethoprim-sulphamethoxazole, Fansidar, or aerosolized pentamidine is recommended.

At the San Francisco General Hospital, we employ an outpatient cyclic chemotherapy combination: cyclophosphamide 1200 mg/m^2 i.v. and vincristine 1.4 mg/m^2 i.v. on day 1; methotrexate 500 mg in a 6-hour infusion with leucovorin rescue (25 mg orally every 6 hours, 6 times on day 8); etoposide 150 mg/m^2 i.v. and arabinosyl cytosine 3.0 g i.v. on day 22. The regimen is then repeated every 3 weeks for six cycles. Intrathecal methotrexate 12 mg weekly for 4 weeks is also given. Patients with primary central nervous system lymphoma are managed by surgery and radiation therapy, but their prognosis is extremely poor.[8]

Pathogenesis

Individuals infected with HIV have marked abnormalities of the B lymphocyte compartment. Peripheral blood B lymphocytes from HIV-infected individuals display a 10-fold increase in spontaneous proliferation, and spontaneous secretion of immunoglobulins.[15] These abnormalities are not corrected by the addition of normal helper T lymphocytes, suggesting that B lymphocytes from HIV-infected individuals have either intrinsic defects or are responding to some proliferative stimulus present *in vivo*. This increased B-cell activity is responsible for the finding of hypergamma-globulinaemia, and more recently the finding of monoclonal and oligoclonal paraproteins in the serum of HIV-infected individuals.[16]

Because of the high prevalence of B-cell lymphoma in AIDS, it is logical to examine the genesis of the vigorous B-cell proliferation that characterizes the earlier clinical stages of AIDS-related complex (ARC) and AIDS. At least four mechanisms have been identified. One is activation of Epstein–Barr virus (EBV), which by itself can 'immortalize' B-cells *in vitro* and is impugned in the genesis of other lymphomas such as Burkitt's lymphoma in Africa and the immunoblastic lymphomas in X-linked immunodeficiency.[15,17] A second mechanism is activation of cytomegalovirus, which is capable of stimulating B-cell proliferation *in vitro*.[18] A third possibility is a direct mitogenic effect of HIV.[19] Finally, HIV infection of CD4 (helper-inducer) lymphocytes and macrophages will induce lymphokines that stimulate B-cell proliferation (including EBV-containing cells).[20] It is not known at present which of these mechanisms predominates in the B-cell proliferation of AIDS. It is clear, however, that with repeated mitosis and a larger pool of B-cells, accidental translocations and other chromosomal errors are more likely to occur, leading to lymphoma development.

Lymphomagenesis in AIDS may be directly related to retroviral replication. In experimental systems, chronic antigenic stimulation has been implicated as a cause of B-cell transformation. For example, the H-2a4bp/wts mouse strain develops high grade B-cell lymphomas after hyperimmunization with sheep red blood cells (SRBC). Analysis of the lymphoma surface immunoglobulins showed them to be directed against SRBC determinants.[21] Similarly, B-cell lymphomas develop spontaneously in BALB/c mice in association with an endogenous retrovirus and display cell surface IgM directed against retroviral gene products.[22] Although the sequence of events leading to B-cell transformation *in vivo* is likely to be complex, it is plausible that transformation in some cases can be initiated through chronic antigenic stimulation, although to date the presence of anti-HIV determinants on B-cell lymphomas in AIDS patients has not been demonstrated.

Human immunodeficiency virus antigens cause B-cell proliferation either in a mitogenic, or antigen specific manner,[19,20] and anti-HIV antibody titres greater than 1:1 000 000 are commonly encountered in HIV-infected individuals.[23] The finding that the macrophage is a principal target for HIV infection and viral expression[24] suggests that this population of HIV antigen expressing cells may serve as a potent stimulus for HIV responsive B lymphocytes *in vivo*. No data are currently available concerning the antigenic specificity of AIDS-associated lymphoma immunoglobulin.

Although the principal retrovirus present in HIV-infected individuals is HIV, retroviral-mediated antigenic stimulation could be caused by another retrovirus. For example, some HIV-infected individuals are co-infected with leukaemia viruses, the human T-cell lympho-trophic viruses (HTLV-I, HTLV-II).[25] Type I has been implicated as the transforming agent, or at least a predisposing agent in adult T-cell leukaemia in HIV-infected individuals,[26] and in B-cell transformation in a subpopulation of patients infected with HTLV-I alone.[27]

Because HTLV-I is a non-cytopathic virus, transformation of B-cells mediated through antigenic stimulation can be envisaged to occur through two separate mechanisms. Figure 10.1 demonstrates that initiation of the transformation cascade could occur with a cell making its own set of antigens (*a*). In this situation the retrovirus-infected transformed cell would express an immunospecific receptor for a retrovirus determinant thereby causing continued rounds of proliferation. Alternatively, (*b*) an antigen-presenting accessory cell chronically producing retroviral antigens could cause antigenic stimulation indirectly, and responding B lymphocytes would be unable to escape the chronic stimulus produced by those infected accessory cells. This model does not exclude any of the previously discussed models of B-cell transformation. After antigen specific activation, any non-lethal mutation including those described previously could contribute to the lymphomagenic process as it occurs *in vivo*.

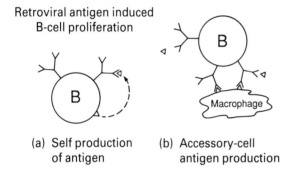

Fig. 10.1 Model for retrovirus-directed lymphomagenesis. (a) Auto-produced antigens. (b) Antigens derived from accessory cells (*see* text).

An extensive essay on the molecular aspects of lymphomagenesis is beyond the scope of this chapter, but several points relative to HIV infection are noteworthy. Oncologists generally agree that non-Hodgkin's lymphomas in AIDS patients are predominantly monoclonal tumours that derive from oligoclonal B-cell proliferation. The precise biochemical events that lead to malignant transformation are unknown but presumably involve a step-wise medley of proto-oncogene activation. A possible scenario is depicted in Fig. 10.2, wherein polyclonal B-cell proliferation leads to 8;14 (or 8;2 or 8;22) chromosome translocation. The *c-myc* proto-oncogene then becomes transcriptionally active in its new environment. Activation of other

transforming proto-oncogenes such as B-*lym*, c-*fgr*, and c-*ras*, may also play a role.[28–30]

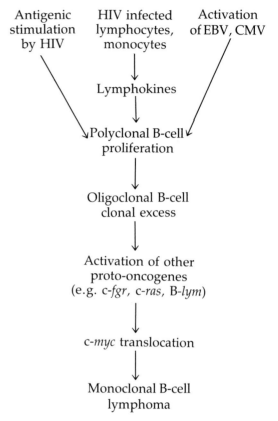

Fig. 10.2 Pathogenesis of non-Hodgkin's lymphoma in AIDS. B-cell proliferation can result from a number of events: direct HIV (or related retrovirus) stimulation; B-cell directed lymphokines from HIV-infected immunocytes; activation of endogenous DNA viruses (*see* text). EBV, Epstein–Barr virus; CMV, cytomegalovirus.

The activation of *c-myc* appears to be an important event in lymphomagenesis. Recent work has demonstrated heterogeneity in the c-*myc* breakpoint that correlates with the stage of differentiation of the transformed B-cell. Thus, tumours from patients with EBV-associated Burkitt's lymphoma (endemic in Africa) display c-*myc* breakpoints 5′ of the first exon of the gene and may be a consequence of errors in the V-D-J joining process. Conversely, tumours from patients with 'sporadic' Burkitt's lymphoma display breaks within the 5′ portion of the gene, and may be a consequence of errors in the heavy chain switching process.[31,32] Since V-D-J joining precedes IgM class switching, these data imply that *c-myc* translocation in endemic (EBV-associated) Burkitt's lymphoma occurs at an earlier stage of B-cell differentiation than in sporadic Burkitt's lymphoma (Table 10.2).

Table 10.2 Pathogenesis of *c-myc* translocation in Burkitt's lymphoma

	Endemic (African)	Sporadic (American)
Breakpoint	Outside *myc*	Inside *myc*
c-myc rearranged	No	Yes
Error	V-D-J joining	Ig class switch
Maturity	Less mature	More mature

In summary, lymphomagenesis associated with HIV infection is undoubtedly a complex, multifactorial process. The common denominator appears to be polyclonal B-cell proliferation, followed by clonal outgrowth of malignant, transformed cells. Clinically, these tumours are difficult to manage and ways must be sought to reverse the immunodeficiency caused by HIV.

References

1. Ziegler JL, Drew WL, Miner RC, *et al. Lancet* 1982; ii, 631.
2. Ziegler JL, Beckstead JA, Volberding PA, *et al. New England Journal of Medicine.* 1984; **311**, 565.
3. Kalter SP, Riggs SA, Canbanillas F, *et al. Blood.* 1985; **66**, 655.
4. Kaplan LD, Volberding PA, Abrams DI. *III International Conference on AIDS*, June 1–5, 1987, 9 (abstract).
5. Kaplan MH, Susin M, Pahwa SG, *et al. American Journal of Medicine.* 1987; **82**, 389.
6. Levine AM, Gill PS. *Oncology.* 1987; **1**, 41.
7. Lowenthal DA, Straus DJ, Campbell SW, Gold JWM, Clarkson BD, Koziner B. *Cancer,* 1988; **61**, 2325.
8. So YT, Beckstead JA, Davis RL. *Annals of Neurology.* 1986; **20**, 566.
9. Ioachim HL, Cooper NC, Hellman GC. *Cancer.* 1985; **56**, 2831.
10. Odajnyk C, Subar M, Dugan M, *et al. Blood.* 1986; **68**, 131A.
11. Bernandez MA, Grant KM, Rodvien R. *Blood,* 1986; **68**, 121.
12. Dugan M, Subar M, Odajnyk C, *et al. Blood.* 1986; **68**, 124A.
13. Samuels BL, Ultmann JE. *Annals of Oncology.* 1987; **3**, 10.
14. Rosenberg SA, Berard CW, Brown CW. *Cancer.* 1982; **49**, 2112.
15. Birx DL, Redfield RR, Tosato G. *New England Journal of Medicine.* 1986; **314**, 874.
16. Heriot K, Hallquist AE, Tomar RH. *Clinical Chemistry.* 1985; **31**, 1224.
17. Hanto DW, Frizzera G, Gajl-Peczalska KJ, Simmons RL. *Transplantation.* 1985; **39**, 461.
18. Yachie A, Tosato G, Straus RA, Blaese RM. *Clinical Research.* 1984; **32**, 510A.
19. Schnittman SM, Lane HC, Higgins SE, Folks T, Fauci AS. *Science.* 1986; **233**, 1084.
20. Yarchoan R, Redfield R, Broder S. *Journal of Clinical Investigations.* 1986; **78**, 439.
21. Bishop GA, Arnold IW, Haughton G. *Critical Reviews in Immunology.* 1986; **6**, 105.
22. McGrath MS, Tamura GS, Weissman IL. *Journal of the National Cancer Institute.* 1987; in press.
23. Nath N, Wunderlich C, Darr FW, *et al. Journal of Clinical Microbiology.* 1987; **25**, 364.
24. Crowe S, Mills J, McGrath MS. *AIDS Research and Human Retroviruses.* 1987; **3(2)**, 46.
25. Robert-Guroff M, Weiss SH, Giron JA, *et al. Journal of the American Medical Association.* 1986; **215**, 3133.
26. Harper ME, Kaplan MT, Marselle LM, *et al. New England Journal of Medicine.* 1986; **315**, 1703.
27. Mann DL, DeSantis P, Mark G, *et al. Science.* 1987; **236**, 1103.
28. Pelicci P-G, Knowles DM, Arlen ZA, *et al. Journal of Experimental Medicine.* 1986; **164**, 2045.
29. Chea MSC, Ley TJ, Tronick SR, Robbins KC. *Nature.* 1986; **319**, 238.
30. Diamond A, Devine JM, Cooper GM. *Science.* 1984; **225**, 516.
31. Pelicci P-G, Knowles DM, Magrath IT, Dalla-Favera R. *Proceedings of the National Academy of Sciences USA.* 83, 2984.
32. Haluska FG, Finter S, Tsujimoto Y, Croce CM. *Nature.* 1986; **324**, 158.

CHAPTER 11

VIRUSES ASSOCIATED WITH NON-HODGKIN'S LYMPHOMAS

Dharam V Ablashi and S Zaki Salahuddin

The first evidence that a virus or filterable agent could cause tumours dates back approximately 80 years to the studies of Rous[1] and Ellerman and Bang[2] in chickens. About 50 years later, Gross showed that viruses could cause leukaemia in inbred mice.[3] Subsequently, Jarrett et al.[4,5] in an experiment with cats, demonstrated for the first time the viral aetiology of naturally occurring leukaemia/lymphoma in an outbred mammalian species.[6,7]

The possibility that a diffuse B-cell lymphoma, which involved the jaws of African children and which was first described by Denis Burkitt in 1958,[8] (Burkitt's lymphoma, BL) might have a viral aetiology, resulted from investigations carried out by Epstein and his associates Achong and Barr in 1964.[9] Electron micrographs (EM) showed that uncultured sections of primary tissues from an African BL tumour were negative for virus particles. However, EM examination of cultured cells in vitro revealed virus particles which morphologically resembled herpesviruses (see Fig. 11.1a and b).[10,11] Following the initial discovery, an identical herpesvirus, later termed Epstein–Barr virus (EBV), was observed in other cell lines established from BL tumours from widely separated parts of the world, and in cell lines established from normal blood donors as well as from patients with infectious mononucleosis (IM). Further investigations by Henle and Henle[12,13] showed that EBV was a new herpesvirus.

Since these initial observations, an immense body of information has accumulated on EBV, one of the few DNA viruses which has been associated with human cancer. Epstein–Barr virus has been shown to cause IM, to be associated with BL and nasopharyngeal carcinoma (NPC)[13–16] and has now been linked to other neoplasms and polyclonal lymphoproliferative disorders in immunocompromised individuals (Table 11.1).[17] A survey by Lenoir et al.[18] showed that, besides the endemic area for this tumour (equatorial Africa and New Guinea), BL is found throughout most of the rest of the world. However, although by definition all BLs, regardless of their geographic origin, are histologically identical, only a minority (20 per cent) of those found outside equatorial Africa and New Guinea are EBV-genome positive. This geographical variation poses a number of questions regarding the role of EBV in the pathogenesis of BL and raises the possibility that, despite uniform histology, BL in different regions differs biologically.

The past few years have been momentous in retrovirology because of the discovery of another family of viruses linked with human neoplasia.[19,20] These viruses, known as human T-cell lymphotrophic viruses, HTLV-I, HTLV-II and HTLV-III or LAV (now called human immunodeficiency virus, HIV), are aetiologically associated with opposite ends of the spectrum of human T-cell diseases. Successful isolation of these viruses came after two important discoveries. The first was the validation of the antithetical notion that DNA can be synthesized

Table 11.1 EBV-associated diseases

Burkitt's lymphoma
Nasopharyngeal carcinoma (undifferentiated
 and well differentiated)
Salivary gland:
 (a) adenoid-cystic carcinoma from Sjögren's
 syndrome
 (b) undifferentiated lymphoepithelial lesion
Carcinoma of the palatine tonsil
Thymic carcinoma
Cervical carcinoma (epithelial cells)
Wiskott–Aldrich syndrome and Chediak–
 Higashi syndrome (EBV detected in
 malignant lymphoproliferative nodes)
Some B-cell lymphomas in AIDS
X-linked lymphoproliferative syndrome
Infectious/chronic mononucleosis
Hairy leucoplakia

Modified from Ablashi *et al.*[17]
Hairy leucoplakia's epithelial cells not only have EBV-DNA, but also replicate EBV, as demonstrated by monoclonal antibodies and electron microscopy.

on an RNA template under the influence of the enzyme reverse transcriptase. The recognition of reverse transcriptase not only shed light on fundamental biological processes, but also provided knowledge about how retroviruses cause disease. The second, the discovery of T-cell growth factor (TCGF), or interleukin-2 (IL-2), in the conditioned medium of lectin-stimulated lymphocyte cultures, permitted the propagation *in vitro* of neoplastic T-cell lines and led to the discovery of HTLV-I in 1978, HTLV-II in 1982 and HIV in 1983–84.[19–22] Human retroviruses show similarities and some important differences from animal retroviruses. Most animal leukaemias are characterized by abundant retroviral replication, and the isolation of such viruses has been easy. Human retroviruses, on the other hand, do not give rise to viraemia, and only the successful culture of the leukaemic cells *in vitro* permitted virus isolation.[21] Since these initial observations many new isolates of human retroviruses have been reported. Moreover, the counterparts of these viruses have also been isolated from non-human primates.[21,22]

In this chapter we review the epidemiology, immunovirology, molecular analysis and animal studies of EBV which link this virus to B-cell lymphomas and to other tumours. We provide, at the same time, approaches of value to laboratory investigations, clinical diagnosis and the determination of the prognosis of EBV- or other herpesvirus-associated diseases. We also briefly describe the new member of the human herpes virus family, human B-cell lymphotropic virus (HBLV), now designated human herpesvirus-6 (HHV-6), which was recently isolated from patients with B-cell lymphoma in AIDS and other malignancies and lympho-proliferative disorders.[23] Because of the importance of human retroviruses to T-cell leukaemia/lymphoma, we also review the epidemiology, immunobiology and molecular analysis of HTLV-I and HTLV-II. Even though the aetiology of tumours is multifactorial, the demonstration of a viral role in the causation of some lymphomas and carcinomas could lead to the prevention of these diseases by means of a vaccine, or to the development of novel therapeutic approaches using immune modulators and/or antiviral drugs.

Herpesviruses

Morphological characterization

Epstein–Barr virus and HHV-6 are herpesviruses (Fig.11.1a and b) which are characterized by the presence of double-stranded linear DNA in the core of the virion, an icosadeltahedron containing 162 capsomers, which is assembled in the nucleus, and an envelope derived from either the nuclear membrane or the cell surface membrane. Even though herpesviruses are highly disseminated in nature, they vary greatly in their biological properties, host range and replication efficiency.

Epstein–Barr virus

Replication, molecular analysis of the EBV genome and the presence of EBV DNA in tumours

Epstein-Barr virus infects cells by attachment to a cell surface receptor, which in lymphocytes is

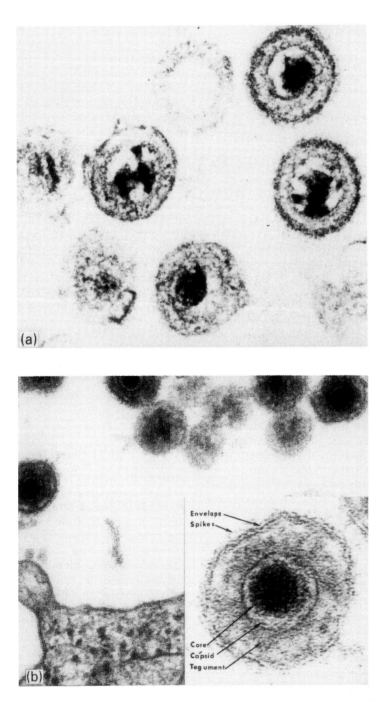

Fig. 11.1 (a) Epstein–Barr virus particles at different stages of replication in a B-lymphoblastoid cell line established from Burkitt's lymphoma from an AIDS patient; (b) enveloped and unenveloped extracellular HHV-6 particles from HHV-6-infected human cord blood mononuclear cells. The insert shows an HHV-6 particle exhibiting typical herpesvirus morphology.

also a receptor for the c3d component of complement.[16] Cells productively infected with virus undergo lysis and do not survive,[16,24] but in some cells, notably mature B-cells, latent infection, in which virion assembly does not occur, can result in immortalization of the cell which then becomes capable of proliferating indefinitely, at least *in vitro*. Pre-B-cells have also been shown to be liable to infection with EBV. The population of B-cells susceptible to transformation has been variably estimated to be between 10 and 100 per cent of circulating B lymphocytes.[16]

The transcription and replication of viral DNA and the assembly of the capsid takes place in the nucleus. The DNA of EBV is a large, double-stranded molecule with a guanine and cytosine content of approximately 59 per cent, a molecular weight of 10^8 daltons and a density of 1.718 g/ml in CsCl.[16] The DNA of EBV has been used as a probe to demonstrate the presence of the virus in BL-derived cell lines,[25,26] as well as in lymphoblastoid cell lines. In such cell lines the viral genomes are predominantly present in a latent form as multiple, extra-chromosomal or episomal circular DNA molecules.[27] Some viral genomes are also believed to be stably integrated into cellular DNA. In the virion the genome is linear, and consists of about 175 000 base pairs.[28,29] The entire genome of the transforming EBV (B95-8) has been sequenced.[28]

The association of EBV with BL, initially demonstrated by immunological assays, was confirmed by molecular hybridization. Using EBV DNA as a probe, hybridization to human tumour biopsies has demonstrated the presence of EBV genomes in BL and anaplastic carcinomas of the nasopharynx, as well as other carcinomas and lymphomas (*see* Table 11.1). In contrast, DNA from other carcinomas of the head and neck region and from other lymphomas were negative for EBV. The DNA of EBV has also been detected in oral hairy cell leucoplakia. In this disease, unlike other EBV-containing epithelial neoplasms, viral replication can be readily demonstrated.[30]

Strains of EBV

Biologically, two strains of EBV have been defined (non-transforming and transforming), based on their abilities to 'transform' peripheral B lymphocytes into cell lines capable of indefinite propagation *in vitro*. One non-transforming strain, P3HR-1, infects, but does not immortalize primary B-cells, although it can induce EBV early antigens in EBV genome-containing B-cell lines, such as Raji.[16,24] Even though non-transforming strains of EBV have been isolated from patients,[31,32] there is as yet no clear-cut association of individual disease with specific virus strains. So far, 99.5 per cent of EBV isolates are of the transforming type. However, both transforming and non-transforming strains have been reported from AIDS patients.[33] The pathological significance of this finding is not known. Strains of EBV differ with regard to the patterns of DNA fragments produced when viral DNA is digested by restriction endonucleases (enzymes which cut double-stranded DNA at specific sites defined by the nucleotide sequence) (Fig. 11.2a).

Humoral immunity: EBV antigens

Immunofluorescence assays (IFAs) have allowed the identification of four major viral antigen complexes in cells infected with the virus, i.e. early antigens (EA), virus capsid antigen (VCA), membrane antigens (MA) and nuclear antigens (EBNA). Based on human sera, approximately 35 polypeptides expressed during the viral replication cycle have been described.[34,35] Recently, with the aid of monoclonal antibodies, major EBV proteins which make up the four major antigen complexes have been characterized. The genomic location of the EBNAs is shown in Fig. 11.2b.

EARLY ANTIGENS (EA)

Early antigens are a group of non-structural polypeptides whose synthesis does not require DNA-synthesis, hence the designation 'early'. Their expression is necessary for virus replication. The serum level of antibody to this antigen has prognostic value in patients with acute or chronic EBV infections and EBV-

(a)

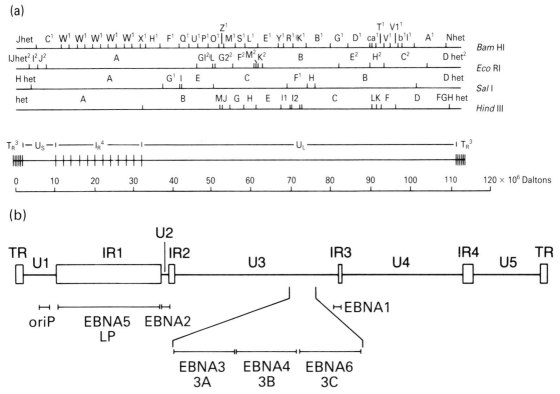

(b)

Fig. 11.2 (a) Linkage map of the B95-8 strain of EBV, showing restriction enzyme sites for BamH1, EcoR1, Sal 1 and Hind 111; repeat unique regions of the genome (T_R terminal repeats; U_S and U_L short and long unique regions; I_R internal repeats); scale is in daltons; modified from Dambaugh *et al*. In Palese A, Roizman B (eds). *Genetic Variations of Viruses*. New York Academy of Sciences **354**, 1980: 309. (b) structural map of EBV genome showing location of regions coding for EBNAs. oriP, origin of plasmid replication; U, unique regions; R, repeat regions; T, terminal; I, internal.

associated malignancies, such as BL and NPC. Human sera were found to possess antibody to the two main components of the EA complex, diffuse (D) or restricted (R), using IFAs, and were also found to immunoprecipitate several polypeptides from cells expressing EA. The major protein of EA-D is a phosphoprotein with a variable size of 50–56 kilodaltons (K), and of unknown function. The 85 K EA-R polypeptide is a component of the EBV ribonucleotide reductase.[36] It has been shown by IFA that EA-R antibodies are found in patients with BL, that the titres of such antibodies correlate with the tumour burden, and therefore prognosis, and that the serum level decreases after treatment.[34,35,37] In NPC patients, anti-EA-D titres are elevated and also have prognostic value. In normal individuals EA antibodies tend to be low or absent, and elevated levels are usually detected only in the acute phase of IM (Table 11.2).

VIRUS CAPSID ANTIGEN (VCA)

This antigen is found within cells producing virus. It was the first EBV antigen to be identified and antibodies against it have long been of predominant importance in seroepidemiological studies. The major polypeptide in EBV nucleocapsids has a molecular weight of 160 K,[35] and most VCA-positive human sera will precipitate it. This protein is partially encoded by the EcoRl 'I' fragment of the genome (*see* Fig. 11.2a). Recent investigations have shown that a glycosylated polypeptide of 125 K found predominantly in the cytoplasm is a major VCA antigen and that the BamH1 'IA' fragment of the viral genome contains the gene encoding this glycoprotein (*see* Fig. 11.2a).[34,35]

Pearson *et al.*[34] have developed a sensitive enzyme-linked immunosorbent assay (ELISA) to measure VCA-IgG and VCA-IgA antibodies to the EBV-specific 125 K protein. A good correlation was found between ELISA and IFA antibody titres, although, in general, the ELISA assay is more sensitive.

MEMBRANE ANTIGENS (MA)

The EBV–MA complex is of particular importance to the efforts to develop a subviral vaccine against EBV.[35] The MA complex consists of four polypeptides.[34,35] Early and late MAs are expressed in the membrane of infected cells and in mature viral particles,[37] and are responsible for eliciting virus-neutralizing antibody. Polyclonal and monoclonal antibodies directed against MA have demonstrable virus-neutralizing effects. Such antibodies also prevent the immortalization of cells by transforming EBV. The gene encoding MA glycoproteins has been mapped to the BamHl 'Z' fragment of EBV DNA. The targets for antibody-dependent cellular cytotoxicity (ADCC) are located on two of the polypeptides of the MA complex, gp 320/350 and gp 240/250.[34,35] Sera from patients in the acute phase of IM contained antibody to gp 85, but not to gp 320/350 or gp 240/250. Since gp 320/350 elicits neutralizing and cytotoxic antibodies, this polypeptide is now being actively investigated as the basis for a subviral vaccine.

NUCLEAR ANTIGENS (EBNA)

Epstein–Barr virus-converted B-cells express EBNA, detectable by anticomplement IFA, as originally described by Reedman and Klein.[38] The synthesis of EBNA occurs prior to viral DNA synthesis (and cellular DNA synthesis is not required). After the appearance of EBNA, cellular DNA synthesis is stimulated, and between 36–48 hours after infection, mitosis is observed. Recent studies have identified six EBNAs (EBNA 1, 2, 3, 4, 5, and 6)[39,40] (*see* Fig. 11.2b). Nuclear antigen 1 is encoded by the BamHl 'K' fragment and EBNA 2 by the BamHl 'Y' and 'H' fragments of the genome. The sequences coding for EBNA 3, the function of which is unknown, include the open reading frames known as BERF-1, 2 and 3. Nuclear antigen 4 is also coded by the 'Y' fragment, differential splicing giving rise to the different RNAs. The coding for EBNA 5 includes the BamHl 'W' internal repeats.[40] Nuclear antigen 1 is responsible for maintaining the plasmid viral DNA in latently infected cells, by transactivating the origin of plasmid replication (OriP) and EBNA 2, and is important in the process of B-cell activation and immortalization by EBV. It induces a surface antigen (CD23) and the latent membrane protein of EBV.

Lymphocyte-detected membrane antigen (LYDMA)

The antigen defined operationally on the surface of latently infected EBV-transformed cells by *in vitro* tests of cell-mediated cytotoxicity has been called LYDMA. Anti-LYDMA reactivity has not been demonstrated in the T-cell fraction of peripheral blood of BL patients. A small number of LYDMA-reactive effector cells have been isolated from EBV-induced tumours in animals or from draining lymph nodes.[41] The presumptive LYDMA polypeptide has not been definitely identified, although it has been suggested that a p60 protein, encoded by the EcoR1 'D' fragment (on the right side of the BamHl 'N' fragment) may be LYDMA. Latent membrane protein (LMP)[42] may comprise all or part of LYDMA. If so, the outer-reverse-turn domains of LMP are probable candidates for T-cell recognition.[43]

Cell-mediated immunity (CMI)

Considerable progress has been made in characterizing cell-mediated immunity (CMI) against EBV in EBV-associated malignancies and lymphoproliferative disorders.[44–46] Using an ADCC assay to investigate the ability of patient sera to mediate ADCC activity specifically, it was shown that high ADCC titres in NPC patients correlated with a good prognosis, while low titres were associated with a poor response to therapy and progression of the disease.[47] In African BL sera, higher ADCC antibody titres also correlated with a better prognosis.[48] Clinical observations in IM, organ transplant recipients and EBV-associated malignancies support the premise that T-cells play an important role in limiting the proliferation of cells infected/transformed by EBV.[49,50] Rickinson described the specific role of helper/inducer T-cells, suppressor T-cells and cytotoxic T-cells in primary and persistent EBV infections.[44] Pope specifically studied the role of NK-cells in EBV infection. One interesting finding, of unknown significance, is the increased sensitivity of cell lines superinfected with EBV to NK-mediated cytotoxicity.[45] An evaluation of the contribution of cell populations other than T-cells to cell-mediated immunity against EBV infected cells remains an important research aim.[37,51] Further knowledge and understanding of EBV cellular immunity will permit better evaluation of the immunogenic properties of vaccines and may be of diagnostic significance.

Clinical application of EBV serology

The pattern of development of EBV antibodies after primary infection is quite characteristic. Immediately after primary infection anti-EBV VCA-IgM antibody develops in all patients. Titres subsequently decline and ultimately reach non-detectable levels, but not before the development of anti-VCA-IgG antibody. In 80 per cent of patients, anti-VCA-IgG subsequently declines slowly. In contrast, early antigen-IgG antibody (EA-D) develops in 70–80 per cent of patients and rapidly declines to undetectable levels. The level of VCA antibody appears to reflect the severity of the primary infection. Several weeks after an acute infection, antibodies to EBNA appear and persist for life. In individuals with X-linked proliferative syndrome (XLP) who develop fatal IM or lymphoma, however, anti-EBNA usually does not appear. In developing countries, EBV infection occurs soon after maternal antibody disappears (at about 6 weeks), probably because of the poor socioeconomic conditions leading to rapid parent-to-child transmission. In chronic infectious mononucleosis or other lymphoproliferative disorders, persistently elevated titres of antibodies against EBV-EA appear to reflect ongoing EBV infection.[16,35–37] In BL, NPC and other EBV-associated B-cell lymphomas, it has been shown that EA antibody titres rise (anti-EA-R in BL and anti-EA-D in NPC) with

the development of the disease, and decline some time after treatment of the tumour.[16,36,37] The serological profile of antibodies directed against EBV-VCA (IgG and IgA) and EBV-EA (R and D) in healthy donors and in IM, BL and NPC patients is shown in Table 11.2.

In a classical, prospective seroepidemiological study in Africa, de Thé and co-workers showed that children with high antibody titres (two or more dilutions greater than the mean titre to EBV-VCA) are at higher risk for the development of BL. They found 14 cases of BL in individuals showing elevated titres of antibody to VCA before the clinical onset of BL.[52] These findings have been interpreted as strongly supporting a causal association between EBV and BL.[53] They could, however, also be interpreted as demonstrating that children destined to develop BL also have a tendency to develop high anti-VCA titres following EBV infection, either because of inherent differences in immune reactivity, or because of differences in their environment leading to a higher EBV inoculum or repeated exposure to EBV.

Induction of tumours in animals with EBV

Since it is not possible to test the pathogenesis and oncogenesis of EBV in man, animal studies are necessary to support Koch's postulates, and also to develop a model for therapy and vaccine trials. Attempts have been made to induce tumours in animals using BL cell lines or freshly obtained BL tumour cells. B-cells, newly transformed by EBV, have been shown to be unable to proliferate as tumours in nude mice, in contrast to the oncogenicity of cell lines established from BL patients[16] (Fig. 11.3a). The histology of the tumours produced in nude mice[54,55] resembles that of poorly differentiated lymphomas in humans (Fig. 11.3b).

Among non-human primates, the cottontop marmoset appears to be the most susceptible to the induction of lymphomas by transforming EBV.[16,14,56,57] Although the peripheral blood lymphocytes of the white-lipped marmoset can be transformed with EBV *in vitro*, it is much more difficult to induce tumours by direct inoculation of EBV *in vivo* in this species.[16,57] Sundar *et al.*[58] however, have successfully induced lymphomas in white-lipped marmosets by inoculation of

Table 11.2 Serological profile of anti-EA, anti VCA-IgG and anti VCA-IgA in healthy donors and EBV-associated diseases[1]

						Antibody titres									
Anti-EA[2]						Anti-VCA(IgG)[3]				Anti-VCA(IgA)[4]					
IM	C	BL	C	NPC	C	BL	C	NPC	C	IM	C	BL	C	NPC	C
20D	<10	80R	<10	320D	<10	640	80	1280	80	<5	<5	<5	<5	20	<5
40D	<10	40R	<10	640D	<10	640	80	2560	160	<5	<5	<5	<5	80	<5
80D	<10	320R	<10	160D	<10	1280	160	2560	160	<5	<5	<5	<5	320	5
160D	<10	640R	10	640D	10	320	40	5120	160	<5	<5	5	5	160	10
40D	<10	640R	<10	320D	10	2560	80	5120	>80	<5	<5	<5	<5	320	5
40D	<10	320R	10	160D	<10	1280	80	2560	80	<5	<5	<5	<5	640	<5
80D	<10	160R	<10	320D	<10	640	>80	1280	>80	<5	<5	<5	<5	640	<5
160D	<10	40R	10	640D	<10	640	>80	640	>80	<5	<5	<5	<5	40	<5

C, controls; IM, infectious mononucleosis; BL, Burkitt's lymphoma; NPC, nasopharyngeal carcinoma

[1]In acute mononucleosis and/or primary EBV infection, VCA-IgM antibody is detected (>1:10). Since it is not an easy assay to perform, the titres are not considered very important; [2]<10 is considered as negative for anti-EA-R or -D; [3]40–160 is considered as a normal VCA-IgG titre in healthy individuals; [4]<5 is considered as negative for anti-VCA-IgA. Some healthy Chinese show detectable VCA-IgA antibody (1:5 to 1:20); R, IF staining is restricted to the nucleus.

The control serum samples were obtained from healthy individuals from the same geographic area as the patients. They were age- and sex-matched. For IM, the samples were from USA; for BL, they were from Africa; for NPC the control samples were obtained from Southern Chinese from Hong Kong, Malaysia and Singapore, presenting non-NPC tumours of the head and neck region. Each number represents an individual patient or healthy individual.

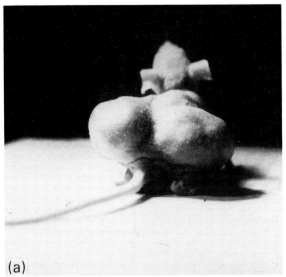

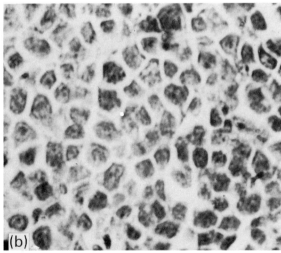

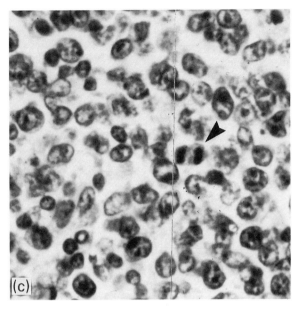

Fig. 11.3 (a) Athymic nude mouse showing tumours after inoculation with EBV genome-containing B-lymphoblastoid cells; (b) histological section of cells from a nude mouse tumour induced by EBV genome-positive B-cells showing starry sky appearance, which is typical of BL tumours; (c) histological section of lymph node from EBV-inoculated white-lipped marmoset, which developed mesenteric lymphoma. Arrow shows a cell undergoing mitosis.

transforming EBV. Epstein–Barr virus can also transform peripheral blood lymphocytes of the common marmoset, owl monkey, squirrel monkey, moustached marmoset and woolly monkey.[16,57] Moreover, fatal lymphoprolifera-tive disease has been observed in squirrel monkeys after inoculation of the AG-876 transforming strain of EBV.[59] Generally, the EBV-induced lymphoproliferative processes in the cottontop marmoset involve the bowel mesentery. Individual cells have large vesicular nuclei and are irregular in size and shape. Cells undergoing mitosis are frequently present (Fig. 11.3c) and numerous small foci of large reticular

histiocytic cells give rise to a 'starry sky' appearance. Similar pathological changes are observed in tumours developing after inoculation of BL cells into nude mice (Fig. 11.3b).[54,55]

Infected non-human primates develop EBV-specific antibodies and EBV DNA has been demonstrated in virus-induced lymphomas. Tumour cells seem to harbour the entire EBV genome.[57] Cleary *et al.*[60] showed that B-cell lym-phoproliferations/lymphomas induced in cottontop marmosets are oligo- or monoclonal in origin and that individual tumours in the same animal arise from different B-cell clones. This is similar to observations in EBV-associated 'lymphomas' in patients with organ transplants, which may not be true lymphomas, but rather, virus-infected cells, whose proliferation is inadequately controlled because of drug-induced immunodeficiency.[53]   However, whether truly neoplastic or not, the protection of cottontop marmosets against EBV-induced B-cell lymphoproliferation with purified gp 340 immunization,[61] strongly supports the use of the cottontop marmoset for the testing of liposomal subunit EBV vaccines.[62]

The ability of EBV to transform lymphocytes *in vitro* and to induce lymphoproliferative syndromes in animals is consistent with a possible causal role for this virus in those BLs associated with EBV, especially endemic BL. However, this is far from being direct proof and at present the role of EBV in BL remains unknown.

Chromosomal translocations and EBV in BL

The most consistent abnormality, seen in 80 per cent of BLs, is the translocation of a portion of chromosome 8, containing the c-*myc* oncogene, to the long arm of chromosome 14, which contains the heavy chain immunoglobulin genes. In the remaining cases, portions of the light chain immunoglobulin regions on chromosomes 2 or 22 are translocated to chromosome 8. Although abnormalities of chromosome 14 have been reported in other lymphoproliferative disorders, specific t(8;14,q24;q32), t(8;22,q24;q11) and t(8;2,q24;q11) are found almost exclusively in BL tumours and BL-type leukaemias.[17,63] These translocations are found in BL regardless of the presence or absence of EBV, and there is little doubt that they are essential to the neoplastic state. Thus EBV, if it has a role in tumorigenesis, either acts as a co-factor, and increases the chance of a translocation developing by increasing the size of the B-cell pool through its ability to transform B lymphocytes, or it may have a direct, and possibly critical role in the induction of neoplasia in concert with a subset of structural changes caused by the translocations. Although there is little to distinguish one 8;14 translocation from another at a cytogenetic level, molecular analysis has clearly shown that at the level of DNA, the location of the chromosomal breakpoints differs. In particular, the breakpoint locations differ in endemic (predominantly EBV associated) BL from sporadic (predominantly EBV unassociated) BL. Thus a formal possibility exists whereby EBV may have a tumorigenic role in the majority of endemic tumours and possibly a fraction of sporadic tumours. This possibility can now be examined through sophisticated experiments in which the effect of EBV gene products on cellular genes can be examined directly. In this regard, the demonstrated trans-activating effect of several EBV genes is of interest. It is entirely possible that such genes may activate cellular genes in addition to their appropriate targets (EBV genes). Indeed, this would appear to be the likely mechanism of cellular transformation, and is probably involved in the induction of CD23 by EBNA 2. The activation of specific oncogenes as a result of chromosomal translocations and their possible role in oncogenesis is addressed in Chapter 6.

Lymphoproliferative disorders and B-cell lymphomas in X-linked lymphoproliferative syndrome (XLP) and organ transplant recipients

Purtilo[64] postulated that EBV may be oncogenic in individuals with inherited or acquired immunodeficiency disorders. This was based on the consequences of EBV infections in males in kindreds with an identifiable immunodeficiency known as XLP. Approximately 70 per cent of such individuals develop fatal mononucleosis or B-cell lymphomas, immunoblastic sarcomas with B-cell characteristics, plasmacytomas or large cell lymphomas. The lesions in the liver and bone marrow are due to EBV-carrying B-cells admixed with suppressor T-cells. The broad spectrum of the morphological appearance of lymphomas in XLP closely resembles herpesvirus-induced lymphoproliferations in animals. Some of these lymphomas have been classified as American BL but the majority are polyclonal. A considerable number of these tumours have been found to be EBV-associated, based on EBV-serology and the presence of EBV DNA.[53,65]

Purtilo has suggested that defective immune surveillance against EBV-infected cells may allow the B-cell lymphoproliferation to persist. If such defects are profound, the individual is likely to succumb from a massive polyclonal B-cell proliferation consequent upon EBV infection. Patients with more subtle immune deficiencies appear to develop a smouldering B-cell proliferation which in some cases may become monoclonal. The increased incidence of polyclonal B-cell lymphoma-like lesions has also been observed in young and old patients with renal allografts, Sjögren's syndrome, AIDS, and in organ transplant recipients.[65,66] The patients show elevated antibody levels to various EBV antigens and the presence of EBV DNA in the tumour cells.

The remarkable similarity between the lymphoproliferative processes of XLP and other lymphoproliferative disorders in immunodeficient individuals strongly suggests that similar pathogenetic mechanisms are operative. The cells participating in the lymphoproliferative process, whether designated as fatal infectious mononucleosis or a malignant lymphoma, are EBV-infected B-cells which are inadequately regulated, (although in some cases a true lymphoma, bearing a clonal cytogenetic abnormality, may be superimposed on the polyclonal process). Therefore, immunodeficient patients provide an opportunity to study specific defects in the control of EBV-infected cells. Whether these observations will prove relevant to the multistep process of lymphomagenesis occurring in EBV-associated BL, or even in lymphomas in general, remains to be seen.[53,65,66]

Human B-cell lymphotrophic virus (HBLV) (human herpesvirus-6 (HHV-6))

Virus isolation, biological and molecular aspects

A novel human herpesvirus (*see* Fig. 11.1b), designated human B-cell lymphotrophic virus, was initially isolated from fresh mononuclear cells of patients with a variety of lymphoid neoplasms and lymphoproliferative disorders.[23,67] It was isolated from AIDS patients with immunoblastic lymphoma, dermatopathic lymphadenopathy or angioimmunoblastic lymphadenopathy, and from patients with B-cell, cutaneous T-cell lymphomas or acute lymphocytic leukaemia.[23] The cells in culture were short-lived, large and refractile. These cells were generally mono- or binucleated and contained inclusion bodies.[23] After mitogen stimulation, the peripheral blood mononuclear

cells from these patients showed large, refractile cells which exhibited nuclear and diffuse staining of the entire cell, using patients' sera in IFA. Originally, the virus obtained from these infected cells was found to possess a narrow host range *in vitro*, and to be highly cytopathic to human cord blood mononuclear cells and to peripheral blood lymphocytes and spleen cells from adults.[23] Recent data show that HHV-6 infected cells from peripheral blood, bone marrow, tonsils and thymus express predominantly T-cell associated antigens (*i.e.* CD7, CD5, CD2, CD4 and to a lesser extent CD8) as detected by immunoprecipitation and by monoclonal antibodies.[68] Thus, there is no doubt that this virus can also infect T-cell subsets. Since the initial report, similar viruses have been isolated from patients with AIDS, chronic fatigue syndrome and other lymphoproliferative disorders (Ablashi *et al.*, unpublished observations).[68–70]

According to the classification of herpesviruses proposed by the International Herpesvirus Nomenclature Committee, human herpesviruses, i.e. herpes simplex 1, (HSV-1), herpes simplex 2 (HSV-2), varicella zoster (VZV), EBV, and cytomegalovirus (CMV) are classified as human herpesviruses (HHV) 1, 2, 3, 4, and 5. It was suggested by a member of the International Herpesvirus Nomenclature Committee, that HBLV should be called HHV-6. Although the HHV designation has rarely been used for any herpesvirus, in the case of HBLV, perhaps because it is a newly identified herpesvirus, the designation HHV-6 has become widely used.

Human B-cell lymphotrophic virions have a uniform shape and size and are produced as abundant extracellular particles (*see* Fig. 11.1b). Like EBV, HHV-6 has an enveloped icosahedral core which consists of 162 capsomeres. The diameter of the enveloped particle is about 200 nm. While morphologically similar to other herpesviruses, HHV-6 differs from known human herpesvirus in that infected cells contain a higher proportion of fully mature virus particles.[71] Recently, several established permanent cell lines which can be productively infected, and produce large amounts of virus (⩾ 2.0–4.0 logs/ml) have been identified.[72] These lines are free of CMV, EBV and HSV DNA.[72] A cell line derived from a glioblastoma has also been abortively infected, and recently, infection of EBV genome-positive B-lymphoid cell lines has been accomplished.[72]

Molecular analysis of HBLV has revealed that the double-stranded genome is more than 170 kbp in size.[67] A molecular clone, designed pZVH-14 (9.0 kb), was obtained from HHV-6 DNA. When used as a probe, this clone specifically hybridized to the DNA of HHV-6 infected cells, and to DNA extracted from peripheral blood lymphocytes obtained from seropositive patients including a patient with acute lymphoblastic leukaemia, two with Sjögren's syndrome and B-cell lymphomas, an African BL and a follicular large cell lymphoma.[73] The African BL also contained EBV DNA. Furthermore, hybridization *in situ* using cytological preparations revealed a small number of HHV-6-positive cells in seven of 10 African BLs. Epstein–Barr virus was also detected in the African tumours carrying HHV-6 (Josephs *et al.*, unpublished observations). Sjögren's syndrome and follicular large cell lymphoma tissues positive for HHV-6 by Southern blot analysis lacked EBV DNA.

Immunology and serology

Human herpesvirus-6 appears to be unrelated to EBV, HSV, VZV, or to simian oncogenic and non-oncogenic herpesvirus. Antisera against other herpesviruses, i.e. of bovine, equine, porcine, feline, murine and avian origin also fail to react with HHV-6 infected cells by IFA and by Western blot analysis (unpublished data – Ablashi). Initial reports suggested that only 4 per cent of the sera collected from healthy individuals contained IgG antibody to HHV-6 as detected by IFA.[23] Since then, however, more data have been collected, using IFA and immunoblots, and it appears that there is considerable geographic variation in the frequency of seropositive individuals. Sera collected from diverse areas in the USA and Europe revealed that at least 60 per cent of healthy donors are seropositive, whereas sera obtained from Africans showed that 87 per cent contained HHV-6 antibody. In contrast, elevated HHV-6 antibody levels have been found in patients with Hodgkin's disease, African

Burkitt's lymphoma, other B-cell lymphomas, acute lymphocytic leukaemia and in HIV-1 antibody-positive AIDS related complex (ARC), persistent generalized lymphadenopathy (PGL) and AIDS (Ablashi *et al.*, unpublished data). Elevated antibody titres to HHV-6 ($\geq$1280) have also been detected in patients with chronic fatigue syndrome, previously referred to as chronic mononucleosis syndrome.[74,75] It is not known, at present, whether HHV-6 has a causal or contributary role in any of these conditions.

More than 67 per cent of sera collected from patients with Sjögren's syndrome, including three serial samples from a patient with a B-cell lymphoma, had elevated HHV-6 antibody levels, suggesting an HHV-6 association with this autoimmune disorder which is characterized by lymphocytic infiltration of the salivary and lacrimal glands. DNA of EBV has also been detected in parotid saliva samples and salivary gland biopsies from patients with Sjögren's syndrome,[76] but since this is the normal location of viral replication, the significance of this is unclear.

The fact that HHV-6, unlike EBV and CMV, can infect B- and T-cells, megakaryocytes and glioblastoma cells[72] means that it could have a potential pathogenic role in a wide spectrum of diseases, including some T-cell leukaemias/lymphomas (Jarrett, personal communication). Since elevated HHV-6 antibody is present in 75 per cent of HIV-1 antibody-positive patients with AIDS, and in light of the cytopathic effect exerted *in vitro* on CD4 positive T-cells, the possibility that HHV-6 could further impair immune function in patients with HIV infection should be considered. The specific role of HHV-6 in malignant and lymphoproliferative diseases, however, remains to be determined.

Human retroviruses

Even though retroviruses have been known to cause cancers in animals for many years,[1–7] attempts to isolate retroviruses from human leukaemia/lymphoma tissues were unsuccessful until the discovery of T-cell growth factor (TCGF) and the development of techniques to culture tumour cells *in vitro*.[21,77] In 1970, Gallo and his co-workers initiated a systematic search for retroviruses associated with human disease.[19,20,22]

Morphology, immunobiology and molecular features of HTLVs

A new family of human retroviruses, human T-cell lymphotrophic viruses (HTLV), thus far includes three different types of viruses, designated as HTLV-I, HTLV-II and HTLV-III/LAV or HIV-1 and 2.[78–83] Type I is aetiologically linked to adult T-cell leukaemia/lymphoma (ATLL) and tropical spastic paraparesis, and has also been isolated frequently from AIDS patients.[84,85] The role of HTLV-II in human cancer is unclear.[80,86] It has, however, been isolated from patients with AIDS, from tumour cells in T-cell hairy cell leukaemia,[80] from a haemophiliac patient with pancytopenia and from intravenous drug abusers.[21,22,86–89] Isolation of HTLV-II consistently from hairy cell leukaemia suggests a pathogenic role for HTLV-II in this malignancy. It is difficult to distinguish serologically between HTLV-I and HTLV-II; this poses difficulties to the study of the epidemiology of HTLV-II. Based on virus isolation, however, it is apparent that HTLV-II is less prevalent than HTLV-I, and no consistent disease association has been found for HTLV-II. The third virus, HTLV-III/LAV, now called HIV, is the causative agent of AIDS, which is a fatal disease involving the severe depletion of helper-T-cells which leads, in turn, to a variety of life-threatening opportunistic infections and/or malignancies, particularly Kaposi's sarcoma and lymphomas.[81,82] The three types differ morphologically (Fig. 11.4). They are similar in the early stages of virion formation, but mature HIV particles have a more compact, cylindrical core (Fig. 11.4, insert).[21,88] All have the typical structure of retroviruses including *gag*, *pol* and *env* genes (Fig. 11.5a). These viruses do, however, have two features in common – their T4-cell tropism and the presence of additional S^1 genes, previously termed LOR (long open reading frame) in a region of the viral genome originally termed Px (1.5 kb) (Fig. 11.5.). Products of this region activate other viral genes and are also able to activate the expression of cellular genes including IL2-R (Table

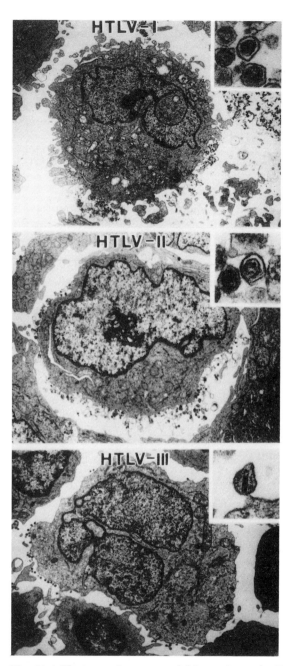

Fig. 11.4 Electron microscopy of thin sections of cells producing HTLV-I, HTLV-II and HTLV-III (HIV-1). Virus-particle budding from the cell membrane and free particles detached from the membrane are shown. Inserts show high magnification of virus particle. The insert for HBLV-III shows the cylindrical core region, which is different from the HTLV-I and HTLV-II virus particles.

Table 11.3. List of accessory genes of human retroviruses

New name	Previous name(s)	Product Size-Kd	Cellular location	Known function
HTLV I and II				
tax_1	x-lor, tat-1 p40X	41, 42	nucleolus	trans-activator of all viral proteins
tax_2	tat-2, TA	38	nucleolus	same as tax_1
rex_1	pp27X, tel	27	nucleolus	regulator of expression of virion proteins
rex_2		25	nucleolus	same as rex_1
HIV-1/HIV-2				
tat	tat-3, TA	14	nucleolus	trans-activator of all viral proteins
rev	art, trs	19, 20	nucleolus	regulator of expression of virion proteins
vif	sor, A, P', Q	23	cytoplasm inner membrane	virus infectivity
nef	3'-orf, B, E', F	27	cytoplasm	negative regulator of virus expression GTP binding
vpr	R	?	18	unknown
vpx (present in HIV-2/SIV)	X	16, 14	cytoplasm	unknown
vpu (present only in HIV-1)		15, 16	?	facilities viral release

11.3).[21,22,86,89] Types I and II have a limited host range and both transform T-cells exclusively.[21] They do not contain oncogenes, nor are they found to be integrated near cellular oncogenes in tumours or transformed cells. Further biological properties of these two viruses are provided in Table 11.4.

Comparative and distinguishing features of HTLVs and mammalian type-C retroviruses

Members of the HTLV family are morphologically similar to other type-C retroviruses (Fig. 11.5) and contain high molecular weight reverse transcriptase.[22,87,88] Several isolates have been completely sequenced. Unlike most mammalian type-C viruses, their reverse transcriptase functions more efficiently in the presence of Mg^{2+}, rather than Mn^{2+}.[21,88] The small size of the core-protein (P24), the glycosylation of the transmembrane protein (gp21 or gp41), the lack of viraemia in infected individuals, the absence of a specific integration site in the tumour and transactivation of long terminal repeat (LTR)-directed transcription[21,22] are other features which distinguish human retroviruses from mammalian type-C retroviruses.[21,22,88] Finally, HTLV-III or HIV env genes differ from other retroviral env genes in that the major exterior glycoprotein (gp 120/160) is large and heavily glycosylated with over 20 potential glycosylation sites.[87] Human T-cell lymphotrophic virus-I is structurally related to bovine leukaemia virus (BLV), which has three major internal proteins, P24, P19 and P15, and to the Simian virus, STLV-I.[22,87] There is much greater structural similarity between HTLV-I and BLV than between HTLV-I and HIV.[22] The small phosphoprotein interposed between the amino-terminal gag protein and the major capsid protein in HTLV-I and BLV is not present in HIV nor in any other known retroviruses. Human immunodeficiency virus shows a number of similarities to the lentiviruses, which include progressive pneumonia virus of sheep and goats, and caprine arthritis virus (CAIV) of sheep.[87,88,90] These similarities include a cytopathic effect *in vitro*, the accumulation of a large amount of integrated viral DNA in the infected cells and the capacity of the virus to infect the brain. In animals, infection by lentiviruses is frequently inapparent, with no obvious pathological sequelae for periods which approximate the normal lifespan of the host.[90] Human immunodeficiency virus also establishes persistent and non-cytopathic infections in normal lymphocytes. In persistently infected cultured lymphocytes, virus production may be absent or limited, in keeping with the definition of latency.[90]

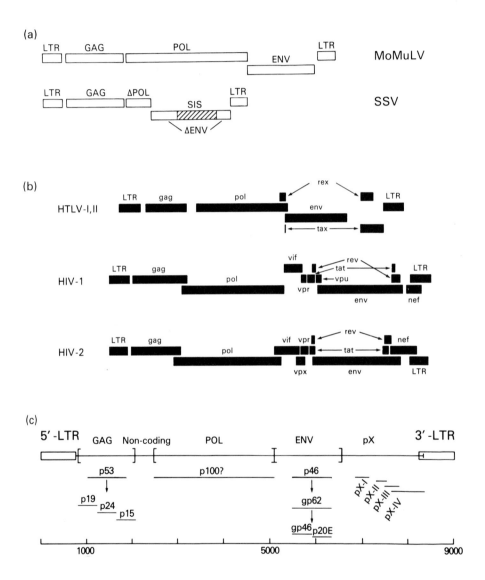

Fig. 11.5 Genetic structures of (a) animal retroviruses, MO MuLV, Moloney murine leukaemia virus; SSV, simian sarcoma virus; (b) human retroviruses, HTLV-I, HTLV-II, HIV-1 and HIV-2; (c) genome of HTLV-I showing some major proteins of *gag*, *pol* and *env* region and the px region. The genome of HTLV-I is 9 kb in size.

Table 11.4 Properties of HTLV-I and HTLV-II

Biological properties	HTLV-I	HTLV-II
1. Host range		
i) *in vivo*	Primarily T4+ T-cell	Primarily T4+ T-cell
ii) *in vitro*	Pan-T-cell types in non-human species	Also infects B-cells and pan-T-cells
2. *In vitro* immortalization	T-cells only	T-cells only
3. Disease association	Causes adult T-cell leukaemia (ATL) HTLV-I associated myelopathy (HAM) (tropical spastic paraparesis (TSP)	Hairy cell leukaemia (HCL) T-cell variant and various lympho-proliferative disorders
4. Receptor	Not known	Possibly OKT-10
5. Transactivation	*tax-I*	*tax-II*/uncertain
6. Induction of IL-2 receptor expression	Strong induction	Moderate induction
7. Induction of cytokine expression	Strong expression of a variety of cytokines	Strong induction of a variety of cytokines
8. Genomic homology	Highly conserved	Possibly some heterogeneity
9. Immunological homology	Strong	Strong
10. Syncytia formation	Frequent	Frequent
11. Transmission		
i) *in vivo*	Breast milk	Not known
ii) *in vitro* by co-culture	Cell associated and cell free	Co-culture and cell free
12. Seroprevalence, endemic population	15–30%	Not known

HTLV-I

This virus is endemic in various parts of the world including Japan, the Caribbean, South and Central America, the southeastern USA and especially in Africa.[91] It was isolated from T-cell lines established from a Black patient with adult T-cell leukaemia/lymphoma (ATLL) in the USA.[77,79] Adult T-cell leukaemia/lymphoma was first described as a specific malignant disease with unusual clinical, pathogenic and epidemiological future by Uchiyama *et al.* in Japan.[85] Patients manifest a lymphoproliferative syndrome characterized by lymphadenopathy, hepatosplenomegaly, hypercalcaemia, skin infiltrates and mature pleiomorphic neoplastic T-cells. Yamaguchi *et al.*[92] have recently described a smouldering form of ATLL with skin erythema and papules or nodules in a few patients, which can undergo blast transforma-tion to more typical ATLL. It was the geographic distribution of ATLL in Japan which originally suggested an infectious agent co-factor. Over 100 isolates have been reported from the USA, the Caribbean, Africa, Japan, UK, Israel and other parts of the world.

The overall incidence of ATLL in Japan is 3.5 cases per 100 000 in persons less than 40 years of age and 5.7 cases per 100 000 in persons more than 40 years of age.[89,91] The Caribbean Basin is also an endemic region of ATLL. In Jamaica there are one to two cases per 100 000 and in Trinidad and Tobago 2.8 cases per 100 000.[89] While Trinidad and Tobago have an ethnic composition of Africans, Asians and Caucasians, all patients with ATLL are of African descent and of low socioeconomic status. A recent study showed that of 95 patients with non-Hodgkin's lymphoma in Kingston, Jamaica, 24 of 27 cases with ATLL had HTLV-I antibodies (88 per cent). Catovsky *et al.*[93] showed that non-Hodgkin's lymphoma in Jamaica and southern Japan, both being HTLV-I endemic areas, consists primarily of T-cell lymphomas, in contrast to B-cell lymphomas found in adults in the USA, UK and other non-endemic areas for ATLL. Antibodies to HTLV-I were found in 89 per cent of sera from patients with T-cell leukaemia/lymphoma from the USA, the Caribbean and Japan.[89,91] In the Caribbean, sera from 5 per cent of normal donors were also antibody positive.[87] The healthy family members of ATLL patients usually exhibited a high incidence of HTLV-I antibody. Tajima *et al.*[94] recently showed that in Tsusjima Island, Japan, the prevalence of HTLV-I antibody in males increased little with age, however, the prevalence in females was distinctly age-related. The HTLV-I antibody prevalence in older females (more than 30 years of age) was higher than in males, and the prevalence of carrier children when the mother was also a carrier, was estimated to be 20 per cent. A 15-year follow-up study in Okinawa, Japan, showed that mother-to-child transmission of HTLV-I was 15.4 per cent. In addition, children born to seropositive mothers had acquired their HLTV-I antibodies by the age of 3 years and were still seropositive at the age of 18 years.[95]

Southern blot hybridization of HTLV-I probes to genomic DNA from fresh leukaemia cells or cell lines of HTLV-positive patients with various T-cell malignancies has demonstrated that these cells contain HTLV provirus. HTLV-I is T-cell tropic and *in vivo* predominantly infects helper T-cell populations (OKT4). A striking feature of HTLV-I positive T-cell leukaemia cell lines is the high constitutive level of expression of IL-2 receptor, and rarely, the simultaneous production of IL-2. Speculation has concentrated on the possibility that the inappropriate expression of these cellular genes, which play an important role in regulating growth, may be involved in the development of ATLL. Whether this is an essential component of oncogenesis, or increases the risk of tumour formation by increasing the size of the target cell population and the risk of the development of genetic abnormalities is not known. The studies of Siekevitz *et al.*,[96] showed that *tax*-1 protein stimulates a three-to-six-fold increase in IL-2R promoter activity in transfected Jurkat T-cells. In contrast, *tax*-1 alone, has no effect on IL-2 promoter activity. The specific effect of the *tax*-1 gene product on the IL-2 receptor promoter suggests the possibility of an autocrine or paracrine mechanism of T-cell growth as an early event in HTLV-I mediated leukaemogenesis.[96] T-cells infected *in vitro* display many properties of transformed ATLL cells, such as altered morphology, increase in growth rate, cell clumping, reduced dependency on exogenous IL-2, a high level of cell surface expression of IL-2 receptors and HLA-/DR-antigens (*see* Table 11.3).

Recently, HTLV antibodies have been detected in macaques in Japan and in baboons from Sukhumi, USSR. Retrovirus has been isolated from the HTLV-antibody-positive baboons. Simian T-cell lymphotropic virus (STLV-I) is closely related to HTLV-I (greater than 95 per cent homology). Simian T-cell lymphotropic virus-positive animals also have a high incidence of malignant lymphomas.[21,91]

HTLV-II

This virus was originally isolated from a single patient with a T-cell variant of hairy cell leukaemia[80] and from leucocytes of an intravenous drug abuser/AIDS patient.[21,86] Although there are many morphological, structural and genomic similarities between HTLV-II and HTLV-I, these viruses are readily distinguishable both by protein serology and by nucleic acid hybridization. Like HTLV-I, HTLV-II has the ability to transform T-cells and to abrogate certain immune functions. Even though the virus has been isolated from malignant cells, HTLV-II is not strongly linked to any disease. Isolates have recently been obtained from a variety of diseases including dermatopathic lymphoadenopathy associated with leukaemia, patients with chronic lymphocytic leukaemia with skin lesions, and from haemophiliacs with or without pancytopenia. All of these patients, however, were also infected with HIV-1. Thus far, the HTLV-II isolates from hairy cell leukaemia have been found to be free of other human retroviruses (HTLV-I or HIV-1 or 2).

Concluding remarks

Human T-cell lymphotrophic virus types I and II cause proliferation and immortalization of T-cells *in vitro*, which is similar to the effect of EBV on B-cells. These viruses also cause immunosuppression. The evidence that HTLV-I and II are causally associated with T-cell malignancies derives from seroepidemiology and the presence of viral genomes in tumour cells. This, again, is comparable to the similar association of EBV with BL and NPC. It is interesting to note that the two human retroviruses HTLV-I and HIV, while having common features, cause an opposite set of effects on T-cells; presumably due to their effects on cellular genes. The former predisposes to T-cell neoplasia, the latter to B-cell lymphomas. The lymphoproliferation of B-cells induced by EBV and of T-cells (via IL-2R) induced by HTLV-I may represent a premalignant process, in which the increased cell turnover and possibly, life span, predisposes to cellular genetic changes, which can ultimately result in neoplasia. Human immunodeficiency virus probably predisposes to B-cell neoplasia because of defective T4 cell-mediated regulation of B-cell proliferation. The possible participation of viral gene products (i.e. in HTLV-I and EBV associated neoplasia) in the production and maintenance of the neoplastic state (presumably in concert with cellular oncogenes) cannot be excluded.

Like *Herpesvirus saimiri* (HVS), HHV-6 is highly cytopathic *in vitro*. *Herpesvirus saimiri* is known to cause tumours in non-human primates (owl monkey and marmoset), and under some conditions can lead to cellular transformation *in vitro*.[97] In contrast, even though HHV-6 is the aetiological agent of *Exanthem subitum* in infants,[98] and 12 per cent of heterophile-negative infectious mononucleosis cases result from primary infection with HHV-6,[99] its role in human tumours is unclear. Infection of some cells with HHV-6 induces a blast-like appearance in the infected cells, which then appear to have a selective growth advantage during the period prior to the release of virus. If the lytic (virion replicative) phase could be prevented, either by mutation or deletion within the viral genome, a direct growth promoting effect could occur, leading to malignant transformation *in vivo*.[100]

Whether human herpesviruses and retroviruses participate directly or indirectly in oncogenesis, it would appear that prevention of infection would be likely to reduce markedly the incidence of the tumours associated with them. Thus an appropriate goal is the development of safe vaccines using viral envelope proteins which elicit neutralizing antibody. In the event that viral products are essential to the neoplastic state, the viral genes provide a potential target for antineoplastic therapy which could permit the development of highly selective treatment approaches. However, drugs which prevent virus replication are likely to be effective only in controlling virus infection, and thus will probably not be effective once a neoplasm has developed. One potentially lucrative research opportunity is the elucidation of the mechanism whereby viral genes regulate cellular genes. Interference with this process could have anti-neoplastic value.

References

1. Rous P. *Journal of Experimental Medicine*. 1911; **13**, 397.
2. Ellermann V, Bang O. *Zentralblatt für Bakteriologie*. 1908; **46**, 595.
3. Gross L. *Proceedings of Experimental Biology and Medicine*. 1951; **76**, 27.
4. Jarrett WFH, Crawford EM, Martin W, *et al*. *Nature*. 1964; **202**, 567.
5. Jarrett WFH, Martin WB, Crighton GW, *et al*. *Nature*. 1964; **202**, 566.
6. Essex M. In: Phillips L (ed). *Viruses Associated with Human Cancer*. New York: Marcel Dekker, 1982: 553.
7. Essex M. In: Magrath IT, O'Conor GT, Ramot B (eds). *Pathogenesis of Leukemia and Lymphomas*. New York: Raven Press, 1982: 315.
8. Burkitt D. *British Journal of Surgery*. 1958; **46**, 218.
9. Epstein MA, Barr YM. *Lancet*. 1964; **i**, 252.
10. Epstein MA, Achong BG, Barr YM. *Lancet*. 1964; **i**, 702.
11. Epstein MA, Achong BG. *Journal of the National Cancer Institute*. 1968; **40**, 609.
12. Henle G, Henle W. *Journal of Bacteriology*. 1966; **91**, 1248.
13. Henle W, Henle G. In: Biggs PM, Thé G de, Payne LN (eds). *Oncogenesis and Herpesviruses*. Lyon: International Association for Research

Against Cancer, 1973: 269.

14. Klein G. In: Epstein MA, Achong BG (eds). *The Epstein–Barr Virus.* Berlin: Springer-Verlag, 1979: 339.

15. de Thé G. In: Epstein MA, Achong BG (eds). *The Epstein–Barr Virus.* Berlin: Springer-Verlag, 1979: 417.

16. Miller G. In: Fields BN, Knipe DM, Chanock RM, Melnick JL, Roizman B, Schope RE (eds). *Virology.* New York: Raven Press, 1985: 563.

17. Ablashi DV. In: Levine PH, Ablashi DV, Nonoyama M, Pearson GR, Glaser R (eds). *Epstein–Barr Virus and Human Diseases.* Clifton, New Jersey: Humana Press, 1987: 415.

18. Lenoir GM, Philip T, Sohier R. In: Magrath IT, O'Conor GT, Ramot G (eds). *Pathogenesis of Leukemia and Lymphomas.* New York: Raven Press, 1984: 283.

19. Gallo RC. *Cancer.* 1985; **55**, 2317.

20. Gallo RC. *Scientific American.* 1986; **225**, 88.

21. Sarngadharn MG, Markham PD, Gallo RC. In: Fields BN, Knipe DM, Chanock RM, Melnick JL, Roizman B, Shope RE (eds). *Virology.* New York: Raven Press, 1985: 1345.

22. Wong-Staal F, Gallo RC. *Nature.* 1985; **317**, 395.

23. Salahuddin SZ, Ablashi DV, Markham PD, *et al. Science.* 1986; **234**, 596.

24. Miller G. In: Klein G (ed). *Viral Oncology.* New York: Raven Press, 1980: 713.

25. Nonoyama M, Huang CH, Pagano JS, *et al. Proceedings of the National Academy of Sciences USA.* 1973; **70**,3265.

26. Zur Hausen H, Schulte-Holthausen H, Klein G, *et al. Nature.* 1970; **228**, 1056.

27. Adams A, Lindahl T. *Proceedings of the National Academy of Sciences USA.* 1975; **70**, 1477.

28. Baer R, Bankier AT, Biggin MD, *et al. Nature.* 1984; **310**, 207.

29. Kieff E, Dambaugh T, Heller M, *et al. Journal of Infectious Diseases.* 1982; **146**, 506.

30. Resnick L, Herbst JS, Ablashi DV, *et al. Journal of the American Medical Association.* 1988; **259**, 384.

31. Aalfieri C, Joncas JH, Raab-Traub N, *et al.* In: Levine PH, Ablashi DV, Nonoyama M, Pearson GR, Glaser R (eds). *Epstein–Barr Virus and Human Diseases.* Clifton, New Jersey: Humana Press, 1987: 260.

32. Glaser R, Takimoto T, Zhana H, *et al.* In: Levine PH, Ablashi DV, Nonoyama M, Pearson GR, Glaser R (eds). *Epstein–Barr Virus and Human Diseases.* Clifton, New Jersey: Humana Press, 1987: 299.

33. Magrath I, Erikson J, Whang Peng J, *et al. Science.* 1983; **222**, 1094.

34. Pearson GR, Luka J, Docherty J. In: Lopez C,

Roizman B (eds). *Human Herpesvirus Infections.* New York: Raven Press, 1986: 211.

35. Pearson GR. *AIDS Research.* 1986; **2**, 549.

36. Goldschmidt W, Luka J, Pearson GR. *Virology.* 1987; **157**, 220.

37. Pearson GR. In: Klein G (ed). *Viral Oncology.* New York: Raven Press, 1979: 739.

38. Reedman B, Klein G. *International Journal of Cancer.* 1973; **23**, 610.

39. Sugden B, Mark W. *Journal of Virology.* 1977; **23**, 503.

40. Dillner J, Kallin B, Alexander H, *et al. Proceedings of the National Academy of Sciences USA.* 1986; **83**, 6641.

41. Jondal M, Svedmyr E, Klein E, *et al. Nature.* 1975; **255**, 405.

42. Wang D, Lebowitz D, Kieff E. *Cell.* 1985; **43**, 831.

43. Lebowitz D, Wang D, Kieff E. *Journal of Virology.* 1986; **58**, 233.

44. Rickinson AB, Strang G, Murray R, *et al.* In: Levine PH, Ablashi DV, Nonoyama M, Pearson GR, Glaser R (eds). *Epstein–Barr Virus and Human Diseases.* Clifton, New Jersey: Humana Press, 1987: 335.

45. Pope JH. In: Levine PH, Ablashi DV, Pearson GR, Kottaridis SD (eds). *Epstein–Barr Virus and Associated Diseases.* Boston: Martinus Nijhoff Publishing Co., 1984: 511.

46. Menezes J, Sundar SK. In: Levine PH, Ablashi DV, Pearson GR, Kottaridis SD (eds). *Epstein–Barr Virus and Associated Diseases.* Boston: Martinus Nijhoff Publishing Co., 1985: 535.

47. Pearson GR, Johansson B, Klein G. *International Journal of Cancer.* 1978; **22**, 120.

48. Pearson GR, Qualtiere LF, Klein G, *et al. International Journal of Cancer.* 1979; **24**, 402.

49. Gaston JS, Rickinson AB, Epstein MA. *Lancet.* 1982; **i**, 923.

50. Sundar SK, Menezes J. *Microbial Pathogenesis.* 1987; **2**, 259.

51. Tosato G, Pike SE, Yuan M, *et al.* In: Levine PH, Ablashi DV, Nonoyama M, Pearson GR, Glaser R (eds). *Epstein–Barr Virus and Human Diseases.* Clifton, New Jersey: Humana Press, 1987: 379.

52. de Thé G, Geser A, Day NE, *et al. Nature.* 1978; **274**, 756.

53. Purtilo TT. In: Levine PH, Ablashi DV, Pearson GR, Kottaridis SD (eds). *Epstein–Barr Virus and Associated Diseases.* Boston: Martinus Nijhoff Publishing Co., 1985: 511.

54. Ablashi DV, Glaser R, Easton JM, *et al. Experimental Hematology.* 1978; **6**, 365.

55. Gurtsevitch VE, O'Conor GT, Lenoir GM. *International Journal of Cancer.* 1988; **41**, 87.

56. Johnson DR, Wolf LG, Levan G, *et al. International*

57. Miller G. In: Klein G (ed). *Viral Oncology*. New York: Raven Press, 1979: 713.
58. Sundar SK, Levine PH, Ablashi DV, *et al. International Journal of Cancer*. 1981; **27**, 107.
59. Ablashi DV, Aulakh GS, Leutzler J, *et al. Comparative Immunology and Microbiology of Infectious Diseases*. 1983; **6**, 151.
60. Cleary ML, Epstein MA, Finery S, *et al. Science*. 1985; **288**, 722.
61. Epstein MA, Morgan AJ, Finery S, *et al. Nature*. 1985; **318**, 287.
62. Gregoriadis G. *Nature*. 1986; **320**, 87.
63. Sandberg A. In: Magrath IT, O'Conor GT, Ramot B (eds). *Pathogenesis of Leukemia and Lymphomas: Environmental Influences*. New York: Raven Press, 1984: 263.
64. Purtilo DT. *Cancer Research*. 1981; **41**, 4226.
65. Purtilo DT. In: Levine PH, Ablashi DV, Nonoyama M, Glaser R (eds). *Epstein–Barr Virus and Human Disease*. Clifton, New Jersey: Humana Press, 1987: 5.
66. Magrath I. In: Schlossberg D (ed). *Infectious Mononucleosis*. New York: Praeger, 1983: 225.
67. Josephs SF, Salahuddin SZ, Ablashi DV, *et al. Science*. 1986; **234**, 601.
68. Lusso P, Salahuddin SZ, Ablashi DV, *et al. Lancet*. 1987; **ii**, 743.
69. Tedder RS, Briggs M, Cameron CH, *et al. Lancet*. 1987; **ii**, 390.
70. Downing RG, Sweankambo M, Swerwadddda D, *et al. Lancet*. 1987; **ii**, 39.
71. Biberfield P, Kramarsky B, Salahuddin SZ, *et al. Journal of the National Cancer Institute*. 1987; **79**, 933.
72. Ablashi DV, Salahuddin SZ, Josephs SF, *et al. Nature*. 1987; **329**, 207.
73. Josephs SF, Buchbinder A, Streicher HZ, *et al. Leukemia*. 1988; **2**, 132.
74. Holmes GP, Kaplan JE, Stewart JA, *et al. Journal of the American Medical Association*. 1987; **257**, 2297.
75. Krueger GRF, Koch B, Ablashi DV. *Lancet*. 1987; **i**, 36.
76. Fox RI, Pearson GR, Vaughan JH. *Journal of Immunology*. 1986; **137**, 3162.
77. Morgan DA, Ruscetti FW, Gallo RC. *Science*. 1976; **193**, 1007.
78. Poisz BJ, Ruscetti FW, Gazdar AF, *et al. Proceedings of the National Academy of Sciences USA*. 1980; **77**, 7415.
79. Poisz BJ, Ruscetti FW, Reitz MS, *et al. Nature*. 1980; **294**, 268.
80. Kalyanaraman VS, Sarngadharan MG, Robert-Guroff M, *et al. Science*. 1982; **218**, 571.
81. Popovic M, Sarngadharan MG, Read E, *et al. Science*. 1984; **224**, 497.
82. Barr-Sinoussi F, Chermann JC, Rey F, *et al. Science*. 1983; **220**, 868.
83. Gallo RC, Salahuddin SZ, Popovic M, *et al. Science*. 1984; **224**, 500.
84. Takatsuki K, Uchiyama J, Sagawa K, *et al.* In: Seno F, Takaku F, Irino S (eds). *Topics in Hematology*. Amsterdam: Excerpta Medica, 1977: 73.
85. Uchiyama J, Yodoi J, Sagawa K, *et al. Blood*. 1977; **50**, 481.
86. Hahn BH, Popovic M, Kalyanaraman VS, *et al.* In: Gotteib MS, Groopman JE (eds). *Acquired Immune Deficiency Syndrome*. New York: Alan R Liss, 1984: 73.
87. Sarin PS, Gallo RC. *Scientific American*. 1986; **225**, 88.
88. Salahuddin SZ, Markham PD, Wong-Staal F, *et al. Progress in Medical Virology*. 1985; **32**, 195.
89. Hinuma Y, Komoda H, Chosa T, *et al. International Journal of Cancer*. 1982; **29**, 631.
90. Haase AT. *Nature*. 1986; **322**, 130.
91. Levine PH, Blattner WA, Biggar RJ, *et al. Viruses and Human Cancer*. New York: Alan R Liss, 1987: 93–103.
92. Yamaguchi K, Nishimura H, Kawano F, *et al. Japanese Journal of Clinical Oncology*. 1983; **13**, 189.
93. Catovsky D, Rosa M, Goolden AWG, *et al. Lancet*. 1982; **i**, 639.
94. Tajima K, Kamura S, Ito S, *et al. International Journal of Cancer*. 1987; **40**, 741.
95. Kusuhara K, Sonoda S, Takahashi K, *et al. International Journal of Cancer*. 1987; **40**, 755..
96. Siekevitz M, Feinberg MB, Holbrook N, Wong-Staal F, Greene WC. *Proceedings of the National Academy of Sciences USA*. 1987; **84**, 5389.
97. Flekenstein B, Desrosiers RC. In: Roizman B (ed). *The Herpesvirus*. New York: Plenum Publishing, 1982: 253.
98. Yamanishi KK, Shiraki T, Kondst A *et al. Lancet*. 1988; **i**, 1065.
99. Bertram G, Dreiner N, Krueger GRF *et al.* In Ablashi DV, Faggioni A, Krueger GRF, Pagano JS, Pearson GR (eds). *Epstein–Barr Virus and Human Disease*. Clifton, New Jersey: Humana Press, 1989: 361.
100. Ablashi DV, Josephs SF, Buchbinder A, *et al. Journal of Virological Methods*. 1988; **21**, 29.

CHAPTER 12

CLINICAL FEATURES AND STAGING

Ian Magrath, Wyndham Wilson, Klara Horvath, Ronald Neumann and Francisco Barriga

The non-Hodgkin's lymphomas (NHLs) encompass a spectrum of neoplasms ranging from indolent tumours, which can occasionally undergo spontaneous regression, to rapidly progressive tumours which may be fatal within weeks if untreated. They are usually generalized diseases and can involve almost any organ or tissue, giving rise to a broad array of possible clinical presentations. Individual lymphomas, however, may differ markedly from one another with regard to their clinical features. These reflect the biological characteristics of the constituent tumour cells, particularly their proliferative capacity and their relative ability to grow in various anatomical locations as a cellular infiltrate or mass. Some of the clinical features may be caused by chemical mediators produced by the lymphoma cells, by metabolic changes consequent upon a high rate of cell death in the tumour, or by secondary events such as opportunistic infections, pyrexia, weight loss, hypercalcaemia, hyperuricaemia, hypoglycaemia, immunosuppression and certain neurological syndromes (e.g. progressive multifocal leucoencephalopathy).

The majority of patients present to a physician because of a tumour mass or its consequences (Table 12.1), but perhaps 10 per cent of patients seek medical advice because of general symptoms such as weight loss, pyrexia or lethargy. Some 39 per cent of all patients have these symptoms at the time of presentation.[1] Even less common presentations include hyperuricaemic renal failure, symptoms caused by hypercalcaemia, paraneoplastic neurological syndromes or severe hypoglycaemia. In patients with an underlying prelymphomatous state, such as a lymphoproliferative syndrome (e.g. alpha heavy chain disease, angioimmunoblastic lymphadenopathy, angiocentric immunoproliferative lesions), an immunodeficiency syndrome (inherited, acquired or iatrogenic) or a chronic inflammatory state (Sjögrens disease, lymphomatoid granulomatosis), there may be an insidious onset of lymphoma with presenting features which hardly differ from those of the underlying disease. In such diseases there is often chronic lymphadenopathy which may wax and wane, and it may be difficult to decide when to undertake a lymph node biopsy, the only means of establishing a definitive diagnosis of NHL. In general, any progressive increase in lymphadenopathy or the development of new, unexplained mass should always lead to a biopsy and the application of all available methods, including cytogenetics, phenotyping and molecular characterization in an attempt to confirm or exclude a diagnosis of NHL.

Anatomical sites of involvement

Patterns of organ and tissue involvement

The anatomical locations characteristic of the various NHLs reflect, to a degree, their phenotypic characteristics, since lymphoid neoplasms tend to occur in the same regions of lymphoid tissue as their normal counterpart cells. B-cell lymphomas of germinal centre cells, for example, often retain a follicular architecture and occur in B-cell zones of lymphoid tissue; mantle zone lymphomas may retain a tendency to surround residual germinal centres and neoplasms of immature T-cells involve the thymus in a high proportion of cases. Other lymphomas have characteristic patterns which do not obviously reflect their phenotypic characteristics, such as small non-cleaved cell

Table 12.1 Possible presentations in patients with non-Hodgkin's lymphomas

Lymphoid system	Lymphadenopathy – peripheral or central Hepatosplenomegaly Thymic (anterior superior mediastinal) mass Waldeyer's ring involvement Bone marrow involvement
Gastrointestinal system	Abdominal or pelvic mass Upper or lower gastrointestinal bleeding Malabsorption Intussusception Perforation Fistula Biliary obstruction Pancreatic mass Ascites Salivary gland swelling
Genitourinary system	Renal mass, ureteric obstruction Testicular mass Ovarian mass Vaginal bleeding
Nervous system	Meningeal involvement Cranial nerve palsies Intracranial mass (extradural or intracerebral) Paraspinal mass Intraorbital, periorbital or ocular mass Peripheral neuropathy Progressive multifocal leucoencephalopathy
Endocrine system	Thyroid mass Adrenal mass
Other	Bone involvement Paranasal sinus involvement Jaw involvement Skin infiltration Venous or (rarely) arterial obstruction Pericardial effusion Cardiac involvement Pleural effusions Pulmonary infiltration
General	Pyrexia/night sweats Weight loss Lethargy

lymphomas which have a predilection for the small bowel, or in Africa, the jaw, and lymphomas of peripheral T-cells which frequently involve the skin and central nervous system (CNS). Although there is considerable overlap, particularly with regard to peripheral lymph node involvement, the overall patterns of organ and tissue involvement of individual NHLs have emerged more clearly as diagnosis and classification have been refined by the use of immunophenotyping, and to a lesser extent (at present), cytogenetics.

The recognition of a new subtype of lymphoma has usually been based initially upon histological criteria, but often the immunological characterization of a tumour, coupled to a reasonably consistent clinical pattern, has confirmed the validity of such a histological distinction. Examples include the separation of lymphoblastic lymphoma from diffuse, poorly differentiated lymphocytic lymphoma,[2] the identification of a lymphoma with a degree of differentiation intermediate between the small lymphocytic cell and small cleaved cell lymphomas (the 'mantle zone' lymphoma)[3] and recognition of adult T-cell leukaemia/lymphoma in Japan.[4] Within histologically homogeneous groups, such as lymphoblastic lymphoma, diffuse mixed or large cell lymphomas, immunophenotyping has led to the recognition of immunological subtypes (T versus B), each of which can then be recognized as having a different, if overlapping, anatomical distribution. Pre-B-cell lymphoblastic lymphomas, for example, preferentially involve lymph nodes, skin or bone rather than the thymus, and diffuse mixed or large cell tumours of T-cell origin preferentially involve T-cell zones of lymphoid tissue and never manifest remnants of a follicular architecture as is often seen in their B-cell counterparts. The converse of this situation: tumours with the same phenotype and similar anatomical distribution, but a range of histological appearances, has also been observed, e.g. the post-thymic T-cell lymphomas (peripheral T-cell lymphomas and adult leukaemia/lymphoma) may be diagnosed histologically as diffuse large cell lymphomas or mixed cell lymphomas.[5]

Knowledge of the characteristic distribution patterns of different types of lymphoma is important to the planning of optimal staging strategies and in some circumstances, e.g. where the possibility of CNS involvement is high, may have an impact on the design of treatment strategies.

Cell surface molecules relevant to organ and tissue distribution

The mechanisms responsible for specific patterns of tissue and organ involvement by lymphomas, although not well elucidated at the present time, are likely to involve cell surface molecules involved in the recognition of receptors on other cells present at particular anatomical locations. Soluble factors, including chemotactic factors, may also have a role in tumour localization. At least two candidate systems of recognition molecules have been identified. These are the molecules involved in the adherence of lymphocytes to the endothelial linings of specialized veins, including the high endothelial venules (HEV) found in organized lymphoid tissues and sites of chronic inflammation,[6] and the family of intercellular adhesion molecules represented by the lymphocyte function-associated molecules LFA-1 and LFA-3. These bind respectively to intercellular adhesion molecule-1 (ICAM-1) and the molecule responsible for sheep red cell rosette formation of T-cells, CD2.[7,8] These molecules have been shown to mediate the adhesion of T lymphocytes to target cells as a necessary component of cellular cytotoxicity, and are likely to play a role in several other effector functions of lymphocytes.[9]

LFA-1 is expressed at very low levels by high-grade lymphomas, such as small non-cleaved cell lymphomas. Recently, a difference in expression of LFA-1, LFA-3 and ICAM-1 was shown between Epstein–Barr virus (EBV)-negative and -positive Burkitt's lymphoma cell lines,[10] the former having lower levels than the latter, and both having much lower levels than EBV-transformed lymphoblastoid cell lines. It is quite possible that such molecules are necessary for the manifestation of a host antitumour response, and low surface levels may hinder or even totally abrogate the regulation of the proliferation or migration of lymphoma cells. As more is learnt about the cell surface molecules which mediate cell–cell adhesion, they may prove to be of value in distinguishing lymphomas with different propensities to invade certain tissues or organs, e.g. the CNS, marrow, etc., and thus be of value in the design of treatment protocols.

Nodal and extranodal sites of involvement

Lymphomas are often divided into those which are confined to lymph nodes and those which involve extranodal sites. Although differences in prognosis between nodal and extranodal presentations can be discerned overall, prognosis is more a consequence of the cell type and tumour bulk, than the nodal or extranodal location of the tumour *per se*. High grade lymphomas, which are the predominant category in children, tend particularly to involve extranodal sites; low grade lymphomas tend to be often nodal, while intermediate grade lymphomas are also intermediate with regard to their involvement of lymph nodes.[11] Just as the frequency of extranodal disease is higher in the NHLs than Hodgkin's disease, so too, the patterns of spread of the NHLs are less predictable, and although contiguous lymphatic spread may be seen (the frequency depending upon how 'contiguity' is defined), involvement of more distant nodal groups occurs with similar frequency.[11] This has important implications for staging strategies, and for the planning (where appropriate) of radiation therapy (*see* Chapter 14).

Staging

Importance of determining the extent of disease

The determination of the extent of disease in patients with NHL serves multiple purposes. It provides information regarding the imminence of potential complications, it gives an indication of prognosis and it is often of critical importance to treatment planning.[12,13] Therapy for patients with limited disease usually differs from treatment for patients with extensive disease, and disease at special sites, such a the CNS, may require therapy components directed specifically at these locations. Precise knowledge, not only of the extent of disease but of the margins of individual lesions, is of particular importance when radiation therapy is contemplated. Finally, in circumstances where surgical resection may be beneficial, (e.g. in small noncleaved cell (SNCC) lymphoma of the abdomen) it is important to determine, as far as possible, whether complete resection is feasible – a decision which can only be made when all sites of disease have been determined.

Staging schemes

At the completion of the 'staging work-up', patients are assigned to a disease stage. In the NHLs this usually includes information obtained from marrow biopsy and sometimes liver biopsy. Technically, when the results of multiple biopsies are included in the determination of stage, the designation of 'pathological stage' as opposed to 'clinical stage' is used. In practice, however, since staging laparotomy, the usual source of biopsy material, is rarely performed today, these designations are not generally used. Staging schemes provide a shorthand notation of the extent of disease, and along with histology, staging is the most widely used criterion to assess comparability of different patient groups (e.g. patients in different clinical trials or in different arms of a randomized study of different treatment approaches).

Unfortunately, since stage usually depends only upon the location and number of disease sites, it is not a true measure of tumour burden, one of the most important prognostic determinants in patients with NHL. Even when tumour size is included as a determinant of stage (e.g. stage III of the St Jude scheme for childhood lymphomas requires that the tumour be 'extensive') (*see* Table 12.2), size criteria are not specified.

Thus a single clinical stage encompasses a range of tumour burdens and disease sites, making it a somewhat unsatisfactory parameter for assessing prognostic comparability of patient

Table 12.2 Staging systems for non-Hodgkin's lymphomas

Staging system	Stage	Definition
Ann Arbor adult NHL	I	Involvement of a single lymph node region or of a single extranodal organ or site (I_E)
	II	Involvement of two or more lymph node regions on the same side of the diaphragm, or localized involvement of an extranodal site or organ (II_E) and one or more lymph node regions on the same side of the diaphragm
	III	Involvement of lymph node regions on both sides of the diaphragm, which may also be accompanied by localized involvement of an extranodal organ or site (III_E) or spleen (III_S) or both (III_{SE})
	IV	Diffuse or disseminated involvement of one or more distant extranodal organs with or without associated lymph node involvement

Fever >38°C, night sweats and/or weight loss >10% of body weight in the 6 months preceding admission are defined as systemic symptoms and denoted by the suffix B. Other patients are denoted by the suffix A.

St Jude childhood NHL	I	Single tumour (extranodal) Single anatomical area (nodal) excluding mediastinum or abdomen
	II	Single tumour (extranodal) with regional node involvement Primary gastrointestinal tumour with or without involvement of associated mesenteric nodes only, grossly completely resected. On same side of diaphragm: a) two or more nodal areas b) two single (extranodal) tumours with or without regional node involvement
	III	On both sides of the diaphragm: a) two single tumours (extranodal) b) two or more nodal areas All primary intrathoracic tumours (mediastinal, pleural, thymic) All extensive primary intra-abdominal disease All primary paraspinal or epidural tumours regardless of other sites
	IV	Any of the above with initial CNS or bone marrow involvement (<25%)
Proposed NCI SNCC	I	Single extra-abdominal tumour
	IR	Resected (<90%) intra-abdominal tumour
	II	Multiple extra-abdominal sites excluding bone marrow and CNS
	III_A	Unresected intra-abdominal tumour Epidural tumour not otherwise in stage IV
	III_B	Intra- and extra-abdominal tumour except bone marrow
	IV_A	Bone marrow involvement without abdominal or CNS tumour
	IV_B	Bone marrow and abdominal tumour
	IV_C	CNS disease (malignant CSF pleiocytosis/cranial nerve palsies)
Proposed NCI LL	I	Single extrathoracic tumour
	II	Multiple extrathoracic tumours excluding bone marrow and CNS
	III_A	Single mediastinal (thymic) tumour
	III_B	Mediastinal tumour with pleural effusion Mediastinal tumour with extrathoracic tumour excluding bone marrow and CNS
	IV_A	CNS disease (malignant CSF pleiocytosis/cranial nerve palsies) without bone marrow involvement
	IV_B	Bone marrow and intrathoracic tumour (without CNS)
	IV_C	Bone marrow and extrathoracic tumour (without CNS)
	IV_D	Bone marrow and CNS disease

(stages IV B, C, and D are probably better diagnosed as ALL) groups. Moreover, in view of the differences in biology and the patterns of anatomical involvement among different lymphomas, it would seem logical to use a staging system designed for each disease rather than the same staging system for all. In practice, however, the most widely used staging system for the NHLs (of all histologies) is the Ann Arbor scheme, which, ironically, was originally designed for Hodgkin's disease! This scheme suffers from the disadvantage that the distinction between stages III and IV, i.e. the presence of involvement of one or more distant extranodal sites (stage IV disease), does not greatly influence treatment approach or outcome in the NHLs, whereas in Hodgkin's disease, because of the much greater emphasis on radiotherapy, this can be an important distinction.

In paediatric lymphomas, which are predominantly extranodal, the most widely used staging scheme is usually referred to as the 'St Jude', or 'Murphy' scheme. The latter is, of necessity, a fairly drastic modification of the Ann Arbor scheme because of the predominant extranodal distribution of the high grade lymphomas. Like the Ann Arbor scheme in adult lymphomas, the St Jude scheme is used for all childhood lymphomas, the major subgroups of which (lymphoblastic and SNCC lymphomas) differ markedly with regard to their predominant sites of involvement. The use of different staging schemes in childhood and adult NHL makes comparison of the results of published treatment approaches to high grade lymphomas in different age groups very difficult. Clearly, there is a need either to incorporate measures of tumour volume into staging schemes (e.g. serum lactate dehydrogenase (LDH))[14,15] or at least to use such information in both the design and analysis of treatment protocols. Staging schemes currently in use, and two proposed schemes designed for SNCC and lymphoblastic lymphomas as examples of disease specific staging systems, are shown in Table 12.2.

Stage distribution

A large study of 473 consecutive patients with NHL treated at the National Cancer Institute (NCI), Bethesda, USA, clearly showed that the majority of patients with NHL have widespread disease. More than 70 per cent of all patients in this study had stage III or IV disease (Ann Arbor).[1] Pathological staging, i.e. the inclusion of information from bone marrow and liver biopsies and, in selected cases, laparotomy, increased the proportion of patients with stage IV disease from 14 to 49 per cent in the follicular lymphomas and from 39 to 56 per cent in the diffuse lymphomas, but the majority of the 'upstaged' patients came from stage III so that the proportion of patients with stages I and II disease, which was in any event very low, was not changed significantly (Table 12.3).

The staging work-up

Knowledge of the type of lymphoma and its characteristic pattern of anatomical distribution is relevant to planning the series of investigations directed towards defining the extent of disease, i.e. the staging work-up.[16,17] To some extent the staging work-up may be tailored to individual diseases, based on the likelihood that various investigations, such as a lymphogram, liver biopsy, etc., will detect disease in different lymphomas, as well as the importance to management of detecting involvement at particular sites. Whether or not specific investigations are included may also depend upon the nature of the institution undertaking care of the patient. In research institutions it may be of importance to document the involvement of as many sites as possible or to compare the advantages and disadvantages of different staging strategies. In such institutions, investigations that are rarely positive may be routinely included in the staging work-up and multiple imaging studies are often performed (e.g. computed tomography (CT), magnetic resonance imaging (MRI), ultrasonography (US) and radionuclide scans). On the other hand, considerations of morbidity, cost, convenience and availability (of specialized procedures) must be given greater weight when planning a staging work-up for patients not entered into a clinical research study. A basic list of investigations

Table 12.3 Proportions of patients with disease at different stages

	I(%)	II(%)	III(%)	IV(%)
Clinical				
All follicular[1]	15 (8.3)	21(11.7)	119(66.1)	25(13.9)
DSC	0	2 (5.1)	23(59.0)	14(35.9)
DSCC	6(18.2)	10(15.6)	22(34.4)	26(40.1)
DMC	6(18.2)	8(24.2)	11(33.3)	8(24.2)
DLC	10(10.9)	18(19.8)	23(25.3)	40(44.0)
SNCC	9(13.6)	19(28.8)	12(18.2)	26(39.4)
All diffuse	31(10.6)	57(19.5)	91(31.1)	114(38.9)
Pathological[2]				
All follicular	11 (6.2)	17 (9.6)	62(34.8)	88(49.4)
DSC	0	2 (5.1)	9(23.1)	28(71.8)
DSCC	6 (9.4)	8(12.5)	11(17.2)	39(60.9)
DMC	7 (7.7)	20(22.0)	16(17.6)	48(52.7)
DLC	3(11.5)	8(30.8)	6(23.1)	9(34.6)
SNCC	24 (7.8)	16(25.0)	9(34.0)	34(53.1)
All diffuse	22 (7.6)	53(18.2)	52(17.9)	164(56.3)

Data from 473 patients evaluated at the National Cancer Institute, Anderson *et al.*[42]
DSC, diffuse small cell lymphoma; DSCC, diffuse small cleaved cell lymphoma; DMC, diffuse mixed cell lymphoma; DLC, diffuse large cell lymphoma; SNCC, small non-cleaved cell lymphoma
[1]There was no difference in the distribution of clinical stages among different histological categories of nodular lymphomas.
[2]Pathological staging included bilateral bone marrow biopsies, peritoneoscopy with multiple directed liver biopsies and laparotomy in selected patients.

usually included in the work-up of lymphoma patients is shown in Table 12.4.

History and physical examination

The clinical history and physical examination are critically important components of staging. Not only can they lead to the detection of the majority of disease sites, but they also provide information which may lead to modifications in the basic staging strategy. Investigations which are not performed routinely (e.g. myelography) may be imperative for confirmation of tumour at a particular site, the presence of which is suggested by the history and physical examination. In addition, the history and physical examination may raise the suspicion of the presence of a potentially serious complication and thus lead to appropriate priorities being assigned to investigations. For example, impending airway obstruction from a pharyngeal mass, respiratory distress from massive mediastinal involvement, pleural effusions or lung involvement, superior or inferior vena caval obstruction, cardiac tamponade, gastrointestinal bleeding or perforation of the bowel, paraparesis, intracerebral tumour, and renal failure from uric acid nephropathy or outflow tract obstruction should be detected or suspected when the patient is first seen by the physician, and appropriate investigations and emergency measures instituted.

The physical examination is also important for the detection of disease sites not always identified by routinely performed staging studies, such as the presence of peripheral lymphadenopathy, including epitrochlear and popliteal nodes, involvement of lymphoid tissue in Waldeyer's ring, cranial or peripheral nerve palsies and the presence of skin or testicular involvement. Other kinds of useful information obtained by physical examination include the consistency of a mass, whether it is fixed or

Table 12.4 Suggested staging studies in NHL

Recommended in all patients	Recommended in selected patients
History and physical exam	ENT examination
Chest X-ray	Chest CT
Electrocardiogram	Echocardiogram
Abdominal/pelvic CT scan	Abdominal/pelvic ultrasound
	Lymphogram
	Contrast radiography of gastrointestinal tract
	Endoscopic examination
	Head CT scan
	Myelogram or CT myelogram
	Magnetic resonance imaging
Technetium-99m-MDP scintigram	Skeletal X-rays
Gallium-67 scintigram	
Biochemical tests of liver and renal function, serum calcium	Liver biopsy
	Renal ultrasound
Serum LDH and uric acid	Other serum tests which correlate with tumour burden
Haematological para-meters	
Bilateral bone marrow aspirates and biopsies	Aspiration of serous effusion for cytological examination
CSF examination	

mobile or has characteristics more often associated with inflammation, the presence of jaundice, pyrexia, petechial haemorrhages or bruising, cardiac arrhythmias or tamponade, or clinical features suggesting a metabolic abnormality such as hypoglycaemia or hypercalcaemia.

Radiological investigations

Unlike Hodgkin's disease, where the sites of involvement are more predictable and orderly, the multiplicity of possible disease locations in NHLs and the variety of clinical patterns which can be encountered preclude the adoption of a single scheme for the radiological work-up.[17] However, once a diagnosis of lymphoma has been established, there are a number of studies which, if not already obtained, should be performed routinely.

Chest

All patients with NHL should have a chest X-ray, which may lead to the detection of a mediastinal mass, hilar adenopathy, parenchymal lung infiltration or pleural or pericardial effusions. Computed tomography of the chest is more sensitive than chest X-ray for the detection of all of these abnormalities, and is far superior to the plain film for the detection of chest wall disease. Since, however, involvement of intrathoracic structures is relatively uncommon, chest CT is not an invariable part of the staging work-up. It is indicated in patients with histologies such as lymphoblastic lymphoma, where involvement of the chest is likely, when radiation therapy is planned, when anatomical detail is required in patients with airway or intrathoracic vascular obstruction or when a finding on the chest radiograph requires clarification.[18–20] Magnetic resonance imaging may also be useful for the detection of chest wall or mediastinal tumour, but is not usually helpful in examination of the lung parenchyma.

Abdomen

Abdominal/pelvic CT should be performed in all patients with NHL, since abdominal or pelvic masses, whether nodal or extranodal, occur frequently (Fig. 12.1) – in up to 90 per cent of patients in some subgroups (e.g. small non-cleaved lymphomas).[21] Patients with lympho-blastic lymphoma rarely have abdominal involvement, although hepatosplenomegaly or involvement of kidneys or pancreas may occasionally be observed. In children or very thin individuals, in whom there is little retroperitoneal fat, intra-abdominal structures are often poorly delineated by CT, and an ultrasonogram should be performed.[22] Detection and follow-up of involvement of the liver or spleen is improved by use of the selective hepatosplenic contrast agent, ethiodized oil emulsion-13 (EOE), when performing upper abdominal CT,[23] but this agent is not widely available. Dynamic CT scanning with water-soluble contrast material promises similar results, but both techniques suffer from the disadvantages that lesions smaller than 0.5 cm and diffuse infiltration cannot be detected.

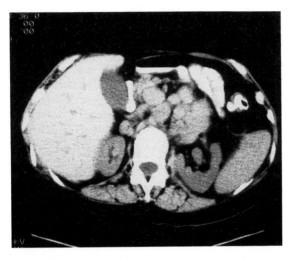

Fig. 12.1 CT scan of abdomen showing gross enlargement of multiple mesenteric lymph nodes. The contrast filled bowel surrounds the periphery of the central nodular mass.

Lymphography is usually performed on patients who have lymphomas which have a high likelihood of involvement of intra-abdominal lymph nodes. In practice this includes the majority of adult NHLs. Lymphography is not usually performed, however, in tumours which are predominantly extranodal, such as the childhood NHLs. An important advantage of the lymphography is that the dye often remains in the nodes for 6 months or more, so that abnormal lymph nodes can be closely monitored with repeated abdominal X-rays during treatment and follow-up. Lymphography is extremely sensitive, detecting the presence of involved para-aortic lymph nodes in nearly 100 per cent of cases. Even when they are not enlarged and therefore not detectable with CT, filling defects may be readily apparent.[24] Occasionally, even enlarged

architecturally abnormal nodes readily apparent on lymphography do not show as definite abnormalities on the CT scan (Fig. 12.2). On the other hand, CT, although not as sensitive as lymphography, will detect extranodal masses, organ involvement, high para-aortic, retro-crural, mesenteric, liver and splenic hilar lymph adenopathy, none of which are detectable by lymphography[25] (Fig. 12.3). In cases where CT shows the same abnormal nodes as the lymphogram, repeat CT is not necessary for follow-up. When CT shows additional extranodal masses, however, or abnormal nodes in sites not opacified by lymphography, then it should be included in the follow-up studies.

Because of the value of the combination of CT and lymphography in detecting both intra- and extranodal masses, contrast radiology of the gastrointestinal tract is not routinely performed. However, this technique is much more sensitive than CT for detection of intrinsic bowel involvement, and is indicated if there is a high index of suspicion for bowel lymphoma, e.g. in the presence of lymphoma of Waldeyer's ring. Often, contrast radiography of the gastrointestinal tract is performed in the evaluation of a patient with unexplained abdominal pain, early satiety or symptoms of peptic ulcer or obstruction, and may therefore lead to the detection of a thickened stomach or bowel wall, with or without ulceration, or a mass lesion.

In children, contrast radiography is often used to demonstrate the presence of intussusception, a common presentation of SNCC lymphoma. In such circumstances, the causal tumour mass is usually too small to be visualized by other imaging modalities.

Endoscopic procedures may be valuable both for diagnosis (biopsies can be obtained under direct visualization) and follow-up in appropriate clinical circumstances, e.g. lymphomas of the stomach and large bowel.

Head and neck

Although CT of the head is not a routine staging procedure, it should be obtained in patients with a facial tumour. Patients with symptoms suggestive of a nasopharyngeal mass or intracranial disease should also undergo CT of the

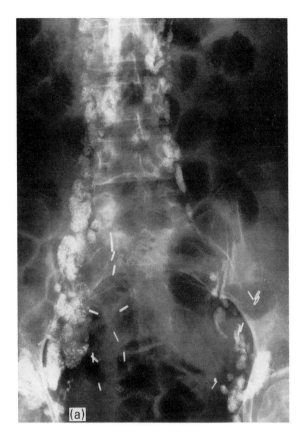

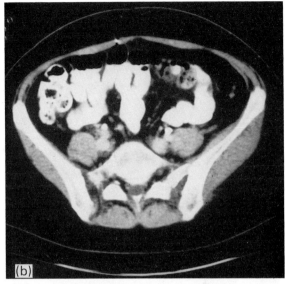

Fig. 12.2 (a) Lymphogram showing significantly enlarged and architecturally abnormal lymph nodes in the lower para-aortic and iliac regions on the right side, the presence of lymphoma was confirmed by needle aspiration; (b) CT performed 2 days later (prior to treatment). No definite abnormality is apparent in this slice which passes through the abnormal node region, and the rest of the CT also failed to reveal any abnormality.

head to delineate the soft tissue masses at the base of the skull or in the paranasal sinuses, or to provide evidence of intracerebral lymphoma.[26–28] In patients with clinical evidence of intraorbital disease or ophthalmic nerve palsies, the presence of an orbital mass is best defined by CT with special orbital cuts, or by MRI,[29] which provides improved contrast between different tissues. In general MRI is significantly more sensitive in detecting intracerebral tumour than CT (Fig. 12.3) and its use will doubtless become more routine when intracranial disease is suspected.[30]

Primary lymphoma of the brain usually presents as a solitary lesion, while secondary dissemination frequently leads to multiple, often smaller masses. The margins of these tumours are usually ill-defined and central necrosis and peritumoural oedema are not typical.[31] Most NHLs of the brain are periventricular and tend to involve the basal ganglia, corpus callosum, thalamus or septum pellucidum, although approximately 10 per cent will diffusely involve the brain parenchyma. Eventually, almost one-third of patients with lymphoma of the brain will develop disseminated disease.

In some circumstances a baseline CT of the brain may be of considerable value, e.g. in the event of neurological complications subsequent to the initiation of treatment, and comparison with an earlier scan may aid the interpretation of subtle findings. Whether or not a baseline CT is performed will depend upon the likelihood of such complications arising. For example, patients with bone marrow or testicular involvement, (the latter typically found in older men) are at high risk of having or developing CNS disease and a baseline CT of the brain is recommended.

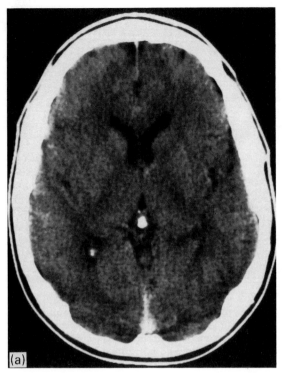 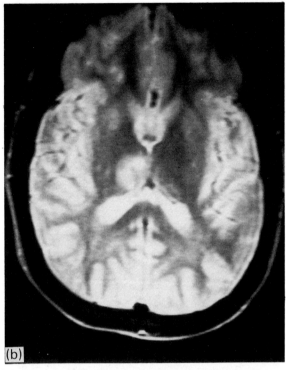

Fig. 12.3 (a) CT and (b) MRI scans of the same patient demonstrating the increased sensitivity of MRI in detecting intracerebral lymphoma. The MRI was a spin echo sequence with T_2 weighted imaging. The CT scan with contrast was normal, while the MRI scan showed obvious increased signal intensity in the right thalamic region. (Case kindly provided by Dr N Patronas, Clinical Center, NIH, Bethesda, MD)

Other sites

Routine X-rays of other sites are not recommended, but should be performed as indicated by the clinical setting, e.g. airway films for pharyngeal tumours, erect and supine abdominal films for suspected intra-abdominal perforation of a viscus or bowel obstruction, sinus films for patients with a suspicion of sinus involvement or with any facial tumour, and bone films in clinically suspicious areas or areas in which a radionuclide scan demonstrates increased uptake. Computed tomography with bone windows or MRI may be more valuable than plain films, or may complement plain films in patients with suspected bone involvement.

Special radiographic procedures are indicated in emergency situations. A myelogram or spinal CT with metrizamide is obligatory in patients with symptoms or signs suggestive of cord compression, both to document the finding and to assist in the planning of emergency treatment. Such studies may, however, soon be replaced by special MRI techniques (*see* below).

Ultrasonography

Ultrasound can be of considerable value in a number of circumstances, particularly for delineating abdominal, hepatic or pelvic tumour,[32] for assessing the size and response to therapy of superficial nodes[33] and for determining the presence of cardiac or pericardial involvement. With the possible exception of small children lacking in retroperitoneal fat, however, ultrasonography is not performed routinely. In situations where the interpretation of a CT scan is in doubt, such as when there is poor filling of the bowel with oral contrast rendering it difficult to distinguish bowel from tumour, abdominal ultrasound examination of the suspected area may resolve the uncertainty. In patients at high risk of renal involvement or obstructive uropathy, renal ultrasound provides an accurate, easily performed and readily repeatable assessment of renal size and the presence of hydronephrosis or intrarenal masses. It is worth noting that lymphomas are usually markedly echopenic, so that lymphomatous masses in the kidney are frequently difficult to distinguish from renal cysts. In patients with suspected pericardial effusions, an echocardiogram is indicated.

Magnetic resonance imaging

Magnetic resonance imaging (MRI), being a new and costly imaging modality, has not been widely used, so that its overall role in the staging of malignant lymphomas is still being assessed. In some cases it provides information similar to that obtained by other imaging modalities, while in other circumstances it may provide unique information. Because of the ability of MRI to distinguish tumour from surrounding soft tissue more readily than CT in some anatomical locations, it may provide a more accurate assessment of the true extent of disease in such sites.[27,34,35] It has also been shown to be an effective means of detecting patchy involvement of the bone marrow in patients with lymphoma (Fig. 12.4), and some studies suggest that it may be more sensitive than radionuclide scintigraphy in this regard.[36-38] The particularly high resolution of magnetic resonance images of the brain and spinal cord offers considerable advantages over CT of these sites (*see* Fig. 12.3). Because of its greater sensitivity to pathological alteration of cerebral tissues MRI is likely to replace CT in brain imaging. Preliminary studies provide evidence that the use of a special

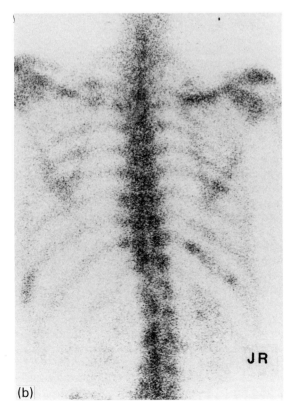

Fig. 12.4 (a) MRI scan (inversion recovery 1500/100, STIR sequence) clearly demonstrating bright signal intensity lesions in the 11th thoracic and 2nd and 3rd lumbar vertebral bodies; (b) bone scan performed in the same patient 2 days later which did not reveal any abnormalities.

contrast material, gadolinium DTPA, a paramagnetic metal ion chelater, will enhance MRI tissue contrast even further.[30,39] Gadolinium DTPA has also been shown to improve the detection of intradural and extramedullary tumour deposits in the spinal canal, and therefore promises to replace myelography and spinal CT in the future.[40]

Radionuclide scans

Radionuclide scans, which are generally nontomographic in nature, are useful whole body screening procedures. Gamma cameras can be used to image radionuclide activity in specific body regions if so desired. The most frequently performed scans are gallium-67 (^{67}Ga) and technetium-99m (^{99m}Tc) methylene diphosphonate (MDP) bone scintigraphy. Traditional ^{99m}Tc sulphur colloid liver/spleen scintigraphy is sometimes helpful, but can rarely add to the information derived from CT or MRI studies, and often provides less information because of scintigraphy's relative lack of sensitivity for small (< 2 cm) lesions.

[67]Ga scintigraphy

Gallium-67 is accumulated by most lymphomas to a greater or lesser extent, while Burkitt's lymphoma invariably shows avid uptake in nearly all lesions (Fig. 12.5)[41] However, there can be significant variation in the accuracy of ^{67}Ga scintigraphy for detecting sites of involvement in patients with NHL. Much of the published data on the utility of radiogallium imaging in lymphoma patients are derived from outdated gallium scintigraphy methodology, i.e. low ^{67}Ga citrate doses in the 2–3 mCi range and scans performed with rectilinear scanners. Data from studies using newer ^{67}Ga scintigraphy techniques, i.e. 10 mCi doses and triple peak scintigraphy with tomography, are impressive, with sensitivity and accuracy figures in the 90–100 per cent range.[42,43] Gallium-67 provides a useful whole body screen for unanticipated lymphoma sites and is usually worth performing as a routine staging procedure. The entry of ^{67}Ga into leukaemic cells *in vitro* is enhanced tenfold[44] by the presence of transferrin, which complexes with gallium and permits the gallium to enter the cell via transferrin receptors. Thus uptake can occur in both tumours (particularly rapidly growing ones with high levels of surface transferrin receptors) and rapidly metabolizing benign or reactive lymphoid tissues such as the infant's thymus (or the thymus of some patients who have recently completed chemotherapy) so that care must be taken when interpreting gallium studies in these settings.[45–47]

Because the physical half-life of ^{67}Ga is approximately 3 days, other required nuclear medicine studies, such as ^{99m}Tc-MDP bone scintigraphy, should be performed prior to ^{67}Ga imaging to avoid complications in the scintigraphic technique caused by ^{67}Ga photon scatter into the ^{99m}Tc windows. And, because ^{67}Ga is excreted in part via the gastrointestinal tract, the requirement for repeated images following mild catharsis should be anticipated for accurate interpretation of ^{67}Ga uptake in the abdominal/pelvic region.

Bone scintigraphy

Bone scintigraphy with ^{99m}Tc-MDP is the best method for performing a skeletal survey to detect bone involvement by NHL. Approximately 10–20 per cent of patients will have bone involvement. Bone scintigraphy is also readily repeated at appropriate intervals to assess the effect of therapeutic regimens, especially in the first few years following diagnosis. Bone abnormalities detected by scintigraphy should be further evaluated with a radiograph, because although scintigraphy is a very sensitive procedure it does not provide specificity in determining the cause of altered radionuclide uptake. Not all abnormal sites in the scintigram will necessarily be caused by lymphoma; degenerative disease, trauma, benign bone lesions, etc. can all give false positive indications of skeletal lymphoma. Comparison with directed radiographs and ^{67}Ga citrate scintigrams can often be helpful in determining the exact aetiology of abnormal sites on the bone scintigram. Patterns of more diffuse increased uptake in the long bones, and particularly increased uptake in the region of the metaphyses, can indicate marrow involvement.

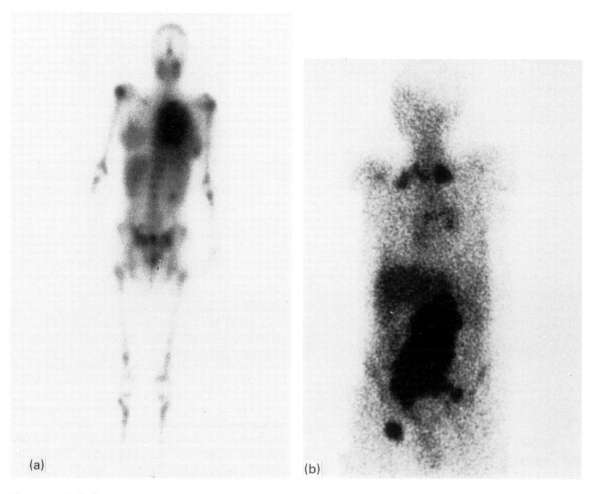

(a)   (b)

Fig. 12.5 67-Gallium scintigrams showing (a) anterior view of a patient with 4-quadrant jaw, chest, breast, abdominal, marrow (long bones, especially femurs) and probable pelvic involvement with Burkitt's lymphoma; (b) anterior view of a patient with a large abdominopelvic mass, supraclavicular, hilar, right femoral and left inguinal node involvement with Burkitt's lymphoma.

Sites of previous marrow biopsy will frequently show increased radionuclide activity for variable periods after the biopsy procedures and should not be misinterpreted. Those patients receiving treatment regimens which include steroids are at increased risk for avascular necrosis, which will be apparent in a bone scintigram, but the pattern of altered bone uptake will change with the evolution of bone necrosis. Finally, areas of bone included in radiation therapy ports can show increased or decreased uptake of skeletal radiopharmaceuticals – both ^{99m}Tc-MDP and ^{67}Ga – so that knowledge of the skeletal areas which received beam irradiation is essential for accurate interpretation of subsequent bone scintigrams.[48]

Positron emission tomography

A potentially exciting area of imaging research is the use of positron emission tomography (PET) with short-lived radiopharmaceuticals for

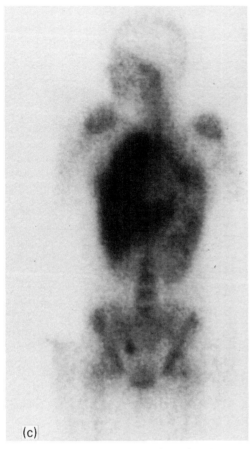

Fig. 12.5 (c) 67-Gallium scintigram showing anterior view of a patient with involvement of the right hemithorax, part of the left chest and pelvis by large cell lymphoma.

physiological imaging of tumours, including lymphomas. The advantage of PET derives from the nature of positron tomography which allows for more precise quantification of radioactivity in small lesions. In addition to positron-emitting isotopes of gallium, there are a number of metabolic-cycle radiopharmaceuticals such as fluorine-18 2-fluoro-deoxyglucose which show potential as PET agents to permit improved imaging of lymphomas.[49]

Radiolabelled monoclonal antibodies

Imaging with radiolabelled monoclonal antibodies holds promise because of the potential specificity of the technique – derived from the specificity of antibodies directed towards tumour-associated antigens on lymphoma cell membranes. Radiolabelled antibody imaging could be used to follow response to treatment and, theoretically, to derive diagnostic information about tumour cell surface antigen type and content when direct tissue biopsy is not feasible or desirable. At present the utility of scintigraphy with radiolabelled monoclonal antibodies is limited by the lack of truly tumour-specific antibodies (with the exception of anti-idiotypes), inconvenience, expense of producing the antibody in radiopharmaceutical form and the high rate of antimouse antibody response which occurs after repeated intravenous administration of available murine monoclonal antibodies. Modulation of the relevant cell surface antigen is also a theoretical problem when multiple antibody administrations are planned.

In most studies published to date, there is considerable variability in the selectivity of radiolabelled antibody uptake in tumours compared to normal tissues. This problem also limits the value of therapeutic approaches using monoclonal antibodies carrying potentially tumoricidal doses of radionuclides. An example of successful scintigraphy using the radiolabelled murine monoclonal antibody T-101 (CD5) in patients with chronic lymphocytic leukaemia/ lymphoma of small lymphocytes is shown in Fig. 12.6.[50] This antibody binds to a pan-T-cell antigen present on normal T lymphocytes but present in much higher concentrations on most T-cell neoplasms and on B-cell chronic lymphocytic leukaemia. Another antibody currently under study is Heffe-1 (CD30), raised against a Hodgkin's lymphoma cell line,[51] which may be of value in CD30 positive lymphomas as well as in Hodgkin's disease. The value of radiolabelled antibody scintigraphy is under active investigation and preliminary trials of tumour therapy with these agents have also been started.

Histological and cytological staging procedures

In some circumstances a biopsy, paracentesis or fine needle aspirate may be necessary to obtain

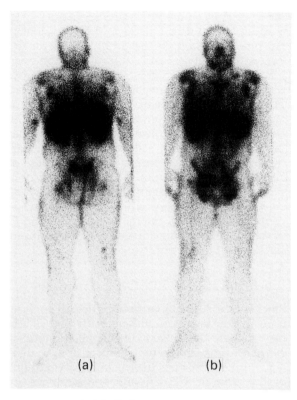

(a)   (b)

Fig. 12.6 Radiolabelled T101 scintigram in a patient with chronic lymphocytic leukaemia showing uptake of the antibody in multiple lymph node regions (cervical, axillary, supraclavicular, supratrochlear, iliac, inguinal and femoral) as well as liver and spleen. (a) Posterior view; (b) anterior view.

definitive information regarding a potential site of involvement by NHL. Bone marrow examination should always be done, and there is no doubt that the rate of detection of marrow involvement is higher when multiple samples are examined, regardless of the tumour type.[52,53,] It is usual, therefore, to perform bilateral iliac crest aspirates, biopsies and clot sections. In the NCI study shown in Table 12.3, 36.1 per cent of all patients were found to have at least one positive bone marrow biopsy, the marrow being the most frequently positive tissue sampling procedure. Most patients with bone marrow involvement will have abnormal haematological parameters. In one study, all patients with thrombocytopenia or granulocytopenia had documented bone

marrow involvement.[54]

The cerebrospinal fluid (CSF) should also be examined at the time of presentation in patients in high risk groups, including all intermediate lymphomas of stages II, III and IV, and all high grade lymphomas. Patients less than 40 years old and patients with stage IV disease, bone marrow, skin, bone or gastrointestinal involvement are particularly at risk from the development of meningeal lymphomatous spread. In such high risk groups, or in patients who fail initial treatment, CFS examination may be repeated at intervals, although in adults the risk of development of CNS involvement is sufficiently low when the initial CSF examination fails to show malignant cells, that in many centres repeat CSF examination is only performed in the presence of suggestive symptoms or signs. In one series of 602 patients,[55] meningeal involvement occurred at some time in some 6 per cent of patients with NHL, in approximately 1–3 per cent of patients with low grade lymphomas and in 4–5 per cent of patients with large cell lymphomas. Patients with high grade lymphomas had a 19–23 per cent rate of meningeal disease, but in this group of patients, the incidence of CNS disease depends upon the efficacy of CNS prophylactic therapy.

Serous effusions should be aspirated and examined cytologically for lymphoma cells. Such preparations are also ideal for performing phenotyping and cytogenetic studies. If lymphoma cells are not detected and the effusion has the characteristics of a transudate, a non-malignant cause should be considered. In the presence of suspicious abnormalities in liver function tests, a biopsy is the most definitive means of confirming the presence of malignant infiltration. However, some patients have involvement of the liver in the absence of abnormal liver function tests or radiological abnormalities and at the NCI, liver biopsy has for some time been a part of the routine evaluation of adult patients with NHL. Patients in whom percutaneous liver biopsy was negative had multiple peritoneoscopy-directed liver biopsies and, in some circumstances, laparotomy with wedge liver biopsies was used to determine the value of these approaches in detecting liver involvement.[52,56] Approximately

60 per cent of all patients, representing all histological types of lymphoma, had a positive liver biopsy. Percutaneous biopsy was positive in 21 per cent of 131 patients, and of those patients who were negative a further 29 per cent were found to be positive after peritoneoscopy-guided biopsy. Of the patients still negative after peritoneoscopy, a further 21 per cent had positive biopsies at laparotomy.[1,52] Of interest was the observation that 57 of 60 patients with positive liver biopsies had positive lymphographies; two were equivocal and only one of 26 patients with a negative lymphogram who underwent biopsy by any of the three routes had a positive result.[52] This suggests that liver involvement is accurately predicted by the lymphogram, and is therefore scarcely justifiable, particularly now that chemotherapy is used in the treatment of almost all patients with NHL.

Staging laparotomy

In general, laparotomy is not a routine staging procedure in patients with non-Hodgkin's lymphoma, although its utility in this regard has been investigated by a number of centres.[56–59] Laparotomy may be necessary to establish the nature of an abdominal mass in the absence of extra-abdominal disease and in patients who present with an acute abdomen or uncontrolled gastrointestinal bleeding. Unlike Hodgkin's disease, the pattern of spread of NHLs is much less predictable and more often involves extranodal sites. This makes radiation therapy an ancillary rather than a primary therapeutic modality, and there is rarely an indication to perform laparotomy either to detect the presence of, or to establish the precise extent of, intra-abdominal disease.

In a study performed at Stanford University Medical Center, 31 per cent of 197 patients subjected to staging laparotomy were upstaged from stage III to stage IV.[58] However, the excellent correlation between a positive lymphogram and the presence of liver disease, the finding that less than 10 per cent of patients with a positive lymphogram had any additional disease detected at laparotomy, and the invariable use of chemotherapy in patients with stage III as well as stage IV disease, obviates the need for laparotomy in stage III patients.[52,56] In a study conducted at the M.D. Anderson Hospital, Houston, Texas, 17 of 28 patients (61 per cent) with stage I and II follicular lymphomas but showing no evidence of bone marrow disease and having a negative lymphogram, had positive abdominal lymph nodes or spleen at laparotomy. In diffuse lymphoma patients the corresponding figure was nine of 40 (22.5 per cent).[57] Patients with stage I lymphomas, particularly if diffuse – some 10 per cent or less of all NHL patients – may therefore be the only groups in whom staging laparotomy may be considered, *if* therapy with radiation alone is contemplated (see Chapter 14). The morbidity of staging laparotomy in patients in the Stanford series was 11 per cent.

Biochemical tests and tumour markers

Biochemical tests have two principal applications in the staging of patients with NHL. They may suggest the presence of hepatic tumour or extrinsic compression of the biliary tree, or they may provide an objective, if indirect, measure of the tumour burden and the presence or likelihood of the development of an acute tumour lysis syndrome. The use of biochemical tests that reflect tumour burden is likely to become of increasing importance as more specific tests are developed. In the presence of a large tumour burden and a rapid tumour cell turnover the serum uric acid level is often elevated and correlates with an increased likelihood of the development of a tumour lysis syndrome (*see* Chapter 15). The serum level of lactate dehydrogenase (LDH) is a more sensitive measure of tumour burden in most lymphomas, since many patients will have an elevated serum LDH in the presence of a normal serum uric acid level. Lactate dehydrogenase has proved to be a valuable prognostic indicator in diffuse large cell lymphomas and SNCC lymphomas.[14,15,60]

Recently the level of serum interleukin-2 receptor (IL-2R) has been shown to have prognostic significance, presumably because it is an indicator of tumour burden in both T-cell and B-cell lymphomas. In SNCC lymphomas, serum IL-2R has been reported to have greater prognostic significance than clinical stage.[61]

Several other biochemical markers in serum have been found to be of value, including β_2-microglobulin, ferritin and deoxythymidine kinase.[62,63] Cerebrospinal fluid β_2-microglobulin and ferritin have also been observed to be elevated in the presence of CNS involvement.[64,65] In African Burkitt's lymphoma patients, the antibody titre against the early antigen of the Epstein–Barr virus (EBV) has been shown to have prognostic significance and, in the context of this predominantly EBV-associated tumour, probably also reflects tumour burden.[66] Unfortunately, these biochemical correlates of tumour burden are not widely used at present as the emphasis remains on anatomical staging. While the latter clearly provides information not obtained by other means, the advantages of being able to obtain an estimate of tumour burden and prognosis with a single biochemical test that can also be used to follow treatment response are obvious. Moreover, if such measures were routinely published, comparison of different treatment regimens would be more meaningful. The development of new serum indicators of tumour burden based upon molecules synthesized by lymphoid cells is likely to be a productive area for future research.

Prognostic indicators

In addition to histology and total tumour burden (as reflected by stage, serum LDH level and the presence of bulky disease)[12,14,67–69] the proliferative potential and the presence of tumour at sanctuary sites are the major predictors of survival. Growth rate correlates with histology (low grade lymphomas grow much less rapidly than the high or intermediate grade lymphomas), as well as with more direct measurements such labelling index and mitotic index. In some studies the labelling index has been shown to predict more accurately initial response and survival than histology and stage.[70] Other factors which have been shown to be of importance in follicular lymphomas include B symptoms, hepatosplenomegaly, anaemia and abnormal liver function tests.[12,67–69,71] Age is an important prognostic variable in both follicular and diffuse lymphomas in adults,[12,68] but the prognostic value of bone marrow involvement, a significant factor in many series, has been questioned.[72] Like all other potential prognostic factors, the prognostic significance of marrow involvement is likely to vary with the treatment protocol being used.

Much more work needs to be done to determine the value of newer diagnostic criteria as prognostic indicators, such as immunophenotype, cytogenetics and molecular characterization. The evaluation of immunophenotype must take into account that each of the two main groups, B- and T-cell tumours, encompass a large number of pathological entities. Thus, comparisons of B-cell versus T-cell tumours are not useful, except perhaps within a single histological, or otherwise identified subgroup.[73,74] Few studies have been conducted to evaluate the prognostic significance of karyotype. Recently it was shown that the presence of chromosomal abnormalities in addition to an isolated 14;18 translocation indicates a worse prognosis in follicular lymphomas.[75] In large cell lymphomas, one study indicated that patients whose tumours had breaks in the short arm of chromosome 2 had a better prognosis, and it appeared that the presence in the tumour of normal metaphases also correlated with a higher complete remission rate and longer survival.[76] It remains to be seen whether large cell lymphomas or small non-cleaved cell lymphomas with 14;18 translocations have a different prognosis from those with 8;14 translocations.

References

1. Anderson T, Chabner BA, Young RC, *et al. Cancer*. 1982; **50**, 2699–707.
2. Nathwani BN, Kim H, Rappaport H. *Cancer*. 1976; **38**, 964–83.
3. Jaffe ES, Bookman MA, Longo DL. *Human Pathology*. 1987; **18**, 877.
4. Uchiyama T, Yodoi J, Sagawa K, *et al. Blood*. 1977;**62**, 401.
5. Jaffe ES. *Cancer Investigation*. 1984; **2**, 413.

6. Streeter PR, Berg EL, Rouse BTN, _et al. Nature._ 1988; **331**, 41–6.
7. Makgoba MW, Sanders ME, Luce GEG, _et al. Nature._ 1988; **331**, 86–8.
8. Shaw S, Luce GGE. _Journal of Immunology._ 1987; **139**, 1037–45.
9. Shaw S, Luce GGE, Quinones R, _et al. Nature._ 1986; **323**, 262–4.
10. Billaud M, Calender A, Seigneurin J-M, _et al. Lancet._ 1987; **ii**, 1327–8.
11. Fuks Z, Glatstein E, Kaplan HS. _British Journal of Cancer._ 1975; **31** (Suppl. II), 286–97.
12. Anderson T, DeVita V, Simon RM, _et al. Cancer._ 1982; **50**, 2708–21.
13. Murphy SB _Developments in Oncology._ 1985; **32**, 627–32.
14. Ridgway D, Smiley S, Neerhout RC. _Journal of Pediatrics._ 1981; **99**, 611–13.
15. Magrath IT, Janus C, Edwards B, _et al. Blood._ 1984; **63**, 1102–11.
16. Neumann CH, Parker BR, Castello RA. In Bragg DG, (ed). _Oncologic Imaging._ New York. Pergamon Press, 1985; 477–500.
17. Braggs DG, Colby TV, Ward J. _Radiology._1986; **159**, 291–304.
18. Tschappeler H. _Pediatric Radiology._ 1983; **18**, 269–80.
19. Khoury MB, Godwin JD, Halvorsen RA, _et al. Radiology._ 1986; **158**, 659.
20. Batra P, Ovenfors CO, Brown K, _et al._ 86th Annual Meeting of the American Roentgen Ray Society. April 14–18, 1986, Washington, DC. 1986; 292–3.
21. Magrath IT, Sariban E. In: Lenoir G, Olweny CL, _Burkitt's Lymphoma – a Human Cancer Model._ Lyon: IARC Publications, 1985: 119–27.
22. Winkler P, Amon O, Bohndorf K. _Monatsschrift Kinderheilklind._ 1985; **133**, 823–7.
23. Thomas JL, Bernardino ME, Vermess M. _Radiology._ 1982; **145**, 629–34.
24. Marglin S, Castellino RA. _Radiology._ 1981; **140**, 351–3.
25. Pera A, Capek M, Shirkoda A. _Radiology._ 1987; **164**, 631–3.
26. Harnsbeger HR, Bragg DG, Osborn AG, _et al. American Journal of Neuroradiology._ 1987; **8**, 673.
27. Cruz J, Karstead K, Wolfman N, _et al._ (1986); _Proceedings of the Annual Meeting of the Americans Society of Clinical Oncology._ **5**, 194.
28. Lee YY, Van Tassal P, Nauert C, _et al. American Journal of Neuroroadiology._ 1987; **8**, 665.
29. Flanders AE, Espinosa GA, Markiewicz DA, _et al. Radiologic Clinics of North America._ 1987; **25**, 601–13.
30. Brant-Zawadzki M. _Radiology._ 1988; **166**, 1–10.
31. Holtas S, Nyman U, Cronquist S. _Neuroradiology._ 1984; **26**, 33–8.
32. Wermecke K, Peters PE, Kruger KG. _British Journal of Radiology._ 1987; **60**, 655.
33. Bruneton JN, Normand F, Balu-Maestro C, _et al. Radiology._ 1987; **165**, 233–5.
34. Anonymous _Magnetic Resonance Imaging 1986:_ 3rd Annual National Symposium. May 5–9, 1986, Orlando, Fl.
35. Weinreb JC, Brateman L, Maravilla KR. _American Journal of Radiology._ 1984; **143**, 1211–24.
36. Porter BA, Shields AF, Olson DO. _Radiologic Clinics of North America._ 1986; **24**, 269–86.
37. Shields AF, Porter BA, Churchley S, _et al. Journal of Clinical Oncology._ 1987; **5**, 225–30.
38. Ling A, Horvath K, Dwyer AJ, _et al._ 73rd Annual Meeting of the Radiological Society of North America. Chicago, Nov 29th–Dec 4th 1987.
39. Runge VM, Schaible TF, Goldstein HA, _et al. Radiographics._ 1988; **8**, 147–59.
40. Sze G, Abramson A, Krol G, _et al. American Journal of Neuroradiology._ 1988; **9**, 153–63.
41. Glass RB, Fernback SK, Conway JJ, _et al. American Journal of Roentgenography._ 1985; **145**, 671–6.
42. Anderson KC, Leonard RCF, Canellos GP, _et al. American Journal of Medicine._ 1983; **75**, 327–31.
43. Tumeh SS, Rosenthal DS, Kaplan WD, _et al. Radiology._ 1987; **164**, 111–14.
44. Chitamber CR, Zivkovik Z. _Cancer Research._ 1987; **47**, 3929–34.
45. Neumann RD, Hoffer PB. In: Freeman L (ed). _Freeman and Johnson's Clinical Radionuclide Imaging._ Orlando: Grune and Stratton, 1984: 1319–64.
46. Hibi S, Todo S, Imashuku S. _Journal of Nuclear Medicine._ 1985; **28**; 293–7.
47. Donahue DM, Leonard JC, Basmadjian GP, _et al. Journal of Nuclear Medicine._ 1981; **22**, 1043–8.
48. King MA, Weber DA, Casarett GW, _et al. Journal of Nuclear Medicine._ 1980; **21**, 22–30.
49. Paul R. _Journal of Nuclear Medicine._ 1987; **28**, 288–92.
50. Carrasquillo JA, Bunn PA, Keenan AM, _et al. New England of Medicine._ 1986; **315**, 673–80.
51. Hecht TT, Longo DL, Cossman J, _et al. Journal of Immunology._ 1985; **134**, 4231–6.
52. Chabner BA, Johnson RE, DeVita VT, _et al. Cancer Treatment Reports._1977; **61**, 993–7.
53. Coller BS, Chabner BA, Gralnick HR. _American Journal of Hematology._ 1977; **3**, 105–19.
54. Bloomfield CD, McKenna RW, Brunning RD. _British Journal of Haematology._ 1975; **32**, 41–6.
55. Ersbll J, Schultz HB, Thomsen BL, _et al. Scandinavian Journal of Haematology._ 1985; **35**, 487–96.
56. Chabner BA, Johnson RE, Chretien PB, _et al. British Journal of Cancer._ 1975; **31** (suppl. II), 242–7.
57. Heifetz LJ, Fuller L, Rodgers RW, _et al. Cancer._ 1980; **45**,2778–86.

58. Goffinet DR, Warnke R, Dunnick NR, *et al. Cancer Treatment Reports.* 1977; **61**, 981–92.

59. Rosenberg SA, Dorfman RF, Kaplan HS. *British Journal of Cancer.* 1975; **31** (suppl. II), 221–7.

60. Csako G, Magrath IT, Elin R. *American Journal of Clinical Pathology.* 1982; **78**, 712–17.

61. Wagner D, Kiwanuka J, Edwards BK, *et al. Journal of Clinical Oncology.* 1987; **5**, 1262–74.

62. Hagberg H, Killander A, Simonsson B. *Cancer.* 1983;**51**, 2220–5.

63. Hagberg H, Killander A, Glimelius B. *Second International Conference on Malignant Lymphomas.* (Astract): 1984: 42.

64. Dillmann E, Lopez-Karpovitch X, Alvarez-Hernandez X, *et al. Revista de Investigacion Clinica.* 1982; **34**, 95–8.

65. Gonzalez Diaz M, Vicente Garcia V, Martin Rodriguez M, *et al. Revista Clinica Espanola.* 1982; **164**, 325–8.

66. Magrath IT, Lee YJ, Anderson T, *et al. Cancer.* 1980; **45**, 1507–15.

67. Cabanillas F, Smith T, Bodey G, *et al. Cancer.* 1979; **44**, 1983–9.

68. Rudders RA, Kaddis M, DeLellis RA, *et al. Cancer.* 1979; **43**, 1643–51.

69. Gospodarowicz MK, Bush RS, Brown TC, *et al. International Journal of Radiation Oncology, Biology and Physics.* 1984; **10**, 489–97.

70. Costa A, Bonadonna G, Villa E, *et al. Journal of the National Cancer Institute.* 1981; **66**, 1–5.

71. Gallagher CJ, Gregory WM, Jones AE, *et al. Journal of Clinical Oncology.* 1986; **4**, 1470–80.

72. Bennett JM, Cain KC, Glick JH, *et al. Journal of Clinical Onocology.* 1986; **4**, 1462–9.

73. Huber H, Thaler J, Greil R, *et al. Onkologie.*1986; **9**, 108–13.

74. Morell A, Hirt A. *Therapeutische Umschau.* 1981; **38**, 854–61.

75. Yunis JJ, Frizzera G, Oken MM, *et al. New England Journal of Medicine.* 1987; **316**, 79–84.

76. Levine EG, Arthur DC, Frizzera G, *et al. Annals of Internal Medicine.* 1988; **108**, 14–20.

CHAPTER 13

PRINCIPLES OF CHEMOTHERAPY

Wyndham Wilson and Ian Magrath

The majority of the non-Hodgkin's lymphomas, being diseases of the immune system, are systemic and nearly always require treatment with chemotherapy. They are among the few malignancies in which the major advances in the development of systemic therapy over the last 25 years have led to significant improvements in patient survival. These advances are a direct consequence of both the expanding armamentarium of anticancer drugs and the increased understanding and application of the principles of chemotherapy which has come from animal experimentation and empirical clinical experience. It is clear from the accumulated clinical experience with the non-Hodgkin's lymphomas that, although as a group they respond to a similar spectrum of drugs, vastly different therapeutic approaches are required for the different subtypes. Of course, selection of the optimal approach can only be determined after accurate diagnosis, careful staging, consideration of the unique features of individual patients, and by the participation of an oncologist experienced in the treatment planning and therapy of these diseases. In this chapter, we provide an overview of the general principles upon which chemotherapy is based and of the various treatment approaches in use today for the treatment of the non-Hodgkin's lymphomas.

General principles

Growth fraction and fractional cell kill

Much of the progress made in the treatment of lymphomas has resulted from an improved understanding of the principles of chemotherapy. Many of the fundamental principles were developed by Skipper from a model system based on the rodent leukaemia L1210 cell line.[1] From this model come a number of observations which illustrate several important interactions between the tumour (L1210) and host. One of the most basic observations was that the survival of CDF1 mice inoculated with L1210 cells was inversely proportional to the tumour cell inoculum. Further experiments revealed that a single tumour cell was capable of causing death, that the time interval to death was proportional to the inoculum and that the interval between injection of cells and death could be calculated from the tumour doubling time and inoculum size. When the effect of chemotherapy in the L1210 model system was investigated, it was found that the fraction of tumour cells undergoing DNA replication, termed the growth fraction, was an important determinant of drug sensitivity. This is a consequence of the temporary resistance demonstrated by tumour cells to many classes of chemotherapeutic agents while in the resting (G_0) phase of the cell cycle, a concept which provides a partial explanation for the resistance of some lymphomas to treatment. The inverse correlation, for example, which is observed between growth fraction and tumour volume probably accounts in part for the prognostic significance of tumour burden and for the lower curability of advanced stage lymphomas.[2] A similar mechanism of drug resistance may be operating in the low grade lymphomas where the tumour cell population has a lower growth fraction compared to higher grade lymphomas.

The greater sensitivity of proliferating tumour cells to chemotherapy may have practical significance for the design of treatment protocols. If methods could be found to increase the tumour growth fraction prior to the administration of chemotherapy, then tumour cell kill could be significantly enhanced. Possible approaches include the selection of appropriate drugs and administration schedules which synchronize the tumour cells and deliver chemotherapy at the height of a new round of tumour replication, and the use of tumour cell mitogenic agents which stimulate the tumour cells to divide. It should be noted, however, that such approaches are theoretical, and that no clinical data exist to substantiate their efficacy.

Another important concept emerging from the L1210 model is that the number of tumour cells killed by a cycle of chemotherapy is limited by first-order kinetics, i.e. a given drug dose kills a constant fraction of cells, independent of cell number.[1,2] Of course, the actual fraction of cells killed is dependent on the sensitivity of the tumour to the chemotherapy agents administered, and this fraction may change during the course of treatment. This finding implies that a single cycle of chemotherapy is unlikely to achieve a cure except in the most sensitive tumours, such as Burkitt's lymphoma, which, when the tumour burden is low, can sometimes be cured by a single dose of cyclophosphamide.[3] This concept may also not be strictly applicable to settings where a single cycle of intensive chemotherapy is administered with autologous bone marrow reinfusion, as this can be an effective treatment in relapsed aggressive lymphomas, albeit in the presence of minimal tumour burden.

The concept of fractional cell kill also implies that surgical resection of tumour may be beneficial if it is of sufficient degree, as illustrated by the excellent prognosis of patients with Burkitt's lymphoma in whom abdominal tumour can be essentially completely resected.[4] Unfortunately, in practice, surgical resection does not significantly improve the outcome in most lymphomas probably because wide dissemination is the rule. For the majority of clinical situations, however, the concept of fractional cell kill suggests that optimal results are likely to be obtained by using high doses of chemotherapy administered over multiple cycles.

Goldie–Coldman hypothesis

Despite the better prognosis of patients with low tumour burdens, not all such patients are cured because the absolute tumour bulk is not the only determinant of treatment outcome. The inability to eradicate all tumour with chemotherapy may be due to a failure of drug to reach the tumour cells and/or to the presence or emergence of tumour cells resistant to the administered chemotherapy. In 1979, Goldie and Coldman proposed a hypothesis to explain the spontaneous development of resistance of cancer cells to chemotherapeutic agents.[5] This hypothesis was derived from the observation, made originally by bacterial geneticists, that the development of resistance by *Escherichia coli* to infection by bacteriophage occurs through the preferential expansion of bacterial clones that have undergone spontaneous mutation to a resistant phenotype.[6] Goldie and Coldman extrapolated this concept to human tumours and correlated the emergence of resistant tumour cells with their spontaneous mutation rate.

For example, the model predicts that if the mutation rate for a drug resistance gene is in the range of 10^{-6} or higher, the possibility of the emergence of at least one resistant cell to a given drug is high, even before the cell population reaches 10^{-6} cells, a tumour size which is orders of magnitude less than can be clinically detected. Other events such as non-random cytogenetic alterations found in many cancers may also contribute to their intrinsic resistance to anticancer drugs.[7] Eventually, resistant subclones predominate in the tumour cell population as a result of the selective pressure of anticancer drug treatment; i.e. resistant cells are able to proliferate under conditions which lead to the death of non-resistant cells.

In addition, the Goldie and Coldman formula predicts that resistance may emerge within a two log increment in cell number which, in the case of rapidly proliferating lymphomas, may occur within several weeks. Consequently, prolonged delays before starting therapy and between cycles of therapy may reduce the chance of cure.

By providing a hypothesis for the emergence of resistant subclones, the Goldie–Coldman model offers an explanation for the inverse relationship observed between curability and cell number, independent of tumour growth kinetics and fractional cell kill.[5] This model has important theoretical implications for the design of chemotherapy protocols, and provides explanations for some of the principles already established through empirical observation.

First, the probability of the existence of cells which are resistant to one or more drugs is high in patients with large tumour burdens, providing one explanation for the greater efficacy of combination chemotherapy over single agents. However, combination chemotherapy has not completely overcome the problem of drug resistance, partly because the likelihood of the emergence of simultaneous resistance to two different classes of drugs is greater than the product of the rate of mutation conferring resistance to each individual drug. This is because a single mutation is capable of inducing resistance to more than one class of drugs.[8,9] Therefore, although combination chemotherapy may induce complete remissions (CR) in the majority of lymphoma patients, the presence of even a small number of resistant cells in a large tumour mass is sufficient to account for the high relapse rate observed in some clinical circumstances.

Second, the growth fraction of a tumour mass will increase as the tumour cells sensitive to the administered chemotherapy are killed, resulting in an increase in the mitotic rate of the remaining tumour cells, including the drug-resistant subclones. Thus, the Goldie–Coldman hypothesis implies that not only is it important to minimize delays between chemotherapy cycles, but that the use of alternating, non-cross-resistant drug combinations is more likely to result in a successful outcome.

Pleiotropic drug resistance

A major obstacle to the cure of lymphomas is the development of simultaneous resistance to multiple classes of anticancer drugs, a phenomenon termed pleiotropic drug resistance.[10,11] Such resistance may occur spontaneously, or it can be induced by exposure to a single drug. One mechanism of pleiotropic drug resistance, which is associated with resistance to the anthracyclines, epipodophyllotoxins, vinca alkaloids and actinomycin D, results from the increased expression or amplification of the multidrug resistance gene (*mdr*-1).[9,12] Increased expression of this gene results in a greater ability of resistant tumour cells, cultured *in vitro*, to decrease intracellular drug levels; a probable unifying mechanism for various types of pleiotropic drug resistance.

The product of the *mdr*-1 gene, the P170 glycoprotein, appears to be an important component of a membrane pump, the function of which, in normal cells, may be to eliminate toxic compounds. It is of interest that a number of chemotherapeutic agents, such as vincristine, are natural products and could be encountered in small quantities during everyday life, and that cells such as colonic epithelium, renal tubules and bile canaliculi, which are involved in excretion and would be predicted to encounter higher levels of such toxins, express the *mdr*-1 gene in increased amounts.[13] If the activity of this membrane pump plays an important role in drug resistance, then mechanisms which overcome its action may play a role in cancer chemotherapy. In fact, possible approaches to interfering with the membrane pump include the use of specific drugs, such as verapamil and quinidine, which bind to the P170 glycoprotein and inhibit binding (and therefore expulsion) of anticancer drugs, and the use of increased doses of chemotherapy or continuous infusion schedules in an attempt to increase intracellular drug levels.[14,15]

A secondary phenomenon of increased sensitivity, termed collateral sensitivity, to other classes of drugs has been observed in pleotropically resistant cell lines.[11] Although the clinical impact of collateral sensitivity on treatment response is unknown at present, the use of drugs to which pleotropically resistant cells become more sensitive, such as cyclophosphamide and glucocorticoids, in concert with or following anthracyclines or vinca alkaloids, could result in increased efficacy of the chemotherapy regimen.

Dose rate

The association between the amount of drug administered over time, termed dose rate, and cell kill is one of the more important principles relevant to the treatment of lymphomas. In animal models of high growth rate tumours, a linear–log relationship between drug dose and tumour cell kill has been demonstrated. For example, doubling drug doses may increase cell kill by as much as 10-fold, while reductions by as little as 20 per cent may decrease the cure rate by 50 per cent.[16] Since fractional cell kill is rarely, if ever 100 per cent, it is not surprising that the dose per unit time is of critical importance to the ultimate outcome, at least in terms of achieving a CR. In fact, recent analyses, such as those performed by Hryniuk *et al.* in patients receiving adjuvant chemotherapy for breast carcinoma, have demonstrated a remarkably linear correlation between relative dose intensity and response.[17,18] This is also likely to be true in lymphomas, where alterations in drug doses often have a profound effect on tumour cell kill. In fact, in an analysis performed in diffuse aggressive lymphomas, DeVita *et al.* demonstrated a significant relationship ($P < 0.001$) between the relative dose intensity (RDI) of the major chemotherapy regimens and their respective disease-free intervals (DFI) Fig. 13.1.[19]

When applying this concept to protocol design, it is important to keep in mind that a steep dose–response curve exists for both the therapeutic and toxic effects of many anticancer drugs. Clearly these must be balanced when determining the dose and rate at which chemotherapy is to be delivered. However, the amount of toxicity for a course of chemotherapy can be altered or reduced by techniques such as autologous or allogeneic bone marrow transplantation, which allow major increases in dose

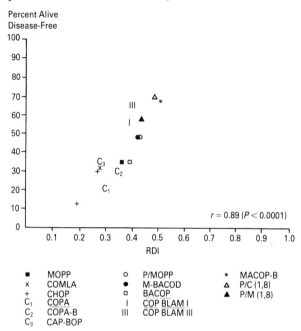

Fig. 13.1. Relation between nine-drug RDI and DFI in diffuse large cell lymphoma. $P < 0.001$, $r = 0.084$. RDI, relative dose intensity; DFI, disease-free interval; MOPP, mechlorethamine, vincristine, procarbazine, prednisone; COMLA, cyclophosphamide, vincristine, methotrexate, leucovorin, cytarabine; CHOP, cyclophosphamide, doxorubicin, vincristine, prednisone; COPA, cyclophosphamide, vincristine, prednisone, doxorubicin; COPA-B, COPA plus bleomycin; CAP-BOP, cyclophosphamide, doxorubicin, procarbazine, bleomycin, vincristine, prednisone; ProMACE-MOPP, prednisone, methotrexate, doxorubicin, cyclophosphamide, etoposide, plus MOPP; M-BACOD, methotrexate, bleomycin doxorubicin, cyclophosphamide, vincristine, dexamethasone; BACOP, bleomycin, doxorubicin, cyclophosphamide, vincristine, prednisone; COP-BLAM 1, cyclophosphamide, vincristine, prednisone, bleomycin, doxorubicin, procarbazine; COP-BLAM 111, same drugs as COP-BLAM 1; MACOP-B, methotrexate, doxorubicin, cyclophosphamide, vincristine, prednisone, bleomycin; ProMACE-CytaBOM, ProMACE plus cytarabine, bleomycin, vincristine, methotrexate. Reproduced by permission from DeVita *et al. The Role of Chemotherapy in Diffuse Aggressive Lymphomas.*[19]

by overcoming the dose–limiting effect of myelosuppression. In the extreme case of marrow transplantation, where only a single cycle of therapy is administered, dose and dose rate are equivalent. However, for multiple cycle regimens, dose rate is not necessarily optimized by giving the largest possible doses. Smaller doses at more frequent intervals could, depending upon the degree and type of toxicity, be superior.

Another approach to increasing the dose rate is through the protection of normal, but not malignant tissues, from the toxic effects of chemotherapy. Experiments in mice have shown that a large, normally fatal dose of a cytotoxic drug can be administered if the animals are pretreated 2–4 days earlier with a priming dose of the same or different cytotoxic drug, such as cyclophosphamide.[20] In this setting, the priming dose exerts a protective effect on normal tissues such as bone marrow, uroepithelium and intestinal epithelium, but less so on malignant tissues, although this differential effect is dependent on the tumour type. Further investigations have demonstrated that such a priming dose can induce a transient resting state (G_0) in highly proliferating tissues, thereby reducing their sensitivity to the subsequent high dose of chemotherapy, and can induce increases in intracellular glutathione transferase which is important for the detoxification of alkylating agents.[21] Although these approaches have yet to be tested in humans, they have exciting possibilities. When specific drug toxicities are dose-limiting, measures which provide regional protection, such as the use of mesna to prevent oxazaphosphorine-induced haemorrhagic cystitis, will also have implications for the achievement of maximal dose rate.

The minimal interval which can be achieved between chemotherapy cycles is dependent upon the rate at which the bone marrow recovers. Unfortunately, delays in drug administration due to haematopoietic recovery may allow regrowth of that fraction of tumour cells not killed by the previous dose of chemotherapy, even though the cells are not necessarily drug resistant. Clearly, this will have the greatest impact on lymphomas with high growth fractions, so that the intervals between cycles are usually kept to a minimum. There are now some potentially exciting new approaches to improving haematopoietic recovery and minimizing cycle length through the use of the recombinant colony stimulating factors, GM-CSF, G-CSF and IL-3, which are necessary for the normal proliferation and differentiation of haematopoietic cells.[22] Preliminary studies have demonstrated that these factors may shorten the period of neutropenia by stimulating bone marrow recovery, and are currently undergoing clinical investigation in the setting of repeated cycles of chemotherapy.[23,24]

It is important to point out that, in clinical practice, there is an unfortunate tendency to reduce drug doses and delay cycles of chemotherapy in order to minimize toxicity, without taking into account the adverse impact this could have on a successful clinical outcome. Clearly, a balance between toxicity and maximization of dose rate must be achieved and in the case of the aggressive lymphomas, significant treatment toxicity will often be incurred in order to achieve an adequate dose rate. Ultimately, however, this balance rests on the clinical experience and judgement of the oncologist.

Principles of protocol design

Even before the basic principles of chemotherapy design were fully appreciated, combination drug therapy had evolved from the need to develop more effective treatment than was provided by single agents. It is now clear that combination therapy is markedly superior to monotherapy for the majority of drug-responsive tumours. However, its success is dependent both on the application of the principles of chemotherapy to protocol design and on the use of effective anticancer drugs. Although early combination chemotherapy protocols were developed in an era when many of these principles were not appreciated, their success can now be partly understood within the context of these principles. For example, the Goldie–Coldman hypothesis provides one explanation for why combination therapy, compared to monotherapy, more effectively overcomes existing tumour cell resistance and slows down or prevents the emergence of additional clones of resistant cells. In addition, the ability of combination therapy to achieve a greater dose rate compared to monotherapy, through its higher therapeutic ratio, is a major contributor to its effectiveness.

The development of an effective combination chemotherapy regimen is dependent on the appropriate selection of drugs and administration schedules, and on the application of the aforementioned principles to the design of new protocols.[16] First, only drugs which have significant single agent activity should be chosen, and although clinically unproven, the selection of drugs which have synergistic activity *in vitro* has a theoretical appeal. It should be emphasized that, although it is not always possible to identify the most active drugs, the use of drugs which have a questionable activity towards the tumour being treated will add toxicity, and will usually lead to a reduction in the dose rate for the effective drugs. Second, drugs with minimal overlapping toxicity should be used whenever possible in order to avoid dose reductions of other drugs in the combination with similar toxicities, and to minimize unacceptable organ toxicity. Third, the choice of dose, rate and route of drug administration (e.g. oral, intravenous bolus or infusion) should be based on the pharmacokinetics of the drug(s) in question and on existing information regarding the maximal tolerated dose(s) for any given schedule. In the setting of aggressive lymphomas, the interval between cycles should be adjusted to achieve the maximum dose rate.

These principles provide a framework for protocol design, but must clearly be applied within the context of both the natural history of the disease and empirical observations made from the results of previous treatment protocols. Ultimately, protocols are judged by results, and since there are so many variables which impact upon the outcome of chemotherapy, it must be recognized that there still remains a large element of empiricism in protocol design.

In specific situations, radiotherapy is used in combination with chemotherapy in protocols written with curative intent. Of course, with the exception of total body irradiation (TBI), radiation is a locoregional modality. Thus, its principal role in combined modality approaches is to treat local sites of bulky disease which might be relatively chemotherapy resistant. When radiotherapy is incorporated into a protocol, it may be viewed as a treatment modality which is generally non-cross-resistant with chemotherapy. It adds a specific spectrum of toxicities which are due to direct tissue interactions, the severity and quality of which will also depend on the type of chemotherapy administered to the patient. It should be pointed out that, with the possible exception of specific types and stages of lymphomas, the value of radiation therapy as a complement to combination chemotherapy protocols remains controversial.

Chemotherapy of lymphomas

For the purposes of treatment, the non-Hodgkin's lymphomas can be classified into a number of clinically distinct groups which are principally defined by histology, despite a rapidly expanding understanding of the immunobiology of lymphomas. Although there are several clinically equivalent classifications, the Working Formulation provides a useful division of low, intermediate and high grade groups.[25] For the purposes of this chapter, we will discuss the therapy of lymphomas within the context of these three divisions, although it is clear that the subtypes within these divisions often require significantly different treatment approaches (Table 13.1). For example, as a group, the low grade lymphomas are often not treated until medically necessary (watch and wait approach),[26] and yet it is clear that at least for the follicular mixed (FM) lymphoma subtype, initial aggressive chemotherapy may achieve durable CRs and is the therapy of choice.[27] Similarly, the aggressive lymphomas which are classified as either intermediate or high grade are always treated with intensive chemotherapy regimens but, depending on the subtype, require treatment approaches which may differ significantly in dose intensity, types of drugs administered and the need for central nervous system (CNS) prophylaxis.[28,29,30] Predictably, as both the therapy and our understanding of these diseases improve, the significance of prognostic

Table 13.1 Selected treatment regimens for advanced stage non-Hodgkin's lymphomas

Lymphoma subtype	Regimens	Reference
Low grade		
FSC, SL	Observation/CVP/M-BACOD	38, 33, 40
FM	ProMACE-MOPP/M-BACOD	68, 66
Intermediate		
FL, DL	ProMACE-CytaBOM/M-BACOD	70, 66
DM, DSC	MACOP-B	69
High grade		
IBL	ProMACE-CytaBOM/MACOP-B	70, 69
LBL (childhood)	LSA$_2$-L$_2$/APO/77-04	75, 77, 29
LBL (adult)	LSA$_2$-L$_2$/77-04/Stanford LBL	75, 29, 73
SNC, (DL) (childhood)	COMP/77-04/LMB0281/BFM-83	74, 29, 79, 80
SNC (adult)	77-04	29

FSC, follicular small cleaved; SL, small lymphocytic; FM, follicular mixed; FL, follicular large cell; DL, diffuse large cell; DM, diffuse mixed; DSC, diffuse small cleaved; IBL, immunoblastic, LBL, lymphoblastic, SNC, small non-cleaved.

factors, such as tumour bulk and histology, which guide the selection of therapy is diminishing.

Low-grade lymphomas

The low-grade lymphomas are unique among the non-Hodgkin's lymphomas because they can be effectively treated, often for years, with non-aggressive treatment approaches such as single alkylating agents. In fact, response rates as high as 80 per cent have been reported with single agents, but the vast majority of responses are only partial, and when CRs are achieved, they are usually of short duration.[31] Predictably, higher CRs can be achieved with combination chemotherapy regimens (such as cyclophosphamide, vincristine and prednisone (CVP)) compared to single agents (37 versus 13 per cent, respectively), but without an improvement in overall patient survival.[32,33] Many trials conducted during the 1970s were designed to examine a variety of therapeutic approaches including radiotherapy, combined modality and aggressive chemotherapy, but no significant improvement in patient survival was demonstrated when the more intensive approaches were compared to therapy with single agents or CVP.[34–37] Trials such as these demonstrated that durable CRs were not only uncommon but, perhaps surprisingly, did not have great prognostic significance. It is the paradoxically excellent response of these tumours to a variety of treatment approaches and yet their resistance to cure, which is so perplexing.

This paradoxical response of the low grade lymphomas led to two radically different treatment approaches. In a conservative approach, investigators at Stanford University managed a selected group of asymptomatic, advanced stage patients without therapy, until this was medically necessary.[38] The rationale behind this trial came from the observation that there is little evidence in asymptomatic patients that initial therapy has any impact on overall survival and patients may remain asymptomatic for significant time periods without treatment. In contrast, in a currently active trial at the National Cancer Institute (NCI) Bethesda, USA, patients with advanced stage, low grade lymphomas are randomized to receive either initial therapy with very intensive ProMACE-MOPP flexitherapy (prednisone, methotrexate, doxorubicin, cyclophosphamide, etoposide, mechloroethamine, vincristine, procarbazine followed by 2200–2500 cGy total nodal irradiation (TNI), as described in Chapter 21), or conservative management until the disease progression requires therapy, at which time the same intensive multi-modality therapy is started.[39] The rationale for this approach is to determine whether an intensive regimen will significantly improve patient survival and the approach is based on trials, such as one conducted at the Dana Farber Cancer Center, Boston, USA, which demonstrated that patients treated with the aggressive regimen M-BACOD (methotrexate, bleomycin, doxorubicin, cyclophosphamide, vincristine, dexamethasone) achieved a significantly higher CR rate (56 per cent) than that obtained with less intensive regimens, raising the possibility that some of these patients may be cured.[40]

The results from the Stanford and NCI trials have yielded important information. The Stanford group reported that, with their conservative approach, the median survival of 11 years did not significantly differ from that in two other prospective trials in similar groups of patients treated at Stanford with standard chemotherapy approaches. Of importance was the observation that patients with FM lymphoma had a more aggressive course with a significantly shorter time to treatment and lower actuarial survival (16.5 months and 60 per cent at 5 years, respectively) than did patients with follicular small cleaved (FSC) lymphoma (48 months and 80 per cent at 10 years, respectively).[38] Although this study provides a persuasive argument for the conservative management of low grade lymphomas and has become a commonly used approach in the community, its non-randomized design, using historical or parallel controls treated with a variety of non-aggressive therapies, still leaves the optimal management of these diseases in doubt.

It is in the setting of resistant disease that the Goldie–Coldman hypothesis predicts that non-cross-resistant combination chemotherapy regimens will be of benefit. The NCI trial is a radical departure from previous studies because of its use of intensive, non-cross-resistant chemotherapy followed by TNI in low-grade lymphomas. The role of radiotherapy in this setting is intriguing because despite its being a locoregional technique, it clearly is effective against disseminated disease; a clinical effect which suggests that poorly understood regulatory mechanisms play an important role in the control of the low grade lymphomas.[41,42] Although this study has yet to reach maturity, there is a significant difference in disease-free survival (DFS) between the treatment arms, favouring the intensive therapy arm.[39] Unfortunately, it is too early to conclude whether the latter treatment approach should be widely adopted for advanced stage low grade lymphomas or whether cures will result, but when completed, this trial should help to define the role of aggressive therapy in these diseases.

The value of aggressive chemotherapy for the treatment of patients with advanced stage FM lymphomas is much less controversial. It is clear from numerous trials that the FM subtype has a significantly more aggressive clinical course and more durable response to chemotherapy compared to the FSC and small lymphocytic (SL) lymphoma subtypes.[43–45] In fact, in patients with advanced stage FM lymphoma treated at the NCI with cyclophosphamide, vincristine, procarbazine and prednisone (C-MOPP) chemotherapy, a 72 per cent complete response rate and a median DFS of over six years was achieved.[27] The results of several other studies were similar, indicating that patients with FM lymphoma should probably be treated with a second or third generation aggressive chemotherapy regimen (*see* Table 13.1).

A number of interesting biological observations can be made from these and other trials which may help to explain the refractoriness of the low-grade lymphomas to cure. These lymphomas retain many of the characteristics of their normal B-lymphoid counterparts, such as tissue distribution, cell surface antigens and sensitivity to regulatory controls which presumably operate via the patient's immune system.[46,47] Clinically, this is reflected in the frequent waxing and waning course of these diseases and by the well-recognized phenomenon of spontaneous tumour regression.[26] It has even been suggested that the low-grade lymphomas could be considered 'pre-malignant' because of their indolent course. In fact, these tumours are rarely the direct cause of patient death, which is usually associated with a transformation to an aggressive subtype.[48–50] Thus, because of its close phenotypic proximity to normal lymphocytes, it may be very difficult to eradicate the follicular lymphoma cell clone without killing the patient. In addition, there may be an increased likelihood of resistant subclones in these patients because of the high tumour burdens which are typical of the low grade lymphomas, although the repeated responses of these tumours to identical chemotherapy render this an ·unsatisfactory explanation for the low cure rate. Indeed, the probable persistence of tumour cells in patients who have obtained a CR has been elegantly demonstrated by Ault *et al.*[51,52] Using a flow cytometric analysis technique, these investigators demonstrated the presence of circulating monoclonal B-cells in 64 per cent of patients with follicular lymphoma 18 months after CRs were achieved. In contrast, no circulating monoclonal B-cells were detected in patients with aggressive lymphomas after CRs were achieved, although monoclonal B-cells could be detected initially in 84 per cent of these patients.

A model based on the presence of two different tumour cell compartments may account for the paradoxical response of the low grade lymphomas to therapy. Clues to the nature of these compartments come from molecular biology. There is substantial evidence that the 14;18 translocations which are present in the majority of these tumours arise very early in the B-cell differentiation pathway: in fact during the process of D-J joining when commitment to the B-cell lineage is in the process of being established (*see* Chapter 3).[53,54] Tumour cells at this early stage of differentiation, probably present in insufficient numbers to be detected, may serve as a stem cell compartment which can replenish the compartment containing the bulk of the more differentiated cells. It is entirely possible that the cells in the latter compartment are very sensitive to chemotherapy, while the stem cell compartment is highly chemotherapy resistant, possibly because such cells are often in a non-proliferative phase, as are many haematopoietic stem cells.

Another paradox seen in the treatment of low grade lymphomas is the high rate of durable remissions achieved with involved field radiation in patients with stage I and II disease,[55] despite the reported presence of circulating monoclonal cells.[51] A model which can account for this has been proposed. In this model the renewable tumour stem cells are restricted to the involved lymph node(s) while the circulating monoclonal cells represent the more differentiated tumour cells, which have a limited proliferative potential. Of course, immunological mechanisms probably also play an important role in this clinical setting.

The higher incidence of durable CRs seen with FM lymphomas, compared to the FSC and SL subtypes indicates that there are significant biological differences between these diseases. Although FM lymphoma is pathologically differentiated from FSC lymphoma by the presence of at least five to 15 large cells per high powered field, the ratio of these two cell types, as well as the ratio of follicular to diffuse architecture, lies on a continuum and can be correlated with the aggressiveness of the tumour.[56] Why these characteristics of FM lymphoma result in a higher rate of durable CR is unclear, but mechanistically they suggest that either the stem cell compartment is sensitive to chemotherapy or that it is not present.

This model of the follicular lymphomas resembles that of chronic myeloid leukaemia and suggests that cure in the FSC and SL subtypes will only be achieved by the total eradication of the malignant clone, including the theoretical stem cell component. In chronic myeloid leukaemia this has been accomplished by very intensive 'marrow ablative' therapy, which eliminates the entire haematopoietic stem cell compartment, followed by 'marrow rescue'.[57] Such approaches have also been attempted in follicular lymphomas, with promising preliminary results.[58]

Intermediate grade lymphomas

Unlike patients with low grade lymphomas, those with intermediate and high grade lymphomas do poorly when treated with non-aggressive chemotherapy, such as CVP and single agents. At best, regimens such as CVP only result in CRs in 25–30 per cent of patients and most patients eventually relapse and die.[59,60] It has become clear that failure to achieve an initial CR as well as relapse are both associated with rapid disease progression and death.[61] Unfortunately, despite the development of chemotherapy regimens which are highly effective at inducing durable CRs, there are no really effective salvage regimens for patients who relapse (10–20 per cent durable CR rate).[62]

It is important to recognize that regimens with equivalent rates of CR do not necessarily have equivalent rates of relapse. In a study comparing C-MOPP and BACOP, (containing bleomycin, doxorubicin, cyclophosphamide, vincristine, prednisone) for the treatment of diffuse large cell (DL) lymphoma, for example, the CR rates were 49 per cent and 51 per cent, respectively, but the relapse rates were significantly different, 52 per cent and 32 per cent, respectively.[63] This suggests that, although both regimens may kill enough cells to produce a remission, the fractional cell kill at some point in the treatment is significantly less with the C-MOPP regimen. Mechanistically, this may be due either to the existence, prior to treatment, of more cell clones resistant to C-MOPP chemotherapy or to the greater likelihood of the development of resistant clones during treatment, or to both.

Theoretically, tumour cells which are resistant to a regimen can be more effectively treated by a combination containing non-cross-resistant drugs, while kinetic problems due to the regrowth of tumour cells between cycles of treatment may be partially overcome by keeping the cycle length as short as possible. In fact, both of these approaches have been applied, to variable degrees, to the development of the newer generations of chemotherapy regimens used for the treatment of aggressive lymphomas and have resulted in apparently improved CR rates and lower relapse rates.[64–66] Unfortunately, there have been few direct comparisons of the many regimens in use, so that comparison of trial results must be viewed circumspectly and could be due to differences in patient groups, follow-up and quality of care rather than intrinsic differences in chemotherapy efficacy.

Many of the clinical improvements in the early chemotherapy regimens were achieved through the addition or substitution of drugs and by changes in drug doses and scheduling. For example, the first generation CHOP regimen (cyclophosphamide, doxorubicin, vincristine and prednisone) was basically derived from CVP by the addition of doxorubicin and by changes in drug dose and schedule, and it achieved a significantly improved rate of survival compared to CVP.[64] Further variations, however, such as CHOP-bleomycin and BACOP (CHOP and bleomycin with different doses and schedules) did not significantly improve on the results obtained with CHOP, probably because the addition of doxorubicin was the most important change.[65,67] Despite these improvements, a major problem with these first-generation regimens was the low rate of cure. An approach found to be effective in second-generation programmes was to increase the number of non-cross-resistant drugs and to administer them in shorter, alternating cycles. This was accomplished in several different ways. For example, in the M-BACOD (methotrexate, bleomycin, doxorubicin, cyclophosphamide, vincristine, dexamethasone) regimen, drugs were administered on days 1 and 14, and repeated every three weeks for 10 cycles.[66] A more novel approach, based on the Goldie–Coldman model, was used at the NCI where ProMACE-MOPP flexitherapy was developed.[68] The NCI group reasoned that if the rate of fractional cell kill by a regimen decreased over time because of the emergence of resistant clones, then the use of a second non-cross-resistant regimen at that time may result in an increased fractional cell kill. Therefore, ProMACE drugs were administered until the rate of tumour shrinkage stabilized, at which time the patients were crossed over to receive the MOPP drugs. However, despite the theoretical appeal of such a novel approach, the key to the apparent improvements achieved by the second-generation regimens probably lies in the increased dose intensity achieved through the use of more non-cross-resistant drugs and shorter cycle lengths.

Only modest improvements in the rate of CR and relapse have been achieved with the third generation regimens.[69,70] In general, the design of these regimens is not conceptually different from that of the second-generation regimens, with the exception of the MACOP-B regimen which was developed at the University of British Columbia.[69] This regimen has several unique features which are theoretically appealing. First, drugs are administered every week for the duration of therapy. This has been achieved by alternating myelosuppressive and myelosparing drugs on a weekly basis. This delivery schedule is appealing because it minimizes the time allowed for the repair of tumour DNA and proteins and hence the regrowth of tumour, before the next cycle of chemotherapy. In addition, the expansion of resistant clones is minimized by alternating non-cross-resistant drugs on a weekly schedule. Second, by rapidly alternating cycle specific and non-specific drugs, this regimen may theoretically increase the number of cells in cycle, thereby increasing the fractional cell kill of the cycle specific drugs. Third, this regimen is completed in 12 weeks whereas most other regimens require from 16 to 40 weeks. The ability to achieve complete tumour eradication in 12 weeks suggests that effective drugs delivered at high-dose intensity are among the most important ingredients of an effective chemotherapy regimen, and that in chemosensitive tumours, long durations of therapy are probably unnecessary. These features of the MACOP-B regimen set it apart as a model approach for the design of future protocols.

The intensive third-generation regimens should be used in patients who have advanced stage disease with intermediate grade and immunoblastic, high grade lymphomas. In specific circumstances where it is felt that a patient cannot tolerate such intensive approaches, usually in elderly patients, less aggressive approaches with regimens such as CHOP may be appropriate. However, most patients will tolerate intensive chemotherapy regimens and the decision not to use such approaches is likely to compromise the chance of a durable CR (*see* Fig. 13.1).

High grade lymphomas

High grade lymphomas occur in both paediatric and adult populations and have unique geographical distributions associated with specific biological behaviours. They are heterogeneous in their cells of origin, being principally of T-cell origin in lymphoblastic lymphomas (LBL), B-cell origin in small non-cleaved (SNC) lymphomas and either of B- or T-cell origin in immunoblastic lymphomas (IBL).[47,71] Clinically, this diversity is reflected by their different patterns of presentation, prognosis and response to chemotherapy.[72–74] In addition, both the staging and definition of LBL have differed from centre to centre, making comparisons of trials difficult. Some investigators, for example, distinguish LBL from T-cell acute lymphoblastic leukaemia (ALL) by the presence of less than 25 per cent bone marrow involvement, while other groups do not make this distinction. This is important to take into consideration when interpreting the results of chemotherapy trials because patients with extensive bone marrow disease may have a poorer prognosis with the same chemotherapy regimens.[75–78]

Despite these problems excellent results can be obtained in the high grade lymphomas in the paediatric age group. Analysis of early chemotherapy trials suggests that LBL responds better to intensive leukaemic-like regimens, while paediatric SNC lymphoma responds better to intensive lymphoma-like regimens with a greater emphasis on alkylating agents.[74] In 1979, Wollner reported a 73 per cent long-term DFS in paediatric non-Hodgkin's lymphomas treated with an intensive 10-drug combination called LSA_2L_2 which principally contains cyclophosphamide, vincristine, daunomycin, vincristine, prednisone, cytosine arabinoside and L-asparaginase.[75] This regimen was based on an ALL treatment approach where patients received intensive induction and consolidation chemotherapy followed by maintenance for one year. The group from Dana-Farber have also reported good results with another ALL-like regimen known as APO Adriamycin (doxorubicin), prednisone, Oncovin (vincristine) in patients with LBL.[76] A number of centres and cooperative groups have subsequently reported similar results with the LSA_2L_2 regimen in patients with disseminated LBL (76 per cent 2-year DFS in one trial) but have reported significantly poorer results with this regimen (26 per cent 2 year DFS) in patients with non-lymphoblastic disease.[74,77] The Children's Cancer Study Group, for example, found that the LSA$_2$L$_2$ regimen was relatively ineffective for non-lymphoblastic lymphomas which responded best to a four-drug regimen of cyclophosphamide, vincristine, methotrexate and prednisone (COMP).[74] It now appears that the success of the ALL-like protocols in lymphoblastic lymphoma is not necessarily a consequence of the 'induction-consolidation-maintenance' design of these protocols. The Pediatric Oncology Group demonstrated no difference in therapeutic outcome in patients with LBL randomized to receive either a four-drug combination called A-COP (doxorubicin, cyclophosphamide, vincristine, prednisone) or the LSA$_2$L$_2$ regimen.[77] In addition, in a study conducted at the NCI, there was no difference in treatment outcome between patients with LBL and SNC lymphomas treated with a lymphoma-like regimen which included cyclophosphamide, doxorubicin, vincristine, methotrexate and prednisone (protocol no. 77-04).[29,78]

Several conclusions regarding the choice of drugs for the high grade lymphomas can be made from these trials. First, anthracyclines are an important drug for the treatment of LBL, and leukaemia-like regimens, in which a complex array of drugs is administered, are probably not necessary. These trials also suggest that L-asparaginase is not an essential component of therapy for LBL, and raise the question as to whether extended maintenance therapy for up to 2 years is really necessary. Second, cyclophosphamide, administered in a dose-intensive fashion, appears to be critically important for the treatment of SNC lymphoma. Its importance was illustrated by the poor results obtained with regimens such as the LSA$_2$L$_2$ and APO protocols which principally deliver vincristine, prednisone and anthracyclines during the induction phase. Agents such as methotrexate, cytosine arabinoside and etoposide also have significant activity and should be considered for inclusion in protocols for the treatment of high grade lymphomas.[79,80] Future protocols should be designed within the context of the above observations and the principles of chemotherapy.

It has now become clear that there is significant overlap in the optimal treatment approaches for both LBL and SNC lymphomas and that, while optimal therapy durations may differ, identical drugs and schedules may be used. Such protocols should at least include cyclophosphamide, anthracyclines, vincristine and prednisone, which are among the most effective drugs for LBL and SNC lymphomas. Although most of these conclusions are based on trials in high grade childhood lymphomas, they are also relevant to the treatment of high grade lymphomas in adults. Unfortunately it is difficult to reach conclusions regarding the differential response of LBL and SNC lymphomas in adults to these different therapeutic approaches, because the paucity of trials with uniformly treated patients makes accurate conclusions impossible at the present time.

It should be emphasized that the high incidence of CNS relapse makes inclusion of CNS prophylaxis essential in protocols for high grade lymphomas. This can be achieved through the direct administration of methotrexate and/or cytosine arabinoside into the CNS or the use of high dose systemic methotrexate. However, there is no evidence that cranial irradiation is superior to drug therapy in the prophylactic setting, and its potential adverse effects on intellectual function argue against its use.[78]

References

1. Skipper HE, Schabel FM, and Wilcox WS. *Cancer Chemotherapy Reports* 1964; **35**, 1.
2. Schabel FM, Simpson-Herren L. *Antibiotics and Chemotherapy* 1978; **23**, 113.
3. Burkitt DP. *Cancer* 1967; **20**, 756.
4. Magrath IT, Lwanga S, Carswell W, Harrison N. *British Medical Journal*. 1974; **2**, 308.
5. Goldie JH, Coldham AJ. *Cancer Treatment Reports*. 1979; **63**, 1727.
6. Luria SE, Delbruck M. *Genetics*. 1943; **28**, 491.
7. Yunis JJ. *Science*. 1983; **221**, 227.
8. Moscow JA, Cowan KH. *Journal of the National Cancer Institute*. 1988; **80**, 14.
9. Gros P, Neriah YB, Croop JM, Housman DE. *Nature*. 1986; **323**, 728.

10. Ling V, Thompson LH. *Journal of Cell Physiology*. 1973; **83**, 103.
11. Bech-Hansen NT, Till JE, Ling V. *Journal of Cell Physiology*. 1976; **88**, 23.
12. Gros P, Croop J, Housman D. *Cell*. 1986; **47**, 371.
13. Fojo AT, Ueda K, Slamon DJ, *et al. Proceedings of the National Academy of Sciences* USA. 1987; **84**, 265.
14. Tsuruo T, Lida H, Kitatani Y, *et al. Cancer Research*. 1984; **44**, 4303.
15. Yalowich JC, Zucali JR, Gross MA, Ross WE. *Cancer Research*. 1985; **45**, 4921.
16. DeVita VT, In: DeVita VT, Helleman S, Rosenberg SA. (eds). Cancer: *Principles and Practice of Oncology*, 2nd ed. Philadelphia: Lippincott, 1987.
17. Hryniuk WM. *Seminars in Oncology*. 1987; **14**, 65.
18. Hryniuk W, Levine MN. *Journal of Clinical Oncology*. 1986; **4**, 1162.
19. DeVita VT, Hubbars SM, Young RC, Longo DL. *Seminars in Hematology*. 1988; **25**, 2.
20. Millar JL, Hudspith BN, Blackett NM. *British Journal of Cancer*. 1975; **32**, 193.
21. Carmichael J, Adams DJ, Ansell J, Wolf CR. *Cancer Research*. 1986; **46**, 735.
22. Rennick D, Yang G, Gemmell L, Lee F. *Blood*. 1987; **69**, 682.
23. Groopman JE, Mitsuyasu RT, DeLeom MJ *et al. New England Journal of Medicine*. 1987; **317**, 593.
24. Vadhan-Raj S, Hittelman WN, Beuscher S, *et al. Proceedings of the American Society of Clinical Oncology*. 1988; (abstract) **639**.
25. Rosenberg SA, Berard CW, Brown SM, *et al. Cancer*. 1982; **49**, 2112.
26. Horning SJ, Rosenberg SA. *New England Journal of Medicine*. 1984; **311**, 1471.
27. Longo DL, Young RC, Hubbard SM, *et al. Annals of Internal Medicine*. 1984; **100**, 651.
28. Skarin AT. *Seminars in Oncology*. 1986; **13**, 10.
29. Magrath IT, Janus C, Edwards BK, *et al. Blood*. 1984; **63**, 1102.
30. Sullivan MP, Boyett J, Pullen J, *et al. Cancer*. 1985; **55**, 323.
31. Jones SE, Rosenberg SA, Kaplan HS, *et al. Cancer*, 1972; **30**, 31.
32. Lister TA, Cullen MH, Beard MEJ, *et al. British Medical Journal*. 1978; **1**, 533.
33. Bagley CM, DeVita VT, Berard CW, *et al. Annals of Internal Medicine*. 1972; **76**, 227.
34. Brereton HD, Young RC, Longo DL, *et al. Cancer*. 1979; **43**, 2227.
35. Ezdinli EZ, Anderson JR, Melvin F, *et al. Journal of Clinical Oncology*. 1985; **3**, 769.
36. Young RC, Johnson RE, Canellos GP, *et al. Cancer Treatment Reports*. 1977; **61**, 1153.
37. Hoppe RT, Kushland P, Kaplan HS, *et al. Blood*. 1981; **58**, 592.
38. Portlock CS, Rosenberg SA. *Annals of Internal Medicine*. 1979; **90**, 10.
39. Young RC, Longo DL, Glatstein E, *et al. Proceedings of the American Society of Clinical Oncology*. 1987; (abstract) **790**.
40. Anderson KC, Skarin AT, Rosenthal DS, *et al. Cancer Treatment Reports*. 1984; **68**, 1343–50.
41. Glatstein E, Fuks Z, Goffinet DR, Kaplan HS. *Cancer*. 1976; **37**, 2806.
42. Carabell SC, Chaffey JT, Rosenthal DS, *et al. Cancer*. 1979; **43**, 994.
43. Lawrence EH, Weiss LM, Hoppe RT, Horning SJ. *Journal of Clinical Oncology*. 1985; **3**, 1183.
44. Ezdinli EZ, Costello WG, Icli F, *et al. Cancer*. 1980; **45**, 261.
45. Osborn CK, Norton L, Young RC, *et al. Blood*. 1980; **56**, 98.
46. Urba WJ, Longo DL. *Seminars in Oncology*. 1985; **12**, 250.
47. Foon KA, Todd RE. *Blood*. 1986; **68**, 1.
48. Hubbard SM, Chabner BA, DeVita VT, *et al. Blood*. 1982; **59**, 1982.
49. Garvin AJ, Simon RM, Osborne CK, *et al. Cancer*. 1983; **52**, 393.
50. Acker B, Hoppe RT, Colby TV, *et al. Journal of Clinical Oncology*. 1983; **1**, 11.
51. Smith BR, Weinberg DS, Robert NJ, *et al. New England Journal of Medicine*. 1984; **311**, 1476.
52. Ault KA. *New England Journal of Medicine*. 1979; **300**, 1401.
53. Siminovitch KA, Jensen JP, Epstein AL, *et al. Blood*. 1986; **67**, 391.
54. Croce CM, Nowell PC. *Blood*. 1985; **65**, 1.
55. Hu E, Weiss LM, Hoppe RT, Horning SJ. *Journal of Clinical Oncology*. 1985; **3**, 1985.
56. Thomas DE, Clift RA, Fefer A, *et al. Annals of Internal Medicine*. 1986; **104**, 155.
57. Takvorian T, Canellos GP, Ritz J, *et al. New England Journal of Medicine*, 1987, **316**, 1499.
58. Paryani SB, Hoppe RT, Cox RS, *et al. Cancer*. 1983; **52**, 2300.
59. Portlock C, Rosenberg S. *Cancer*. 1976; **37**, 1275.
60. Jones SE, Fuks Z, Bull M, *et al. Cancer*. 1973; **31**, 806.
61. Fisher RI, DeVita VT, Johnson BL, *et al. American Journal of Medicine*. 1977; **63**, 177.
62. Cabanillas F, Hagemeister FB, Bodey GP, Freireich EJ. *Blood*. 1982; **60**, 693.
63. Dupont J, Caray G, Scaglione C, *et al. Second International Conference on Malignant Lymphomas*, Lugano, Switzerland. Martinus Nijhoff. 1984; 475.
64. Armitage JO, Fyfe MAE, Lewis J. *Journal of Clinical Oncology*, 1984; **2**, 898.
65. Schein PS, DeVita VT, Hubbard S, *et al. Annals of*

Internal Medicine. 1976; **85**, 417.

66. Skarin AT, Canellos GP, Rosenthal DS, *et al. Journal of Clinical Oncology.* 1983; **1**, 91.
67. Rodriguez V, Cabanillas F, Burgess MA, *et al. Blood.* 1977; **49**, 325.
68. Fisher RI, DeVita VT, Hubbard SM, *et al. Annals of Internal Medicine,* 1983; **98**, 304.
69. Klimo P, Connors JM. *Annals of Internal Medicine.* 1985; **102**, 596.
70. Fisher RI, DeVita VT, Hubbard SM, *et al. Proceedings of the American Society of Clinical Oncology.* 1984; **3**, 242.
71. Jaffe ES. *Seminars in Oncology.* 1986; **13**, 3.
72. Ziegler JL. *New England Journal of Medicine.* 1981; **305**, 735.
73. Coleman CN, Cohen JR, Burke JS, Rosenberg SA.

Blood. 1981; **57**, 679.

74. Anderson JR, Wilson JF, Jenkin RD, *et al. New England Journal of Medicine.* 1983; **308**, 559.
75. Wollner N, Exelby PR, Lieberman PH. *Cancer.* 1979; **44**, 1990.
76. Weinstein HJ, Cassady JR, Levey, R. *Journal of Clinical Oncology.* 1983; **1**, 537.
77. Hvizdala EV, Callihan BT, Falletta J, *et al. Journal of Clinical Oncology.* 1988; **6**, 26.
78. Magrath IT. *Hematologic and Oncologic Clinics of North America.* 1987; **1**, 577.
79. Patte C, Philip T, Rodary C, *et al. Journal of Clinical Oncology.* 1986; **4**, 1219.
80. Muller-Weihrich ST, Ludwig R, Reiter A, *et al. Proceedings of the Third International Conference on Malignant Lymphomas* (abstract). 1987; **42**, 43.

CHAPTER 14

RADIATION THERAPY IN THE NON-HODGKIN'S LYMPHOMAS

Jane Grayson and Eli Glatstein

Ionizing radiation has been an important therapeutic agent in the treatment of the non-Hodgkin's lymphomas for many decades. Data from patients treated as early as the 1930s with orthovoltage equipment suggest that 'some lymphoma patients may have been cured by adequate radiation therapy'.[1] The application of single and multiagent chemotherapy to the malignant lymphomas has also resulted in dramatic responses. The use of combination chemotherapy in the non-Hodgkin's lymphomas during the past several decades now appears to offer the potential for cure to many patients with disseminated disease, at least to those with aggressive histology. In the 1980s emphasis on combined modality therapy has led to efforts to integrate radiation therapy and chemotherapy in the curative approach to malignant lymphomas. However, the enthusiasm for even more aggressive approaches to treatment must be tempered by the potential for late complications and second malignancies. The deleterious as well as beneficial effects of these multiple agents make it critical to establish the roles of radiotherapy and chemotherapy in the treatment of the non-Hodgkin's lymphomas and to study their use in prospective, carefully controlled trials.

This chapter is confined to an evaluation of radiation therapy in the treatment of non-Hodgkin's lymphomas in adults; in childhood, the efficacy of multiagent chemotherapy is enough that radiotherapy is usually used today for local palliation or as part of transplantation programmes with total body irradiation. Rather than present treatment approaches to specific diseases, which are covered in other chapters, this discussion considers general principles of radiation therapy as they relate to these lymphomas.

Hodgkin's disease and the non-Hodgkin's lymphomas

'The current temporary terminology of "non-Hodgkin's lymphomas" reflects somehow the contemporary provisional concepts in terms of natural history and correct approach to therapeutic problems.'[2]

Unfortunately, now more than a decade after this statement, significant confusion still remains regarding the classification, staging and treatment of the non-Hodgkin's lymphomas. Even the designation of 'non-Hodgkin's lymphomas' to this heterogeneous group of malignant lymphoid tumours reflects the confusion of early investigators. Most of our treatment strategies for the lymphomas other than Hodgkin's lymphomas were derived from the successful therapy of Hodgkin's disease. However, investigators soon realized that the natural histories and responses to therapy of these non-Hodgkin's lymphomas were significantly different from Hodgkin's disease.

In the 1950s and 1960s, various concepts regarding the treatment of patients with Hodgkin's disease were established. These patients tended to be young and otherwise healthy. Their malignancy tended to have a predictable mode of lymphatic spread and relatively infrequent extranodal extension.[3] Epitrochlear, mesenteric and Waldeyer's ring nodes were infrequently involved. The pioneering studies of Dr Henry Kaplan and his colleagues at Stanford University helped to identify treatment options for Hodgkin's disease patients in the era of megavoltage radiation therapy. Their philosophy of treatment evolved from data which demonstrated that high dose irradiation could result in greater than 90 per cent local control in nodal groups.[4] High dose irradiation, administered to large volumes of nodal tissue and consistent with the orderly progression of Hodgkin's lymphoma, resulted in the cure of many patients with early stages of the disease. The concepts of staging which evolved at the Rye[5] and the Ann Arbor[6] meetings were consistent with the emerging clinical understanding of Hodgkin's disease.

Unfortunately, the malignant lymphomas other than Hodgkin's disease did not demonstrate the same high rate of curability when treated with involved or extended field radiotherapy. Investigators became aware that the natural histories of these lymphomas were markedly different. Central nodal irradiation would be unlikely to play the same curative role in these non-Hodgkin's lymphomas as it did in Hodgkin's disease.

Many characteristics distinguish these lymphomas from Hodgkin's disease. As a group, in contrast to Hodgkin's disease, they have a remarkable propensity to spread beyond the lymphatic system. There are marked increases in the frequency of involvement of bone marrow, mesenteric node, Waldeyer's ring and the central nervous system (CNS). Although the most common sites of recurrence are in lymph nodes, extranodal involvement at the time of relapse is almost as frequent. Patients with non-Hodgkin's lymphomas tend to be two to three decades older than Hodgkin's disease patients; as a consequence they manifest more organ dysfunction unrelated to lymphoma. In contrast, they are less likely to have systemic symptoms at diagnosis related to their malignancy (B symptoms) than Hodgkin's

patients (10–15 per cent versus 30–35 per cent). Patients with Hodgkin's disease frequently present when the disease is still localized; 60–70 per cent have stage I or II lymphoma at presentation. In contrast, the majority of non-Hodgkin's lymphoma patients present with advanced stage disease (III or IV). In patients with nodular histology, fewer than 20 per cent of patients present with pathological stage I or II disease. In patients with diffuse histology lymphomas, between 30 and 50 per cent of patients have early stage disease, but less than 15 per cent have stage I.[7–10] One needs to determine for which stages and which histological subtypes radiation therapy is an appropriate treatment option. One of the difficulties in evaluating the literature addressing these issues is the problem encountered by pathologists in classifying these tumours.

Over the past three decades, at least six major histopathological classification systems for the non-Hodgkin's lymphomas have evolved. The confusion and controversy regarding the categorization of the malignant lymphomas have resulted in difficulty in evaluating the efficacy of various treatment programmes. Comparing the results of various clinical studies is complicated and often impossible.

The development of the 'Working Formulation for Clinical Usage' of the Non-Hodgkin's Lymphomas Pathologic Classification Project[11] was an important step in encouraging communication among pathologists. It has provided a means for translating clinical trials from different institutions into common terminology. Another important result was the demonstration of clinical relevance of the classification systems. It is critical that the categories carry prognostic importance relative to modern therapeutic modalities and that the categorization process be reproducible. The study demonstrated that the recognition of the follicular pattern, one of the major prognostic variables in predicting natural history and determining therapy, was a highly reproducible observation (95 per cent probability).[12] There was considerable variation in identification of many of the other histological subtypes. This wide range in reproducibility was true for individual pathologists reviewing a single slide twice and for two pathologists evaluating the same slide. It is apparent that there is still need for improvement in the classification of the non-Hodgkin's lymphomas. The application of new immunological and molecular data should help to distinguish further the subtypes of malignant lymphomas.

In addition to the inherent complexity in distinguishing the histopathology of a single subtype of lymphoma is the problem of multiple subtypes existing in an individual patient. Divergent histologies may be present during the initial staging either in the same or different lymph nodes.[13–15] In a review from the National Cancer Institute,[16] 101 patients had multiple tissue sites biopsied at presentation; 33 had more than one histological subtype identified. Other patients will have a second histology documented at the time of a repeat biopsy months after the initial diagnosis, or at autopsy.[17–19]

All of these issues add to the confusion regarding the classification of the non-Hodgkin's lymphomas and to the difficulty in planning optimal therapy. It is apparent that the issues concerning histology are extremely difficult even for expert pathologists. Clinicians must have realistic expectations and appreciate the uncertainties involved.

Radiation dose and local control

The era of megavoltage radiotherapy began in the 1950s. Radiation oncologists were no longer limited by the toxicity associated with kilovoltage irradiation where maximal dose was delivered to the skin surface. The devices capable of providing beams with energies of millions of electron volts included Van de Graaff generators, radioactive cobalt-60 teletherapy units, Betatrons, and linear accelerators. These high energy machines allowed for treatment of all lymphoid tissue in the body with acceptable normal tissue toxicity. This led to encouraging results in the treatment of Hodgkin's disease.

The curative potential of radiation therapy in Hodgkin's disease had been recognized by several groups prior to the 1950s.[20,21] However, the depth dose characteristics of kilovoltage X-ray beams with maximal surface dose and rapid attenuation in tissue hampered these early investigators' attempts to deliver curative doses to adequate volumes. Modern radiation therapy techniques utilizing high energy machines and complex, multifield treatment planning, optimized dose distribution. This allowed for tumoricidal doses to be delivered to involved areas with tolerable doses to normal tissues. Additionally, dose fractionation was recognized as a highly significant factor in tumour control and normal tissue damage. Early radiation therapists often employed single high dose therapy. Trial and error and unacceptable normal tissue complications led to protracted fractionation schemes. A daily dose of 180–200 cGy delivered in five fractions per week ultimately proved to be highly effective and to have tolerable side-effects.

Another major issue for the radiation oncologist, related to both tumour control and complications, is the volume to be irradiated. If radiation is to be used as a single agent, the irradiated field must include clinically apparent tumour as well as microscopic disease. When defining a course of radiation therapy for a specific patient, the probability of acute and chronic complications must be weighed against tumour control. Optimal therapy is that which provides maximal probability of cure with minimal adverse effects.

The deposition of energy in tissue from radiation is a random event, as is the cell injury which results. The dose–cell death relationship is exponential, i.e. for every increment of radiation dose, the same proportion, not the same number, of cells is killed. Therefore, the total number of surviving cells will be proportional to the initial number present and the fraction killed with that dose of radiation. Thus, various total doses of radiation (assuming comparable fractionation) will result in a different probability of local tumour control based on the inherent radiosensitivity of the tumour, the number of clonogenic cells present in each tumour, and the number of sites involved in each patient. Curves can be generated describing tumour control as a function of radiation dose. Likewise, similarly shaped curves often define the probability of normal tissue damage as a function of radiation dose. The therapeutic ratio is the comparison between tumour control and complication frequency.

Fortunately for most of the lymphomas, the therapeutic ratio is relatively favourable, i.e. the curve for tumour control is to the left of that for normal tissue damage. Kaplan compiled data from numerous studies on the recurrence rates of Hodgkin's disease as a function of radiation dose. At a dose of approximately 4400 cGy delivered in 4–4.5 weeks, only 1.3 per cent true local recurrence was documented. At 1000 cGy or less, 80 per cent probability of local recurrence was documented.[22] There appeared to be no relationship to the risk of failure and the histological subtype of Hodgkin's disease.

In contrast, the non-Hodgkin's lymphomas must be examined by individual histological diagnosis to evaluate dose–response relationships. Even the early report of Peters[1] based on kilovoltage as well as megavoltage data, documented that the diffuse lymphomas, particularly diffuse histiocytic lymphomas, required a considerably higher dose for local control. Peters reported the tumour dose ranges which were successful in preventing local recurrence as follows:

1. 2500 cGy in 2 weeks to 3000 cGy in 4 weeks for 'giant follicular lymphoma'
2. 1500 cGy in 1 week to 4500 cGy in 4 weeks for 'lymphosarcoma'
3. 5000 cGy in 4 weeks for 'reticulum cell sarcoma'.

Substantial data have been published since that time confirming many of these early observations. Dose–response data for the non-Hodgkin's lymphomas have been reviewed by numerous authors.[23–25] Using the histopathological classification of Rappaport, Fuks and Kaplan[26] reported on dose–response relationships in all of the subtypes of the non-Hodgkin's lymphomas. Recurrence was defined as 'the appearance of lymphadenopathy or other evidence of tumour growth in a previously treated involved field as the first new manifestation of lymphoma following an initial course of radiotherapy.'[26]

Evaluating the nodular histologies, at doses of 1500–3500 cGy, recurrence rates were 50 per cent for nodular lymphocytic, poorly differentiated (NLPD), 15 per cent for nodular mixed lymphoma (NML), and 45 per cent for nodular histiocytic lymphoma. At greater than or equal to 4400 cGy, the control was excellent for all of the nodular lymphomas: 94 per cent for NLPD, 97 per cent for NML, and 100 per cent for nodular histiocytic lymphoma. Dose–response data for all of the nodular lymphoma are shown in Fig. 14.1.

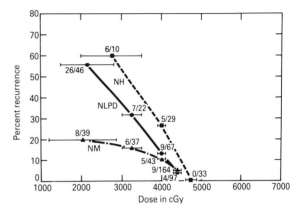

Fig. 14.1 Nodular lymphomas: recurrence rate in radiation treated areas.

Bush and Gospodarowicz[27] confirmed the excellent local control rates in nodular lymphomas. In their pooled data for indolent histology lymphomas treated at the Princess Margaret Hospital, Toronto, local control was compared for fields receiving doses equal to or less than 3450 cGy (average 2715 cGy) and greater than 3450 cGy (average 3787). The control rate was 90 per cent in both low and high dose subgroups except in patients aged 60 years or older with a tumour mass of 2.5 cm or more. Because of the small numbers of failures at any dose level, they did not construct dose–response curves. It is difficult to compare this with the Stanford University data since very few patients at the Princess Margaret Hospital were treated with less than 2000 cGy.

The Stanford University data for local control in diffuse lymphomas are shown in Fig. 14.2.[26] Fuks and Kaplan could not demonstrate a clear

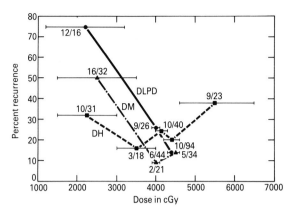

Fig. 14.2 Diffuse lymphomas: recurrence rate in radiation treated areas.

dose–response curve in the diffuse histiocytic lymphomas (DHL). With doses ranging between 1500 and 6500 cGy, recurrence rates were between 21 and 37 per cent . However, many of these patients had advanced disease (stage III and IV). Evaluating patients with stages I and II DHL, the recurrence rate was 19.2 per cent with high dose radiation (greater than 3500 cGy). An increase in local failure was seen with increasingly higher doses (5000–6500 cGy); this paradox relates to a group of particularly unresponsive tumours which were given additional radiation treatment despite failure to respond at a lower dose (4000 cGy). Although they had not responded at 4000 cGy, the majority of such self-selected cases were controlled by administering doses up to 6500 cGy; in chemotherapeutic parlance, they were non-responders. Data from the Princess Margaret Hospital[27,28] show a dose–response curve for DHL with a suggestion of a plateau above 4000–4500 cGy. In stages IA–IIA, they reported control rates of 75–80 per cent with doses of 4000 cGy or greater. It is apparent that DHLs require higher doses for local control, and there are clearly some that are not controlled even with doses greater than 6000 cGy.

Data from Fuks and Kaplan[26] on diffuse lymphocytic, poorly differentiated (DLPD) demonstrated a dose–response curve with a relatively low recurrence rate at 4400 cGy or greater (15 per cent), consistent with the Bush and Gospodarowicz data[29] on DLPD which was

included with their indolent lymphoma group. Bush and Gospodarowicz suggested that although 2500–3000 cGy result in 90 per cent local control in the involved site, the chance of tumour control falls to 81 per cent ($0.9 \times 0.9 \times 100$) when two regions are involved with lymphoma. They therefore recommended a higher dose, approaching normal tissue tolerance, to maximize the chance of control of multiple sites in each patient. This is consistent with the theoretical arguments of Kaplan in his discussion of Hodgkin's disease.[22]

Given the above information on dose–response in the non-Hodgkin's lymphomas, one can better evaluate published data on local control of these tumours when treated with radiation therapy. Data from Fuks *et al.*[30] reveal a high percentage of local control in all histological subtypes except DHL (69 per cent) and nodular histiocytic lymphomas (74 per cent) (Table 14.1). This study involved a review of patients with stages I, II and III lymphomas, all of whom were treated with radiation alone as initial treatment. There are a number of other studies reviewing early stage patients from which one can evaluate the risk of local failure after irradiation. In reviewing the treatment of stages I and II nodular lymphomas with radiation therapy, many studies confirm the high rate of local control. In six major studies reviewing 493 patients with early stage nodular lymphomas[27,30–34] the frequency of local recurrence was only 7 per cent in areas treated with doses ranging from 2000 to 5000 cGy. The majority of patients were treated with 3500 cGy or greater. Six studies evaluating patients with stages IA and IIA DHL and DML included 614 cases.[29,30,35–38] Local failure was 21 per cent with doses ranging from 2500 to 5600 cGy. In 323 patients who received treatment with 4000 cGy or greater, local failure occurred in approximately 11 per cent.

Several papers address the issue of bulky disease and the probability of local control in areas of massive tumour treated with radiation therapy alone. In patients with aggressive histology tumours, predominantly DHL, several studies suggest that relapse is strongly related to size of the tumour in patients treated with radiation therapy. Bush and Gospodarowicz[29]

Table 14.1 Local control of lymph node involvement in patients with malignant lymphoma treated with radiotherapy (3500 cGy or more)

	I	II	III	Total	No. failures in irradiated nodes	Local control of nodal disease(%)
NLPD	11	16	22	49	1	98
NM	9	16	31	56	3	95
NH	4	10	5	19	5	74
DLPD	6	12	7	25 }	5	89
DM	5	9	6	20 }		
DH	13	33	19	65	20	69
	48	96	90	234	34	85

NLPD, nodular lymphocytic poorly differentiated; NM, nodular mixed; NH, nodular histiocytic; DLPD, diffuse lymphocytic poorly differentiated; DM, diffuse mixed; DH, diffuse histiocytic
(Adapted from Fuks *et al.* 1975[29])

reported that local recurrence in DHL less than 2.5 cm is approximately 17 per cent in contrast to 45 per cent in tumours greater than this size. Mauch *et al.*[36] reported no local failures in patients with tumours less than 10 cm in contrast to 43.5 per cent (10/23) in tumours greater than this. Patients in this study received 3500–5600 cGy, with a median of 5000 cGy. There is still considerable controversy about the issue of bulk of tumour as a prognostic factor for survival in DHL patients treated with chemotherapy,[39] but most investigators believe that larger tumour masses inversely correlate with outcome in the aggressive lymphomas.

Correlation with bulk of tumour and local recurrence is more difficult in the favourable histology non-Hodgkin's lymphomas. In data from Princess Margaret Hospital Toronto,[29] relapse-free survival was changed when comparing patients with tumours less than or greater than 2.5 cm (diffuse lymphocytic, well differentiated (DLWD), diffuse lymphoma, intermediate differention (DLID), NLPD, mixed cell (MC), nodular histiocytic (NH)). However, there appeared to be minimal impact on local control. A review of nodular and favourable histology lymphomas, stages I and II, treated with megavoltage irradiation at Stanford University Hospital,[34] reported no difference in survival or freedom from relapse at 5 years in comparing patients with tumours greater than or less than 5 cm.

The issues of dose–reponse, local control, number of sites of disease, and bulk of tumour are all critical in planning radiation therapy for patients with non-Hodgkin's lymphomas. They are essential issues to evaluate when comparing specific protocols. The ability of multiagent chemotherapy to achieve local control of lymphatic involvement is a subject that has been neglected by medical oncologists. Making some assumptions which appear reasonable, one can use the data of Anderson *et al.*[40] to make an estimate of chemotherapy's ability to control disease locally. This estimate is projected to be approximately 35 per cent of all patients who were treated (Table 14.2), although it should be acknowledged that the regimens used belonged to the first and second generations of chemotherapy protocols for non-Hodgkin's lymphomas. Nonetheless, it should also be noted that long-term data showing a clear superiority for today's regimens over these are lacking. It is precisely because local control with drugs alone is so low and because the typical sites of failure in irradiated patients are outside the portals of treatment that the authors believe more studies of combined modality treatment are indicated.

Table 14.2 Local control of lymph node involvement in patients with malignant lymphoma treated with C-MOPP, CVP or BACOP

	No.	No. CR	No. not relapsed	
NLPD	49	33	12	81% of relapses (37 of 46) occurred only in lymph nodes, virtually always previously involved
NM	31	24	20	
NH	4	3	0	
DLWD	11	7	2	
DLPD	25	7	1	Estimate of local lymph node control in this series is 61 + 9 = 70 patients of 199 patients (35%)
DM	10	1	1	
DH	62	29	23	
DU	7	3	2	
	199	107 (54%)	61	

NLPD, nodular lymphocytic poorly differentiated; NM, nodular mixed; NH, nodular histiocytic; DLWD, diffuse lymphocytic well differentiated; DLPD, diffuse lymphocytic poorly differentiated; DM, diffuse mixed; DH, diffuse histiocytic; DU, diffuse undifferentiated; C-MOPP, cyclophosphamide, vincristine, procarbazine, prednisone; CVP, cyclophosphamide, vincristine, prednisone; BACOP, bleomycin, adriamycin, cyclophosphamide, vincristine, prednisone (Adapted from Anderson *et al.* 1977[38]).

Dose fractionation

Dose fractionation has been studied in many patients with Hodgkin's disease.[41–43] Several groups have reported similar results. The method involved plotting a scatter diagram, each point representing an instance of local control or recurrence of lymphoma in a field treated with a specified dose in a specified number of days. From such diagrams, regression curves may be described to obtain an estimate of the lowest total dose of irradiation, delivered over a defined time interval, at which few local recurrences would be expected. The curves for Hodgkin's disease indicate greater than 95 per cent probability for local control with doses of 4000–4300 cGy in 40 days. Other fractionation schemes yielded the same probability of control: 2500–3200 cGy in 10 days, 2900–3900 in 30 days. These data were consistent with clinical studies demonstrating high rates of local control with 4000–4400 cGy.

There are fewer dose fractionation data available for the non-Hodgkin's lymphomas. Time–dose scattergrams were reported by Cox *et al.*[44] for 131 patients with lymphoreticular malignancies. They described isoeffect lines as essentially flat at 2200 cGy for the nodular and 4200 cGy for the diffuse lymphomas. They noted that small tumours were as likely to recur as large at a given dose level and that fractionation did appear to be critical. These and other time–dose data on the non-Hodgkin's lymphomas suggest that total dose was the most important variable in control of these malignancies. The problems in determining optimal dose with these retrospective data are that:

1. fractionation schemes have generally been disregarded.
2. lower doses have generally been used only when regression of the tumour mass was marked.
3. quantification of tumour bulk has generally been neglected. Obviously persistent disease has usually received additional doses.

Local control has been reported with radiation schemes ranging from single fractions of 800–1000 cGy, to multiple 15 cGy fractions, to a total of 150 cGy as delivered with total body irradiation. As discussed under issues of dose–response, excellent local control can be obtained in both the nodular and diffuse lymphomas with treatment of 3500–5000 cGy. One of the major issues in deciding on a fractionation scheme is normal tissue tolerance. Normal tissue damage is greatly influenced by varying fractionation schemes. Late sequelae appear to be substantially more severe in patients receiving a large dose per fraction. Standard therapy regimens utilize 180–200 cGy per fraction delivered five times per week. These have proved to be highly effective in the treatment of the non-Hodgkin's lymphomas, especially of non-large cell histologies, with excellent local control and acceptable normal tissue toxicity.

Radiation volume

The non-Hodgkin's lymphomas have been treated with radiation therapy fields ranging from small fields delivered to sites of clinically apparent disease to total body irradiation. One must consider the histological subtype, the stage of disease, and obviously whether the goal is curative or palliative when determining the extent of the treatment fields. As a palliative modality, irradiation may be extremely effective when delivered to sites of tumour involvement causing symptoms. One must consider whether contiguous sites of disease might require palliative radiation therapy in the future and plan for potential match areas between radiation fields. If prior treatment dose has been low, one can also consider re-irradiation of previous fields. In the curative approach to the non-Hodgkin's lymphomas with radiation, considerable controversy still exists with respect to the volume to be treated.

Definition of terms is essential in evaluating the literature on irradiation of lymphomas. Involved field radiotherapy refers to treatment limited only to involved lymph node chains. Extended field includes treatment of any apparently uninvolved lymphatic regions which are contiguous to sites of involvement. Therapy to all major lymph node areas is referred to as total nodal irradiation. Total lymphoid

irradiation will cover additional areas such as Waldeyer's ring, the spleen, and mesenteric nodes. Total body irradiation can be given by a number of techniques to deliver treatment to all body tissues, using low doses of radiation as a 'spray'.

Critical to the theoretical approach to field size is evaluation of sites of relapse in the non-Hodgkin's lymphomas. Fuks *et al.*[30] reviewed 234 patients with stages I, II, and III non-Hodgkin's lymphomas treated initially with radiation therapy alone. Patients received either involved field or extended field irradiation for stages I and II. Total nodal irradiation was most commonly used in the management of stage III disease. In spite of a significant pattern of involvement of contiguous lymph node areas at presentation (79 per cent), relatively few patients failed only in adjacent nodal sites (32 per cent). Eighty per cent of initial failures of the stages I and II nodular lymphoma patients were in lymph nodes with 47 per cent failing in non-contiguous nodes and 33 per cent in contiguous nodes. Thirteen per cent failed in extralymphatic sites and 7 per cent involved both lymphatic and extralymphatic extension. In the diffuse histology lymphomas, 43 per cent of patients failed in extralymphatic sites: 21 per cent failing in extralymphatic sites alone and 22 per cent in conjunction with lymphatic sites. Fifty-seven per cent failed in lymphatic sites; 30 per cent failed in contiguous nodal areas and 27 per cent non-contiguous. Thus, unlike Hodgkin's disease, where 80 per cent of nodal relapses occurred within contiguous nodal areas, non-Hodgkin's lymphomas showed a more random pattern of relapse. Obviously extranodal extension was an important pattern of relapse, but nodal relapse was even more frequent in the Stanford series.

Other data have confirmed a relatively moderate risk of contiguous spread in patients treated with radiation therapy. In data from Yale University, Chen *et al.*[31] reported on 114 patients with clinically staged I and II non-Hodgkin's lymphoma. Contiguous nodal relapse was not documented in any patient with nodular histology. There were four true recurrences in the patients with diffuse histologies and no other contiguous nodal relapses. Non-contiguous nodal disease accounted for 75 per cent (six of eight) of the relapses in nodular lymphoma patients and 13 per cent (four of 30) in diffuse histology patients. Sixty-three per cent of all failures involved extralymphatic sites. Part of the discrepancy in these data may be explained by the fact that transdiaphragmatic spread via the thoracic duct was considered non-contiguous by Chen *et al.* and contiguous by Fuks *et al.*, if the left neck was felt to be involved. The critical issue to the radiotherapist is whether increasing the volume of irradiated nodal tissue can result in improved survival in these patients. To a large degree, the answer depends on histology, because chemotherapeutic efficacy with curative intent is dramatically histology dependent.

Early stage low grade lymphomas

In a retrospective review of data from Stanford University, Paryani *et al.*[34] evaluated 124 patients with stages I and II favourable histology (low grade) lymphomas who were treated with involved, extended, or total lymphoid irradiation. Dose ranged from 3500 to 5000 cGy. With a median follow-up of 5.5 years, there were no significant differences in survival among the three treatment groups. Total lymphoid irradiation demonstrated significantly better freedom from relapse than either involved field or extended field. More prolonged follow-up is certainly needed to evaluate long-term results in these patients, but follow-up to 15 years showed an actuarial freedom from relapse at 50 per cent.

Attempting more precisely to define optimal treatment volume in early stage favourable histology patients, investigators at Stanford are presently conducting a prospective randomized study. Patients in this trial have stages I and II NLPD or NML and are surgically staged. They are randomized to receive involved field or total lymphoid irradiation. Data on the first 20 patients entered on this protocol reveal no statistical difference in survival or freedom from relapse. It is apparent that the issue of volume to be irradiated is still unresolved.

There are a number of reports evaluating laparotomy-staged I and II nodular lymphoma

patients treated with radiation therapy to only one side of the diaphragm which confirm the Stanford 5-year survival in these patients: Stanford – 84 per cent;[34] Toonkel *et al.* – 87 per cent;[38] McLaughlin *et al.* – 74 per cent;[45] Lawrence *et al.* – 78 per cent;[33] Monfardini *et al.* – 62 per cent;[46]. Other studies reveal similarly high 5-year survival rates in clinically staged I and II favourable lymphoma patients: Chen *et al.* – 83 per cent;[31] Bush *et al.* – 72 per cent;[28] Reddy *et al.* – 91 per cent;[47] Timothy *et al.* – 77 per cent;[48] Peckham *et al.* – 75 per cent.[49] Because of the retrospective nature of most of these reports, the variability in staging procedures, the differences in treatment fields and dose, and the limited follow-up, it is difficult to determine the optical treatment volume for irradiation in the indolent lymphomas. Nonetheless, there are considerable data to suggest that treatment of involved nodal regions and contiguous clinically uninvolved areas is curative in approximately one-half of the patients with indolent histology lymphomas of stage I and II extent. It remains to be established whether total nodal irradiation or the addition of chemotherapy, as suggested by several authors, will ultimately improve the survival in this group of patients. It is important to realize that at present, no curative chemotherapeutic regimen has been demonstrated for these histologies.

Early stage, intermediate and high grade lymphomas

The issues of radiation volume in early stage aggressive lymphomas are also unresolved. With a greater percentage of aggressive histology patients presenting with stages I and II than in the indolent lymphomas, it is particularly important in this subset of patients to determine if irradiation alone is an appropriate treatment option. Several studies have evaluated radiation therapy in pathologically staged patients with stages I and II diffuse aggressive lymphomas.

Sweet *et al.*[36] reported on 28 pathologically staged patients; 14 were stage I or I$_E$, 14 were stage II or II$_E$. Treatment varied from involved field to total nodal irradiation. Patients with stage I supradiaphragmatic lymph node disease achieved a 93 per cent 11-year actuarial disease-free survival. Patients with stage II or II$_E$ achieved a 33 per cent 11-year actuarial disease-free survival. Toonkel *et al.*[38] reviewed a small number of pathologically staged patients: nine of 12 patients with stage I or I$_E$ DHL remained disease free in contrast to one of three with stage II or II$_E$. Because of the apparent differences in stage I and stage II patients, it is more difficult to interpret data in which these patients are considered as a single group. In a more recent report from the M.D. Anderson Hospital, Houston, Texas, Lester *et al.* reviewed 31 patients with large cell lymphoma (23 with stage I or I$_E$, eight with II or II$_E$) who were treated with radiation therapy alone.[50] Disease-free survival was 62 per cent and overall survival after salvage was 88 per cent. Kaminski *et al.*[51] reviewed 121 patients treated with primary radiation therapy; 38 per cent had stage I or I$_E$ and 62 per cent had stage II or II$_E$. Of this series, 72 patients received limited field irradiation, defined as treatment to one side of the diaphragm, either involved or extended field. Five-year survival was 35 per cent and five-year freedom from relapse was 25 per cent. With extensive irradiation, either subtotal or total lymphoid, five-year survival and freedom from relapse were both 67 per cent. These results were similar to comparable patients treated at Stanford during the same time period receiving limited irradiation plus adjuvant chemotherapy with survival and freedom from relapse at 68 per cent and 65 per cent respectively.

There are numerous reports of clinically staged patients with aggressive lymphomas, predominantly diffuse histiocytic, describing survival after treatment with radiation therapy alone. In six studies in which stage I and stage II patients were evaluated separately,[31,32,35,47,49,52] relapse-free survival in stage I patients ranged from 35 to 65 per cent with an average of approximately 58 per cent. In stage II patients, the data revealed relapse-free survival ranging from 0 to 47 per cent with an average of 26 per cent. These data must be compared with studies evaluating chemotherapy alone or in combination with radiation. Three studies have addressed this in a randomized fashion with a mixed population of stage I and II patients and reported improvement in relapse-free as well as survival data in patients treated with combination irradiation and chemotherapy when compared to irradiation alone.[46,52,53] Several studies have also demonstrated excellent disease-free and overall survival in patients treated with chemotherapy alone.[54,55] With the controversy concerning prognostic factors and the difficulty in stratifying patients, comparison among trials has been problematic. Ongoing trials may further define optimal treatment strategies for these early stage aggressive lymphoma patients. At the present time, however, it appears reasonable to treat patients with aggressive histology lymphomas of stage I or II with chemotherapy. The case for radiation as well is suggestive but not clearly established.

Advanced stage low grade lymphomas

Defining the radiation volume has been primarily of concern in the early stage non-Hodgkin's lymphomas where irradiation has played a major role in the curative approach to treatment. However, for the nodular lymphomas, a significant percentage of advanced stage patients have lymph node failure as their only site of relapse. In these initially stage III patients, perhaps radiation to the majority of lymph node areas may also have curative potential. In 1976, Glatstein *et al.*[56] and Cox *et al.*[23] evaluated the role of total lymphoid irradiation in patients with stage III indolent lymphomas. With a median follow-up of 80 months, the series from Stanford University demonstrated 75 per cent survival at five years and 68 per cent at 10 years. The relapse-free survival rates were 43 per cent and 33 per cent at five and 10 years respectively. These figures appear to compare favourably with chemotherapy, since 10-year figures, free of relapse, are virtually impossible to find in the literature. Interestingly, of the 28 patients with nodular lymphomas who failed after total nodal irradiation radiation therapy, 64 per cent (18/28) had their initial relapse confined to lymph nodes; five were intra-abdominal and six were epitrochlear or brachial. This would suggest that increasing the volume of treatment to include these areas might improve results. Cox's total central lymphatic irradiation included whole abdomen but not epitrochlear nodes. As in the Stanford technique, Waldeyer's ring was treated in most of the patients. Survival and relapse-free survival as reported by Cox were 78 per cent and 61 per cent respectively, with a 6-year median period of observation. Because of the long natural history of these lymphomas (median survival of 8 years), additional follow-up is necessary to determine whether this approach will result in cure of some stage III nodular lymphoma patients. Certainly with the excellent complete response (100 per cent and 97 per cent) and local control rates obtained with irradiation, new treatment modalities for this subset of patients must compare favourably with patients treated with total lymphoid irradiation.

Advanced stage, intermediate and high grade lymphomas

For stages III and IV aggressive histology patients, the main thrust of treatment is chemotherapy alone, with radiotherapy presently reserved for dealing with symptomatic local problems that do not respond to multi-agent drug therapy.

Total body irradiation

The final issue regarding volume of radiation to be discussed is that of total body radiation therapy. Because of the extreme sensitivity of the lymphomas to radiation, the possibility of using radiation as a 'systemic agent', i.e. total body radiation, was considered. Early reports of response of lymphomas to this therapy,[57] led the National Cancer Institute to initiate a randomized prospective study in 1968 comparing extensive radiation therapy (11/49, extended total nodal irradiation and 38/49, total body irradiation) to combination chemotherapy (cyclophosphamide, vincristine, prednisone (CVP) or cyclophosphamide, vincristine, procar-

bazine, prednisone (C-MOPP) for poorly differentiated lymphocytic lymphomas. The complete response rate for nodular lymphomas treated with radiation (33 patients: 25 NPDL, eight NML) was 85 per cent and for diffuse lymphomas (eight DPDL) was 69 per cent. For chemotherapy-treated patients, the complete response rate for nodular and diffuse lymphomas were 62 per cent and 13 per cent respectively. Long-term survival and relapse-free survival were almost identical for patients treated with either radiation or chemotherapy. In spite of the excellent response of these tumours to radiation, only 20 per cent of patients remained continuously free of disease at four years. A second NCI trial compared C-MOPP alone to C-MOPP and total body irradiation. Both regimens had an excellent response rate without an advantage to the combined modality arm, but only 50 per cent of patients were disease free at two years, data which are similar to most series reported with multiagent chemotherapy.

Numerous other studies have evaluated total body irradiation in advanced non-Hodgkin's lymphoma. The data from all of these reports are similar. The complete response rate was approximately 81 per cent in nodular lymphomas and 70 per cent in the diffuse lymphomas.[58-61] Five-year survival is 68 per cent in the nodular lymphoma patients and 50 per cent in diffuse lymphoma patients and corresponding relapse-free survival is 25 per cent and 16 per cent. Stanford University data[62] comparing total body irradiation with either single agent or combination chemotherapy, revealed no significant advantage to any approach in the favourable histology lymphomas. There appeared to be no plateau on the survival curve even at 10 years.

It is unlikely that total body irradiation represents a curative approach to favourable or unfavourable histology lymphomas. In indolent lymphomas, it has been successful in obtaining complete responses and offering survival comparable to chemotherapy regimens. Thus, it may have a role in initial treatment of such patients who are not good candidates for chemotherapy or decline chemotherapy. In advanced stage aggressive histology lymphomas, combination chemotherapy offers cure to many patients, and combined modality protocols are being investigated.

Summary

The role of radiation therapy in management of the non-Hodgkin's lymphomas remains largely undefined. Other chapters in this book discuss the specific subtypes of these lymphomas and the therapeutic options available for them. We have tried to discuss the critical issues related to the use of radiation in these lymphomas: dose–response and local control, time-dose-fractionation, and radiation volume.

It is apparent that simple extrapolation from the therapy approaches for Hodgkin's disease will not be effective in this heterogeneous group of nodal and extranodal lymphomas with multiple histological subtypes. Even the staging system used for the non-Hodgkin's lymphomas was developed for Hodgkin's disease and may not be relevant with respect to the prognostic indicators in the non-Hodgkin's lymphomas.

Virtually all the non-Hodgkin's lymphomas are sensitive to ionizing radiation; local control rates are excellent. Relapse is almost exclusively in untreated areas when doses above 3500–5000 cGy are delivered. This is in marked contrast to patients treated with multiagent chemotherapy where nodal failure in sites of previous disease is common. Additional investigation of combined modality treatment seems a critical issue.

There are relatively few tumours as sensitive to both radiation therapy and chemotherapy as the non-Hodgkin's lymphomas. Future studies may better define the optimal sequencing and integration of these agents in the curative approach to these tumours.

References

1. Peters MV, *American Journal of Roentgenology*. 1963; **5**, 956–67.
2. Veronesi U, Musumeci R, Pizzetti F, Gennari L, Bonadonna G. *Cancer* 1974; **33**, 446–59.
3. Rosenberg SA, Kaplan HS. *Cancer Research*. 1966; **31**, 1225–31.
4. Kaplan HS. *Cancer Research*.1966; **26**, 1221–4.
5. Rosenberg SA. *Cancer Research*. 1966; **26**, 1310.
6. Carbone PP, Kaplan HS, Smithers DW, Tubiana M. *Cancer Research*. 1971; **31**, 1860–1.
7. Castellani R, Bonadonna G, Spinelli P. *et al. Cancer*. 1977; **40**, 2322–8.
8. Chabner BA, Johnson RE, Young RC, *et al. Annals of Interal Medicine*. 1976; **85**, 149–54.
9. Goffinet DR, Castellino RA, Kim H, *et al. Cancer*. 1973; **32**, 672–81.
10. Non-Hodgkin's Lymphoma Pathologic Classification Project. *Cancer*. 1982; **49**, 2112–35.
11. National Cancer Institute Non-Hodgkin's Classification Project Writing Committee. *Cancer*. 1985; **55**, 91–5.
12. Kim H, Hendrickson MR, Dorfman RF. *Cancer*. 1977; **40**, 959–76.
13. Mead GM, Kushlan P, O'Neil M, Burke JS, Rosenberg SA. *Cancer*. 1983; **52**, 1496–1501.
14. Warnke RA, Kim H, Fuks Z, Dorfman RF. *Cancer*. 1977; **40**, 1229–33.
15. Fisher RI, Jones RB, DeVita VT, *et al. Cancer*. 1981; **47**, 2022–5.
16. Acker B, Hoppe RT, Colby TV, Cox RS, Kaplan HS, Rosenberg SA. *Journal of Clinical Oncology*. 1983; **1**, 11–16.
17. Garvin AJ, Simon RM, Osborne CK, Merrill J, Young RC, Berard CW. *Cancer*. 1983; **52**, 393–8.
18. Hubbard SM, Chabner BA, DeVita VT, *et al. Blood*. 1982; **59**, 258–64.
19. Easson EC, Russell MH. *British Medical Journal*. 1963; **1**, 1704–97.
20. Peters MV. *American Journal of Roentgenology*. 1950; **63**, 299–311.
21. Kaplan HS. In: *Harvey Lectures 1968–1969*. New York: Academic Press, 1970.
22. Cox JD, Komaki R, Kun LE, Wilson JF, Greenberg M. *Cancer*. 1981; **47**, 2247–52.
23. Newall J, Freidman M. *Radiology*. 1970; **94**, 643–7.
24. Seydel HG, Bloedorn FG, Wizenberg M. *et al. Radiology*. 1971; **98**, 411–18.
25. Fuks Z, Kaplan HS. *Radiology*. 1973; **108**, 675–84.
26. Bush RS, Gospodarowicz M. *Radiation Therapy*. 1982; **28**, 485–502.
27. Bush RS, Gospodarowicz M, Sturgeon J, Alison R. *Cancer Treatment Reports*. 1977; **61**(6), 1129–36.
28. Bush RS, Gospodarowicz M. In: Rosenberg SA, Kaplan HS (Eds). *Malignant Lymphomas*. London: Academic Press, 1982; 485–502.
29. Fuks Z, Glatstein E, Kaplan HS. *British Journal of Cancer*. 1975; **31**, 286–97.
30. Chen MG, Prosnitz LR, Gonzalez-Serva A, Fisher DB. *Cancer*. 1979; **43**, 1245–54.
31. Hagberg H, Glimelius B, Sundstrom C. *Acta Radiologica*. 1972; **21**, 145–50.

32. Lawrence T, Urba W, Steinberg S, Sundeen J, Cossman J, Young R, Glatstein E. *Prognostic Factors for Stage I and II Indolent Lymphomas.* (unpublished data)
33. Paryani SB, Hoppe RT, Cox RS, *et al. Cancer.* 1983; **52**, 2300–7.
34. Kun LE, Cox JD, Komaki R. *Radiology.* 1981; **141**, 791–94.
35. Mauch P, Leonard R, Skarin A, Rosenthal D, Come S, Chaffey J, Hellman S, Canellos G. *Journal of Clinical Oncology.* 1985; **3** (10), 1301–8.
36. Sweet DL, Kinzie J, Gacke ME, Golomb HM, Ferguson DL, Ultmann JE. *Blood.* 1981; **58**, 1218–23.
37. Toonkel LM, Fuller LM, Gamble JF, *et al. Cancer.* 1980; **45**, 249–60.
38. Anderson T, Bender RA, Fisher RI, *et al. Cancer Treatment Reports.* 1977; **61**, 1057–66.
39. Friedman M, Pearlman AW, Turgeon L. *American Journal of Roentgenology.* 1967; **99**, 843–50.
40. Scott RM, Brizel HE. *Radiology.* 1964; **52**, 1043–9.
41. Seydel HG, Bloedorn FG, Wizenberg MJ. *Radiology.* 1967; **89**, 919–22.
42. Cox JD, Koehl RH, Turner WM, King FM. *Radiology.* 1974; **112**, 179–85.
43. McLaughlin P, Fuller LM, *et al. Cancer.* 1986; **58**, 1596–1602.
44. Monfardini S, Banfi A, Bonadonna G, *et al. International Journal of Radiation, Oncology, Biology and Physics.* 1980; **6**, 125–34.
45. Reddy S, Saxena VS, Pellettiere EV, Hendrickson FR. *Cancer.* 1977; **40**, 98–104.
46. Timothy AR, Lister TA, Katz D, Jones AE. *European Journal of Cancer.* 1979; **16**, 799–807.
47. Peckham MJ, Guay JP, Hamlin ME, Lukes RJ. *British Journal of Cancer.* 1975; **31**, 413–24.
48. Lester JN, Fuller LM, Conrad FG, Sullivan JA, Velasquez WS, Butler JJ, Shullenberger CC. *Cancer.* 1982; **49**, 1746–53.
49. Kaminski MS, Coleman CN, Colby TV, Cox RS, Rosenberg SA. *Annals of Internal Medicine.* 1986; **104**, 747–56.
50. Nissen NI, Ersboll J, Hansen HS, Walbom-Jorgensen S, Pedersen-Bjergaard J, Hensen MM, Rygard J. *Cancer.* 1983; **52**, 1–7.
51. Landberg TG, Hakansson LG, Moller TR, *et al. Cancer.* 1979; **44**, 831–8.
52. Cabanillas F, Bodey GP, Freireich EJ. *Cancer.* 1980; **46**, 2356–9.
53. Miller TP, Jones SE, *Blood.* 1983; **62** (2), 413–18.
54. Glatstein E, Fuks Z, Goffinet RD, Kaplan HS. *Cancer.* 1976; **37**, 2806–12.
55. Cox JD. *International Journal of Radiation, Oncology, Biology and Physics.* 1976; **1**, 491–6.
56. Young RC, Johnson RE, Cannellos GP, Chabner BA, Brereton HD, Berard CW, DeVita VT. *Cancer Treatment Reports.* 1977; **61**; 1153–9.
57. Brereton HD, Young RC, Longo DL, *et al. Cancer.* 1979; **43**, 2227–31.
58. Chaffey JT, Hellman S, Rosenthal DS, Moloney WC. *Cancer Treatment Reports.* 1977; **61**, 1149–52.
59. Chaffey JT, Rosenthal DS, Moloney WC, Hellman S. *International Journal of Radiation, Oncology, Biology and Physics.* 1976; **1**, 399–405.
60. Hoppe RT, Kushlan P, Kaplan HS, Rosenberg SA, Brown BW. *Blood.* 1981; **58** (3), 592–8.
61. Thar TL, Million RR, Noyes WD. *International Journal of Radiation, Oncology, Biology and Physics.* 1979; **5**, 171–6.
62. Choi NC, Timothy AR, Kaufman SD, Carey RW, Aisenberg AC. *Cancer.* 1979; **43**, 1636–42.
63. Glatstein E, Donaldson SS, Rosenberg SA, Kaplan HS. *Cancer Treatment Reports.* 1977; **61**, 1199–1207.

CHAPTER 15

COMPLICATIONS IN THE MANAGEMENT OF NON-HODGKIN'S LYMPHOMA

Francisco Barriga, Ian Magrath and Wyndham Wilson

As for all cancer, the management of the non-Hodgkin's lymphomas (NHL) entails the administration of specific therapy and the treatment of the multiple complications which may arise, either from the disease itself or as unwanted side-effects of treatment. Complications may arise acutely – before or during therapy – or may occur months or years after treatment. Familiarity with such complications is essential if they are to be prevented or treated effectively. The greater the likelihood of long-term survival, the more important become delayed effects such as impaired or uneven growth in children, effects on reproductive function and second malignancies. Although the NHLs comprise a diverse group of tumours, with respect to both their biological and clinical behaviour, they share many of the same complications, since sites of involvement and treatment approaches to the various lymphomas frequently have much in common. Moreover, while NHLs differ from many other cancers with regard to their more rapid growth rate, particularly in the case of intermediate and high grade lymphomas, many of the complications encountered occur in cancer patients in general.

The complications of cancer management can be divided into four broad categories:

1. those related to space-occupying lesions, i.e. complications arising from tumours with the potential to compress or invade surrounding structures, or to cause bleeding or exudation into a cavity (e.g. superior vena caval obstruction, gastrointestinal bleeding, meningeal lymphomatosis)
2. those resulting from 'distant' effects of the tumour on the host (e.g. metabolic complications, paraneoplastic syndromes)
3. acute consequences of therapy (e.g. the rapid tumour lysis syndrome or side-effects of chemotherapy or radiation)
4. late complications of therapy (e.g. growth abnormalities, infertility and second tumours).

This chapter deals primarily with complications that are pertinent to NHL, and will not address the immediate complications of chemotherapy and radiotherapy, or the late complications of specific drugs.

Complications related to space-occupying lesions

An important characteristic of lymphomas is their rapid growth rate, which often leads to the acute onset and rapid progression of complications arising from space-occupying lesions. Since lymphomas can arise in essentially all organs and tissues, and can progress very rapidly, the diagnosis of NHL must be entertained and established (or refuted) as rapidly as possible, particularly in the presence of a tumour mass in a vulnerable site such as the mediastinum or central nervous system (CNS). However, even emergency treatment should not be commenced, except in life-threatening situations, without obtaining adequate material for diagnostic purposes, since a rapid response to therapy could lead to failure to establish the correct diagnosis, thus depriving the patient of optimal therapy. Sites of disease that are easily accessible (i.e. lymph nodes, subcutaneous tumours, serous effusions, bone marrow and cerebrospinal fluid) should be biopsied or aspirated, thus avoiding risky surgical procedures that could create additional complications.

In addition, and partly because of their higher than average growth rate, lymphomas differ from most other malignancies in that they are extremely sensitive to chemotherapeutic agents and/or radiation. The choice of the most appropriate therapeutic modality to deal with mass lesions on an emergency basis can thus be difficult, and is dependent upon the nature of the complication and the type of tumour. Radiation therapy has been traditionally used to treat space-occupying lesions and the recognition that this modality has a limited role in modern lymphoma therapy, coupled with the very high response rate of untreated lymphomas to chemotherapy – the major component of all treatment regimens – and the additional toxicity incurred by combined modality therapy, has led to a greater willingness to use chemotherapy rather than radiotherapy in emergency situations. There is no evidence that the rapidity of response to chemotherapy differs from that to radiation.

CNS involvement

Lymphomatous infiltration or compression of nervous tissue by a discrete mass can occur in all parts of the nervous system including the leptomeninges, cranial nerves, brain, spinal cord and peripheral nerves. Lymphomatous masses arising from extradural locations (e.g. skull, orbit, nasopharynx, paraspinal) may also impinge upon adjacent nervous tissue. The signs and symptoms of nervous system involvement can therefore be extremely diverse and include relatively non-specific, though potentially serious symptoms, such as headache, backache or seizures. Sometimes, more definite features of raised intracranial pressure such as papilloedema, bradycardia and vomiting are present, and localizing signs such

as motor weakness and sensory changes may also be observed.

Examination of the cerebrospinal fluid (CSF) is especially helpful in establishing a diagnosis of meningeal lymphoma and should always be performed at the commencement of treatment except in the presence of an intracranial lesion which may have the potential to induce herniation of intracranial structures through the tentorium cerebelli or foramen magnum. Primary diffuse infiltration of the cerebral parenchyma can be difficult to diagnose and often presents with generalized neurological deterioration and seizures, although there may also be localizing signs. The possibility that these symptoms and signs could be due to intracranial haemorrhage, particularly in a patient who deteriorates neurologically while undergoing therapy (especially if thrombocytopenic), should be considered, since the management of such a patient would be quite different. Lymphomatous leptomeningitis usually responds well to intrathecal chemotherapy (via lumbar puncture or Ommaya reservoir) with methotrexate or cytarabine, or to high dose systemic administration of these drugs. Cranial irradiation may also be used in some circumstances and high dose corticosteroids are given in the presence of raised intracranial pressure.

Spinal cord compression

Although spinal cord compression from epidural lymphoma is not a common complication of NHL, the malignant lymphomas are one of the most common causes of spinal cord compression. In 15 of 96 patients who underwent laminectomy for spinal cord compression in a recent series,[1] the underlying tumour was lymphoma. All 15 cases were previously untreated and four had disease confined to the epidural region. This complication has been reported as a late manifestation of NHL but is more often a presenting feature; in a series of 72 patients with spinal cord compression from NHL, 85 per cent were undiagnosed before the compression occurred.[2] Patients may have rapidly or more slowly progressive symptoms, depending upon the growth rate of the lymphoma and may present with back pain, paraesthesias and/or weakness of the lower extremities, with complete paralysis and loss of sphincter control in the most severe cases. Patients with the most rapidly growing tumours can develop painless paraplegia within hours, and delays in treatment may result in irreversible neurological damage, so that suspected paraspinal disease requires immediate evaluation and treatment. Occasionally, infarction of the cord may occur, due to compression of the spinal arteries, and such patients are unlikely to recover function.

Metrizamide myelography is currently the preferred procedure for the evaluation of patients with spinal cord compression (CSF can be obtained at the same time as the procedure). Although magnetic resonance imaging (MRI), particularly with gadolinium DTPA, may eventually replace contrast myelography as the method of choice for accurate determination of the level of the block. In the absence of other sites of tumour, laminectomy is required to establish a histological diagnosis.

Radiotherapy to the spine is the most commonly employed therapy for spinal cord compression. High dose steroids (dexamethosone) are given to reduce local oedema and hopefully lessen the degree of compression, and they may also exert a lympholytic effect. Therapeutic laminectomy may be necessary in some patients when there is recurrence in a previouly irradiated region.[3] Chemotherapy has also been used to treat spinal cord compression[4] and is probably as effective or more effective than radiotherapy in tumours which are highly chemosensitive, such as Burkitt's lymphoma (which is also relatively radioresistant), lymphoblastic lymphoma and intermediate grade lymphomas. The avoidance of radiation, where possible, has the advantage of not adding to myelosuppression because of irradiation of vertebral bone marrow. This is not a minor consideration in tumours where chemotherapy provides the only real chance of a cure. Usually, systemic chemotherapy is commenced during spinal column irradiation in patients with lymphoma who present with spinal cord compression.

Superior vena caval obstruction and mediastinal masses

Obstruction of the superior vena cava (SVC) is a well-recognized complication of lymphomas of the anterior superior mediastinum. In adults, NHL is the second most frequent cause of SVC obstruction after bronchogenic carcinoma. A review of three large series of patients with SVC obstruction caused by a malignant neoplasm[5-7] showed that 12–21 per cent of the 215 patients had lymphoma. Conversely, 3–8 per cent of patients with lymphoma present with SVC obstruction and most of these will have NHL.[8] Among children, NHL is the most frequent neoplastic cause of SVC obstruction. The anatomy of the SVC, with its thin wall and close apposition to the vertebral column, makes it particularly vulnerable to compression or invasion by malignancies arising in the mediastinum. Prolonged compression and invasion frequently result in thrombosis and complete occlusion of the vein, although lymphomas, being less invasive and more rapidly growing than carcinomas, more often cause compression without thrombosis.[9] The degree and rapidity of obstruction determine the severity of the symptoms and signs, while these are offset by the development of an effective collateral circulation. The wide spectrum of clinical features include swelling of face, neck and arms with prominence of collateral veins, shortness of breath, orthopnoea, dizziness, headache, dysphagia, epistaxis, altered mental status and syncope associated with bending.[5,9-11] The appearance of a pleural effusion often indicates simultaneous obstruction of the thoracic duct, although direct involvement of the pleura is also likely. The presence of laryngeal and/or cerebral oedema has often been stated to indicate a poor prognosis in patients with SVC obstruction,[5,6] but these complications are rare and have not been clearly shown to be an immediate consequence of SVC obstruction rather than of direct invasion of airways or brain by tumour.[12] In addition, the prognosis of patients with SVC obstruction relates more to the nature of the causal neoplasm than to the magnitude of symptomatology.

Diagnostic procedures should include a chest

X-ray to demonstrate a mediastinal mass or mediastinal widening. A peripheral venogram or technetium-99m flow study may be performed to determine the patency of the venous system as well as the development and efficiency of collateral circulation, but this is likely to be of limited practical value. A computed tomographic (CT) scan of the chest may be performed to determine more accurately the extent of the tumour as well as to plan the best approach for a biopsy and, where appropriate, the radiation fields to be employed. It is wise to avoid biopsy of a mediastinal mass if possible because of the relative inaccessibility and the potential for complications.

When present, more accessible sites of disease, such as peripheral lymph nodes or a pleural effusion, should be sought for diagnosis, and the bone marrow should be examined. If the tumour is confined to the mediastinum, however, then biopsy via a mediastinoscope or parasternal mediastinotomy is warranted. Mediastinoscopy provides better access to paratracheal masses, while mediastinotomy is the procedure of choice for anterior mediastinal tumours.[9] Patients with mediastinal masses are at higher risk of developing complications during the induction of anaesthesia or the surgical procedure itself, increased bleeding and occasional fatalities have occurred. In consequence, some authors have recommended therapy with corticosteroids (which may induce only minimal shrinkage) or mediastinal radiotherapy before performing a biopsy.[13] However, complications of biopsy of a mediastinal mass are rare, occurring in six patients among 132 subjected to thoracotomy or mediastinoscopy in collected series from the literature.[12] Since treatment prior to biopsy may prevent the establishment of a definitive diagnosis and therefore the employment of optimal therapy, the institution of therapy without the establishment of a definitive tissue diagnosis can be justified only in life-threatening situations, e.g. when there is respiratory obstruction.

Clearly, in patients with a lymphoma causing SVC obstruction, it is appropriate to institute treatment expeditiously. It is worth pointing out, however, that the presence of SVC obstruction itself does not appear to be life-threatening. Ligation of the SVC in dogs is not fatal, and symptoms abate in one week.[12] Fatalities due to the venous obstruction *per se*, have not been indisputably demonstrated in the literature and patients have survived for as long as 28 years with unrelieved SVC obstruction.[12] Indeed, autopsy evidence in a series of almost 2000 cases with malignant SVC obstruction treated by radiotherapy, and the observation of spontaneous resolution in 44 patients not treated with radiotherapy,[14] strongly suggest that in the SVC syndrome overall resolution of symptoms is frequently, if not most often, due to the development of a collateral circulation rather than relief of the SVC obstruction itself. These large series, however, contain few patients with lymphomas (only three were included in the latter series) and caution is required in applying the lessons learned from SVC obstruction caused by carcinomas to SVC obstruction caused by lymphomas, because of the difference in growth rate of these tumours. Nevertheless, these observations do suggest that emergency treatment is not indicated simply because of the presence of SVC obstruction, and that an uncomplicated SVC syndrome does not represent sufficient grounds for immediate irradiation without the establishment of a pathological diagnosis. In the case of lymphomas, specific therapy should be instituted as soon as a diagnosis has been established and sufficient information for treatment planning has been obtained.

Chemotherapy can bring about rapid resolution of SVC obstruction caused by NHL and is emerging as the treatment of choice in this situation. This is already the case in aggressive, high grade lymphomas, where a considerable reduction of tumour bulk can be achieved with a single cycle of chemotherapy, and is particularly relevant in children where the commonest NHL which causes SVC obstruction is lymphoblastic lymphoma, in which overall survival is not improved by the addition of mediastinal radiation to chemotherapy[10] (*see* Chapter 16). Radiotherapy should thus be reserved for tumours that are less likely to respond quickly to chemotherapy or for the rare lymphoma that is relatively chemoresistant.

When radiotherapy is utilized, the field should include all gross tumour plus a tumour-free margin. The mediastinal, hilar and supraclavicular lymph nodes are also usually irradiated.[11] The total radiation dose and rate of administration are dependent on the type of tumour, the patient's condition and the degree of local disease extension.

Pleural involvement

Non-Hodgkin's lymphoma presenting in the chest can result in malignant pleural or pericardial effusions. Leukaemias and lymphomas account for approximately 13 per cent of malignant pleural effusions while 16 per cent of patients with lymphoma will develop a pleural effusion in the course of their disease.[15,16] Pleural effusions provide an excellent source of malignant cells for cytological and immunophenotypic diagnosis.[17] The most effective therapy for a malignant effusion is treatment of the underlying lymphoma. Repeated therapeutic thoracentesis or an indwelling chest tube is occasionally necessary for symptomatic relief while awaiting response to chemotherapy. Because rapid response to therapy is the rule, pleurodesis with a sclerosing agent (e.g. tetracycline) after complete drainage of the pleural fluid is only indicated for palliation of tumours refractory to chemotherapy.

Pericardial involvement

Although less common than pleural effusions, pericardial effusion is far more serious because of the risk of life-threatening cardiac tamponade. Thus, suspicion of a malignant pericardial effusion demands rapid evaluation and, depending on the severity of symptoms, urgent treatment. M-mode or two dimensional echocardiography is the procedure of choice for the detection of fluid in the pericardial sac, and should be performed whenever a pericardial effusion is suspected because of the presence of a pericardial rub, characteristic ST segment elevation in an electrocardiogram or suggestive radiological findings. When there are signs of cardiac tamponade such as pulsus paradoxus, hypotension or elevated venous pressure, pericardiocentesis should be performed without delay. This procedure both relieves tamponade and provides fluid for diagnostic cytology. As with pleural effusions caused by lymphoma, pericardial fluid usually stops accumulating after chemotherapy. Radiotherapy should be avoided if possible because of the potential for cardiac damage, particularly if an anthracycline is included in the planned drug regimen. Continuous drainage of the pericardium with a catheter or surgical construction of a pericardial window may be necessary while awaiting a response to chemotherapy if reaccumulation of fluid is rapid after periocardiocentesis, or for palliation in patients with refractory lymphomas. In the latter circumstance, instillation of tetracycline into the pericardial sac has successfully prevented the accumulation of pericardial fluid without causing constrictive pericarditis.

Involvement of the gastrointestinal tract

Primary gastrointestinal lymphoma can present as a medical or surgical emergency due to obstruction, haemorrhage or perforation of the involved viscus. The most frequent site of involvement varies with age and histology. In the first two decades of life, the most frequent lymphoma involving the gastrointestinal tract is the small non-cleaved cell lymphoma, which commonly involves the small bowel, particularly the terminal ileum, and the caecum. This tumour often presents with bowel obstruction, either by compression of the bowel lumen, or by serving as the lead point for an ileo-ileal or ileocolic intussusception. Non-Hodgkin's lymphoma should be considered in the child that develops an intussusception after the first year of life. In such cases the diagnosis is made at laparotomy, at which time the tumour can be completely resected in about 25 per cent of patients. Definitive chemotherapy should be given within days of surgery, since regrowth can be rapid and the advantage of reduction of tumour bulk may quickly be lost. In the Middle East small intestinal lymphoma is more frequent than stomach involvement, even in adults, because of the high incidence of the immunoproliferative syndrome of the small intestine/α-heavy chain disease (IPSID) *see* Chapter 23.

Ninety per cent of children with small non-cleaved cell lymphomas present with abdominal disease which is usually intrinsic to the bowel. However, primary gastrointestinal lymphoma is rare in adults, and when it does occur, the commonest site of involvement is the stomach. In fact, gastric lymphoma is the second most common malignancy of the stomach after adenocarcinoma. Weingrad et al.[18] found 104 cases of gastrointestinal lymphoma among over 4000 patients with NHL treated at the Memorial Sloan-Kettering Cancer Center of which 73 per cent were gastric, the majority being diffuse large cell lymphomas. In this series the rate of acute complications was not specified.

Fleming et al.[19] reported their experience in the management of 32 cases of gastric lymphoma. Of these, two presented with bleeding and perforation and the diagnosis was made at laparotomy. Of interest is the fact that in five patients the diagnosis was made preoperatively and chemotherapy was given without surgical resection. Four of these patients developed massive gastrointestinal bleeding, a complication that did not occur in the patients that underwent resection prior to chemotherapy and/or radiation to the remaining tumour.

The potential complication of serious bleeding or perforation in gastric NHL, the excellent results achieved with complete surgical resection followed by chemotherapy such as C-MOPP (cyclophosphamide, vincristine, procarbazine, prednisone), BACOP (bleomycin, doxorubicin, cyclophosphamide, vincristine, prednisone) or CHOP (cyclophosphamide, doxorubicin, vincristine, prednisone) in some studies (e.g. 17 of 18 patients disease free at a median of 41 months after surgery, including eight patients with tumours over 10 cm in diameter[20]) and the relatively poor results in patients in whom tumour was not resected or in whom tumour was resected but no further therapy was given, have led some oncologists to advocate surgical resection followed by chemotherapy as standard therapy for gastric NHL.[20,21] However, although this approach can avoid the complications of haemorrhage and perforation and produces excellent results, the incidence of these complications is variable in different series, not all patients are amenable to surgery, and in some series the mortality rate of surgery is as high as 18 per cent. It may be possible to use endoscopic examination to predict which patients are more likely to develop massive haemorrhage or perforation when chemotherapy is commenced (e.g. extent of involvement of the stomach wall, degree of ulceration and necrosis). Recent results suggest that a similar rate of overall survival may be obtained by using intensive chemotherapy, either with no surgery, or with surgery in selected patients only e.g. those with very large (over 10 cm diameter) but resectable tumours, or those considered at high risk for massive haemorrhage or perforation.

Metabolic complications

Hyperuricaemia and the tumour lysis syndrome

Hyperuricaemia is a well recognized occurrence at presentation in patients with extensive haemopoietic neoplasms, particularly NHLs,[22,23] and is a consequence of the rapid turnover of tumour cells rich in nucleic acids, especially DNA. The degree of hyperuricaemia is proportional to the tumour burden, and elevated serum uric acid at presentation is, therefore, also associated with a worse prognosis. Metabolic complications occur predominantly in diffuse lymphomas with a high growth fraction, such as small non-cleaved cell lymphomas, lymphoblastic lymphomas and large cell lymphomas. In this setting there is both hyperuricaemia and a marked increase in uric acid excretion – from two to five times the normal rate.[24,25] The hyperuricaemia is usually asymptomatic and rarely causes gouty arthritis or renal stones. The major complication is the development of acute uric acid nephropathy which may occur before therapy, or as an immediate consequence of therapy if adequate measures are not taken to prevent it. Uric acid nephropathy results from the saturation of the urine with poorly soluble uric acid. This results in the formation of urate crystals in the distal tubules, where urine becomes acid, causing intrarenal obstruction and precipitating acute azotaemic renal failure.

This can be further aggravated by lymphomatous infiltration of the kidneys and/or ureteric compression by tumour masses in the kidney or retroperitoneum (Fig. 15.1). Acidosis accompanying renal failure further compounds the problem by reducing the solubility of uric acid in urine.

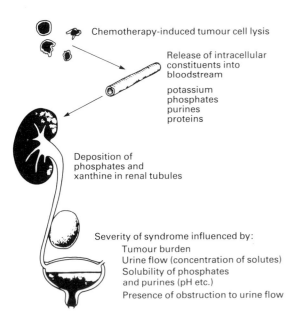

Chemotherapy-induced tumour cell lysis

Release of intracellular constituents into bloodstream

potassium
phosphates
purines
proteins

Deposition of phosphates and xanthine in renal tubules

Severity of syndrome influenced by:
Tumour burden
Urine flow (concentration of solutes)
Solubility of phosphates and purines (pH etc.)
Presence of obstruction to urine flow

Fig. 15.1 Diagrammatic depiction of the acute tumour lysis syndrome and compounding factors.

Rapid tumour destruction as a result of chemotherapy is accompanied by the release of large amounts of metabolites into the circulation from the tumour cells, the most relevant being potassium, oxypurines and phosphorus. These compounds must be excreted by the kidneys. The potentially catastrophic complications resulting from this are often collectively known as the acute tumour lysis syndrome, which occurs most frequently in patients who present with hyperuricaemia and an elevated lactate dehydrogenase.[26,27] Without preventative measures, oliguric renal failure associated with azotaemia, hyperuricaemia, acidosis, hyperphosphataemia, hypocalcaemia and hyperkalaemia rapidly results from the deposition of uric acid and phosphates in the kidney. Hyperkalaemia, which can occur within hours of the start of therapy, particularly in the setting of oliguria, can result in cardiac arrhythmias and arrest. In fact, the acute tumour lysis syndrome was originally recognized because of death from hyperkalaemic cardiac arrest. Hypocalcaemia may also occasionally be responsible for cardiac arrhythmias. The setting in which this dramatic picture was seen most frequently was the poorly hydrated patient with a large tumour burden, receiving chemotherapy to which the tumour was extremely sensitive.

The occurrence of tumour lysis and its complications is frequent enough to warrant intensive prophylactic measures in patients with intermediate or high grade lymphomas and moderate or large tumour burden, or in any patient with an elevated serum uric acid. The highest risk patients are usually best managed in a critical care unit because of the intensive monitoring required. Vigorous hydration with half normal saline (or equivalent sodium content) in the region of 4500–5500 ml/m^2 of body surface area every 24 hours (250 ml/m^2 per hour), liberal use of diuretics when necessary, and allopurinol (initially 10 mg/kg per day in three divided doses) should be commenced immediately, and at least 24 hours before chemotherapy is administered, with the objective of correcting hyperuricaemia. Alkalinization is also usually carried out at this time. If severe pre-existing hyperuricaemia persists, e.g. because a diuresis cannot be established due to renal obstruction, haemodialysis must be commenced prior to, and continued after, the administration of chemotherapy, since an extremely severe lysis syndrome will result when chemotherapy is initiated. In the hope of lessening the biochemical complications of rapid tumour lysis, some authors have advocated a reduction in the dose of chemotherapy at the time of first administration in order to allow a more gradual lysis of tumour cells, but there is no definite evidence to support this approach.[25]

Vigorous hydration should be continued after chemotherapy has begun as long as there is an appropriate urine output, and until the biochemical changes have significantly improved. Once chemotherapy has been commenced, however, further alkalinization is best avoided because phosphate is less soluble in alkaline urine and its deposition in the kidneys is as deleterious as oxypurine deposition. Peak excretion of phosphorus and uric acid occurs at between 2–3 days in the small non-cleaved cell lymphomas,[28] so that if significant biochemical changes have not occurred before this time it is very unlikely that they will develop subsequently, and hydration can be reduced. In the event of oliguria unresponsive to diuretics, biochemical abnormalities are likely to deteriorate rapidly, and in this circumstance haemodialysis should be instituted urgently. Haemodialysis may also be indicated in the presence of severe hyperkalaemia, rapidly increasing serum creatinine or phosphorus, or symptomatic hypocalcaemia. Hypocalcaemia should not be treated with intravenous calcium, except as an emergency measure, because of the risk of precipitating calcium phosphate in the kidneys or soft tissues.

Allopurinol is a strong inhibitor of the enzyme xanthine oxidase, which markedly reduces the conversion of xanthine and hypoxanthine into uric acid, resulting in the excretion of purines in three forms that are independently soluble in urine. Alkalinization of the urine to a pH of about 7 will increase the solubility of uric acid and xanthine. At this pH, uric acid is some 10–12 times more soluble than at pH 5 (solubility is approximately 150 mg/litre of urine at pH 5, 2000 mg/litre at pH 7) and xanthine more than twice as soluble (solubility at pH 5 is some 50 mg/litre, 120 mg/litre at pH 7). The solubility of hypoxanthine in urine differs little at either pH (1400–1500 mg/litre).[29] High dosage allopurinol will ensure that a significant proportion of the purine metabolites is excreted as xanthine and hypoxanthine, although there should be no attempt to prevent uric acid production completely, because it is more than 10 times as soluble in urine than xanthine and slightly more soluble than hypoxanthine at pH 7. The objective of allopurinol therapy, therefore, is to increase the total amount of oxypurine that can be excreted in a given volume of urine rather than to prevent uric acid formation.

Hypercalcaemia

Hypercalcaemia is an uncommon complication of malignant lymphoma, but is encountered quite frequently in human T-cell lymphotrophic virus (HTLV)-1 associated adult T-cell lymphoma (*see* Chapter 22). It can be caused by a variety of mechanisms, most associated with bone resorption. Bone involvement by tumour is usually present. Secretion by the tumour cells of a molecule with parathormone-like effects, or of an osteoclast-activating factor[31] has been implicated in the pathogenesis of hyperalcaemia caused by lymphomas. Hypercalcaemia most often occurs in patients with large tumour burdens and may be precipitated by dehydration or by immobilization. Hypercalcaemia itself causes renal dysfunction, with a decrease in the glomerular filtration rate and concentrating ability of the kidneys, resulting in dehydration and consequent worsening of the hypercalcaemia. It also has effects on the gastrointestinal tract, causing nausea, vomiting and constipation, and on the CNS, leading to weakness, somnolence and lethargy, a symptom complex which can be mistaken for intracerebral involvement by lymphoma. Potentially fatal cardiac arrhythmias may be precipitated.[32] Clearly, acute hypercalcaemia should be aggressively treated in an effort to prevent its deleterious consequences. Vigorous hydration and induction of a saline diuresis with frusemide may provide adequate control while definitive treatment for the lymphoma is being initiated. If hydration alone provides inadequate control, agents such as prednisone (40–100mg daily) calcitonin (3–8 MRC units/kg i.m. every 6 hours), mithramycin (25 μg/kg i.v.), or diphosphonates (e.g. etidronate, 7.5 mg/kg i.v.) that inhibit bone reabsorption by osteoclasts, may be considered.[32,33] Serum calcium, creatinine and electrolytes should be monitored frequently, and the patient mobilized within tolerated limits. Haemodialysis may be necessary in unresponsive cases. Chronic hypercalcaemia may be treated with oral phosphates, weekly doses of mithramycin or, in the case of lymphomas, corticosteroids. These measures provide only temporary amelioration; control of the underlying lymphoma is clearly the treatment of choice.

Late complications

In recent years, the improved treatment of NHL has resulted in an increase in the number of patients who achieve long-term survival. Consequently, late complications of treatment have become a much more important consideration. Clearly, now that long-term survival of a high proportion of the patients is achievable, efforts to increase survival rates even further by means of more aggressive therapy must be weighed not only against the additional risk of immediate toxicity, but also against the risk of long-term complications which may decrease the quality of subsequent survival. On the other hand, reductions in therapy for 'good risk' patients in order to minimize toxicity may also decrease survival rates – an equally unacceptable situation. Nonetheless, it is particularly important in good risk patients to examine treatment protocols critically, for components which add little to therapy but which may significantly increase toxicity. One area of current controversy in this regard is the use of combined chemotherapy and radiotherapy – a combination that has a particular propensity to give rise to late complications. In the era prior to combination drug regimens, the only NHL patients with a significant chance of cure were those with limited stage disease treated with radiotherapy. Thus it has been particularly difficult to abandon the use of radiation therapy for this subgroup, even now that combination chemotherapy alone has become routine for patients with more extensive disease, and has increased the survival rate of patients with limited disease, especially in children.[34]

The development of late complications represents a particularly serious problem in children, since growth and development are often affected and there is a potentially greater loss to society in terms of man-years of useful life. Thus, in spite of good evidence that children with limited disease had an excellent prognosis when treated with chemotherapy alone[35,36] some investigators felt it necessary to perform a randomized trial to evaluate the contribution of radiation therapy in children with limited disease treated with chemotherapy. This trial demonstrated that radiation adds only toxicity to effective drug combination regimens in such patients, and has no therapeutic advantage.[37]

Although the toxicities of radiation and chemotherapy are sometimes additive, late complications often differ markedly, since radiation causes toxicity in the radiation field such as pulmonary fibrosis, constrictive pericarditis, intellectual dysfunction and endarteritis of a variety of tissues. These complications of radiation can result in chronic renal and bowel disease, hypothyroidism and the impairment of growth of bone and soft tissues. Chemotherapy, on the other hand, may affect any organ or tissue, although late effects are often associated with a specific drug, such as busulfan, which can cause pulmonary fibrosis, or high dose methotrexate which may cause leucoencephalopathy.

Effects on growth and development

Delay or arrest in somatic growth of children is a well recognized complication of cancer therapy. Lymphomas in children and adolescents are virtually always diffuse and high grade, and chemotherapy is the primary therapeutic modality. Although most children will have some degree of growth impairment as a result of chemotherapy itself, and the sometimes attendant poor nutritional state, they usually recover their normal growth rate after treatment has been discontinued.[38,39] Radiation therapy, on the other hand, produces permanent damage to growing bones and soft tissues. For example, radiation to the spine (e.g. for treatment of a mediastinal lymphoma or as therapy for CNS disease) will cause a shortening of the trunk as a result of damage to the growth plates of the vertebral bodies, and a radiation field including one lateral half of the spine will produce severe scoliosis (and hence should never be used). The effects on growth are most dramatic when long bones are irradiated, and unequal limb length will result from unilateral irradiation. Such side-effects should be completely avoidable today, since there is no evidence that radiation therapy has a primary role in the treatment of childhood NHL.

Apart from its direct effects, irradiation of the brain, or scatter from radiotherapy to a neck or face mass, can damage the hypothalamic–pituitary axis, causing a deficit in growth hormone (GH). This complication is more prevalent in children treated for brain tumours, but it has an estimated 15 per cent incidence in all children receiving cranial radiation for any form of cancer.[39] Thus, children who fail to grow normally after cranial irradiation should be evaluated for GH deficiency since replacement therapy can be highly effective.[40] Because effective CNS prophylaxis can be achieved without the use of radiotherapy in children with NHL, this complication should be avoided in the vast majority of patients.

Endocrine dysfunction

Germ cells are very sensitive to the effects of chemotherapy and/or radiotherapy. The damage is most frequently restricted to infertility, but can also present as hormonal dysfunction.[41] In children, the degree of dysfunction induced is influenced by the stage of pubertal development. In the prepubertal female, cancer therapy can result in failure of secondary sexual characteristics to develop, with high gonadotrophin levels indicating ovarian failure. In the postmenstrual female, chemotherapy will often produce amenorrhoea and consequently infertility, although the ovaries usually recover their function after therapy has been stopped, particularly in younger women.[41,42] A clear exception to this are patients who receive even quite small doses of radiation to the pelvis, and in which the incidence of sterility is very high unless the ovaries have previously been removed from the radiation therapy field at laparotomy.[43,44]

The prepubertal testicle is relatively resistant to chemotherapy compared to the postpubertal testis, and boys treated with alkylating agent therapy such as MOPP can develop normal sperm counts after adolescence.[45,46]

Recently, a retrospective cohort study of long-term survivors of childhood and adolescent cancer showed a 60 per cent fertility deficit among males treated with various alkylating agents when compared to their siblings.[47] In females participating in this study, there was no apparent effect of alkylating therapy alone on

fertility, but radiation therapy below the diaphragm reduced the fertility by 25 per cent in both sexes. Even radiation scatter of 414 cGy or less, to the prepubertal testis, particularly when coupled with chemotherapy, can cause azoospermia.[46] In adults, oligo-/azoospermia, loss of libido and decreased sexual function may result from alkylating agent chemotherapy. Infertility is almost invariable in males treated with the MOPP regimen for Hodgkin's disease.[47] While the Leydig cells are more resistant to both chemotherapy and radiation, they can also be affected, giving rise to a resultant decrease in serum testosterone and increase in gonadotrophin levels. Delayed puberty can also be induced by irradiation of the hypothalamo–pituitary axis. Irradiation to the neck frequently results in hypothyroidism.[48]

Second tumours

Nowhere has the occurrence of second tumours been better studied than in the survivors of malignant lymphoma. Although most of the available information pertains to Hodgkin's lymphoma, the occurrence of both acute non-lymphocytic leukaemia (ANLL) and NHL has also been described after therapy for NHL.[49–51] In a recent review of second cancers in 1507 patients with Hodgkin's disease treated at Stanford University Medical Center since 1968, the relative risk of developing a second neoplasm was four to six times higher than the rate of cancer in the general population. The mean risk (actuarial) of all second cancers at 15 years was 17.6 ± 3.1 per cent of which 13.2 ± 3.1 per cent was due to solid tumours. The risk of leukaemia appeared to increase with time.[50]

The clinical characteristics of secondary ANLL are independent of the primary tumour. Patients have usually received intensive chemotherapy, including alkylating agents for their primary tumour, with or without radiotherapy. The leukaemia appears, on average, 4–6 years after treatment, and is usually preceded by pancytopenia and a myelodysplastic syndrome. Chromosomal abnormalities are frequent in leukaemic cells, mainly involving chromosomes 3, 5, 7, and 17. Typically the leukaemia is unresponsive to therapy and survival is short.[52]

Cases of ANLL have occurred after most forms of therapy for NHL, including single agent chemotherapy, combination chemotherapy, radiotherapy alone and combined modality therapy.[50–54] However, in Hodgkin's disease the excess risk of leukaemia is much greater (100-fold) after chemotherapy or chemotherapy and radiation therapy, than after radiotherapy alone (11-fold).[50] It is likely that the same applies in NHL, although the MOPP regimen appears at present (numbers are still small) to be more leukaemogenic than some others, such as PAVe (procarbazine, melphalan and vinblastine) or ABVD (doxorubicin, bleomycin, vinblastine and dacarbazine) when used in combination with radiation.[50] In NHL, all chemotherapy regimens that have been associated with secondary leukaemia contain an alkylating agent, although no single chemotherapeutic regimen or drug has been clearly associated with a higher incidence of secondary ANLL.[51–53]

There is some evidence that the use of more than one alkylating agent correlates with the risk of developing a second malignancy. In a study conducted at Roswell Park Memorial Cancer Institute three different alkylating agents were used and there was a high incidence of secondary ANLL.[52] However, in a study carried out by the Tumor Registry at Manitoba in which only a single alkylating agent was used, there were no cases of secondary leukaemia among 630 patients treated for NHL.[53] The total dose of alkylating agent received may also be important, but at present there is insufficient evidence to be sure of this. Most of the cases of ANLL reported after radiotherapy alone received wide field (total nodal, hemibody) or total body irradiation.[54] The age of the patient at the time of therapy can influence the incidence and type of second malignancy. Sullivan *et al.*[55] for example, observed eight cases of second malignancies among 228 children treated for Hodgkin's disease, which included thyroid carcinoma (3), large cell lymphoma (2), small round cell tumour (1), osteosarcoma (1) and malignant fibrous histiocytoma (1), but no cases of ANLL. The children who developed second tumours in this study were at least 8 years old and all of them had received radiotherapy, either alone or with chemotherapy that included alkylating agents.

In the Stanford series of patients with Hodgkin's disease there was an increased cumulative risk for the development of leukaemia in patients over 50 years of age at the time of diagnosis, but no increase in the relative risk.[50] Recently, splenectomy, performed at staging laparotomy, was shown to be associated with an increased risk of secondary ANLL in patients treated with MOPP-type chemotherapy for Hodgkin's disease, especially in patients over the age of 40 years.[56,57]

For some time, carcinoma of the urinary bladder, and less often of the ureter and renal pelvis, has been implicated as a late complication in patients treated with cyclophosphamide, but the risk of this complication in a cohort of patients followed for a long period has, until recently, not been defined. In a study of 471 patients with NHL treated in Copenhagen, seven developed transitional cell carcinoma of the bladder, with a relative risk for the patient cohort of 6.8.[58] The cumulative risk of developing this complication was 3.5 ± 1.8 per cent 8 years after the start of treatment and 10.7 ± 4.9 per cent after 12 years – similar to the risk of ANLL. The cumulative risk of haemorrhagic cystitis was 11.8 ± 2.1 per cent after five years, but the development of bladder cancer was not significantly related to previous haemorrhagic cystitis. This potentially serious complication (most of the patients died from their bladder cancer) occurred exclusively in patients treated with cyclophosphamide, and it is worth pointing out that all patients had been treated with oral cyclophosphamide for at least 22 months. Based on studies in a rat model, in which sodium 2-mercaptoethane-sulphonate (mesna) can prevent bladder cancer after cyclophosphamide,[59] it is likely that this complication may be avoidable by administration of the same agent in humans. Mesna also provides effective protection against haemorrhagic cystitis.[60]

Non-Hodgkin's lymphoma has been reported as a secondary malignancy following the treatment of Hodgkin's lymphoma,[61,62] and it is theoretically possible that some apparently recurrent NHLs, particularly those arising late, truly represent second malignancies. The NHLs following Hodgkin's disease usually present with diffuse histology, generally of undifferentiated or large cell type, frequently involve the gastrointestinal tract and have an extremely poor prognosis. The risk of secondary NHL at 10 years after therapy for Hodgkin's lymphoma has been calculated as 4.4 per cent, increasing to 15.2 per cent in patients treated with combined modality therapy. Unlike ANLL, the incidence of which appears to decline after 10 years off therapy, there is no evidence so far for a similar reduction in incidence of NHL as the time off therapy increases.

References

1. Grant JW, Kaech D, Jones DB. *Histopathology*. 1986; **10**, 1191.
2. Haddad P, Thaell JF, *et al*. *Cancer*. 1976; **37**, 1485.
3. Friedman M, Kim TH, Panahon AM. *Cancer*. 1976; **37**, 1485.
4. Oviatt DL, Kirshner HS, Stein RS. *Cancer*. 1982; **49**, 2446.
5. Lochridge SK, Knibbe WP, Doty DB. *Surgery*. 1979; **85**, 14.
6. Parish JM, Marschke RF, *et al*. *Mayo Clinic Proceedings*. 1981; **56**, 407.
7. Perez CA, Presant CA, Van Amburg A. *Seminars in Oncology*. 1978; **5**, 123.
8. Shimm DS, Logue GL, Rigsby LC. *Journal of the American Medical Association*. 1981; **245**, 951.
9. Nieto AF, Doty DB. *Current Problems in Cancer*. 1986; **10**, 441.
10. O'Brien RT, Matlak ME, *et al*. *Western Journal of Medicine*. 1981; **135**, 143.
11. Levitt SH, Jones TK, Kilpatrick SJ. *Cancer*. 1969; **24**, 447.
12. Ahmann FR. *Journal of Clinical Oncology*. 1984; **2**, 961.
13. Halpern J, Chatten J, *et al*. *Journal of Pediatrics*. 1987; **102**, 407.
14. Little AG, Golomb HM, *et al*. *Annals of Thoracic Surgery*. 1985; **40**, 285.
15. Mckenna RJ, Khalil M, *et al*. *Current Problems in Cancer*. 1985; **9**, 1.
16. Kline IK. *Cancer*. 1972; **29**, 799.
17. Salyer WR, Eggleston JC, *et al*. *Chest*. 1975; **67**, 536.
18. Weingrad DN, Decosse DJ, *et al*. *Cancer*. 1982; **49**, 1258.
19. Fleming ID, Mitchell S, Dilawari RA. *Cancer*. 1982; **49**, 1135.
20. Sheridan WP, Medley G, Brodie GM. *Journal of Clinical Oncology*. 1985; **3**, 495.
21. Paulson S, Sheehan RG, Stone MJ, Frenkel EP. *Journal of Clinical Oncology*. 1983; **1**, 263.
22. Lynch E. *Archives of Internal Medicine*. 1962; **109**, 43.
23. Sandberg A, Cartwright G, Wintrobe M. *Blood*. 1956; **11**, 154.
24. Primikirios N, Stutzman L, Sandberg A. *Blood*. 1961; **17**, 701.
25. Hande KR. In: McKinney TD (ed). *Renal Complications of Neoplasia*. Praeger Scientific, 1986; 134–56.
26. Krakoff I, Meyer RL. *Journal of the American Medical Association*. 1965; **193**, 89.
27. Cohen LF, Balow JE, *et al*. *American Journal of Medicine*. 1980; **68**, 486.
28. Tsokos G, Balow J, *et al*. *Medicine*. 1981; **60**, 218.
29. Hande KR, Hixson CL, Chabner BA, *et al*. *Cancer Research*. 1981; **41**, 2273.
30. Muggia FM, Heinemann HO. *Annals of Internal Medicine*. 1981; **73**, 281.
31. Mundy GR, Rick ME, *et al*. *American Journal of Medicine*. 1978; **65**, 600.
32. Bull FE. In: Yarbo JW, Bornstein RS (eds). *Oncologic Emergencies*. New York: Grune and Stratton, 1981; 197–214.
33. Jacobs TP, Gordon AC, Silverberg SJ, *et al*. *American Journal of Medicine*. 1987; **82**, 42.
34. Jenkin RDT, Anderson JR, Chilcote PF, *et al*. *Journal of Clinical Oncology*. 1984; **2**, 88.
35. Müller-Weihrich St Henze G, Odenwald E, Riehm H. In: Cavalli F, Bonadonna G, Rozencweig M (eds). *Malignant Lymphomas and Hodgkin's Disease: Experimental and Therapeutic Advances*. Boston: Martinus Nijhoff, 1985; 633.
36. Janus C, Edwards BK, Sariban E, Magrath IT. *Cancer Treatment Reports*. 1984; **68**, 599.
37. Link MP, Donaldson SS, Berard CW, Shuster JJ, Murphy SB. *Third International Conference on Malignant Lymphoma*. Lugano, Switzerland, 1987; (abstract). 43.
38. Sunderman CR, Pearson HA. *Journal of Pediatrics*. 1969; **75**, 1058.
39. D'Angio GJ. *Cancer*. 1978; **42**, 1015.
40. Romshi CA, Zipf WB, Miser A. *Journal of Pediatrics*. 1984; **104**, 177.
41. Byrd R. *Pediatric Clinics of North America*. 1985; **32**, 835.
42. Schilsky RL, Sherins RJ, *et al*. *American Journal of Medicine*. 1981; **71**, 552.
43. Stillman RJ, Schinfield JS, *et al*. *American Journal of Obstetrics and Gynecology*. 1981; **139**, 62.
44. Shalet SM, Beardwell CG, *et al*. *British Journal of Cancer*. 1976; **33**, 655.
45. Sullivan MP, Jaffe N, Boren H, *et al*. *Proceedings of the Annual Meeting of the American Association of Cancer Research*. 1985; **26** (abstract), 182.

46. Whitehead E, Shalet SM, *et al. Cancer.* 1982; **49**, 418.
47. Byrne J, Mulvihill JJ, Myers M, *et al. New England Journal of Medicine.* 1987; **317**, 1315.
48. McHenry C, Jarosz H, *et al. Archives of Surgery.* 1987; **122**, 684.
49. Dorr FA, Coltman CA. *Current Problems in Cancer.* 1985; **9**, 1.
50. Tucker MA, Coleman CN, Cox RS, *et al. New England Journal of Medicine.* 1988; **318**, 76.
51. Coltman CA. In: Bloomfield CD (ed). *Adult Leukemias.* The Hague: Martinus Nijhoff, 1982: **1**, 61.
52. Gomez GA, Aggarwal KK, Han R. *Cancer.* 1982; **50**, 2285.
53. O'Donnell JF, Brereton HD, *et al. Cancer.* 1979; **44**, 1930.
54. McDougall BK, Weinerman BH, Kemel S. *Cancer.* 1981; **48**, 1299.
55. Sullivan MP, Ramirez I, Ried HL. *Proceedings of the American Association of Cancer Research.* 1983; **24** (abstract), 633.
56. Van Leeuwen FE, Somers R, Hart AAM. *Lancet.* 1987; **ii**, 210.
57. Rosenberg SA. *Journal of Clinical Oncology.* 1988; **6**, 574.
58. Pedersen-Bjergaard J, Ersboll J, Hansen VL, *et al. New England Journal of Medicine.* 1988; **318**, 1028.
59. Habs MR, Schmähl D. *Cancer.* 1983; **51**, 606.
60. Brade W, Herdrich K, Varini M. *Cancer Treatment Reviews.* 1985; **12**, 1.
61. Krikorian JG, Burje JS, *et al. New England Journal of Medicine.* 1979; **300**, 452.
62. Armitrage JO, Dick FR, *et al. Archives of Internal Medicine.* 1983; **143**, 445.

CHAPTER 16

LYMPHOBLASTIC LYMPHOMA

John Sandlund and Ian Magrath

Definitions and general description

The lymphoblastic lymphomas consist of several phenotypically similar diseases that are morphologically indistinguishable. Lymphoblastic tumours now characterized by the NCI Working Formulation[1] represent at best a small subset of those designated lymphoblastic in the first half of this century (*see* Chapter 1) and were originally included in the diffuse, poorly differentiated category of Rappaport.[2] The characteristic morphology and clinical pattern of this lymphoma led to its identification as a discrete entity by Lukes and Collins,[3] who referred to it as a tumour of convoluted lymphocytes, and by Nathwani and Kim,[4] who first used the term 'lymphoblastic' in describing the tumour. In European classification schemes (the Kiel classification and the British Lymphoma Investigation) the term lymphoblastic is used more broadly and includes the small non-cleaved cell lymphomas. This chapter deals only with those tumours classed as lymphoblastic in the NCI Working Formulation.

Lymphoblastic leukaemia versus lymphoblastic lymphoma

Lymphoblastic lymphomas are histologically and cytologically indistinguishable from the lymphoblasts of acute lymphoblastic leukaemia (ALL). Because they have the immuno-phenotypic characteristics of lymphocyte precursor cells, lymphoblastic lymphomas never have a follicular cytoarchitecture, although occasionally the patterns of adjacent normal lymphoid tissue may result in a mistaken impression of nodularity.[5]

The cytological, histological and phenotypic similarities between lymphoblastic lymphoma and ALL compel arbitrary criteria to distinguish between these diseases. In some patients there may be no bone marrow involvement at all, so that a diagnosis of leukaemia cannot be entertained; in others the clinical presentation is one of marrow failure, with or without generalized lymphadenopathy, and a mediastinal mass, so that the patient falls naturally into a clinical category of leukaemia. In many patients the distinction is less clear.

Some paediatric oncologists have used an arbitrary criterion of less than or greater than 25 per cent of blast cells present in bone marrow aspirates to differentiate between lymphoblastic lymphoma and ALL, respectively. This is purely an operational definition. Clinical studies comparing disease-free survival rates among patients who were segregated on this basis must be viewed with scepticism because the observed differences could be a consequence of other variables (e.g. the total tumour volume). Moreover, the criterion itself is imperfect because of the potential for sampling error in the assessment of marrow infiltration by tumour cells. Multiple marrow samples taken at the same time or at different times from a single patient frequently show variation in malignant cellularity. This issue must be borne in mind when one analyses the results of treatment protocols. Only when authors have provided their criteria for inclusion of patients can the results of clinical trials be compared with confidence.

There is no doubt that the lymphoblastic leukaemias and lymphomas are neoplasms arising from precursor cells at various stages of differentiation in both the T- and B-cell lineages. Cells at different stages of differentiation are located in different anatomical regions, and their malignant counterparts tend to mirror these topographical differences in their clinical presentations. Thus, pre-B-cells reside primarily, but not exclusively, in the bone marrow, so that neoplasms of these cells usually present as leukaemias. T-cell precursors arise in the bone marrow, migrate to the thymus, and travel to the secondary lymphoid organs, which include the bone marrow. It is not surprising, then, that T-cell neoplasms may present as either leukaemias or lymphomas. Because the cells of a given tumour usually represent more than one developmental stage, individual patients may have clinical features of both leukaemia and lymphoma concurrently or consecutively in the course of the disease (e.g. bone marrow involvement at relapse of lymphoma). These considerations indicate that our concepts of leukaemia and lymphoma are artificial, in that they do not designate distinct pathological entities any more than involvement of the bone marrow by solid tumours. These terms have been in the vocabulary of clinicians and pathologists for more than a century and are unlikely to fall into disuse in the near future. This is unfortunate, as they hinder the understanding and treatment of lymphoid neoplasia, particularly that originating in T-cell precursors.

Histology

A detailed description of the histology of lymphoblastic lymphoma has been given in Chapter 2. The essential cytological features include a high nuclear to cytoplasmic ratio, variably basophilic cytoplasm (usually less than in the small non-cleaved lymphomas), clearly discernible nuclear envelope, finely stippled nuclear chromatin and multiple nucleoli that are usually poorly discernible or imperceptible (Fig. 16.1). Cytoplasmic vacuoles are occasionally seen. A subset of cells is defined morphologically by an irregular nuclear outline and the appearance of nuclear 'folds' (sometimes referred to as crow's feet[5]) due to nuclear convolutions. The degree of convolution varies from tumour to tumour, but this feature is not required for the diagnosis. It is often better perceived on cytocentrifuged preparations and is readily seen by electron microscopy, which also demonstrates abundant free ribosomes but scanty rough endoplasmic reticulum. When the nuclei are predominantly convoluted, a greater variation in nuclear and cell sizes occurs. In this situation, the smallest cells have a hyperchromatic pattern of chromatin and are quite mature in appearance, but they can still be distinguished from normal lymphocytes by their nuclear convolutions. Neither the cytomorphology in general nor the nuclear convolutions in particular have been shown to correlate with phenotype.

The most characteristic cytochemical finding is the presence of focal areas of strong acid phosphatase activity, which are often localized in the region of the Golgi apparatus. The acid non-specific esterase reaction and the β-glucuronide reaction give a similar staining pattern. There may occasionally be isolated clumps of periodic acid-Schiff-positive material that tends to be diastase resistant. These special stains have largely been superseded by immunophenotyping, which is strongly recommended for confirmation of the diagnosis of lymphoblastic lymphoma.[5]

Immunopathology

Although the immunophenotypes of lymphoblastic lymphoma show considerable diversity, the T-cell phenotype is clearly dominant.[6–10] Regardless of phenotype, almost all lymphoblastic lymphomas express the enzyme terminal deoxyribonucleotidyl transferase.[11] This property is consistent with a lymphocyte precursor cell origin, because this enzyme is

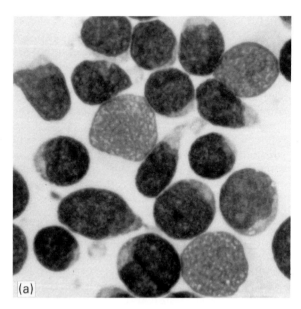

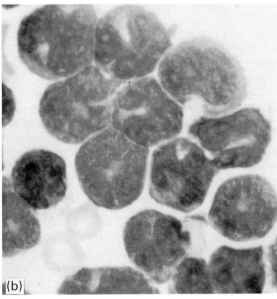

Fig. 16.1 Cytological appearance of lymphoblastic lymphoma. (a) Needle aspirate from a peripheral tumour; (b) cytocentrifuge preparation of cerebrospinal fluid from the same patient, showing nuclear convolutions. The tumour cells demonstrate a high nuclear to cytoplasmic ratio, variably basophilic cytoplasm, clearly discernible nuclear envelope, finely stippled nuclear chromatin and multiple nucleoli that are usually poorly discernible or imperceptible. Cytoplasmic vacuoles are occasionally seen.

involved in the generation of antigen receptor diversity in both B- and T-cells (*see* Chapter 3).

Lymphoblastic lymphoma of thymic origin

The T-cell marker most frequently present on the surface of neoplasms derived from thymocytes is the glycoprotein known as gp40 (function undetermined), which is recognized by the monoclonal antibodies 4H9 (Leu-9), 3A1 and WT-1 (CD7).[12–14] Demonstration of the presence of this antigen may be the best single test for identifying T-cell precursor neoplasms[12–14] and is often present when the receptor for sheep red cells, T11 (CD2),[12,14] formerly the most widely accepted marker of the T-cell lineage, is absent.

Other T-cell markers vary according to stage of thymocyte differentiation. Cells of early thymocyte origin express the transferrin receptor (T9, CD unassigned) and an antigen also present on activated T-cells and plasma cells (T10).[15] When they reach intermediate stages of differentiation, thymocytes express T6 (CD1), T4 (CD4) and T8 (CD8), the antigens expressed by T-cells activated in the presence of class II and class I HLA antigens, respectively.[15] As differentiation continues, the thymocytes express either T4 or T8, as well as the T-cell receptor for antigen coupled to the T3 (CD3) molecule. It has been shown that all of the T-cell receptor subunits, α, β, δ and γ, as well as the T3 molecule, are expressed in the cytoplasm of early and intermediate thymocytes, but are not expressed on the cell surface until the late thymocyte stage.[15–17] The γ and δ chains are the first to be rearranged, followed by β then α, which together form the antigen receptor molecule expressed on the cell surface in proximity to T3.[18]

In Europe and the USA, the phenotype of T-cell lymphoblastic lymphoma corresponds in the majority of cases to the phenotype of intermediate or late thymocytes,[7,8] although atypical patterns may be seen.[8,10,17,19] In contrast, a high percentage of T-cell ALL cases are characterized by early thymocyte marker expression, CD7, T9, and T10, with a lack of T6, T4, T8, and T3,[7,20] although there is overlap in the phenotypes of T-cell ALL and T-cell lymphoblastic lymphomas. The division between intermediate and late stages is controversial, particularly with regard to whether T3 is expressed on intermediate thymocytes. This problem is not of major significance, because the designations of intermediate and late are artificial, and such divisions in lymphoblastic lymphomas probably do not have prognostic significance.[10]

Lymphoblastic lymphoma of non-T origin

Lymphoblastic lymphoma infrequently expresses a pre-B (Ia+, CALLA+, cytoplasmic μ-chain positive) or common ALL (Ia+, CALLA+) phenotype.[6,21–23] Such cases usually present with peripheral lymphadenopathy, isolated bone involvement, or subcutaneous tumour without mediastinal masses.

Sheibani *et al.*[24] reported a series of six patients with lymphoblastic lymphoma whose blast cells expressed antigens associated with natural killer (NK) cells. They all expressed T11 (CD2) receptors and reacted positively with anti-Leu-11b and anti-leu-7 – antibodies that react with a subset of lymphocytes with NK activity. The most common immunophenotype in their series was Leu-11b+, T11+, Leu-7+, Leu-3a+, Ia+, without evidence of cytoplasmic or surface immunoglobulin. Their patients were primarily non-white females.

Cytogenetics and molecular characterization

Non-random chromosomal abnormalities specific for all lymphoblastic lymphomas, or even for phenotypic subsets of lymphoblastic lymphomas, have not been observed.[25] However, in T-cell lymphoblastic leukaemias and lymphomas, a number of translocations involving genes associated with T-cell differentiation have been described.

Chromosomal breakpoints are particularly frequent at the location of the T-cell receptor α chain (TCR-α) and δ chain genes located on chromosome 14q11. The translocations most frequently described in T-cell malignancies have been between chromosomes 11 (p13/15) and 14 (q11).[26–33] Le Beau *et al.* studied a cell line (RPMI-

8402) containing an 11(p14);14(q11) translocation derived from a patient with T-cell ALL.[31] The breakpoint at 14q11 occurred within the variable region of the TCR-α gene and the breakpoint at 11p15 occurred between the HRAS1 gene and the genes for insulin and insulin-like growth factor 2. Their observations suggest that the acivation of one of these genes, or of another between them, may result from their juxtaposition to the T-cell-receptor sequences, a hypothesis reminiscent of the proposed c-*myc* activation in small non-cleaved lymphomas by an enhancer element within the Ig-constant region.[34]

Even greater similarity with the small non-cleaved cell lymphomas resides in those translocations that involve the TCR-α locus and the c-*myc* locus. Mathieu-Mahul *et al.*[30] studied a cell line with an 8(q24);14(q11) translocation derived from a patient with T-cell leukaemia. They demonstrated that the breakpoint on chromosome 8 was located on the 3' side of the third exon of c-*myc*. The breakpoint on chromosome 14 was located at q11, within the TCR-α locus. McKeithan *et al.*[33] described a similar translocation in the Molt-16 cell line, which also was established from a patient with T-cell ALL. The q11 breakpoint on chromosome 14 was close to a joining (J) sequence of the gene encoding the α chain of the T-cell receptor. The constant region and part of the joining region were translocated 3' of the third exon of c-*myc* on chromosome 8. These translocations may result in c-*myc* activation. The translocation of TCR-α sequences distal (3') to c-*myc* parallel the variant translocations occurring in the small non-cleaved lymphomas, in which immunoglobulin light-chain sequences are translocated to a similar position with respect to c-*myc*.

A recent report described the cytogenetic findings in a series of T-cell ALL patients seen at St Jude Children's Research Hospital (SJCRH).[35] Twenty-three patients were classified as stage I thymocyte development (CD7+; CD5+ or CD2+; CD1−; CD3−; CD4−; CD8−); 25 as stage II (CD1+ or CD1− plus CD4+ and CD8+); and nine as stage III (CD3+; CD4+ or CD8+; CD1−). Consistent breakpoints were located at chromosome 7q32-q36 (the TCR-β locus) in eight patients, chromosome 14q11–q13

(TCR-α locus) in six, chromosome 9p21-p22 in nine, and chromosome 6q in nine. In this study it was found that breakpoints involving the T-cell receptor genes occurred in 50 per cent of the translocations regardless of stage of development. There was no relationship between the chromosomal abnormalities and the stage of thymocyte differentiation represented by the blast-cell phenotype.

Epidemiology

Compared with information on the small non-cleaved lymphomas, few epidemiological data are available on lymphoblastic lymphomas. Lymphoblastic lymphomas occur throughout the world, with a considerably higher incidence than Burkitt's lymphoma in certain countries, such as India. The statistics may be somewhat misleading, because the arbitrary distinction between lymphoblastic lymphoma and ALL vary from one country to another.

Unlike the bimodal age-incidence curve seen in Hodgkin's disease, there is a steadily increasing incidence of non-Hodgkin's lymphoma (NHL) throughout life. Although only 3 per cent of the cases occur in persons younger than 16,[36] lymphoblastic lymphoma is generally considered a disease of children and young adults, with a peak incidence in the second decade of life. An exception to this was reported by Nathwani[37] in a review of 97 patients with this disease; 50 per cent of the patients were older than 30, with a median age of 27 years in males and of 50 years in females. The male:female raio was 2:1. Males demonstrated a bimodal age distribution, with peaks in both the second and seventh decades. These findings may be skewed, in that the patient population of the Repository Center for Lymphoma Clinical Studies, from which the data were obtained, consists primarily of adults.

In children younger than 15 years of age, non-Hodgkin's lymphomas account for less than 10 per cent of all childhood malignancies in industrialized countries, following acute leukaemias and brain tumours in frequency. Between 1973 and 1982 the SEER surveillance/epidemiology programme of the NCI[38] reported that in the USA non-Hodgkin's lymphoma accounted for 7 per cent of all cancers in White children (annual incidence, 9.1 per million) and 4 per cent of all cancers in Black children (annual incidence, 4.6 per million) younger than 15 years old.

The lymphoblastic lymphoma subtype accounts for approximately one-third of the cases of NHL in children. Unlike the small non-cleaved and immunoblastic lymphomas, lymphoblastic lymphoma does not occur at increased frequency in patients with an underlying immunodeficiency syndrome,[5] nor does radiation play a significant role in pathogenesis. Unlike acute leukaemia, there was no early lymphoma peak in children who survived the atomic bomb explosions in Nagasaki and Hiroshima. Although there was an increased incidence of NHL in individuals who were exposed to no greater than 200 or 100 cGy at Nagasaki and Hiroshima, respectively, there was no significant increase in incidence at higher exposure levels.[39]

Clinical features and staging

Patients with lymphoblastic lymphoma most commonly present with a mediastinal mass (50–70 per cent); in many cases a pleural effusion may also be present (Fig. 16.2). The associated symptoms may include dyspnoea, dysphagia and pain. In the event of superior vena caval obstruction, swelling of the neck, face and upper extremities may also occur. Lymphadenopathy, usually located in the neck, axilla, or supra-clavicular region, occurs in 50–80 per cent of all patients. Abdominal involvement is very unusual, but when it does occur it is found primarily in the liver and spleen. Occasionally, intra-abdominal lymph nodes, kidneys, or other retroperitoneal structures may be involved, but bowel involvement has not been described in a well-documented case. Occasionally, sites of involvement include bone, skin and testes.

Bone marrow and central nervous system involvement

Bone marrow involvement is common in lymphoblastic lymphoma,[40,41] but in view of the arbitrary and controversial distinction between

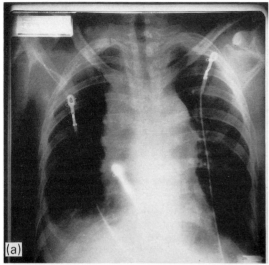

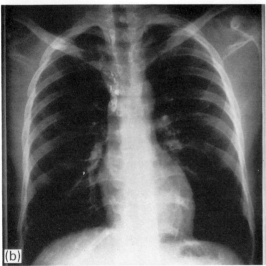

Fig. 16.2 Chest X-ray demonstrating a mediastinal mass in a patient with lymphoblastic lymphoma (a) before and (b) 10 days after chemotherapy.

T-cell ALL and lymphoblastic lymphoma, estimates depend upon the definition used to distinguish these conditions. Central nervous system (CNS) involvement is uncommon at presentation, but is more likely in patients who have bone marrow involvement. Central nervous system involvement may consist of meningeal infiltration, intracerebral disease, cranial nerve infiltration (ophthalmic or facial

nerves), paraspinal mass or some combination of these, most commonly meningeal and cranial nerve involvement.[42,43]

If CNS prophylaxis is not given, CNS disease is likely to occur during therapy, particularly in patients with primary sites in the head and neck. Intracerebral disease is a very unusual finding. It may occur as a consequence of extension from adjacent structures, such as involvement of the skull, and can be seen in patients who have had CNS infiltration that has not been eradicated over a long period.[44]

Staging systems and procedures

The most commonly used staging system for childhood lymphoblastic lymphoma is one developed at St Jude Children's Research Hospital.[45] It is described in Chapter 12 and is modified from the Ann Arbor system which was originally devised for Hodgkin's disease to reflect the non-contiguous nature of disease spread, the predominant extranodal involvement, involvement of CNS and the tendency for leukaemic transformation in childhood NHL. There is room for improvement, however. The use of the diaphragm as a means of defining spread of disease is arbitrary, and use of the term 'primary intrathoracic tumour' as a criterion for stage III disease invites ambiguous interpretation. Unfortunately, in adult patients with lymphoblastic lymphoma, the Ann Arbor system is still widely used. A staging system that takes account of these shortcomings and can be applied to lymphoblastic lymphoma at all ages is suggested in Chapter 12.

Before starting treatment, it is imperative that a definitive tissue diagnosis be made. Generally, biopsy of an easily accessible node or examination of pleural fluid is required. A bone marrow examination may also help in making the diagnosis. If disease is limited to the mediastinum, mediastinoscopy or biopsy via a parasternal incision is indicated.

Appropriate studies for determining the extent of tumour have been described in Chapter 12. In lymphoblastic lymphomas, a careful examination of the chest is mandatory, and computed tomographic scanning[46] is usually performed. An echocardiogram ultrasonogram may be helpful in examining tumour in relation to the heart, but echolucent tumour can easily be mistaken for a pericardial effusion. Gallium-67 is much less avidly taken up in the lymphoblastic lyphomas than in small non-cleaved cell lymphomas, but is worth including in the routine scanning procedures. Bone scan should be performed to detect the presence of occult bone disease and, if positive, X-rays of involved bones should be performed. Bone marrow examination is mandatory and in some circumstances can determine treatment. There is evidence that multiple sampling and bone marrow biopsy, even in lymphoblastic lymphoma, increases the detection rate of marrow involvement. These procedures have not been performed routinely in paediatric centres. Magnetic resonance imaging of the bone marrow is likely to be of value in detecting occult disease in these patients, as it has been in other lymphomas.

A staging laparotomy is not indicated in patients with lymphoblastic lymphoma. Not only is intra-abdominal tumour rare, but because chemotherapy is administered for all disease stages, pathological staging is not indicated.

Treatment and prognosis

Emergency management

Patients with lymphoblastic lymphoma may present with tumour-associated problems that require immediate attention. The most common complications are those which develop secondary to a large mediastinal mass, including superior vena caval syndrome, dyspnoea, dysphagia and, rarely, cardiac arrhythmias or tamponade. There is also an increased risk for anaesthesia-related complications, cardiac arrest, and bleeding from engorged mediastinal vessels in patients with mediastinal primaries.[47] Pleural effusions are common in lymphoblastic lymphoma, and pericardial effusions are sometimes seen. Both may need immediate attention. Airway obstruction by pharyngeal tumour is a rare occurrence. Uric acid-induced nephropathy may also occur, although not as commonly as in B-cell tumours, which have a higher growth fraction. Management of these problems is dealt with in Chapter 15.

It is worth emphasizing that the role of radiation therapy (RT) in the management of superior vena caval obstruction is questionable in this disease, particularly since radiation appears to confer no prognostic advantage and will increase toxicity if anthracyclines are used in treatment.[48,49] In the rare instance in which no response to chemotherapy is attained, RT may be indicated. It may also be indicated if the degree of compromise is deemed immediately life-threatening (e.g. there is also respiratory obstruction) and the added security of combined modality treatment is desired. In these situations, relatively low-dose therapy (e.g. 120 cGy) is preferable.

Central nervous system involvement at diagnosis may require the immediate addition of RT to the therapeutic regimen since chemotherapy is unlikely to be curative. In patients who present with cranial nerve involvement or intracerebral extension of tumour, full doses of cranial irradiation (3000 cGy) are indicated. Most patients with paraplegia are also treated with radiation, but paraspinal tumour is accessible to systemic chemotherapy, and no advantage of radiotherapy over chemotherapy alone has even been demonstrated. However, the potential neurological consequences of an inadequate response of a paraspinal tumour persuade many oncologists to irradiate such tumours when paraparesis is advanced, in addition to administering chemotherapy.

Specific therapy

The primary treatment modality in lymphoblastic lymphoma is chemotherapy. The use of surgery or radiation alone has yielded poor overall results, although a small proportion of patients with localized disease have achieved long-term survival. Surgery has no role in lymphoblastic lymphoma except in establishing the diagnosis. The role of RT is presently controversial, and the most recent successful treatment programmes have not employed it. A recent prospective randomized trial conducted by the

Pediatric Oncology Group demonstrated that RT provided no therapeutic benefit to patients with localized disease (SJCRH stages I and II).[49] A similar conclusion was reached in patients with more extensive disease (SJCRH Stages III and IV) studied at SJCRH.[48] The special situations in which RT may be indicated are almost exclusively limited to patients presenting or recurring with testicular tumour or with CNS involvement.

Chemotherapy

Chemotherapy for lymphoblastic lymphoma currently differs quite markedly in children and adults. The most widely used chemotherapeutic regimens for the treatment of lymphoblastic lymphoma in children have originated from protocols designed for ALL,[50–57] whereas adult patients with lymphoblastic lymphoma are usually treated with regimens similar to those used for the intermediate grade lymphomas (*see* Chapter 21). This approach appears to be a consequence of tradition, rather than scientific method, and is an issue that should be confronted.

During the last 15 years, impressive progress has been made in improving the treatment of childhood lymphoblastic lymphoma, resulting in a much better long-term survival. As recently as 1973, Watanabe *et al.*[40] at the M. D. Anderson Tumor Institute, Houston, Texas, reported the results of treatment of children with lymphoblastic lymphoma with a regimen then in use for ALL. This therapy included RT to the primary site of disease and chemotherapy (one or more of the following agents: mechlorethamine hydrochloride, cyclophosphamide, corticosteroid analogues, dactinomycin, or 6-mercaptopurine). Ten (91 per cent) of 11 children with mediastinal presentations developed bone marrow involvement and five (50 per cent) of these also developed meningeal involvement. There were no long-term survivors reported. Similarly, Wollner[58] reported no long-term survivors among patients with mediastinal NHL treated before 1976 with single agent chemotherapy and RT. In 1974, Glatstein *et al.*,[59] using localized, high-dose (minimum 3500 cGy) RT found that stage I, II, and III patients with

mediastinal involvement were highly likely to develop leukaemia. Studies at SJCRH demonstrated that children with mediastinal primaries who were also leukaemic at presentation had an especially high risk for treatment failure (< 30 per cent survival rate at two years) when treated according to the total VIII protocol.[53] The NHL-75 regimen (SJCRH)[48,57] which employed multiagent systemic chemotherapy and CNS prophylaxis (Table 16.1) resulted in only a 40 per cent disease-free survival (median follow-up of seven years) for patients with advanced stage lymphoblastic lymphoma (SJCRH stage III and IV).

The first encouraging therapeutic results for lymphoblastic lymphoma were obtained with a protocol based on another treatment regimen used in ALL, the LSA_2L_2 protocol designed at the Memorial Sloan-Kettering Cancer Center and first reported in 1976 by Wollner *et al.*[58,60] It is an intensive 10-drug regimen that includes induction, consolidation and maintenance phases (Fig. 16.3). In patients with extensive disease, long-term disease-free survival rates of 60–80 per cent are projected. In patients with limited disease, a cure rate of approximately 90 per cent is anticipated (*see* Table 16.1).[55,56,58,61–63]

Another highly successful protocol is the Berlin–Frankfurt–Münster (BFM) cooperative group protocol used in Germany for the treatment of patients with ALL (Fig. 16.4).[54] This regimen produces excellent results regardless of ALL phenotype. Patients with stage III and IV lymphoblastic lymphoma have achieved a 78 per cent disease-free survival, with a 48+-month median follow-up.

The reasons for the success of the latter two protocols are not evident, but both are intensive and include more drugs than standard leukaemia protocols. A recent study at SJCRH examined the merits of 'early' and 'intermittent' use of tenoposide (VM-26) plus cytarabine (ara-C) before and after remission induction with prednisone, vincristine and asparaginase and during the first year of maintenance therapy.[57] Anthracyclines, high dose methotrexate (MTX), alkylating agents and involved-field RT were not included (Fig. 16.5). Excellent results were obtained: 22 (96 per cent) of 23 evaluable patients

Table 16.1 Treatment protocols

Protocol	Chemotherapy	RT to bulk	CNS prophylaxis	Stage	No. patients	CR(%)	Survival	Median follow-up	Reference
NHL-75 (SJCRH)	VCR, PDN, CTX, ADR, 6MP, MTX	Randomized in stage III and IV	CR RT IT MTX 12 mg/m²	III and IV	20	88	40% (DFS)	7 years	48, 57
LSA₂L₂ (MSK)	CTX, VCR, PDN, DNR, MTX, ARA-C, TG, ASP, BCNU, HU	Yes	IT MTX 6.25 mg/m²	III	9	88	88% (DFS)	70+ months	58, 61
LSA₂L₂ (modified) POG-7615	As above (with modifications)	Yes	IT MTX 6.25 mg/m²	III	24	96	57% (FFS)	3 years	62
LSA₂L₂ (modified) CCG-551	As above (with modifications)	Yes	IT MTX 6.25 mg/m²	III and IV	31	NR	76% (FFS)	2 years	60
BFM	PDN, VCR, DNR, ASP, ARA-C, MTX, 6MP	No	CR RT IT MTX 12 mg/m²	III and IV	42	?	78% (FFS)	4+ years	54
X-H (SJCRH)	VM-26, ARA-C, PDN, VCR, ASP, MTX, 6MP	No	CR RT IT MTX 12 mg/m²	III and IV	22	96	73% (DFS)	4 years	57
APO (Dana Farber)	VCR, ADR, PDN, ASP, 6MP MTX	Yes	CR RT IT MTX 12 mg/m²	III and IV	21	95	58% (DFS)	3 years	52
77-04 (NCI)	CTX, ADR, VCR, PDN, HD MTX	No	IT MTX 12.5 mg/m² HD MTX	III	10	100	70% (FFS)	4 years	67, 68
COMP (CCG)	CTX, VCR, ID MTX, PDN	Yes	IT MTX 6.25 mg/m²	III and IV	24	NR	26% (FFS)	2 years	64, 60
A-COP+ (POG)	ADR, VCR, PDN, CTX MTX, HC	Yes	CR RT IT MTX 15 mg/m²	III	33	NR	54% (DFS)	3 years	69

RT, radiotherapy; CNS, central nervous system; VCR, vincristine; PDN, prednisone; CTX, cyclophosphamide; ADR, doxorubicin, Adriamycin; 6MP, 6-mercaptopurine; MTX, methotrexate; ID MTX, intermediate dose methotrexate (300 mg/m²); HD MTX, high dose methotrexate (2.7 g/m²); IT MTX, intrathecal methotrexate; DNR, daunomycin; ARA-C, cytarabine; TG, thioguanine; ASP, asparaginase; HU, hydroxyurea; CR, complete response; NR, not reported; DFS, disease-free survival; FFS, failure-free survival; CR RT, cranial irradiation.

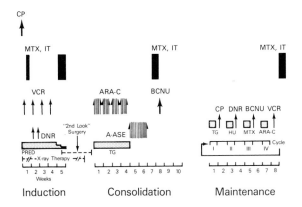

Fig. 16.3 Scheme of original LSA$_2$L$_2$ protocol used by the POG for childhood non-Hodgkin's lymphoma.[56] CP, cyclophosphamide; MTX IT, intrathecal methotrexate; VCR, vincristine; DNR, daunomycin; PRED, prednisone; ARA-C, cytarabine; A-ASE, asparaginase; TG, thioguanine; BCNU, bis-chloroethyl nitrosurea; HU, hydroxyurea. Reproduced with permission from[62]

achieved a complete remission, with a projected four-year continuous complete remission rate of 73 per cent for all patients and 79 per cent for the 19 patients who presented with mediastinal involvement at diagnosis. These data validate the effectiveness of adding VM-26 and ara-C to an otherwise conventional ALL protocol in the management of lymphoblastic lymphoma. VM-26 and ara-C were also included in the successful BFM protocol, although it also contained an anthracycline.

Protocols designed for the treatment of ALL are now accepted as standard regimens for lymphoblastic lymphoma. This development was the result of a randomized trial performed by the Children's Cancer Study Group (CCSG)[60] in which a protocol, (COMP)[64] based on the successful treatment of Burkitt's lymphoma, was compared with the LSA$_2$L$_2$ regimen. COMP, adapted from the work of Zeigler[65] and of Djerassi and Kim,[66] combined pulsed high-dose cyclophosphamide, vincristine, moderate-dose methotrexate, and prednisone (*see* Chapter 17). The LSA$_2$L$_2$ regimen was a modification of the Memorial Sloan-Kettering 10-drug regimen. Both the histological sybtype of disease and the therapeutic regimen (LSA$_2$L$_2$ versus COMP) influenced the clinical outcome of patients with

extensive disease. The modified LSA$_2$L$_2$ regimen was significantly more effective than the COMP regimen in patients with extensive lymphoblastic lymphoma (two-year disease-free survival

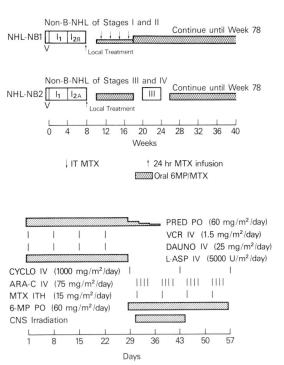

Fig. 16.4 Scheme of the Berlin–Frankfurt–Münster (BFM) cooperative study protocol 1981/3 for the treatment of patients with lymphoblastic (non-B) lymphomas.[54] V, Vorphase-cytoreductive phase with cyclophosphamide and prednisone; I, protocol I; III, protocol III – reinduction therapy similar to protocol I. (The subscripts designate the protocol phase.) CNS irradiation is given during phase I2$_A$ only. Down arrows, intrathecal methotrexate; under 1 year, 6 mg; 1-2 years 8 mg; 2–3 years 10 mg; above 3 years 12 mg. Up arrows, 25-h infusion of methotrexate (500 mg/m²) with leucovorin rescue after 48 h. Shaded area, oral 6-mercaptopurine and methotrexate. Thymic tumours were only irradiated in the presence of residual tumour after completion of protocol I.
IT MTX, intrathecal methotrexate; CYCLO, cyclophosphamide; IV, intravenous; ARA-C, cytarabine; MTX, methotrexate; ITH intrathecal; 6-MP, 6-mercaptopurine; PO, orally; PRED, prednisone; VCR, vincristine; DAUNO, daunomycin; L-ASP, L-asparaginase. Reproduced, with permission, from[54]

rate, 76 per cent versus 26 per cent, respectively, $P = 0.008$).

Although there is now a preference for protocols based on ALL therapy, protocols such as LSA$_2$L$_2$ may not represent optimal therapy for lymphoblastic lymphoma. For example, in the Pediatric Oncology Group (POG) study of a modified version of LSA$_2$L$_2$,[62] only 40 per cent of patients with mediastinal lymphoblastic lymphoma were long-term survivors. At least one treatment regimen not based on an ALL protocol (NCI Pediatric Branch 77-04[67]/Fig. 16.6) has been successful, particularly in patients with large mediastinal masses, although the number of patients in this study is small. The estimated long-term disease-free survival for patients with lymphoblastic lymphoma without marrow involvement treated according to this protocol is 70 per cent. This regimen, which contains both an anthracycline and a high-dose methotrexate infusion with leucovorin rescue, also provides effective therapy for patients with small non-cleaved cell lymphomas. The addition of doxorubicin to a COMP-like regimen was also shown to be effective in the A-COP + (doxorubicin, cyclophosphamide, vincristine, prednisone) regimen. The POG performed a randomized trial comparing LSA$_2$L$_2$ with the A-COP + therapeutic regimen.[69] After adjusting for stage

(I and II, III, IV) there was no statistically significant difference ($P = 0.19$) between A-COP and LSA$_2$L$_2$ regimens on the basis of three-year survival and disease-free survival (62 versus 72 per cent and 53 versus 58 per cent respectively, for the two treatment regimens) however, the ability to detect a clinically meaningful difference in the outcome with the two regimens was limited by the small number of patients.

Limited disease

The prognosis for long-term survival in patients with limited stage lymphoblastic lymphoma (SJCRH stage I or II) is excellent, with a projected 85–90 per cent long-term disease-free survival in all recent regimens of intensive multidrug therapy with or without RT. In the CCSG study,[60] early results suggested that the COMP and LSA$_2$L$_2$ regimens were equally effective; however, recent analysis[49] of the data suggests a survival advantage for LSA$_2$L$_2$.

Because of the associated consequences of therapy (e.g. growth retardation, infertility and second malignancies) Murphy *et al.* designed a treatment regimen with the intent of preserving the high cure rate while lowering the intensity of therapy.[70] Compared with their prior regimen, NHL-75, they reduced the total doses of cyclophosphamide and RT, shortened treatment time and curtailed prophylactic treatment of the CNS, except in patients with a primary head or neck tumour. All 28 patients attained a CR and 24 of 28 remain disease-free at 4+ months to 4 years from diagnosis (median, 24+ months). Murphy *et al.* concluded that a reduction in the therapy of patients with stage I or II lymphoblastic lymphoma is feasible without compromise in cure rate a current POG protocol is as short as two months.

CNS prophylaxis

The CNS is very seldom overtly involved at presentation of lymphoblastic lymphoma. At one time it was a very frequent (approximately 50 per cent) site of relapse,[40,41] but since the advent of effective CNS prophylaxis isolated CNS recurrence has been encountered only rarely.[54,60,66,71]

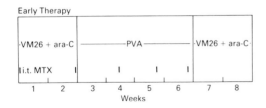

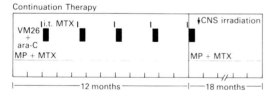

Fig. 16.5 Scheme of the SJCRH protocol for the treatment of non-Hodgkin's lymphoma. ara-C, cytarabine; VM-26, tenoposide; PVA, prednisone, vincristine and asparaginase; MTX, methotrexate; MP, 6-mercaptopurine. Reproduced with permission from.[57]

Various methods of prophylaxis are in use. Some regimens specify cranial irradiation and intrathecal methotrexate (IT MTX);[54] in others, IT MTX and/or intrathecal cytarabine (IT ara-C) are administered with intermediate- or high-dose MTX.[60,66,67] The optimal regimen for CNS prophylaxis is not known, but the adverse effects of cranial irradiation on the CNS argue against its use. Intrathecal chemotherapy (established doses and schedules of agents) coupled with intermediate or high dose (HD) MTX infusions appears to be the treatment of choice for CNS prophylaxis.

Treatment in adults

Recent approaches to the management of adults with lymphoblastic lymphoma have been variably successful. Coleman *et al.*[72] reported a 56 per cent disease-free survival rate with a three-year follow-up in a pilot study of CHOP (cyclophosphamide, doxorubicin, vincristine, prednisone), HD MTX, L-asparaginase, IT MTX, 6-MP (mercaptopurine) and MTX treatment for stage I–IV (Ann Arbor staging) lymphoma. This represented a clear gain over the short median survival they had obtained in the past with

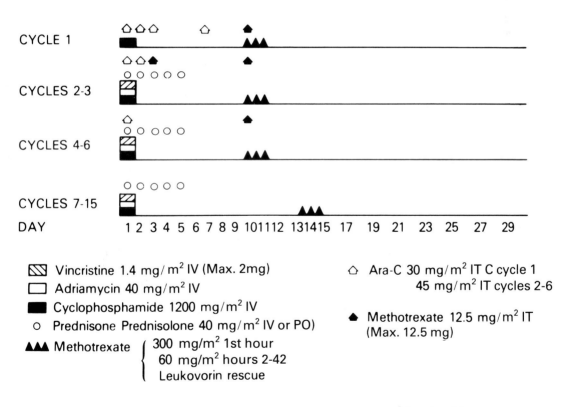

Fig. 16.6 Scheme of the NCI protocol (77–04) for the treatment of non-Hodgkin's lymphoma.[67]

lymphoma-type pulse chemotherapy without CNS prophylaxis. Levine et al.[73] treated 15 patients with lymphoblastic lymphoma using a modified LSA_2L_2 regimen (2000 cGy to the mediastinum, cranial RT and IT MTX). The survival rate at five years was less than 40 per cent. Slater et al.[74] at Memorial Sloan-Kettering Cancer Center summarized the results of therapy for 51 patients with lymphoblastic lymphoma who were enrolled in one of five successive intensive chemotherapy programmes for ALL since 1971. The five-year survival rate for leukaemic and non-leukaemic patients was 45 per cent.

Although more intensive chemotherapy combined with CNS prophylaxis has extended the long-term survival of patients with lymphoblastic lymphoma, the treatment results in adults fall short of those in children. This may reflect differences in the clinical and biological characteristics of adult versus paediatric lymphoblastic lymphoma as first proposed by Nathwani et al.[37] who reported differences in the incidence of mediastinal masses, numbers of mitotic figures and incidence of leukaemic conversion between younger patients and those older than 30 years.

Factors in prognosis

The tumour burden at diagnosis is the most reliable indicator of treatment outcome in NHL.[75] Clinical staging may, in part, reflect tumour burden; however, not all staging systems are based on stepwise increases in tumour burden. Serum levels of molecules, either secreted by tumour cells or accumulated as a result of cellular breakdown, may be more indicative of tumour burden.[66,75-80] Examples include lactic dehydrogenase (LDH), β_2-microglobulin, lactic acid and polyamines. A molecule that has recently been studied is the soluble interleukin-2 receptor (SIL-2R). Wagner et al.[76] performed multivariate analyses of patients with NHL treated with the NCI protocol 77-04 and found that SIL-2R levels were superior to all other prognostic variables examined. A similar study done by Pui et al.[80] demonstrated a correlation between SIL-2R levels and both serum LDH levels ($P = 0.0001$) and disease stage: B-cell ALL > stage III or IV diffuse small non-cleaved cell NHL > stage III or IV lymphoblastic NHL > stage I or II NHL. The findings of their multivariate analysis, like those of Wagner et al., identified SIL-2R levels as a better predictor of treatment response than either disease stage or serum LDH levels.

Biochemical correlates of prognosis are important because they provide the most objective measure of tumour burden, thereby facilitating risk group assignment and subsequent selection of appropriate therapy. These molecules may be important markers of both treatment response and disease recurrence, much as the carcinoembryonic antigen is in patients with carcinoma of the colon. Also, molecules such as SIL-2R may have implications in therapeutic regimens incorporating biological response modification, which often include the use of lymphocyte-synthesized molecules (e.g. IL-2 and gamma interferon). Negative interactions of the therapeutic agent and the lymphoma-cell product may occur either directly or secondary to opposing effects of the molecules derived from normal cell populations (usually lymphocytes) involved in the therapeutic response.

Other prognostic factors associated with specific treatment protocols for T-cell lymphoblastic disease have been reported. As part of the POG study of LSA_2L_2 in T-cell ALL patients, a multivariate analysis of potential risk factors (age at diagnosis, presenting white count, platelet count, haemoglobin level, per cent of E-rosetting cells, sex and race) indicated that only the presenting white blood cell count (WBC) (< or > 50×10^9/l), a reflection of tumour burden, was predictive of the duration of continuous complete remission and of the duration of CNS remission.[81] Interestingly, T-cell ALL patients with less than 50×10^9/l WBC at diagnosis had approximately the same long term CR rate as did mediastinal NHL patients treated with the same protocol (modified LSA_2L_2), suggesting that the lower WBC T-ALL patients are more clinically similar to the T-NHL patients than are the higher WBC T-ALL patients.[82]

Late effects

Recommendations to reduce the long-term complications of therapy for lymphoblastic lymphoma in children are evolving. With results from SJCRH[48] demonstrating no therapeutic benefit from adjuvant involved-field radiation in the treatment of patients with advanced disease, RT has begun to play a smaller role in overall treatment regimens. This is likely to reduce the associated injury to heart, oesophagus and lungs. However, with improved survival obtained with newer, more aggressive chemotherapy regimens, follow-up studies are expected to reveal additional long-term sequelae.

There are three problem areas for patients who have completed therapy: reproductive dysfunction, risk of second malignancies and the psychological implications of experiencing a life-threatening illness.

The reproductive function of males is much more severely impaired than that of females. Alkylating agents, in particular, have caused reproductive dysfunction in men; however, their toxicity is less in prepubertal boys undergoing treatment.[83] Women who are treated before the age of 20 and have not received abdominal radiation will usually maintain normal reproductive function throughout life.[84] Men and women treated with regimens developed to treat patients with ALL seldom experience subsequent reproductive dysfunction, perhaps because of the absence of alkylating agents in most of these regimens. The risk of a second malignancy for patients treated for lymphoblastic lymphoma is not as great as in children with a solid tumour or Hodgkin's disease.[85] Patients who are at a higher risk are again those who have received alkylating agents.

The psychological problems that may develop in patients with a chronic illness are varied. A multidisciplinary late-effects team, including psychologists, social workers, physical therapists, nurses and doctors, is important during off-therapy follow-up to evaluate the complex sequelae of cancer and its treatment.

Future considerations

The treatment of patients with lymphoblastic lymphoma has improved greatly over the past 15 years, primarily because of the use of more intensive multidrug regimens incorporating effective CNS prophylaxis. The development of additional active single agents or new ways of using presently available active drugs for incorporation into aggressive multiagent chemotherapy programmes provides the most likely immediate possibility for improved treatment. Molecularly cloned haematopoietic growth factors (e.g. granulocyte or granulocyte-macrophage colony stimulating factors) that minimize or eliminate myelosuppression, may permit investigators to increase the dose intensity of existing regimens, but these molecules could also stimulate tumour cell growth. The benefit of autologous or allogeneic transplant in these patients has yet to be clarified. Other possibilities for therapy include the use of biological response modifying agents (e.g. interleukin-2, interferons or monoclonal antibodies) alone or in combination with chemotherapy.

As the understanding of the biology of these malignancies improves, so will our ability to target effective therapy, with less associated morbidity.

References

1. Non-Hodgkin's lymphoma pathologic classification project. *Cancer*. 1982; **49**: 2112.
2. Rappaport H. In: *Atlas of Tumor Pathology*, Section 3, Fascicle 8. Washington, DC: US Armed Forces Institute of Pathology, 1966.
3. Lukes RJ, Collins RD. *British Journal of Cancer*. 1975; **31** (suppl. II), 1–28.
4. Nathwani BW, Kim H, Rappaport H. *Cancer*. 1976; **38**, 964–83.
5. Magrath IT. In: Levine AS (ed). *Cancer in the Young*, New York: Masson Pub., 1981, 473–4.
6. Cossman J, Chused TM, Fisher RI, *et al. Cancer Research*. 1983; **43**, 4486.
7. Bernard A, Boumsell L, Reinherz EL, *et al. Blood*. 1981; **57**, 1105.
8. Roper M, Crist WM, Metzger R, *et al. Blood*. 1983; **61**, 830.

9. Crist WM, Kelly DR, Abdelsalam HR, *et al. Cancer*. 1981; **48**, 2070–5.

10. Crist WM, Shuster JJ, Falletta J, *et al. Blood*. 1989; (in press).

11. Braziel RM, Keneklis T, Donlon JA, *et al. American Journal of Clinical Pathology*. 1983; **80**, 655–9.

12. Vodinelich L, Tax W, Bai Y, Pegram S, Capel P, Greaves MF. *Blood*. 1983; **62**, 1108–13.

13. Haynes BF. *Immunobiology*. 1981; **159**, 14.

14. Link M, Warnke R, Finlay J, *et al. Blood*. 1983; **62**, 722.

15. Reinherz EL, Kung PC, Goldstein G, Levey RH, Schlossman SF. *Proceedings of the National Academy of Sciences USA*. 1980; **77**, 1588–92.

16. Royer HD, Acuto O, Fabbi M, *et al. Cell*. 1984; **39**, 261–6.

17. Royer HD, Ramarli D, Acuto O, *et al. Proceedings of the National Academy of Sciences USA*. 1985; **82**, 5510–14.

18. Meuer SC, Acuto O, Hussey RE, *et al. Nature*. 1983; **303**, 808–10.

19. Bernard A, Boumsell L. *Progress in Cancer Research and Therapy*. 1982; **21**, 93.

20. Reinherz EL, Nadler LM, Sallan SE, Schlossman SF. *Journal of Clinical Investigation*. 1979; **64**, 392–7.

21. Bernard A, Murphy SB, Melvin S, *et al. Blood*. 1982; **59**, 549.

22. Link MP, Roper M, Dorfman RF, *et al. Blood*. 1983; **61**, 838.

23. Grogan T, Spier C, Wirt DP, *et al. Diagnostic Immunology*. 1986; **4**, 81–8.

24. Sheibani K, Winberg DC, Burke JS. *Leukaemia Research*. 1987; **11**, 371–7.

25. Kristoffersson U, Heim SW, Heldrug J. *Hereditas*. 1985; **3**, 77.

26. Smith SD, Morgan R, Link MP, *et al. Blood*. 1986; **67**, 650.

27. Denny CT, Yoshikai Y, Mak TW, *et al. Nature*. 1986; **320**, 549–51.

28. Levine EG, Arthur DC, Frizzera G, *et al. Blood*. 1985; **66**, 1414.

29. Dube ID, Raimondi SC, Pi D, Kalousek DK. *Blood*. 1986; **67**, 1181–4.

30. Mathieu-Mahul D, Sigaux F, Zhu C, *et al. International Journal of Cancer*. 1986; **38**, 835–40.

31. Le Beau MM, McKeithan TW, Shima EA, *et al. Proceedings of the National Academy of Sciences USA*. 1978; **83**, 9744–8.

32. Smith SD, Morgan R, Link MP, *et al. Blood*. 1986; **67**, 650–6.

33. McKeithan TW, Shima EA, Le Beau MM, *et al. Proceedings of the National Academy of Sciences USA*. 1986; **83**, 6636–40.

34. Croce CM, Erikson J, Ar-Rushdi A, *et al. Proceedings of the National Academy of Sciences USA*.

1984; **81**, 3170–4.

35. Raimondi SC, Behm FG, Pui C–H, *et al. Blood*. **20** (suppl. 1), 207a, (abstract 683).

36. West R. *World Health Statistics*. 1984; **37**, 98.

37. Nathwani B, Diamond L, Winberg C. *Cancer*. 1981; **48**, 2347–57.

38. Young JL, Ries LG, Silverberg E, Horm JW, Miller RW. *Cancer*. 1986; **58**, 598–602.

39. Finch S. *Pathogenesis of Leukemias and Lymphomas: Environmental Influences*. New York: Raven Press, 1984: 207–223.

40. Watanabe A, Sullivan MP, Sutow WW, Wilbur JR. *American Journal of Diseases of Children*. 1973; **125**, 57–61.

41. Hutter JJ, Favara BE, Nelson M, Holton LP. *Cancer*. 1975; **36**, 2132–7.

42. Ziegler JL, Magrath IT. In: Iochim HL (ed). *Pathobiology Annual*. 1974; New York: Appleton-Century-Crofts, 129–42.

43. Sarban E, Janus C, Edwards B, Magrath IT. *Journal of Clinical Oncology*. 1983; **11**, 677–81.

44. Magrath IT, Mugerwa J, Bailey I, Olweny C, Kiryabwire Y. *Quarterly Journal of Medicine*. 1974; **43**, 489–508.

45. Murphy SB. *Seminars in Oncology*. 1980; **7**, 332.

46. Krudy AD, Dunnick NR, Magrath IT, Shawker TH, Doppman JL, Spiegel R. *American Journal of Radiology*. 1981; **136**, 747–54.

47. Carabell SC, Goodman RL. In: DeVita V, Hellman S, Rosenberg S (eds). *Principles and Practice of Oncology*, 2nd ed, Philadelphia: Lippincott, 1985: 1855–60.

48. Murphy SB, Hustu HO. *Cancer*. 1980; **45**, 630–7.

49. Link MP, Donaldson S, Berard C, *et al.* In: *Proceedings of the Third International Conference on Malignant Lymphomas*. 1987.

50. Murphy SB, Hustu O, Rivera G, Berard CW. *Journal of Clinical Oncology*. 1983; **1**(5), 326–30.

51. Berard A, Boumsell L, Patte C, *et al. Medical and Pediatric Oncology*. 1986; **14**, 148.

52. Weinstein HJ, Cassady JR, Levey R. *Journal of Clinical Oncology*. 1983; **1**, 537.

53. Murphy S. *Cancer Treatment Reports*. 1977; **61**, 1161.

54. Müller-Weihrich ST, Henze G, Odenwald E, *et al.* In: *Malignant Lymphomas and Hodgkin's Disease: Experimental and Therapeutic Advances*. Boston: Martinus Nijhoff, 1985; 633.

55. Pichler E, Jurgenssen OA, Radaszkiewicz T, *et al. Cancer*. 1982; **50**, 2740.

56. Bogusawska-Jaworska J, Koscielniak E, Sroczynska M, *et al. American Journal of Pediatric Hematology and Oncology*. 1984; **6**, 363.

57. Dahl GV, Rivera G, Pui CH, *et al. Blood*. 1985; **66**, 1110.

58. Wollner N, Burchenal JH, Liebermann PH, *et al. Cancer.* 1976; **37**, 123.

59. Glatstein E, Kim H, Donaldson SS, *et al. Cancer.* 1974; **34**, 204–11.

60. Anderson JR, Wilson JF, Jenkin RD, *et al. New England Journal of Medicine.* 1983; **308**, 559.

61. Wollner N, Exelby PR, Liebermann PH. *Cancer.* 1979; **44**, 1990–9.

62. Sullivan MP, Boyett J, Pullen J. *Cancer.* 1985; **55**, 323–36.

63. Miser J, Miser A, Pendergrass T, *et al. American Journal of Pediatric Hematology and Oncology.* 1980; **2**, 317–20.

64. Meadows A, Jenkin R, Anderson J, *et al. Medical and Pediatric Oncology.* 1980; **8**, 14–24.

65. Zeigler J. *New England Journal of Medicine.* 1977; **297**, 75–80.

66. Djerassi I, Kim JS. *Cancer.* 1976; **38**, 1043–51.

67. Magrath I, Janus C, Edwards B, *et al. Blood.* 1984; **63**, 1102.

68. Magrath I. In: Pizzo, Poplack (eds). *Principles and Practice of Pediatric Oncology.* New York: Lippincott, 1988; 415–455.

69. Hvizdala E, Berard C, Callihan T, *et al. Journal of Clinical Oncology.* 1988; **6**, 26–33.

70. Murphy SB, Hustu HO, Rivera G, *et al. Journal of Clinical Oncology.* 1983; **1**, 326–30.

71. Gadner H, Muller-Weihrich S, Riehm H. *Onkologie.* 1986; **9**, 126.

72. Coleman CN, Cohen JR, Burke JS, Rosenberg SA. *Blood.* 1981; **57**, 679–84.

73. Levine AM, Forman SJ, Meyer PR, *et al. Blood.* 1983; **61**, 92–8.

74. Slater DE, Mertelsmann R, Koziner B, *et al. Journal of Clinical Oncology.* 1986; **4**, 57–67.

75. Magrath IT, Lee YJ, Anderson T, *et al. Cancer.* 1980; **45**, 1507–15.

76. Wagner D, Kiwanuka J, Edwards B, *et al. Journal of Clinical Oncology.* 1987; **5**, 1262–74.

77. Hagberg H, Killander A, Simonsson B. *Cancer.* 1983; **51**, 2220–5.

78. Csako G, Magrath I, Elin R. *American Journal of Clinical Pathology.* 1982; **78**, 712–17.

79. Desser H, Woldner R, Klaring W. *Advances in Polyamine Research.* 1983; **4**, 49–58.

80. Pui C–H, Ip S, Kung P, *et al. Blood.* 1987; **70**, 624–8.

81. Boyett JM, Pullen DJ, Sullivan MP. *Proceedings of the American Society of Clinical Oncology.* 1985; **4**, C-636 (abstract).

82. Pullen JD, Sullivan MP, Falletta JM, *et al. Blood.* 1982; **60**, 1159–68.

83. Sullivan MP, Jaffe N, Boren H, *et al. Proceedings of the Annual Meeting of the American Association of Cancer Research.* 1985; **26**, 182.

84. Hall BH, Green DM. *Proceedings of the Annual Meeting of the American Society of Clinical Oncology.* 1983; **2**, C-272.

85. Meadows AT, Baum E, Fossati-Bellani F, *et al. Journal of Clinical Oncology.* 1985; **3**, 532–8.

CHAPTER 17

SMALL NON-CLEAVED CELL LYMPHOMAS

Ian Magrath

Definitions and general description

The small non-cleaved cell (SNCC) lymphomas are rare tumours which have a number of synonyms in various classification schemes,[1] including undifferentiated lymphomas (which encompasses Burkitt's and non-Burkitt's subtypes) in the modified Rappaport classification[2] and lymphoblastic lymphomas (Burkitt type) in the Kiel classification.[3] These terms are purely descriptive and provide little insight into the cellular origins of the tumours, although the term small non-cleaved was originally used by Lukes and Collins because of the morphological resemblance of these tumours to a cell seen by them in the germinal centres of secondary lymphoid follicles.[4] Small non-cleaved cell lymphomas are invariably of B-cell origin,[5,6] but it remains unclear as to whether any or all SNCC lymphomas arise from germinal centre cells.

The clinical behaviour of SNCC lymphomas is quite distinct from the behaviour of the majority of tumours which are believed to arise from the germinal follicles and, although selective involvement of germinal follicles in the bowel has been described in young people,[7] SNCC lymphomas are always diffuse and never have a follicular architecture. Selective involvement of germinal follicles appears to result from the migration of the cells to this location from an adjacent tumour mass, and sequentially involves the mantle zone followed by the germinal centre.[8] This finding indicates

a tendency of SNCC lymphoma cells to home to the germinal follicle, and is not *prima facie* evidence of an origin from the germinal centre itself.

The majority of SNCC lymphomas contain non-random chromosomal translocations which involve the chromosome band (q24) on chromosome 8 on which a proto-oncogene involved in cellular proliferation, c-*myc*, normally resides.[6] However, a proportion of SNCC lymphomas (up to 50 per cent) in individuals above the age of 40 years have been reported to contain 14;18 translocations, a translocation which occurs predominantly in follicular lymphomas.[9] Rare tumours, and at least one derived cell line, containing both 8;14 and 14;18 translocations have also been described.[9,10] Thus a subset of tumours morphologically designated as SNCC lymphomas and arising in older individuals is closely related to germinal centre neoplasia, and in some cases such SNCC lymphomas may arise from pre-existing follicular centre cell neoplasms. However, there is evidence that the chromosomal translocations in follicular lymphomas occur during the process of V-D-J joining of immunoglobulin genes, i.e. at a very early stage of B-cell differentiation. This means that transformation from a follicular lymphoma to an SNCC lymphoma might be more akin to blast transformation in chronic myeloid leukaemia, i.e. transformation represents an additional degree of failure of differentiation such that the predominant cell type in the malignant clone becomes a more immature cell.

While it is apparent that the histological category of 'SNCC lymphoma' is heterogeneous, the most frequently encountered tumour of this type occurs primarily in the first two decades of life, has a B-cell phenotype (nearly always expressing surface IgM) and possesses a translocation involving chromosome 8 at band q24 and one of chromosomes 14, 22 or 2 at bands q32, q11-2 and p11 respectively. Thus, an absolute and objective diagnosis is possible when phenotype and karyotype are examined in addition to histology; their routine employment in diagnosis is strongly recommended. Because of the predominance of the SNCC lymphomas in children and young adults, most of the information in this chapter is derived from this age group.

Histology

A detailed description of the histological appearance of SNCC has been given in Chapter 3. The essential features are a lack of any evidence of differentiation towards plasma cells or mature lymphocytes, a high nuclear to cytoplasmic ratio, a round or oval nucleus with a coarse or 'open' chromatin pattern (i.e. giving the appearance of being able to see through the network of chromatin) and multiple (usually two to five) readily discernible nucleoli (occasionally a single large nucleolus, *see* below). The narrow rim of cytoplasm is very basophilic (staining intensely with methyl-green pyronine) because of the abundant free ribosomes, which are seen readily on electron microscopy. The cytoplasm almost invariably contains lipid vacuoles which stain with oil-red O, the significance of which is unknown. Histological sections usually demonstrate the presence of macrophages, scattered among the tumour cells, in which nuclear debris is discernible, and which give rise to the oft quoted 'starry sky' appearance. This pattern is not pathognomonic and may be seen in any rapidly proliferating tumour.

Although the SNCC lymphomas can be subdivided into Burkitt's and non-Burkitt's lymphomas, the distinction between these two histological entities is subjective, depending upon the degree of pleomorphism and the proportion of cells with single nucleoli, consistent with a diagnosis of Burkitt's lymphoma is ill-defined, but the greater the degree of either, the more likely is a diagnosis of 'non-Burkitt's' lymphoma. However, in different sections from the same tumour, or even in the same section, the degree of pleomorphism may vary so that the same tumour could have some areas consistent with Burkitt's lymphoma and others consistent with non-Burkitt's lymphoma. On occasion this is due to histological artefact, e.g. to improper fixation, but this does not always appear to be the explanation. Hence, in the absence of clear guidelines, such cases may be arbitrarily included as either Burkitt's or non-Burkitt's lymphoma. Less often there is difficulty in distinguishing between SNCC lymphomas and large cell lymphomas. This may be pertinent to the finding that a proportion of large cell lymphomas contain the same chromosomal translocations as SNCC lymphomas.[9,11]

Because of the subjective difficulties inherent in a purely histological distinction between subcategories of SNCC lymphomas it is not surprising that, at least in children, the morphological categories of Burkitt's lymphoma and non-Burkitt's lymphoma do not appear to correlate with differences in prognosis.[12-14] However, it is probably true that non-Burkitt's lymphomas are more often diagnosed in older individuals, and also that older individuals have a worse prognosis (possibly because of the use of different chemotherapy regimens), so that failure to take into account such factors as age and treatment could lead to erroneous conclusions in this regard.[15] In older individuals the non-random 8;14 and 14;18 translocations in SNCC neoplasms do not correlate with morphology,[9] while attempts to determine the influence of cytogenetics on clinical behaviour and response to therapy have yet to be made. In all, there would appear to be little value in attempting to make a histological distinction between Burkitt's lymphoma and non-Burkitt's lymphoma.

Immunopathology

Small non-cleaved cell lymphoma is always of B-cell origin and always expresses surface immunoglobulin, which is IgM in more than 90 per cent of cases.[6,16,17] Sporadic tumours also secrete IgM, which may be detectable in the serum of patients with high tumour burdens.[18,19] A single light chain type which reflects the monoclonal origin of these tumours is present, as are several other B-cell restricted antigens, including B4 (CD19), B1 (CD20), CD22 (usually) as well as B-cell associated antigens, including BA-1 (CD24) and HLA-DR, which are expressed on the cell surface.[6,16,20–22] The common ALL antigen (CD10) is also expressed on almost all SNCC lymphomas *in vivo*, but this antigen is frequently lost during cultivation *in vitro* of derived cell lines, particularly in Epstein–Barr virus (EBV)-positive tumours,[23] leading to differences in phenotype between sporadic and endemic SNCC lymphomas.[20–22] B2 (CD21), which incorporates in a single molecule the receptors for both the C3d component of human complement and EBV is expressed to a variable extent, usually being found in higher numbers on the surface of African Burkitt's lymphoma cells[21,24,25] than on SNCC lymphomas occurring outside this region. The SNCC lymphomas almost invariably fail to express the enzyme terminal deoxyribonucleotide transferase (TdT), unlike lymphoblastic lymphomas,[6] although rare cases of L3 leukaemia bearing 8;14 translocations and expressing TdT have been reported.[10,26]

It is likely that the normal counterpart cell of the majority of SNCC lymphomas is at an antigen-independent stage of B-cell differentiation,[5] but a fraction of tumours (*see* above) may arise from germinal follicle cells, i.e. B-cells undergoing antigen-dependent differentiation. The ontogenetic origins of these lymphomas are further discussed in Chapter 3.

Cytogenetics

Small non-cleared cell lymphomas possess non-random chromosomal translocations which always involve the q24 region on the terminal portion of chromosome 8 and one of the immunoglobulin loci on chromosomes 14 (q32, heavy chains), 22 (q12, λ light chains) or 2 (q13, κ light chains).[5,27,28] The 8;14 translocation is the most frequently observed, accounting for 75–80 per cent of the translocations in SNCC lymphomas among those studied so far.[29] This translocation has also been observed in a small fraction of large cell lymphomas as well as the L3 type of acute lymphoblastic leukaemias.[9,11]

L3 leukaemias appear to represent SNCC lymphomas which present with marrow failure because of diffuse bone marrow infiltration.[30] It would seem reasonable to consider the chromosomal translocations involving chromosome 8, band q24, and one of the immunoglobulin gene loci on chromosomes 14, 22 or 2 as defining a specific pathological entity, or a group of closely related pathological entities, since abundant evidence points towards them being of pathogenetic significance[5] (*see* Chapter 6). These characteristics define a tumour, or group of tumours, containing genetic abnormalities which result in altered expression of the c-*myc* oncogene[5] (*see* Chapter 6). Although it is theoretically possible that the same end result could be produced by a genetic rearrangement which is not manifested as a chromosomal translocation (as has been described in rare mouse plasmacytomas which bear homologous chromosomal translocations,[31] an SNCC lymphoma which lacks one of these chromosomal translocations is likely to be of different pathogenetic origin. The histologically defined SNCC lymphomas observed in adults which bear 14;18 translocations without an 8;14 translocation fall into this category. Since the chromosomal translocations appear to develop during the early stages of B-cell differentiation (*see* Chapter 6), such tumours presumably represent malignant clones in which the stage of cellular differentiation when the tumour is manifested is earlier than the more usual tumours bearing a 14;18 translocation. This is similar to acute lymphoblastic leukaemia (ALL) bearing the same translocations, 9;22 (but often differing at a molecular level), as chronic myeloid leukaemia. It remains to be seen, however, whether the 14;18 translocations in follicular and SNCC lymphomas are identical at a molecular level. Tumours with both 8;14 and 14;18 translocations presumably represent the development of a SNCC lymphoma in a pre-existing (detected or undetected) follicular lymphoma. This is perhaps analagous to the development of 8;14 bearing lymphomas in hyperplastic B-cell clones in patients with AIDS,[32–34] or to blast crisis developing in chronic myeloid leukaemia. This presumption is supported by reports of morphological transformation from follicular lymphoma to diffuse 'Burkitt-like' lymphomas or even L3 leukaemia of pre-B phenotype.[10,35–37] However much more information will be required before these observations can be fully elucidated.

Molecular biology

Since SNCC lymphomas are of B-cell origin, they invariably have evidence of structural immunoglobulin gene rearrangements, i.e. a deviation from the 'germ-line' pattern present in germ cells and non-lymphoid tissue (*see* Chapter 6). Using the technique of Southern blotting, which enables such rearrangements to be recognized, the rearranged fragments can be used as clonal markers (*see* Chapter 6). An additional and even more useful clonal marker is the rearrangement of the c-*myc* gene (a proto-oncogene necessary for cellular proliferation), which is a consequence of the 8;14 chromosomal translocation.[38,39] However, not all SNCC lymphomas with 8;14 translocations have rearranged c-*myc* genes, since the breakpoint on chromosome 8 can be some distance away from the gene, although in this case structural changes within the regulatory region of the gene appear invariably to be present.[40] Moreover, as mentioned above, some SNCC lymphomas in adults carry 14;18 translocations, in which case rearrangements of the *bcl*-2 gene, as is more usually seen in follicular lymphomas,[41,42] are found. Of considerable interest is the recent finding that the structural changes in the c-*myc* gene segregate according to the geographic location of the tumour. In endemic tumours the breakpoint nearly always lies some distance away from the gene itself regardless of the type of chromosomal translocation, while in sporadic tumours, except in the variant translocations, the breakpoint usually lies within the regulatory

region of the gene.[40]

The combination of immunoglobulin and c-*myc* gene rearrangements is pathognomonic of SNCC lymphomas, and in an appropriate histological or cytological setting it provides definitive confirmation of the diagnosis. These structural genetic changes have much greater significance than their use as diagnostic tests, however, since there is little doubt that the chromosomal translocations, which serve to juxtapose immunoglobulin sequences to the c-*myc* gene, lead to dysregulation of c-*myc*. The inappropriate expression of c-*myc*, with resultant inappropriate cellular proliferation, appears to be a critical step in the pathogenesis of SNCC lymphomas (Fig. 17.1) although it is likely that the mechanism whereby the gene is deregulated differs in endemic and sporadic

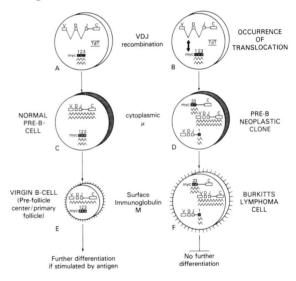

ᴧᴧᴧ gene expression

VDJC variable, diversity, joining and constant immunoglobulin gene regions.

Fig. 17.1 Hypothetical scheme depicting the pathogenesis of Burkitt's lymphoma. On the left the normal series of differentiation steps (including V-D-J joining) for the earliest stages of B-cells, resulting in first cytoplasmic μ chains (c) then surface IgM (e), are shown. Note that the earliest cells expressing surface IgM (virgin B-cells) are resting cells, unlike their more immature counterparts, and have switched off expression of c-*myc*. On the right, chromosomal translocation and deregulation of c-*myc* has occurred, with resultant indefinite proliferation of the cells containing the translocation.

tumours. The probable mechanisms leading to the presence of genetic abnormalities in these tumours, their consequences and pathogenetic significance at a molecular level are discussed in Chapter 6.

Epidemiology

In the USA and Europe, SNCC lymphomas account for only 1–2 per cent of all lymphomas, but 33–50 per cent of childhood lymphomas.[9,43] The incidence is age dependent, being much commoner in the first two decades of life, but occurring at all ages except below the age of two. The incidence of SNCC lymphomas differs dramatically in different parts of the world. In so-called 'endemic' regions, which include equatorial Africa and Papua, New Guinea,[44] there is a relatively high incidence of some 5–10 cases per 100 000 children below the age of 16 years (rather higher than that of acute lymphoblastic leukaemia in the USA and Europe), while in the non-endemic, or 'sporadic' regions, the incidence is two or three cases per million children.[5,16] North Africa and South America appear to be regions of intermediate incidence, but precise figures are difficult to obtain. In both endemic and sporadic regions the male:female ratio is between 2 and 3:1.[16] The difference in incidence between the endemic and sporadic forms of SNCC lymphomas is accompanied by other differences in the biological and clinical features of these two forms of the disease (Table 17.1).

Epstein–Barr virus DNA has been shown to be present in the tumour cells of some 95 per cent of the SNCC lymphomas in endemic regions, and about 85 per cent of the tumours in North Africa. In the USA and Europe, only about 15–20 per cent of tumours contain EBV DNA.[16] The frequency of EBV association in South America has not been determined. Virus particles are not seen in the tumour cells, indicating that the viral genome is harboured in a latent state. Its contribution, if any, to pathogenesis in those tumours which harbour it is unknown. However, it is likely that a major contribution of the virus is to increase the size of the target cell population, thus increasing the possibility that 'random' chromosomal breaks will generate the appropriate chromosomal translocation in a single cell clone. The location of these chromosomal breaks is probably not completely random, since it is likely that the im-

Table 17.1 Differences between endemic and sporadic Burkitt's lymphoma

	Endemic	Sporadic
Average annual incidence (children below 16 years)	10/100 000	0.2/100000
Occurrence	Climatically determined	Not climatically determined
Association with EBV[1]	95%	15%
Chromosome 8 breakpoints	Upstream of c-*myc*	Within c-*myc*
Immunological features	'Blast' Ags CALLA−, Tü1+, B2+ No IgM secretion	Few 'blast' Ags CALLA+, Tü1−, B2− Secretion of IgM
Common sites of tumour	Jaw (58%) Abdomen (58%) Paraspinal (17%) Orbit (11%) Bone marrow (7%) Pleura (3%) Pharynx (0%)	Abdomen (91%) Bone marrow (20%) Pleura (19%) Lymph nodes (13%) Pharynx (10%) Paraspinal (2%) Orbit (1%)

[1]Presence of Epstein–Barr viral DNA in tumour cells

munoglobulin loci are more fragile near the time that rearrangement of immunoglobulin genes is occurring, while band q24 of chromosome 8 contains fragile sites susceptible to mutation.[45] An alternative hypothesis, that EBV is responsible for 'immortalizing' cells which already contain a chromosomal translocation, has been proposed.[46]

The role of environmental factors other than EBV in the endemic region of Africa is unknown. A particularly intriguing observation, however, is the climatic dependency of the distribution of the tumour, which corresponds closely to that of holoendemic malaria[16,29,46] (*see* also Chapter 8). Whether there is a direct relationship between malaria and Burkitt's lymphoma is unknown, but it has been postulated that T-cell supression and B-cell stimulation by malaria may participate in pathogenesis. It has also been shown that there is defective T-cell regulation of EBV infected B-cells in patients with acute malaria.[47] This finding supports the possibility that there is an increased pool of the appropriate population of B-cells or pre-B-cells in African children, which predisposes to the occurrence of non-random chromosomal translocations.

Small non-cleaved cell lymphomas occur with increased frequency in patients with an underlying immunodeficiency. They occur particularly in individuals infected with the human immunodeficiency virus (HIV) (*see* Chapters 9 and 10) and occasionally in families with the X-linked lymphoproliferative syndrome.[48] It seems probable that, like the environmental factors in Africa, such conditions induce an increase in the size of target B-cell populations with a resultant increased likelihood that chromosomal translocations will develop.

Cytokinetics

Small non-cleaved cell lymphomas are rapidly growing neoplasms with very high growth fractions (approaching 100 per cent in some cases) and potential doubling times (i.e. calculated doubling times which do not take into account spontaneous cell death in the neoplasm) ranging from 12 hours to a few days.[49] In practice, the measured (actual) doubling time is several days (in one study the mean doubling time of three skin tumours was 66 hours[49]), although there is considerable variation from patient to patient and between different tumour sites in the same patient. The actual doubling time depends upon the spontaneous cell death rate, which in turn varies according to tumour size (being greater in larger tumours). It is quite probable that the nature of the tissue in which the tumour resides is also important, although only clinical information can be brought to bear on this issue. For example, the marked predisposition of African tumours to sites at which cellular proliferation (and doubtless a high local concentration of growth factors) is occurring, such as the developing molars, ovaries and breast tissue in pubertal or lactating females, suggests that factors external to the cell may be of importance to tumour cell growth. The spontaneous cell death rate has been measured in African Burkitt's lymphoma to be about 70 per cent of all progeny cells.[49] Up to 27 per cent of the cells may be in the S-phase (by flow cytometry).[50,51] These observations have relevance to management. The high spontaneous cell turnover rate in untreated tumours is the immediate cause of pretreatment hyperuricaemia, which occurs frequently in patients with a high tumour cell burden. The short actual doubling times mean that patients should be 'worked up' rapidly and treatment commenced at the earliest possible time. Any delay will increase both the chance of complications and worsen the prognosis, since tumour burden is perhaps the single most important prognostic factor.[52–54] The high growth fraction of SNCC lymphomas is, however, in some respects also beneficial, since it is likely that this is an important factor in the excellent response and frequent cure of these lymphomas when treated with chemotherapy.

Clinical features and staging

Presentation and anatomical distribution of tumour

Although SNCC lymphomas can involve almost any organ or tissue in the body, in the USA and

Europe a high proportion of patients (as high as 90 per cent) have an abdominal tumour at the time of presentation.[54–57] This may be manifested as abdominal pain or swelling, and is frequently accompanied by a symptom complex caused by intussusception, a change in bowel habits, nausea and vomiting, evidence of gastro-intestinal bleeding or, rarely, intestinal perfora-tion.[57] Presentation with a right iliac fossa mass is quite common and can be confused with an inflammatory appendiceal mass. Abdominal involvement may be associated with disease at other sites, such as pleural effusions, peripheral lymphadenopathy, bone marrow involvement, skin, bone, breast, central nervous system disease, pharyngeal disease or testicular in-volvement.[16,54,55] These sites may also be involved in the absence of abdominal disease. In patients with SNCC lymphoma (Burkitt's lymphoma) in equatorial Africa, jaw involvement, affecting multiple jaw quadrants in a high proportion of cases, is the most frequent site of involvement, although it is age dependent, occurring much more frequently in young children. In an early series, 70 per cent of children below the age of 5 years who had Burkitt's lymphoma had jaw involvement, compared with 25 per cent of patients above 14 years.[5,58] In very young children orbital involvement is often present if jaw tumours are absent although at least some of these orbital tumours arise in the maxilla. Jaw involvement in sporadic Burkitt's lymphoma occurs in about 15–20 per cent of patients at presentation, frequently involves a single jaw quadrant and is not age related.[16,59]

Abdominal involvement is also frequent in endemic Burkitt's lymphoma, being present in a little more than half the patients, although the intra-abdominal sites of involvement differ to some extent in endemic versus sporadic dis-ease.[16,54] Involvement of the right iliac fossa (appendiceal/caecal region) is very common in sporadic SNCC lymphomas, occurring in almost half of all patients and being localized to that region (and completely resectable) in about 25 per cent of patients.[60] Presentation with a resectable right iliac fossa mass is very uncommon in African patients.

Nasopharyngeal involvement and peripheral lymphadenopathy are rare in the African patient but central nervous system involvement is more common[16,54] than in American patients.

These differences in the frequency of involvement of various anatomical sites at the time of presentation in equatorial African and North American SNCC lymphomas are accompanied by a series of other epidemiological and biological differences. These differences probably reflect a slightly different cell of origin and differences in pathogenesis (*see* Table 17.1). Patients in North Africa appear to have a spectrum of organ involvement which more closely approximates that of the sporadic disease rather than the endemic form,[61] while patients in South America and Asia are poorly charac-terized.

Bone marrow involvement

In small non-cleaved lymphomas bone marrow involvement occurs in about 20 per cent of patients at presentation,[16,30,54] although there is evidence from the culture and karyotyping of microscopically uninvolved bone marrow that occult involvement occurs in approximately another 20 per cent of patients.[62] Some patients present with a clinical syndrome consistent with leukaemia without any solid lymphomatous masses, apart from lymphadenopathy and hepatosplenomegaly. This is usually referred to as the 'L3' subtype of acute lymphoblastic leukaemia (ALL) (after the French–American–British classification, FAB) or Burkitt's cell leukaemia, and differs from other subtypes of ALL in that it expresses surface immunoglobulin and carries one of the non-random chromosomal translocations seen in SNCC lymphomas in chil-dren.[63,64] It has become clear, however, that not all leukaemias which conform to the criteria of L3 morphology express surface immunoglobulin and have 8;14 translocations,[65,66] – both of which confirm that the neoplasm is a small non-cleaved cell tumour. The true B-cell acute leukaemia of this type responds poorly to standard acute lym-phoblastic leukaemia therapy,[67] and should be considered and treated as a small non-cleaved cell lymphoma.[68] Such neoplasms constitute 2–5 per cent of most large series of patients with ALL and thus have a similar incidence to SNCC lymphomas which present with solid masses, with or without bone marrow involvement (perhaps two cases per year per million children under 16 years of age). Viewed from this perspective, bone marrow involvement occurs at presentation in over two-thirds of patients with SNCC neoplasms in the USA and Europe! This is not the case in African patients with Burkitt's lymphoma, where marrow involvement is uncommon, occurring in only about 8 per cent of patients at presentation.[30] There are, however, no estimates of the proportion of patients who have occult bone marrow involvement in Africa, nor has the frequency of B-cell leukaemia been determined. Bone marrow involvement is also rare at the time of relapse in African patients, even after multiple relapses,[30] whereas in North America almost all patients who die with progressive tumour have bone marrow involvement at some time in the course of their disease,[16,54] indicating again that the frequency of bone marrow involvement in these two regions is very different.

Central nervous system involvement

Involvement of the central nervous system can include meningeal infiltration, cranial nerve involvement, intracerebral disease, a paraspinal mass or some combination of these. The most frequently involved sites are the meninges and cranial nerves.[16,54,69–71] Central nervous system involvement is uncommon at presentation although it is distinctly more common in the presence of bone marrow disease.[30] In the absence of CNS prophylactic therapy, however, CNS spread will occur in a high proportion of patients, particularly those with extensive disease or head and neck primaries. Intracerebral involvement is extremely uncommon at both presentation and relapse, but it is occasionally seen in patients with persistant CNS disease.[70] Any cranial nerve can be affected by tumour, but ophthalmic and facial palsies are the most common. Very rarely the optic nerve can be infiltrated, with resultant blindness. Central nervous system involvement, particularly paraspinal involvement, is distinctly more common in patients with endemic Burkitt's lymphoma. Paraplegia occurs in some 15 per

cent of equatorial African patients at the time of presentation, but in less than 5 per cent in patients in the USA.[16,54,71]

Staging systems and staging procedures

Staging systems in SNCC lymphomas predominantly reflect the tumour volume. The most widely used – those of St Jude and the National Cancer Institute – have been described in Chapter 12. The former system is modified from the system proposed at Ann Arbor for Hodgkin's disease. It is applicable to all histological types of childhood lymphoma and separates patients with limited stage disease (one or two masses on one side of the diaphragm, stage I or II) from those with extensive intrathoracic or intra-abdominal disease (stage III). The meaning of the term 'extensive' is not defined, but clearly covers a relatively broad range of tumour burdens. Patients with bone marrow infiltration but with less than 25 per cent tumour cells seen on a marrow aspirate, and patients with CNS involvement are separated into the worst prognostic group (stage IV).

The system used at the National Cancer Institute was originally devised as a staging system for African patients with Burkitt's lymphoma,[71,72] and reflects the rarity of marrow involvement and the high curability (50 per cent) of patients with CNS disease in Africa. It has recently been modified to take into account the poor prognosis of patients with marrow and CNS disease in the USA.[56] This staging system includes a separate stage that reflects the advantage of complete surgical resection of abdominal disease[60,71] and does not incorporate the use of the diaphragm as a determinant of disseminated disease.

Staging laparotomy is not advocated in patients with non-Hodgkin's lymphoma since chemotherapy is the primary therapeutic modality. Moreover, in non-lymphoblastic lymphomas, abdominal involvement is so frequently present that a high proportion of patients will have had a laparotomy in order to make the diagnosis. Appropriate studies for determining the extent of disease have been described in Chapter 12, but it is worth pointing out that gallium-67 is avidly taken up by SNCC lymphomas and gallium-67 scanning provides a useful whole body screen, often detecting occult disease. Lymphangiography is rarely used because of the high frequency of extranodal tumour. A bone scan is the most sensitive means of detecting bony involvement, but may add little to a gallium scan in this regard. Radionuclide liver and spleen scans also appear to add little to computed tomography (CT) and ultrasound images,[73,74] and the role of magnetic resonance imaging (MRI) and positron emission tomography is not sufficiently well defined for these imaging techniques to be used routinely, although MRI has been shown to be useful for detecting patchy bone marrow involvement[75]. Bone marrow and CSF examination are an essential part of staging, although when prophylactic intrathecal drug administration and systemic therapy are initiated simultaneously, the initial CSF examination can be performed at the start of treatment. Bilateral bone marrow aspirates and biopsies are necessary if the rate of detection of marrow involvement is to be maximized.[76] An acceptable list of investigations to determine the extent of tumour is shown in Table 17.2.

Clinical and, where performed as part of the diagnostic evaluation, pathological staging provides both an abbreviated designation for the approximate volume and extent (i.e. distribution) of disease, and also an indicator of prognosis. Although clinical examination and imaging studies are essential for the determination of the sites of disease, quantitative biochemical or immunochemical measurements may provide simpler and more objective measurements of tumour volume. Measurement of serum lactic dehydrogenase (LDH), interleukin-2 receptor and, in African patients, the titre of antibodies directed against the early antigen of EBV, have been shown to correlate extremely well with prognosis[16,52,53,77] (Figs. 17.2 and 17.3). Such measurements should be included in the evaluation of the patient at initial presentation, and with time may become accepted as being as important as clinical staging.

Table 17.2 Investigations required for accurate staging

Physical examination

Complete blood count
Liver and renal serum chemistries
Serum LDH
Serum uric acid
Serum calcium and phosphorus
Serum lactate (optional)
Serum IL-2-R (optional)

Chest X-ray
Chest CT scan (if chest X-ray abnormal or suspiciously abnormal)
Abdominal ultrasound examination (liver/spleen; kidneys; abdomen; pelvis)
Whole body gallium-67 scan
Abdominal CT scan
Bone scan (optional or if gallium scan suggests bone involvement)
MRI (research)

Bone marrow examination (biopsies and aspirate samples)
CSF examination (cytocentrifuge)

Other studies as indicated

LDH, lactate dehydrogenase; IL-2R, interleukin-2 receptor; CT, computed tomography; MRI, magnetic resonance imaging.

Treatment and prognosis

Immediate considerations

Patients with SNCC lymphomas are prone to develop a number of the complications described in Chapter 15 and these frequently require urgent attention at the time of presentation. They include intestinal obstruction (most commonly from intussusception), perforation or haemorrhage, airway obstruction from pharyngeal tumour, pleural effusions, pericardial effusions and vena caval obstruction.[16,57,60] Among the most common complications at presentation, however, are those related to the high turnover of oxypurines. The likelihood of uric acid nephropathy before chemotherapy or of the development, immediately after chemotherapy, of biochemical abnormalities which can result in renal failure and even death, and which have collectively become known as the 'acute tumour lysis syndrome', correlates directly with the tumour burden.[16,78,79] Because of the short doubling time of small non-cleaved lymphomas and the considerable risks associated with rapid tumour lysis, the initiation of therapy should be considered a medical emergency and staging procedures should be completed as expeditiously as possible.

Prior to commencing therapy, however, it is essential to ensure that the serum uric acid level is not elevated and that the patient is well hydrated and able to maintain a high urine flow. If a period of biochemical correction is necessary it should not exceed 24–48 hours at most. The reduction of serum uric acid to normal levels can usually be accomplished within this period by alkaline diuresis and allopurinol administration, except in those patients with additional renal compromise such as ureteric obstruction or, less commonly, massive involvement of the kidneys by tumour. In such circumstances there may be no alternative to instituting haemodialysis prior to chemotherapy, since to proceed directly with chemotherapy would lead to an extremely acute

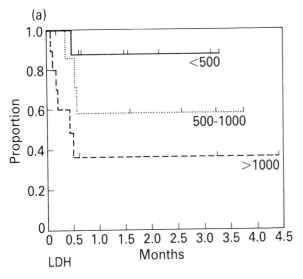

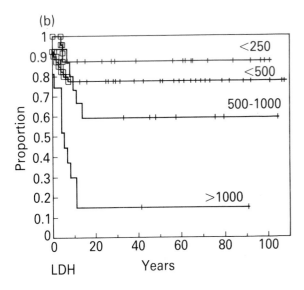

Fig. 17.2 Comparison of total therapy B protocol from St Jude (a), with the NCI 77-04 protocol (b), when failure-free survival is plotted according to lactate dehydrogenase (LDH) level. (a) Reproduced with permission.[86]

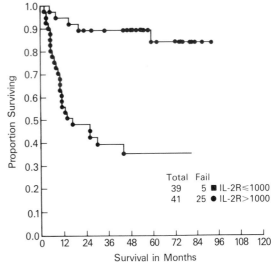

Fig. 17.3 Disease-free interval (failure-free survival) of patients with non-Hodgkin's lymphomas according to serum interleukin-2 (SIL-2R) level. The patients were treated at the NCI with the 77–04 protocol. All patients, even those not achieving a complete response, are shown. The latter are counted as having a disease-free interval of zero.

and probably fatal tumour lysis syndrome. In such cases chemotherapy should be commenced after the completion of a period of haemodialysis when biochemical parameters are close to normal, in order to minimize the possibility of removing drugs (e.g. cyclophosphamide) by dialysis.

In all patients with a large tumour burden it is imperative to maintain a high urine output (as much as 250 ml/m²/h in the patients at highest risk) for the first few days after the initiation of chemotherapy. This ensures that the high solute burden from tumour lysis is accommodated without the onset of potentially fatal hyper-kalaemia[80] or the development of acute renal failure from intratubular deposition of oxypurines and/or phosphates – a consequence of exceeding their solubility in urine.[81] Potassium should not be included in the intravenous solutions and, because of relatively poor solubility of phosphate in an alkaline urine, it is preferable not to administer bicarbonate during chemotherapy. Electrolyte abnormalities are an important consequence of rapid tumour lysis. Hyperkalaemia is most unlikely to occur as long as a high urine output can be maintained. Hypocalcaemia, a consequence of hyperphos-phataemia should not be treated unless symptomatic, and intravenous calcium chloride should be given with great caution, if at all, because of the risk of extra-osseous calcification in the presence of a high serum phosphate level. Systemic alkalinity increases the possibility of symptomatic hypocalcaemia, including tetany – an additional reason to limit alkalinization of the urine to the pretreatment period. Rarely, haemodialysis may be required for symptomatic hypocalcaemia.

The key to the management of acute tumour lysis is the maintainance of a high urine output. As long as this can be achieved, other interventions are unlikely to be needed. If it cannot be achieved rapid progression of biochemical abnormalities will occur, necessitating urgent haemodialysis. Difficulty in maintaining urine output is most likely to occur when there is a tendency for fluids to collect in a third space, as for example when serous effusions or limb oedema from venous and/or lymphatic obstruction are present. In such patients vigorous hydration is complicated by weight gain and an inappropriately low urine flow. This situation can usually be managed by the judicious use of diuretics. Some form of central vascular pressure monitoring, e.g. central venous pressure or pulmonary wedge capillary pressure is extremely helpful in this circumstance, and if an acceptable urine output cannot be maintained haemodialysis must be commenced immediately. It is clear that patients at high risk for the acute tumour lysis syndrome are best managed in a critical care unit.

Specific therapy

Although the extent of disease may govern, to a degree, the choice of treatment protocol, the primary therapeutic modality for SNCC lymphomas is chemotherapy. This is based not only on the belief that these lymphomas are generalized diseases, but also on clinical experience. In a review of eight series of patients with localized non-Hodgkin's lymphomas who were treated with radiation therapy, with or without surgical resection, and single agent chemotherapy published between 1966 and 1978,[82-89] Jenkin *et al.* reported long-term survival in only 18 per cent of 370 patients.[90] In only one of these series did more than 50 per cent of children achieve long-term survival, and that series contained only eight patients.[84] If only patients with gastrointestinal disease are included, in order to be confident that only SNCC lymphomas are considered, still only 15 of 37 patients achieved prolonged survival.[84,85] This contrasts dramatically with the results obtained when children with localized disease are treated with combination chemotherapy, with or without radiation. Ninety per cent or more can be expected to enjoy long-term survival.[13,60,68,91-94] Furthermore, there is good evidence that radiation adds no therapeutic benefit in this situation, but increases both short-term and long-term toxicity.[93] In patients with extensive disease, radiotherapy can, at best, subserve only an ancillary role, i.e. as emergency treatment for involvement of the nervous system, or for testicular involvement.[95] When used as a component of primary therapy in conjunction with an effective chemotherapy regimen, as in the case of localized disease, radiation adds toxicity without overall therapeutic benefit.[96] These findings are consistent with the relative radioresistance of African Burkitt's lymphoma to conventionally fractionated radiation therapy[97] (although they also apply to the more radiosensitive lymphoblastic lymphoma). Suggestions that hyperfractionation of radiation dose may be useful have not been systematically explored beyond the original study conducted in Nairobi.[97]

Although local irradiation may be of little therapeutic benefit, this is not the case with surgery. Patients with bulky abdominal disease in whom tumour can be completely resected prior to chemotherapy have an excellent prognosis – better than that of patients with unresected abdominal disease.[13,60,72] The additional benefits of surgery include prevention of gastrointestinal bleeding and bowel perforation as well as lessening the chances of an acute tumour lysis syndrome.

Chemotherapy of SNCC lymphomas

Small non-cleaved cell lymphomas respond to a wide range of chemotherapeutic agents. This wide response profile is probably due in part to the high growth fraction. Response rates in African Burkitt's lymphoma are shown in Table 17.3. Sporadic tumours appear to have a similar spectrum of sensitivity to chemotherapeutic agents as well as a demonstrable response to high dose methotrexate.[98] Previous experience has clearly indicated that the results of drug combination therapy are far superior to treatment with single agents, although a fraction of patients with SNCC lymphomas can be cured by single agents,[99–102] an almost unique situation in oncology. Another feature of treatment protocols for the SNCC lymphomas is that there appears to be no indication for prolonged therapy. In early trials at the NCI as few as three cycles of a combination of cyclophosphamide, methotrexate and vincristine resulted in disease-free survival in some 40 per cent of patients.[103,104] Although the therapy duration need not be prolonged, it is important to ensure that cycles are delivered with as short an intercycle interval as possible because of the rapid tumour cell

doubling time and the potential for tumour regrowth before bone marrow recovery.

It has been clearly shown in several different studies that treatment protocols based upon the principles shown to be effective for acute lymphoblastic leukaemia, such as the LSA_2L_2, the BFM 1976–81 or the APO regimens, are suboptimal for the treatment of small non-cleaved cell lymphomas.[105–108] However, several protocols using cyclical cyclophosphamide-including combinations coupled with intermediate or high-dose methotrexate (Figs. 17.4–17.8) have been shown to be highly effective for all patients with SNCC lymphomas, except those with bone marrow disease. With such protocols overall survival rates of 50 – 75 per cent have been reported (Table 17.4).[13,91,92,105,106,109,110]

Because of differences in the patient populations (recognized and unrecognized) it is not clear whether any one of these protocols is better than another. Differences may be due to variations in patient characteristics, particularly

Table 17.3 Single agent activity in African Burkitt's lymphoma

Drug	No.[2]	CR[3]	R[4]	%R[5]
Cyclophosphamide	163	43	132	81
Nitrogen mustard	61	10	44	72
Melphalan	26	8	16	61
Chlorambucil	12	3	10	83
Procarbazine	6	0	0	0
Orthomerphalan	14	?	14	100
BCNU (carmustine)	5	0	4	80
Vincristine	21	10	17	81
Vinblastine	2	0	0	0
Methotrexate	45	11	26	58
6-Mercaptopurine	3	0	0	0
Cytosine arabinoside	3	2	2	0
Epipodophyllotoxin	2	2	2	0
Actinomycin D	4	1	4	0
Terephthalanilide	18	1	14	78

[1]*See* reference 53
[2]Number of patients tested
[3]Complete response
[4]Complete and partial responses
[5]Percentage of patients responding

with regard to the spectrum of tumour burdens (the most important prognostic factor) or simply to random variability. Within each stage there may be significant differences in tumour burden, so that similarity of distribution by stage of study populations does not necessarily confirm similarity of tumour burden. The ability to compare the results of different trials would be considerably enhanced by the routine reporting of other measures of tumour burden such as

COMP

Repeat Every 28 Days

■ CTX 1.2 g/m² IV (Induction), 1.0 g/m² (Maintenance)
▨ VCR 2.0 g/m² IV (Induction), 1.5 g/m² (Maintenance) Max.2.0 mg
▲ MTX 300 mg/m² IV (60% Push, 40% 4 h infusion)
○ Prednisone 60 mg/m² PO (Max.60 mg) in 4 divided doses
↑ IT MTX 6.25 mg/m². Omit first maintenance cycle

Total duration 18 months from day 1

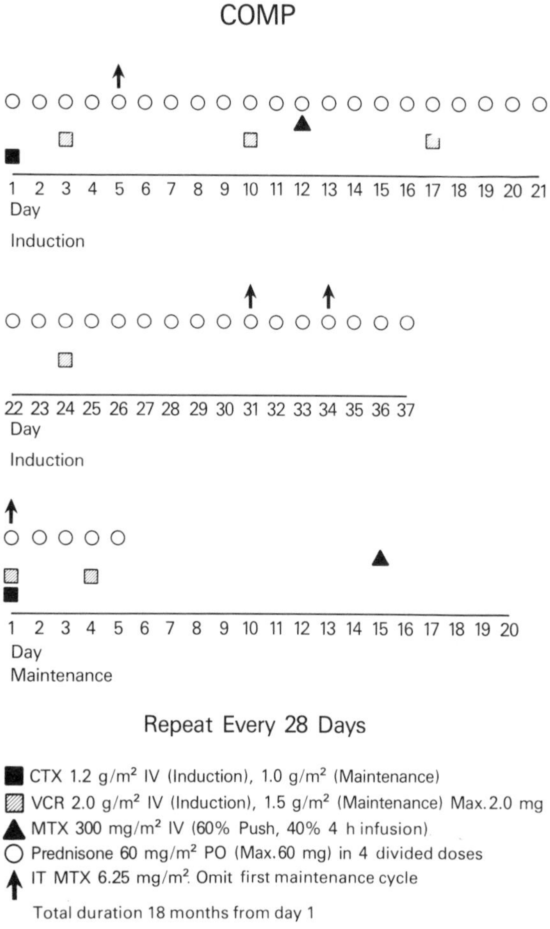

Fig. 17.4 The cyclophosphamide, oncovin (vincristine), methotrexate, prednisone (COMP) protocol used by the CCG. This protocol includes radiation to sites of bulk disease. Scheme prepared according to information provided.[91] CTX cyclophosphamide; VCR, vincristine; MTX, methotrexate; IV, intravenous; PO, by mouth; IT, intrathecal.

LDH and SIL-2R (or even serum uric acid level) and their correlation with disease-free survival.[13,109] The value of the inclusion of such factors in the analysis is shown in Fig. 17.2, which depicts a comparison of the results of the total therapy B and the NCI 77-04 protocols according to serum LDH level. When compared in this way, the results are remarkably similar, although the disease-free survival for stage III patients in the two protocols differed by about 20 per cent (Table 17.4).

The possible influence of age on prognosis should also be considered. For example the median age of patients treated according to NCI protocol 77-04 was 16 years, while that in the French LMB-02 protocol was eight years.[13,92] There is a suggestion in some studies (e.g. NCI protocol 77-04) that children below 10 years of age have a better prognosis, but this has not been confirmed. It is also often considered that adults have a worse prognosis than children. In protocol NCI 77-04, however, there was no difference in outcome between patients less than 16 or between 16 and 35 years of age.[13] Further, this protocol was used at Stanford University Medical Center in an older population with very similar results to those achieved at the NCI.[110]

Adult patients with SNCC lymphomas are often treated with chemotherapy regimens designed for diffuse aggressive lymphomas (primarily of intermediate grade),[111,112] but it is difficult to determine whether such protocols provide optimal therapy since: (1) the number of patients with this histology included in such studies is small; (2) staging systems differ from those used in childhood lymphomas so that direct comparisons are difficult; (3) overall results which include many histologies, or those of diffuse large cell lymphomas alone, are presented, and even if survival in different histological groups is examined, the proportions of patients with various prognostic factors within the subgroup can rarely be discerned; and (4) cytogenetic data are rarely available, so that the proportion of SNCC lymphomas with 8;14 or variant translocations versus those with 14;18 translocations is unknown. To date, the prognostic importance of the type of chromosomal translocation in SNCC lymphomas in adults remains unknown. In some protocols there is no significant correlation between disease-free survival and histology (*see* Chapter 21) and some patients with SNCC lymphoma do well when treated on such protocols. For example in a French protocol, LNH-80 designed for diffuse aggressive adult lymphomas, 53 per cent of 19 patients with SNCC lymphoma were alive at five years.[112] Unfortunately, in the absence of more information regarding the distribution of prognostic factors in this subgroup, this result is largely uninterpretable.

Clearly, more information is required regarding optimal treatment of SNCC lymphomas in adults, but in the absence of a clinical trial to examine the relative efficacies of the various available protocols, it would seem most logical to use one of the proven treatment regimens in children, or a protocol such as 77-04 which appears to have similar results in children and adults.[13] Since none of these protocols is clearly superior to another, the decision as to which one to use should be based on familiarity with the drug regimen used, or considerations

PROTOCOL 77-04

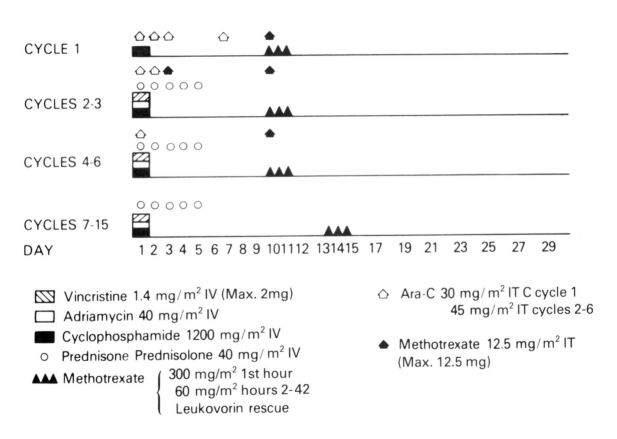

Vincristine 1.4 mg/m² IV (Max. 2mg)
Adriamycin 40 mg/m² IV
Cyclophosphamide 1200 mg/m² IV
Prednisone Prednisolone 40 mg/m² IV
Methotrexate 300 mg/m² 1st hour
60 mg/m² hours 2-42
Leukovorin rescue

Ara-C 30 mg/m² IT C cycle 1
45 mg/m² IT cycles 2-6

Methotrexate 12.5 mg/m² IT
(Max. 12.5 mg)

Cycles commence as soon as granulocytes over 1500/mm³ (or day 28 cycles 7-15)

Fig. 17.5 The 77-04 protocol of the NCI. Radiation therapy was not routinely given. (Adriamycin = doxorubicin.)

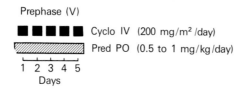

Prephase (V)

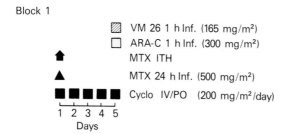

Block 1

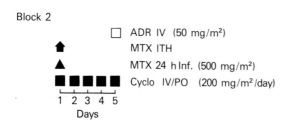

Block 2

Fig. 17.6 The BFM protocol for B-cell lymphomas. The scheme for administration of initial cytoreductive therapy (V) and blocks 1 and 2 are shown with the drugs included in these components. Prophylactic CNS therapy was restricted to patients with advanced stage. In patients with non-resectable abdominal disease a second-look laparotomy was initially performed after the second or third therapy block and radiation given if residual disease was detected. Because of the low yield of this procedure, it was subsequently abandoned, and abdominal irradiation given only for residual disease detected by non-invasive procedures. Cyclo, cyclophosphamide; Pred, prednisone; VM 26, tenoposide; ARA-C, cytarabine; ADR, doxorubicin; IV, intravenous, PO by mouth; IT, intrathecal; Inf., infusion. From: *Malignant Lymphomas and Hodgkin's Disease: Experimental and Therapeutic Advances.* Cavalli R, Bonadonna G and Rosencweig M (eds). Boston: Martinus Nijhoff, 1984; 633–42. Reproduced with permission.

of toxicity or therapy duration. It is worth emphasizing, however, that if continued progress is to be made, as many patients as possible should be entered into research protocols. All reported successful protocols include cyclophosphamide in doses of at least 1 g/m² and either intermediate or high dose methotrexate (300 mg/m²–5 g/m²). Most also include an anthracycline (exceptions are the Childrens Cancer Group (CCG) 'COMP' protocol[105] and a trial carried out at the M.D. Anderson Hospital, Houston, Texas,[113]) the role of which is being examined at present in a randomized trial conducted by the CCG (Protocol CCG-503.)[94]

Limited disease

Patients with limited disease, i.e. localized or completely resected intra-abdominal disease (stages I and II, St Jude, and A and AR, NCI) have an excellent prognosis (at least 90 per cent cure rate) and require less intensive treatment than patients with more extensive disease (all other stages). In the BFM protocols 81/83 and 83/86 these patients receive only eight and six weeks of therapy respectively,[114] while six cycles are given in the NCI 77-04 protocol,[13,60] and six months in CCG-551 and 501 studies.[94] In the CCG trials, six months of therapy gave similar results to 18 months.[94] The preliminary results of the POG study examining the role of radiation to local sites of disease do not support a role for this modality, a conclusion that is in concert with the comparable results obtained in protocols which included local irradiation, for example the CCG protocols,[94,105] and those which did not.[13,60,68,92]

Abdominal disease

Patients with unresectable abdominal disease without bone marrow or CNS involvement (the majority of patients) have an expectancy of cure which is between 60 and 80 per cent in all major protocols (*see* Table 17.4). Abdominal irradiation appears to have no role in therapy, although in the presence of testicular involvement, local treatment (either irradiation or possibly surgery) is probably needed.[95] However, this point has

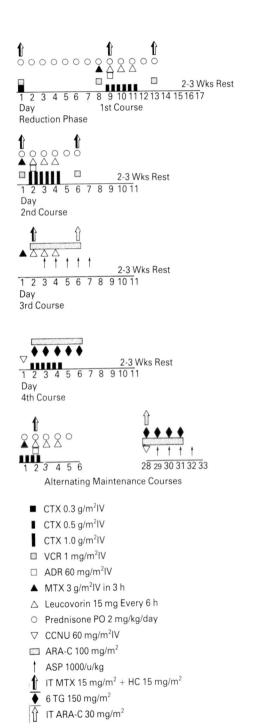

- ■ CTX 0.3 g/m²IV
- ▌ CTX 0.5 g/m²IV
- ▍ CTX 1.0 g/m²IV
- □ VCR 1 mg/m²IV
- □ ADR 60 mg/m²IV
- ▲ MTX 3 g/m²IV in 3 h
- △ Leucovorin 15 mg Every 6 h
- ○ Prednisone PO 2 mg/kg/day
- ▽ CCNU 60 mg/m²IV
- ▭ ARA-C 100 mg/m²
- ↑ ASP 1000/u/kg
- ⇑ IT MTX 15 mg/m² + HC 15 mg/m²
- ◆ 6 TG 150 mg/m²
- ⇑ IT ARA-C 30 mg/m²

Fig. 17.7 The LMB-02 protocol of the SFOP for B-cell lymphomas stage I and II (large nasopharyngeal

primaries in stage II are included). Cyclophosphamide (CTX) is given at the doses shown daily in two fractions. Maintenance courses are given monthly. During maintenance cytarabine (ara-C) is given as two s.c. fractions, otherwise it is given as a continuous i.v. infusion. Radiation therapy was not routinely given. Scheme prepared from ref.[92] VCR, vincristine; ADR, doxorubicin; MTX, methotrexate; ASP, asparaginase; CCNU, cis-chloroethyl nitrosurea; 6 TG, thioguanine IT, intrathecal.

---

not been examined critically with controlled studies.

Bone marrow and CNS disease

In contrast to patients with limited disease, patients with bone marrow involvement have a poor prognosis, ranging between 10 and 50 per cent prolonged survival in most reported studies.[13,106,109] An exception appears to be the French LMB-0281 protocol, where 76 per cent of 21 patients with bone marrow disease (but without CNS involvement) achieved long-term survival.[92] In this study, no difference in survival was apparent between patients with less than or more than 25 per cent of tumour cells in the bone marrow. It is not certain at present whether the apparent advantage to the LMB-02 protocol reflects a true superiority over other protocols in this subgroup of patients, or differences in the patients themselves. In all protocols, even earlier protocols with only three cycles of therapy which gave overall worse results, some patients with bone marrow involvement survived,[103,104] so that there is the potential for misleading results when numbers are small.

All patients with CNS disease (meningeal or cranial nerve involvement) at diagnosis, though representing only a small proportion of patients, have a poor prognosis regardless of the protocol used and improved treatment approaches are clearly required in such patients. Some patients however, particularly African children, have achieved long-term cure when treated with only intrathecal and systemic chemotherapy.[69,102] In France, such patients are often treated by high dose therapy followed by autologous bone marrow rescue, with good results obtained so

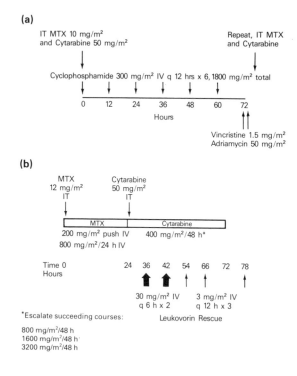

(a)

IT MTX 10 mg/m²   Repeat, IT MTX
and Cytarabine 50 mg/m²   and Cytarabine

Cyclophosphamide 300 mg/m² IV q 12 hrs x 6, 1800 mg/m² total

0   12   24   36   48   60   72
                  Hours

Vincristine 1.5 mg/m²
Adriamycin 50 mg/m²

(b)

MTX   Cytarabine
12 mg/m²   50 mg/m²
IT   IT

MTX   Cytarabine
200 mg/m² push IV   400 mg/m²/48 h*
800 mg/m²/24 h IV

Time 0   24   36   42   54   66   72   78
Hours

30 mg/m² IV   3 mg/m² IV
q 6 h x 2   q 12 h x 3
            Leukovorin Rescue

*Escalate succeeding courses:

800 mg/m²/48 h
1600 mg/m²/48 h
3200 mg/m²/48 h

Fig. 17.8 The total therapy B protocol used at St Jude
Hospital. Successive cycles (a) followed by (b) are
given as soon as haemopoietic recovery (18 – 21 days)
has occurred to a total of four cycles each of A and B;
5–6 months are required for completion. In succeeding
courses after the first, the second intrathecal (IT)
treatment in cycle A is omitted and the infusion dose
of cytarabine (ara-C) in cycle B is escalated to a total of
3200 mg/m². Radiation therapy was not routinely
given. MTX, methotrexate. Reproduced with
permission of the *Journal of Clinical Oncology*[86].

far in a small number of patients.[115] Intracerebral
disease is very uncommon at presentation and
standard approaches to its therapy have not
been developed.[70] In spite of the relatively poor
response of the SNCC lymphomas to radiation
therapy, it may be justified to treat such patients
with cranial irradiation because of the limited
number of drugs which are effective in this
situation. However, alternative approaches
worthy of consideration include high doses of
methotrexate or cytarabine (ara-C) administered
intravenously.

Patients with paraspinal disease presenting
with paraplegia are uncommon except in
equatorial Africa. It is of interest that in such
countries access to radiation therapy is rare, and
almost all patients are treated with chemotherapy alone. Excellent results, both with
regard to survival (such patients often have
disease confined to the paraspinal region, and
therefore have an excellent prognosis) and
ambulation are obtained and there is no reason
to believe that these would be better if
radiotherapy were available. Some patients with
permanent severe neurological deficits have
been shown, at post-mortem, to have sustained
an infarction of the spinal cord.[116] These results,
and the known rapidity of response to treatment
suggest that there is likely to be no advantage
to added radiation in such patients in other parts
of the world, but in the absence of definitive
information many oncologists in Europe and the
US are reluctant to administer chemotherapy
without radiation to the spine. In small children
there is likely to be a definite disadvantage to
this because of the effect of radiation on bone
growth, and if a significant region of the
vertebral column is included in the radiation
field, additional myelosuppression may be
incurred with subsequent chemotherapy.

Other sites of disease

Specific treatment approaches are not required
for patients with other sites of disease except in
so far that this impacts upon emergency
management. This applies to the treatment of
patients with disease sites traditionally treated
with local therapy in addition to chemotherapy,
such as those with localized bone involvement.
A recent review of the NCI series indicated that
bone lesions respond well to chemotherapy.
Even in patients with multiple lesions, overall
survival was approximately 70 per cent in
patients treated with chemotherapy alone,
except in the presence of bone marrow
involvement.

CNS prophylactic therapy

Central nervous system prophylaxis is indicated
in those patients with SNCC lymphomas. Since

Table 17.4 Response rates in advanced childhood B-cell NHL with current regimens

Protocol	Local radiation	CNS prophylaxis	Stage[1]	No. patients	FFS[2] (%)	Follow-up[3] (months)	Reference
COMP	3000 cGy	CI/IT[4]	III	32	62	>18	82
(CCG-551)		IDMTX[5]	IV	6	33	>18	
NCI 7704	None[6]	IT	III	38	60	48	7
		HDMTX[8]	IV	9	28	48	
Total B	None	IT	III	17	81	24	86
		HDMTX/AC[9]	IV	12	17	24	
BMF trials[10]							
81	None	IT	III	29	62	>36	114
		IDMTX	IV[11]	5	20	>36	
			B-ALL[12]	22	45	>36	
83	None	IT	III	47	83	>24	
		IDMTX	IV	12	83	>24	
			B-ALL	24	53	>24	
81/83[13]	None	IT	III	75	73	21	
		HDMTX	IV	15	57	21	
SFOP trials							
LMB-0281	None	IT	III	72	73	>20	71
		HDMTX	IV	42	48[14]	>20	
LMB-84[15]	None	IT	III	126	74	2–14	16
		HDMTX	IV[17]	34	65	2–14	

[1]St Jude staging system except that stage IV includes patients with any degree of bone marrow involvement unless otherwise stated
[2]Failure-free survival. Includes all patients
[3]Median follow-up
[4]Cranial irradiation and intrathecal methotrexate and/or ara-C
[5]Intermediate dose methotrexate (MTX) infusion (less than 1 g/m^2)
[6]Radiation not used routinely
[7]Recent unpublished update of the series reported in ref.[13]
[8]High dose MTX (more than 1 g/m^2)
[9]High dose MTX and ara-C
[10]Data from Müller-Weihrich ST, Ludwig R, Reiter A *et al.*, (1987) *Third International Conference on Malignant Lymphoma*. Cavalli F, Bonadonna G, Rozenczweig M (eds), abstract 43, and Müller-Weihrich, personal communication
[11]Patients with <25% tumour cells in the bone marrow
[12]Patients with >25% tumour cells in the bone marrow
[13]Both trials, 81/83 and 83/86 are combined here. The protocols were similar except the substitution of dexamethasone for prednisone, delivery of MTX and ara-C by Ommaya reservoir for patients with CNS disease at diagnosis, and a reduced duration of therapy in the later trial
[14]No difference between patients with <25% or >25% blasts in the marrow
[15]This protocol includes a randomization between five and eight courses of therapy for stage IV patients who achieve complete remission. Preliminary analysis shows no difference between the arms
[16]Zucker JM, Patte T, Philip T *et al.* (1987). *Third International Conference on Malignant Lymphoma*. Cavalli F, Bonadonna G, Rosenczweig M (eds), abstract 42
[17]Excluding patients with CNS disease.

effective prophylaxis has been achieved without the use of cranial irradiation,[13,92,106] a combination of intrathecal therapy with intermediate or high dose methotrexate represents appropriate treatment. Craniospinal irradiation was shown to have no value in preventing CNS disease in African patients or in patients with L3 leukaemia.[68,117] It has been suggested that patients with completely resected abdominal disease do not require intrathecal prophylaxis. This is based on the observed low frequency of this complication in such patients. However, much depends upon the type of patient subjected to debulking surgery, and the risk of CNS disease may depend upon the bulk of tumour resected. If this is so, patients in whom a large mass of tumour is resected may not be totally without risk. Because of the minimal increase in toxicity associated with the administration of intrathecal therapy, but the very poor prognosis of patients who develop CNS recurrence, it seems appropriate to continue to treat such patients with a small number (e.g. four to six) of intrathecal injections of methotrexate and ara-C until more definitive information is available.

Duration of therapy

The optimal duration of therapy is an important issue which should be addressed. Although in early protocols adopted in Africa and the NCI, only one to three courses of treatment were administered,[102,118,119] in most subsequent protocols therapy has been administered for periods of 12–18 months. There is an increasing realization that with modern, intensive, combination drug protocols, shorter therapy duration may be equally effective, although randomized trials designed to study this aspect of treatment in high risk patients have not been reported. In the SNCC lymphomas relapse occurs predominantly in the first eight months and is almost unknown after 10 months.[16,92,106,109] Treatment protocols with short duration therapy (e.g. the BMF 86 protocol in which even high risk patients receive only 12 weeks of therapy[114]) do not have a survival disadvantage compared to those with a treatment duration of 12–18 months.[16,92,105] The

attendant advantages with regard to toxicity, convenience, psychological impact and cost of short duration protocols provide a strong incentive to reduce treatment to a few months at most.

Future prospects for high risk and relapsing patients

Only patients with stage IV SNCC lymphomas fall into a high risk disease category today, but there is still room for improvement in patients with stage III disease. Such improvements are likely to come from further refinements in combination drug therapy. Agents such as high dose ara-C,[120] ifosfamide and the epipodophyllotoxins have been used to a limited extent and it is possible that incorporation of these agents into treatment regimens will be advantageous to patients with both stage III and stage IV disease. The latest BFM study[86] includes ifosfamide at a dose of 800 mg/m^2 instead of cyclophosphamide in block 1 (referred to as block AA) as well as increased doses of ara-C and VM-26 for patients with CNS disease and bone marrow involvement. Novel intrathecal therapies in patients with CNS disease have also been reported recently.[121,122]

The possible impact of the use of cloned colony stimulating factors such as CSF-GM[123–125] in lessening toxicity, as well as the duration of the period of marrow hypoplasia following each therapy cycle, will be important to assess, particularly in the SNCC lymphomas because of their rapid growth rate and the need to repeat therapy cycles as rapidly as possible. The role of bone marrow rescue after high dose therapy has yet to be formally assessed as a component of primary therapy (e.g. after remission induction) in very high risk patients, although following the demonstration of long-term survival in a proportion of patients with recurrent disease treated with very high dose chemotherapy with or without bone marrow rescue[126–129] (*see* also Chapters 24 and 25), this approach has been adopted with promising early results in a small number of patients in France.[115]

Little information exists in SNCC lymphomas with regard to the value of biological response modifiers. However, one patient was reported to have had a partial response to α-interferon in a study conducted at St Jude Children's Research Hospital.[130]

Follow-up

Appropriate intervals between follow-up studies for SNCC lymphomas can never be optimal because of the very rapid growth rate of these tumours, such that the detection of recurrence before it has become clinically apparent would probably require weekly staging studies. Because of this, it could be argued that routine restaging studies after the cessation of treatment are of questionable value, although frequent follow-up visits are useful; the development of symptoms should precipitate appropriate investigations to determine their origin. The relatively short period during which patients with SNCC lymphomas are 'at risk' for relapse should also be taken into account when deciding on the timing of appropriate follow-up visits. Imaging studies are most unlikely to be of value after the patient has been free of disease for 10 months from the date of presentation. It would seem reasonable to follow known sites of disease with an appropriate imaging study, or studies, at monthly intervals for the first three months while on therapy, to follow serum LDH carefully at frequent intervals (daily to fortnightly, depending how far the therapy has progressed) to perform CSF surveillance during every therapy cycle or monthly for the first 8 months and to perform a gallium scan and examine the bone marrow at two-monthly intervals, once complete remission has been achieved, until 8 months to one year have passed. Thereafter the patient should be seen every 6 months to one year to ascertain that no long-term side-effects have developed[131,132] (*see* also Chapter 15) and to ensure that accurate records are kept of survival duration.

References

1. National Cancer Institute sponsored study of classification. *Cancer* 1982; **49**, 2112–35.
2. Rappaport H, Braylan RC. In: Rebuck JW, Berard CW, Abell MR (eds). *The Reticuloendothelial System; International Academy of Pathology*. Baltimore: Williams and Wilkins Co, 1976; 1–19.
3. Lennert K, Mohri N, Stein H, Kaiserling E. *British Journal of Haematology*. (suppl. II); **31**, 193.
4. Lukes RJ, Collins RD. *British Journal of Cancer*. 1975; **31** (suppl. II), 1–28.
5. Magrath IT. In: Pochedly C (ed). *Pediatric Hematology Oncology Reviews*. Westport: Praeger. 1985: 1–51.
6. Magrath IT. In: Ford RJ, Fuller L, Hagermeister FB (eds). *New Perspectives in Human Lymphoma*. New York: Raven Press, 1984: 201–212.
7. Mann RB, Jaffe E, Braylan RC, *et al. New England Journal of Medicine*. 1976: **295**, 85–91.
8. Palleson GO. In: Mollander D (ed). *Diseases of the Lymphatic System. Diagnosis and Therapy*. Heidelbert: Springer Verlag, 1984: 89–102.
9. Fifth International Workshop on Chromosomes in Leukemia–Lymphoma. *Blood*. 1987; **70**, 1554–64.
10. Gauverky C, Haluska FG, Tsujimoto Y, *et al. Proceedings of the National Academy of Sciences USA*. 1988; **85**; 8548.
11. Bloomfield CD, Arthur DC, Frizzera G, *et al. Cancer Research*. 1983; **43**, 2975–84.
12. Kelly DR, Nathwani BN, Griffith RC, *et al. Cancer*. 1987; **59**, 1132–7.
13. Magrath I, Janus C, Edwards B, *et al. Blood*. 1984; **63**, 1102.
14. Miliauskas JR, Berard CW, Young RC, *et al. Cancer*. 1982; **50**, 2115–21.
15. Grogan TM, Warnke A, Kaplan H. *Cancer*. 1982; **49**, 1817–28.
16. Magrath IT. In: Mollander D (ed). *Diseases of the Lymphatic System Diagnosis and Therapy*. Heidelberg: Springer–Verlag, 1984: 103–39.
17. Gunven P, Klein G, Klein E, *et al. International Journal of Cancer*. 1980; **25**, 711–19.
18. Benjamin D, Magrath IT, Maguire R, *et al. Journal of Immunology*. 1982; **129**, 1336.
19. Magrath I, Benjamin D, Papadopoulos N. *Blood* 1983; **61**, 726.
20. Ehlin-Henriksson B, Manneborg-Sandlund A, Klein G. *International Journal of Cancer*. 1987; **39**, 211–18.
21. Favrot MC, Philip I, Philip T, *et al. Journal of the National Cancer Institute*. 1984; **73**, 841–7.
22. Favrot M, Philip I, Comparet V, *et al.* In: Cavalli F, Bonnadonna G, Rosenczweig M, (eds). *Third International Conference on Malignant Lymphoma*. abstract.
23. Rowe M, Rowe DT, Gregory DC, *et al. EMBO Journal*. 1987; **6**, 2743–51.
24. Magrath IT, Freeman CB, Pizzo P, *et al. Journal*

of the National Cancer Institute. 1980; **64**, 477–83.

25. Freeman CB, Magrath IT, Benjamin D, *et al. Clinical Immunology and Immunopatholgy.* 1982; **25**, 103–13.

26. Secker-Walker L, Stewart E, Norton J, *et al. Leukemia Research.* 1987; **11**, 155–61.

27. Zech L, Haglund U, Nilsson K, *et al. International Journal of Cancer.* 1976; **17**, 47.

28. Bernheim A, Berger R, Lenoir G. *Cancer Genetics and Cytogenetics.* 1981; **3**, 307.

29. Lenoir G, Philip T, Sohier R. In: Magrath IT, O'Conor G, Ramot B (eds). *Pathogenesis of Leukemias and Lymphomas: Environmental Influences.* New York: Raven Press, 1984: 283–95.

30. Magrath IT, Zeigler JL. *Leukemia Research.* 1980; **4**, 33–59.

31. Wiener F, Ohno S, Babonito M, *et al. Proceedings of the National Academy of Sciences USA.* 1984; **81**, 1159–68.

32. Whang-Peng J, Lee EC, Sieverts H, *et al. Blood.* 1984; **63**, 818–22.

33. Chaganti RSK, Jhanwar S, Kozinar B, *et al. Blood.* 1983; **61**, 1269–72.

34. Pelicci PG, Knowles DM, Arlin ZA, *et al. Journal of Experimental Medicine.* 1986; **164**, 2049–60.

35. Catovsky D, Pitman S, Lewis D, *et al. Lancet,* 1977; **ii**, 934.

36. Mintzer DM, Andreeff M, Filippa DA, *et al. Blood.* 1984; **64**, 415–21.

37. Garvin AJ, Simon RM, Osborne CK, *et al. Cancer.* 1983; **52**, 393.

38. Taub R, Kirsch I, Morton C, *et al. Proceedings of the National Academy of Sciences USA.* 1982; **79**, 7837.

39. Dalla-Favera R, Bregni M, Erikson J, *et al. Proceedings of the National Academy of Sciences USA.* 1982; **79**, 7824.

40. Pellici P-G, Knowles D, Magrath I, *et al. Proceedings of the National Academy of Sciences USA.* 1986; **83**, 2984.

41. Tsujimoto Y, Finger LR, Yunis J, *et al. Science.* 1984; **226**, 1097–9.

42. Bakhshi A, Jensen JP, Goldman P, *et al. Cell.* 1985; **41**, 899–906.

43. Philip T, Lenoir GM, Byron PA, *et al. British Journal of Cancer* 1982; **45**, 670–8.

44. Burkitt DP. In Burkitt DP, Wright DH (eds.) *Burkitt's Lymphoma.* Edinburgh, Livingstone, 1970; 186–97.

45. Yunis JJ, Soreng AL, Bowe AE. *Oncogene.* 1987; **1**, 59–69.

46. Lenoir GM, Bornkamm GW. *Advances in Viral Oncology.* 1987; **7**, 173–206.

47. Whittle HC, Brown J, Marsh K, *et al. Nature.* 1984; **312**, 449–50.

48. Purtilo D, Harada S, Bechtold T, *et al.* In: Magrath IT (ed.) *Pathogenesis of Leukemias and Lymphomas: Environmental Influences.* New York, Raven Press: 1984; 235–57.

49. Iverson U, Iverson OH, Ziegler JL, *et al. European Journal of Cancer.* 1972; **8**, 305–10.

50. Braylan RC, Fowlkes BT, Jaffe ES, *et al. Cancer.* 1978; **41**, 201–9.

51. Murphy SB, Melvin SL, Mauer AM, *et al. Cancer Research* 1979; **39**, 1534–8.

52. Wagner D, Kiwanuka J, Edwards B, *et al. Journal of Clinical Oncology.* 1987; **5**, 1262–74.

53. Magrath IT, Lee YJ, Anderson T, *et al. Cancer.* 1980; **45**, 1507–15.

54. Magrath IT, Sariban, E. In: Olweny C, Lenoir G (eds) *Burkitt's Lymphoma: A Human Cancer Model.* 1985; Lyon: IARC Publications, 119–127.

55. Levine PH, Kamaraja LS, Conelly RR, *et al. Cancer.* 1982; **49**, 1016–22.

56. Magrath IT. In: Pochedly C (ed) *Medical Clinics of North America.* 1989. (In press).

57. Meyers PA, Potter VP, Wollner N, Exelby P. *Cancer.* 1985; **56**, 259–61.

58. Burkitt DP. In: Burkitt DP, Wright DH (eds). *Burkitt's Lymphoma.* London: Livingstone, 1970.

59. Sariban E, Donahue A, Magrath IT. *Cancer* 1984; **53**, 141–6.

60. Janus C, Edwards BK, Sariban E. *et al. Cancer Treatment Reports.* 1984; **68**, 599–605.

61. Ladjadj Y, Philip T, Lenoir GM *et al. British Journal of Cancer.* 1984; **49**, 503–12.

62. Benjamin D, Magrath IT, Douglass EC, Corash LM, *et al. Blood.* 1983; **61**, 1017–19.

63. Roos G, Nordenson I, Osterman B, *et al. Leukemia Research.* 1982; **6**, 27–31.

64. Ganick DJ, Finlay J. *Blood.* 1980; **56**, 311–13.

65. Mangan KF, Rauch AE, Bishop M. *American Journal of Clinical Pathology.* 1985; **83**, 121–6.

66. Walle AJ, Al-Katib A, Wong GY, *et al. Leukemia Research.* 1987; **11**, 73–83.

67. Kersey JH, Lebien TW, Hurwitz R, *et al. American Journal of Clinical Pathology.* 1979; **72** (suppl.) 746–52.

68. Muller-Weihrich ST, Ludwig R, Reiter A, *et al.* In: Cavalli F, Bonnadonna G, Rosenczweig M (eds). *Third International Conference on Malignant Lymphoma.* 1987: Abstract.

69. Sariban E, Janus C, Edwards B, *et al. Journal of Clinical Oncology.* 1983; **11**, 677–81.

70. Magrath IT, Mugerwa J, Bailey I, *et al. Quarterly Journal of Medicine.* 1974; **43**, 489–508.

71. Ziegler JL, Magrath IT. In: Ioachim H, (ed). *Pathobiology Annual.* New York: Appleton-Century-Crofts, 1974; 129–42.

72. Magrath IT, Lwanga S, Carswell W, *et al. British*

Medical Journal. 1974; **2**, 308–12.

73. Krudy AD, Dunnick NR, Magrath IT, *et al. American Journal of Radiology.* 1981; **136**, 747–54.

74. Shawker TH, Dunnick NR, Head GL, *et al. Journal of Clinical Ultrasound.* 1979; **7**, 279–83.

75. Shields AF, Porter BA, Churchley S, *et al. Journal of Clinical Oncology.* 1987; **5**, 225–30.

76. Haddy TB, Parker RI, Magrath IT. *Medical and Paediatric Oncology.* 1989; in press.

77. Csako G, Magrath IT, Elin R. *American Journal of Clinical Pathology.* 1982; **78**, 712–17.

78. Cohen LF, Balow JE, Magrath IT. *American Journal of Medicine.* 1980; **68**, 486.

79. Tsokos GE, Balow JE, Spiegel RJ. *Medicine.* 1981; **60**, 218.

80. Arseneau JC, Bagley CM, Anderson T, Canellos GP. *Lancet.* 1973; **i**, 10–14.

81. Hande KR, Hixson CL, Chabner BA. *Cancer Research.* 1981; **41**, 2273–9.

82. Glatstein E, Kim H, Donaldson S, *et al. Cancer.* 1974; **34**, 204.

83. Aur RJ, Hustu HO, Simone JF, *et al. Cancer.* 1971; **27**, 1328–31.

84. Jenkin RDT, Sonley MJ, Stephens CA, *et al. Radiology.* 1966; **92**, 763–7.

85. Nelson DF, Cassady JR, Traggis D, *et al. Cancer* 1977; **39**, 89–97.

86. Murphy SB, Frizzera G, Evans AE, *et al. Cancer.* 1975; **36**, 2121–31.

87. Cebrian-Bonesana A, Schvartman E, Roca-Garcia C, *et al. Cancer.* 1978; **41**, 2372–8.

88. Jenkin RDT. In Deeley TJ (ed). *Modern Radiotherapy and Oncology – Malignant Diseases in Children.* London Butterworths, 1969; 319–59.

89. Murphy SB, Hustu HO, Rivera G, *et al. Journal of Clinical Oncology.* 1983; **1**, 326–30.

90. Jenkin RDT, Anderson JR, Chilcote RR. *et al. Journal of Clinical Oncology.* 1984; **2**, 88–97.

91. Anderson JR, Jenkin RDT. *New England Journal of Medicine* 1983; **309**, 311.

92. Patte C, Philip T, Rodary C, *et al. Journal of Clinical Oncology.* 1986; **4**, 1219.

93. Link MP, Donaldson S, Berard C *et al.* In: Cavalli F, Bonnadonna G, Rosenczweig, M (eds). *Third International Conference on Malignant Lymphoma.* 1987; Abstract.

94. Siegel S, Chilcote R, Coccia P, *et al.* In: Cavalli F, Bonnadonna G, Rosenczweig M (eds). *Third International Conference on Malignant Lymphoma.* 1987; Abstract.

95. Haddy T, Sandlund JT, Magrath IT. *American Journal of Pediatric Hematology and Oncology.* 1988; **10**, 224.

96. Murphy SB, Hustu HO. *Cancer.* 1980; **45**, 630–7.

97. Norin T, Clifford P, Einhorn J. *et al. Acta Radiologica* 1971; **10**, 545–57.

98. Djerassi I, Kim JS. *Cancer.* 1976; **38**, 1043–51.

99. Burkitt D. *Cancer.* 1967; **20**, 756–9.

100. Clifford P. UICC Monograph Series 1967; **8**, 77–93.

101. Arseneau JC, Canellos GP, Banks PM, *et al. American Journal of Medicine.* 1975; **58**, 314–321.

102. Ziegler J, Magrath IT, Olweny CLM. *Lancet.* 1979; **ii**, 936–8.

103. Ziegler JL. *New England Journal of Medicine.* 1977; **297**, 75–80.

104. Ziegler JL, Magrath IT, Deisseroth AB, *et al. Cancer Treatment Reports.* 1978; **62**, 2031–4.

105. Anderson JR, Wilson JF, Jenkin RD, *et al. New England Journal of Medicine.* 1983; **308**, 559.

106. Gadner H, Muller-Weihrich SI, Riehm H. *Onkologie.* 1986; **9**, 126.

107. Muller-Weihrich SI, Henze G, Langermann HJ, *et al. Onkologie.* 1984; **7**, 205.

108. Weinstein H, Vance Z, Jaffe N, *et al. Blood.* 1979; **53**, 687–97.

109. Murphy S, Bowman WP, *et al. Journal of Clinical Oncology.* 1986; **4**, 1732.

110. Bernstein JI, Coleman CN, Strickler JG, *et al. Journal of Clinical Oncology.* 1986; **4**, 847–58.

111. Skarin AT, Canellos GP, Rosenthal DS, *et al. Journal of Clinical Oncology.* 1983; **1**, 91–8.

112. Coiffier B, Byron P-A, French M, *et al. Blood.* 1987; **70**, 1394–9.

113. Sullivan M, Ramirez I. *Journal of Clinical Oncology.* 1985; **3**, 627–36.

114. Muller-Weihrich ST, Ludwig R, Reiter A, *et al. Third International Conference on Malignant Lymphomas.* abstract.

115. Philip T, Biron P, Philip I, *et al.* In: Cavalli F, Bonnadonna G, Rosenczweig M (eds). *Third International Conference in Malignant Lymphoma.* abstract.

116. Wright DH. In Burkitt DP, Wright DH, (eds). *Burkitt's Lymphoma.* Edinburgh, E and S Livingstone, 1970; 64–81.

117. Olweny CLM, Katongole-Mbidde E, Otim D. *et al. Acta Radiologica* 1977; **16**, 225–31.

118. Burkitt DP. *Cancer.* 1967; **20**, 756–9.

119. Ziegler JL, *New England Journal of Medicine.* 1981; **305**, 734–45.

120. Jones GR, Ettinger LJ. *Seminars in Oncology.* 1985; **12** (suppl. 3), 150.

121. Arndt C, Colvin M, Balis F, *et al. Proceedings of the Annual Meeting of the American Association of Cancer Research.* 1987; **28**, 439.

122. Hertler A, Schlossman D, Lester C, *et al. Proceedings of the American Society of Clinical Oncology.* 1987; **6**, A989.

123. Magrath IT (ed). *New Directions in Cancer*

Treatment. Heidelberg, Springer, 1989; 1–29.

124. Wong GG, Temple PA, Leary AC, *et al. Science* 1987; **235**, 1504–8.

125. Giardyina SL, Fooy KA, Beatty SM, Morgan AC Jr. *Immunobiology*. 1986; **172**, 205–12.

126. Appelbaum FR, Deisseroth AB, Graw RG Jr, *et al. Cancer*. 1978; **41**, 1059.

127. Philip T, Biron P, Philip I, *et al. European Journal of Cancer and Clinical Oncology*. 1986; **22**, 1015–27.

128. Philip T, Pinkerton R, Hartmann O, *et al. Clinical Haematology*. 1986; **15**, 205–17.

129. Appelbaum F, Sullivan K, Thomas E, *et al. Journal of Clinical Oncology*. 1987; **5**, 1340–7.

130. Ochs J, Abramowitch M, Rudnick S, *et al. Journal of Clinical Oncology*. 1986; **4**, 883–7.

131. Sullivan MP, Jaffe N, Boren H, *et al. Proceedings of the Annual Meeting of the American Association of Cancer Research*. 1985; **26**, C-182.

132. Meadows AT, Baum E, Fossati-Bellani F. *et al. Journal of Clinical Oncology*. 1985; **3**, 532–8.

CHAPTER 18

LARGE CELL LYMPHOMAS IN CHILDREN

Ian Magrath and Marshall Kadin

Definitions and general description

The large cell lymphomas comprise 15–30 per cent of childhood non-Hodgkin's lymphomas and have an incidence of less than 1 per million per annum in children aged below 15 years.[1,2] Fifteen per cent is probably an underestimate because of the difficulty in classifying some large cell lymphomas and in distinguishing them from anaplastic non-lymphoid tumours. This problem has been lessened by the more frequent use of methods of characterization beyond the simple light microscopic level, including immunopathology and molecular genetics.

Large cell lymphomas are relatively heterogeneous and poorly understood, both with regard to pathology and behaviour, compared to the more frequent small non-cleaved lymphomas and lymphoblastic lymphomas in childhood. This presents a problem with regard to determining optimal treatment, since not only is it likely that different subcategories within the large cell group require different therapies, but it is also probable that patient series from different centres contain different proportions of these subgroups which, in the absence of detailed characterization, renders meaningful comparison difficult or impossible. The rarity of these tumours also greatly increases the difficulty in performing clinical studies. It is easy to see why there is much conflicting information in the literature, and it is appropriate at present that major

emphasis should be given to attempting to characterize the large cell lymphomas in childhood in as much detail as possible. Only when the different subgroups have been clearly defined will it be possible to attempt to determine optimal therapeutic approaches. Until then, treatment must, of necessity, be based upon standard approaches to other types of childhood lymphomas.

Histology

In a recent study carried out by the Pediatric Oncology Group,[2] large cell lymphomas were divided according to the NCI Working Formulation and the Lukes and Collins classification (Table 18.1). Two major categories emerged from this analysis: large non-cleaved or cleaved lymphomas (Fig. 18.1), which probably arise from cells in the germinal centres of secondary lymphoid follicles and are therefore of B-cell origin; and immunoblastic lymphomas. The latter, which accounted for 40 of the 72 tumours studied (56 per cent), were further subdivided into plasmacytoid, clear cell and polymorphous types. The plasmacytoid type corresponds to Lukes immunoblastic lymphoma of B-cell origin, while the other types appear to correspond to immunoblastic lymphoma of T-cell origin (Fig. 18.2). Occasionally the polymorphous appearance leads to a diagnosis of mixed cell lymphoma.

A small and rather uncertain number of large cell tumours are probably of true histiocytic or tissue macrophage origin,[3-5] the differentiation of these from the histiocytoses becomes arbitrary and based more on semantics than biology. Tumours of true histiocytic origin are comprised of cells with large nuclei and abundant dark blue cytoplasm (Fig. 18.3) and can be differentiated from lymphoid tumours by the presence of tumour cell erythrophagocytosis (Fig. 18.4) and diffuse cytoplasmic staining for non-specific esterases. Staining for alpha naphthyl acetate or butyrate esterases or, where available, the use of isoelectric focusing, which can distinguish monocyte/histiocyte esterases from those of other cell types, are currently the best available means of identifying tumours of true histiocytic origin.[6] Recently, monoclonal antibodies apparently specific for cells of histiocytic origin have also been identified, these may prove to be of considerable value in the characterization of histiocytic tumours.[7,8]

Immunopathology

The heterogeneous cellular origins of the large cell lymphomas are readily confirmed by the use of monoclonal antibodies to detect differences in phenotype.[9-11] Some of these antibodies work well in paraffin-embedded tissues.[7] The large cell lymphomas of follicular centre cell origin express, as expected, B-cell antigens, including B1 (CD20), B4 (CD19) and LN-1 (Fig. 18.5).

Surface immunoglobulin (SIg) may, however, be absent in up to one-third of these tumours[9] – a finding which is consistent with the observation that a proportion of large, rapidly proliferating cells in normal germinal centres fails to express SIg.[12] It has been proposed that the temporary absence of SIg occurs during the process of somatic mutation of immunoglobulin gene variable regions (*see* Chapter 3). Mutated immunoglobulins are subsequently expressed on the cell surface and cells bearing immunoglobulins with the highest affinity for antigen are selected, by virtue of the greater likelihood that they will bind and be activated by antigen.[12] If this sequence of events is correct, large cell lymphomas of this type may have a particular propensity to mutate their V region genes, a characteristic which should be definable. In any event, it appears highly probable that lymphomas with the characteristics of large follicle centre cells are the neoplastic counterpart of antigen stimulated B lymphocytes. In children, however, lymphomas with a true follicular pattern are extremely rare (a very small number have been described in older teenagers and young adults[13-15]). Thus large cell lymphomas arising in germinal follicles appear to do so *de novo*, rather than in a follicular lymphoma undergoing histological transformation, a mechanism which occurs quite frequently in adults (*see* Chapters 19 and 21).

Table 18.1 Morphological subdivision of 72 diffuse 'histiocytic' lymphomas collected by POG[2] according to National Cancer Institute (NCI) Working Formulation and Lukes and Collins classification

Rappaport classification	No. of patients	Working Formulation classification	No. of patients	Lukes and Collins classification	No. of patients
Histiocytic	72	Large cell	32		
		large cleaved	3	Large cleaved*	3
		large non-cleaved	29	Large non-cleaved*	29
		Immunoblastic	40	Immunoblastic B	17
		plasmacytoid	17	Immunoblastic T	21
		clear cell	19	Immunoblastic NOS	2
		polymorphous	2		
		NOS†	2		

Reprinted with permission from *Cancer* and Dr BN Nathwani
*Follicular centre cell. †NOS: not otherwise specified.

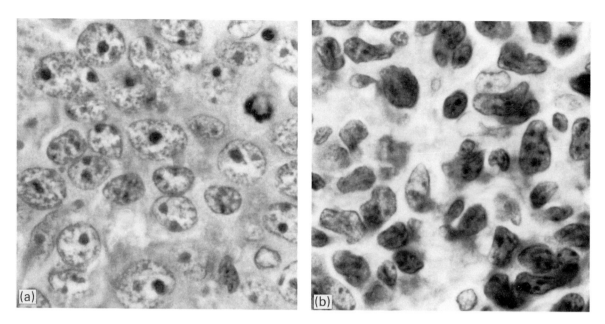

Fig. 18.1 Large cell lymphoma. (a) Large non-cleaved type; (b) Large cleaved cell type. Haematoxylin and eosin stain × 1100. Reprinted from ref.[1] with permission of WB Saunders & Co., Philadelphia.

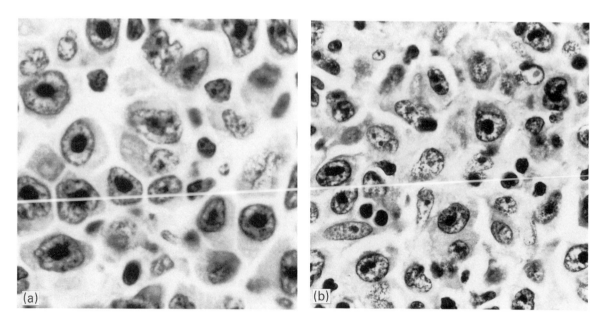

Fig. 18.2 Large cell lymphoma. (a) B-immunoblastic type. The cells have plasmacytoid features; (b) T-immunoblastic type. In addition to the large cells there are smaller lymphocytes with irregular nuclei. Haematoxylin and eosin stain × 1100. Reprinted from ref.[1] with permission of WB Saunders & Co., Philadelphia.

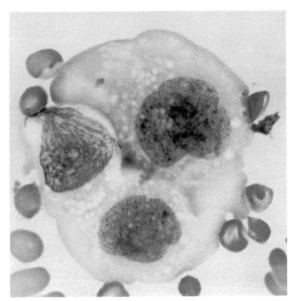

Fig. 18.3 Imprint of large cell lymphoma, histiocytic type. Notice the abundant cytoplasm and nuclei with monoctyoid features. The cells were strongly positive with non-specific esterase stain. Wright's stain, × 1100. Reprinted from ref.[1] with permission of WB Saunders & Co., Philadelphia.

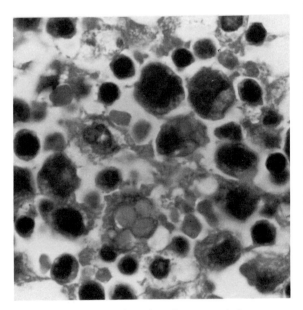

Fig. 18.4 Tumour cell erythrophagocytosis in malignant histioctyosis. Haematoxylin and eosin, × 990.

The characteristics of B-cell immunoblastic lymphomas have not been well defined. Some, or all B-cell lymphomas arising in the thymus may originate in a unique B-cell subpopulation that was recently detected in the thymic medulla. Such cells, which were readily detected with a monoclonal antibody called L26 (which reacts with all B-cells), tended to cluster round Hassall's corpuscles and insinuate between epithelial cells.[16] These cells also stained strongly with antibodies of CD groups 19, 20 and 22 and many express surface IgM. However, they stained negative with antibodies of CD groups 21 and 35, both of which stain mantle zone and follicle centre cells. To date, thymic B-cell tumours have not been sufficiently characterized to determine whether they have a similar phenotype to thymic B-cells.

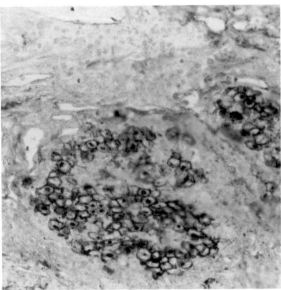

Fig. 18.5 Follicular B-cell lymphoma stained with antibody LN-1. Immunoperoxidase stain, × 200.

Some large cell lymphomas, particularly the clear cell and polymorphous immunoblastic types, express T-cell markers, most commonly T4 (CD4), T11 (CD2) and T1/Leu1 (CD5). A few express antigens characteristic of monocyte/histiocytes, although α-1-antitrypsin, α-1-antichymotrypsin and lysozyme (the enzymes detected) are probably not as reliable markers of a histiocytic origin as was originally thought.[10] New, promising monoclonal antibodies thought to be specific for this lineage have been described, the specificity of these awaits more extensive studies.[7] It seems likely that eventually a panel of monoclonal antibodies, able to discriminate between different subtypes of large cell lymphomas by virtue of the pattern of reactivity, will be established.

Recently, use of the monoclonal antibody Ki-1 (CD30) has shed considerable light on the origins of some large cell lymphomas.[17–19] Many cases formerly classified as malignant histiocytosis, true histiocytic lymphoma or anaplastic carcinoma have been shown to be large lymphoid cell neoplasms by use of this antibody. In addition, many cases classified morphologically as clear cell or polymorphous immunoblastic lymphoma also express the CD30 antigen. Thus morphology is clearly inadequate to differentiate between subgroups of large cell lymphomas. CD30 lymphomas characteristically involve the paracortical and peripheral sinus regions of lymph nodes (Fig. 18.6) and are believed to arise from large activated lymphoid cells (of both B and T phenotype) around the perimeter of follicle centres.[17] It has been suggested that whereas both virgin B-cells (i.e. cells which have not previously encountered antigen) and memory B-cells undergo initial activation by antigen on dendritic cells in the perifollicular area, only memory cells (undergoing a second or subsequent cycle of activation) can subsequently enter the germinal follicle under normal circumstances.[12] Whether CD30-positive lymphomas of B-cell origin can arise from cells undergoing either primary or secondary immune activation is not clear, but if the above hypothesis is correct they are the neoplastic counterparts of cells undergoing an earlier (primary) phase of activation rather than of those within germinal follicles. It is apparent, however, that the majority (70–80 per cent) of CD30 lymphomas are of T-cell origin, and represent antigen activated T-cells (i.e. are peripheral T-cell lymphomas) clearly differing from the T-cell lymphoblastic lymphomas which arise from T-cells undergoing antigen independent differentiation in the thymus.[17,18] However, as is also the case with CD30 lymphomas of B-cell origin, surface markers clearly identifying the lineage are often absent. In such cases, molecular genetics may provide the only method of identifying the cell

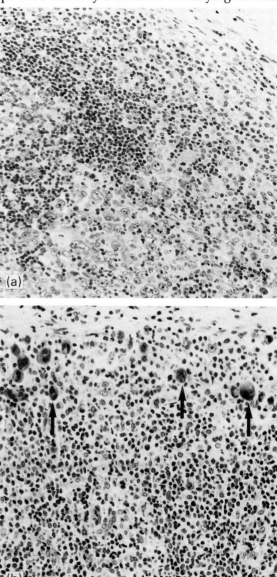

Fig 18.6 Ki-1 (CD30-positive) large cell lymphoma. The tumour cells infiltrating paracortex (a) and subcapsular sinus (b) of lymph node. Haematoxylin and eosin stain, × 200. Reprinted[44] with permission from Grune and Stratton, New York.

lineage. Finally, some CD30 lymphomas have a mixed B- and T-cell phenotype, the significance of which is not clear.[20] It is possible that only one of these components is malignant.

Cytogenetics

At present very little cytogenetic information exists in childhood large cell lymphomas, and to date non-random chromosomal translocations have not been identified, although cytogenetic abnormalities are usually detected. The exceptions to this are 'lymphomas' arising in iatrogenically suppressed patients (usually immunoblastic lymphomas), in whom karyotypic abnormalities are not usually observed.[20] About 38 per cent of all immunoblastic lymphomas are currently determined to be cytogenetically normal,[21] but it is not clear how many of these are arising in immunosuppressed individuals. As discussed below, lymphoproliferation in the immunosuppressed patient probably represents unbridled proliferation of normal cells in an abnormal host environment and would therefore be expected to be cytogenetically normal. In large cell lymphomas in patients of all ages, several different cytogenetic abnormalities have been observed, as discussed in Chapter 5. These include 8;14 translocations, abnormalities of 1p (usually associated with a T-cell phenotype), deletion of 6q (an abnormality which occurs in all histologies), trisomy of 12 (usually associated with a B-cell phenotype) and both 11;14 and 14;18 translocations.[21–23] The range of cytogenetic abnormalities confirms the heterogeneity of these tumours. Moreover, since the translocations observed are characteristically seen in other tumours, including small non-cleaved cell lymphomas (t8;14), small lymphocytic cell lymphomas (t11;14) and follicular lymphomas (t14;18), it is clear that large cell lymphomas are often closely related, or even represent 'transformations' of other lymphomas. This particularly applies to lymphomas arising in follicular centre cells, all of which are of B-cell origin, and in which the breakpoint on chromosome 14 is usually in the q32 region where the immunoglobulin heavy chain genes reside. However, 11;14 and 14;18 translocations have not been observed to date in large cell lymphomas in childhood. In immunoblastic lymphomas translocations involving the q11–13 region of chromosome 14 (the site of the Tα and Tδ genes) have been described.[24] These tumours, as expected from the site of the breakpoint, are of T-cell origin.

Molecular genetics

Another tool which has permitted progress to be made in the identification of the cellular origins of the large cell lymphomas in childhood has been the ability to determine the configuration of the antigen receptor genes of both B-cells (Ig genes) and T-cells. Since neoplasms of lymphocytes are usually clonal (*see* Chapter 3 for discussion), Southern blotting permits the detection of genes which have been rearranged from the germ line state, as a necessary component of lymphocyte differentiation in both T and B lineages. In some cases the examination of Ig or T-cell receptor genes in this way has permitted the identification of tumours (usually immunoblastic lymphomas expressing the CD30 antigen) whose phenotype remained unclear after immunohistochemistry and electron microscopy.[25]

The identification of genes adjacent to chromosomal breakpoints is likely to provide new probes for establishing the subtype of large cell lymphoma at a molecular genetic level, but will doubtless also provide insights into pathogenesis[26] (*see* Chapters 5 and 6).

Epidemiology

Because large cell lymphomas encompass a number of neoplasms of quite different cellular origins, the epidemiological features of these tumours are equally diverse. For the most part there is little available information, and although large cell lymphomas in children have been

described from all parts of the world, areas of particular high and low incidence have not been identified. Lymphomas arising in lymphocytes undergoing antigen-induced activation (particularly lymphomas derived from follicular centre cells) are uncommon in childhood, and almost never occur in young children, perhaps because long periods of antigen stimulation are normally required for neoplasia to result. This could be one of the reasons why the incidence of lymphomas increases with age and why lymphomas of germinal centre cells, if they arise at all in childhood, do so in older children. Neoplasia of activated lymphocytes can be superimposed, however, on underlying immunological abnormalities, including in-herited immunodeficiency syndromes, immunodeficiency resulting from viral infection (e.g. human immunodeficiency virus (HIV) and human T-cell lymphotrophic virus 1 (HTLV-I)) and iatrogenic immunodeficiency as in organ transplant recipients, especially when such individuals have been treated with a monoclonal antibody directed against the CD3 (T3) antigen. The epidemiology of these conditions has been discussed in detail in Chapters 8, 9 and 10, and they account for only a small percentage of childhood lymphomas.

The majority of lymphomas arising in patients with an immunological deficiency are of immunoblastic histology and are nearly always of B-cell origin. They frequently manifest considerable variability in cellular morphology, hence the terms originally used by Frizzera: 'polymorphic diffuse B-cell hyperplasia' or 'polymorphic B-cell lymphoma'.[27] The pathological lymphoproliferative syndromes occurring in immunosuppressed individuals appear to result, in most cases, from the unbridled proliferation of Epstein–Barr virus (EBV)-containing B lymphocytes which show a range of differentiation stages ranging from immunoblasts to plasma cells.[20,27] There is considerable debate as to what constitutes a true neoplastic process in such circumstances, for the majority of such syndromes are polyclonal and do not contain specific cytogenetic abnormalities. Moreover, acute EBV infection in an immunosuppressed patient who has not previously been infected by this virus can result in death from massive proliferation of the same EBV-containing cells which, in a normal individual, would be readily controlled by immune mechanisms.[20] The X-linked lymphoproliferative syndrome is one of the best known of the immunodeficiency syndromes that predisposes to fatal infectious mononucleosis but affected males can also suffer from aggressive lymphomas of immunoblastic or small non-cleaved type, and fatal infectious mononucleosis can occur in females with no family history.[20] The possibility that some apparently spontaneous immunoblastic lymphomas are the consequence of an unrecognized immunodeficiency syndrome should be considered.

The syndromes arising in immunodeficiency states appear to depend to a considerable degree upon the type and extent of immuno-suppression.[20, 24] Localized tumours which may regress upon withdrawal of immunosup-pressive therapy are sometimes seen. On the other hand, chronic lymphoproliferation can ultimately result in the emergence of aggressive lymphoma, probably as a consequence of a genetic change occurring in a single cell, leading to the emergence of a monoclonal neoplasm. Some of these lymphomas, particularly those arising in patients with HIV infections are, in fact, of the small non-cleaved cell type and bear the characteristic 8;14 or variant chromosomal translocations of these lymphomas (*see* Chapters 10 and 17), although such tumours are rarely associated with HIV in children.

Clinical features and staging

Unlike the lymphoblastic and small non-cleaved cell lymphomas of childhood, the clinical features of large cell lymphomas are not particularly characteristic. These tumours may arise in almost any tissue, both nodal and extranodal (e.g. Waldeyer's ring, bone, skin) and involve the abdomen (bowel, mesentery and retroperitoneum) as well as the mediastinum. Large cell lymphomas account for essentially all the non-lymphoblastic non-Hodgkin's lymphomas arising in the mediastinum and almost all of them have im-munoblastic histology (20 out of 24 in a recently published study[28]). Based on histology alone, it would appear that about half of the immunob-lastic tumours arising in the mediastinum are of T-cell origin (peripheral T-cell lymphomas), and half of B-cell origin, but very few immunological data are available. Lymph node involvement is also common, particularly when developing in a patient with an underlying immunological disorder, whether inherited, acquired or iatrogenic. Immunoblastic lymphomas arising in such patients also involve the brain much more frequently than spontaneously arising lymphomas. This is reminiscent of the ability of EBV-transformed lymphoblastoid cell lines to grow readily in the brains of nude mice, but not in the subcutaneous tissues.[29] Large cell lymphomas may also involve the meninges, producing malignant pleocytosis and, like other lymphomas, can involve the bone marrow and single or multiple bones. Large cell lymphomas occur more frequently in 'atypical sites' than small non-cleaved cell lymphomas and lymphoblastic lymphomas. Although such sites are not exempt from involvement by other lymphomas, the chance that the lymphoma is of large cell type is much greater when, for example, the lung parenchyma, skin, subcutaneous tissues or muscle are involved. This is an additional reason why some large cell tumours have been misdiagnosed in the past, since such sites of involvement are not usually equated with lymphomas. Other unusual features including vascular (arterial and venous) obstruction have been observed.

The unusual anatomical distribution of large cell lymphomas has implications for staging studies. Clearly, with so wide a spectrum of possibilities, very extensive studies would be necessary to determine the precise distribution of tumour. In addition, clinical examination is of particular importance because of the possibility of involvement of lymph nodes, skin and soft tissues.[30] Radiological studies should include a chest X-ray, and, wherever possible, computed tomographic (CT) scans of the chest and abdomen. Ultrasound examination is often helpful to evaluate the abdomen, particularly in small children with little retroperitoneal fat. A head CT scan or a magnetic resonance imaging (MRI) scan of the head are valuable studies in immunoblastic lymphomas, in view of the propensity of these tumours to involve the brain parenchyma. Spinal fluid should be examined for malignant cells, preferably after the head has been imaged in order to detect and avoid the imminent possibility of pressure coning in the presence of brain involvement. Gallium-67 and bone scans provide useful whole body screening and, where possible, both studies should be performed (bone should be studied first as gallium-67 will obscure the technetium image). A bone marrow examination, consisting of bilateral biopsies and aspirates, is necessary to determine whether marrow involvement is present. Recently, the value of MRI scanning for detecting patchy lymphomatous involvement of the marrow has been recognized.[31–33] Lymphangiography has not been evaluated sufficiently in children with large cell lymphomas to determine its value. Because of the potential for widespread involvement of multiple organs and tissues, however, it seems unlikely that a lymphangiogram would be a valuable asset.

The value of more objective tumour markers, such as lactate dehydrogeuase (LDH) and interleukin-2 (Il-2) receptors for large cell lymphomas in children has not been extensively analysed and more studies of these measurements are needed to determine their value. It seems likely however, that as in other childhood lymphomas and adults with large cell lymphomas, serum LHD broadly correlates with prognosis.

No staging systems have been devised specifically for large cell lymphomas. In children the staging systems used for small non-cleaved cell lymphomas and lymphoblastic lymphomas are used (*see* Chapters 12, 16 and 17). Perhaps the most widely used staging system is the St Jude system, which is applied to all histologies. Because of the more unusual distribution patterns which can arise in large cell lymphomas, the validity of this and other standard staging systems is difficult to assess. However, there is no doubt that patients with more extensive disease, stages, III and IV, have a worse prognosis in the clinical trials performed so far (*see* below). Until sufficiently large numbers of patients have been treated uniformly a specific staging system cannot be devised. Since there is good evidence that prognosis is dependent upon tumour burden, an appropriate objective is to devise the best way of determining this. Staging systems have the disadvantage that each staging category must, of necessity, include patients with a range of tumour burdens. It is therefore probable, as has been shown for small non-cleaved cell lymphomas,[34-37] that objective biochemical measures such as LDH or Il-2 receptor levels will prove to be more useful. Central nervous system (CNS) disease may be in a separate category, presumably because therapeutic approaches are more limited against tumours at this site. A possible exception to this is brain involvement in patients with underlying immunosuppressive syndromes since some patients with isolated brain parenchymal involvement have achieved prolonged survival with local irradiation alone.

Treatment and prognosis

The optimal treatment of children with large cell lymphomas has not been generally agreed upon, doubtless because of the rarity and heterogeneity of these tumours. As with the development of therapeutic approaches to any tumour, treatment has been based upon that of related lymphomas, namely Hodgkin's disease (particularly in earlier years), small non-cleaved cell lymphomas or lymphoblastic lymphomas. The nature of pediatric lymphomas has been clarified only in the last 20 years, while effective treatment for patients with disseminated disease has been available for an even shorter period. Thus the importance of histology as a prognostic factor, and consequently as a determinant of treatment, could not be investigated until recently. Modern treatment protocols for childhood NHL were initially open to patients with lymphomas of all histologies and were, of course, intended to provide information on possible prognostic factors, including histology. Unfortunately, because large cell lymphomas represented a minority of the tumours, and because detailed characterization of the lymphomas was not always possible (and in fact rarely undertaken) available information regarding response to treatment and long-term outcome in patients with large cell lymphomas should be viewed with caution. There can be no doubt, however, that long-term survival can be obtained with several apparently philosophically different approaches to treatment, including protocols now primarily used for small

non-cleaved lymphomas as well as those used for lymphoblastic lymphomas, which are based on the treatment approaches used for acute lymphoblastic leukaemia.

Treatment of large cell lymphomas with regimens used for lymphoblastic lymphoma

Two main chemotherapy regimens based on protocols designed for acute lymphoblastic leukaemia and successfully used for lymphoblastic lymphomas have also been used for the treatment of large lymphomas. These are the APO regimen, originated at the Dana Farber Cancer Institute,[38] and the LSA$_2$L$_2$ (*see* Chapter 16) regimen designed originally at the Memorial Sloan Kettering Cancer Center but used in modified form by the Childrens Cancer Group (CCG)[39] and the Pediatric Oncology Group (POG)[40] in the USA.

Twenty-nine patients were treated with APO, a regimen which utilizes doxorubicin (A), prednisone (P) and vincristine (Oncovin) (O) induction, consolidation and maintenance for a total of 2 years of therapy. The protocol also includes radiation (3000–4000 cGy) to regional disease given at week eight of therapy in patients with stage I and II tumours (Murphy system), but not in patients with disseminated disease. Patients with primary bone involvement were treated with 5000–5400 cGy over 5–6 weeks. Cranial irradiation (2400 cGy) and intrathecal therapy were given as prophylaxis against spread to the central nervous system in all patients, except those with stage I or II disease, and patients with totally resected gastrointestinal tumour. It should be noted that 13 of the 29 patients had localized disease, mostly involving lymph nodes, Waldeyer's ring, or bone. Patients with disseminated disease predominantly had abdominal involvement. Only one patient had bone marrow disease at diagnosis. Twenty-eight of the 29 patients achieved complete remission, one only after radiation therapy to regional disease. Only two patients relapsed, both had presented with disseminated disease and both had isolated central nervous system relapses. Both were alive and disease-free for more than a year after the last relapse (one of them had two CNS relapses). Two patients with localized disease died in complete remission. With a median follow-up of four years, 76 per cent of patients were estimated to be alive and disease-free at 6 years. Toxicity was acceptable. These results were not further broken down according to histological subtype. Even though this is a small group of patients, it is clear that the APO regimen can be highly successful. A role for radiation has not been established, particularly since patients with disseminated disease who received no radiotherapy did very well, and none relapsed in sites of previous bulk disease.

The CCG used LSA_2L_2 as one of the arms of a randomized study for all children with non-Hodgkin's lymphoma. The other arm consisted of a combination of cyclophosphamide, vincristine, methotrexate and prednisone, known as COMP. A schema for LSA_2L_2, a complex protocol which includes 10 drugs, is shown in Chapter 16 (*see* Fig. 16.3) and that for COMP in Chapter 17 (*see* Fig. 17.4). An attempt was made to irradiate all sites of bulk disease greater than 3 cm, by giving 2000 or 3000 cGy, depending upon the radiation volume (the smaller volumes receiving the larger dose). In the CCG trial, 28 patients in all were diagnosed as having 'histiocytic' (large cell) lymphoma, but further histological subcategorization was not attempted. Seven of these patients had localized disease and five were treated with LSA_2L_2. Although the outcome of these five patients is not discernible from the published results, the total of 32 patients with localized disease treated with LSA_2L_2 had a failure-free survival of 84 per cent. Only nine of the 20 patients with disseminated histiocytic lymphoma included in the study were treated on the LSA_2L_2 arm. These were analysed with 24 other patients who had lymphomas other than lymphoblastic lymphoma. Twenty-three of these had undifferentiated (small non-cleaved cell) lymphomas, and one a non-Hodgkin's lymphoma not further specified. Overall, 26 per cent of these 33 patients were failure-free at 24 months. In a subsequent report, 46 patients with histiocytic lymphomas (large cell) were analysed separately. A higher percentage of thirty patients treated on the COMP arm were failure-free at one and two years compared to the 16

patients treated with LSA_2L_2, but by three years 46 per cent and 44 per cent of patients were failure-free in the respective groups.[41] Thus there was no clear advantage to either regimen in this trial. Severe haematological toxicity was observed in a high proportion of the patients.

The POG trial, in which another slightly modified LSA_2L_2 regimen was used for patients who had neither lymphoblastic lymphomas nor Burkitt's lymphoma, included 28 patients with large cell lymphomas. Thirteen of these patients had stage I or II disease. In this trial, radiation was given only for compressive mediastinal disease and residual disease after induction therapy. Twenty-three of the patients (82 per cent) achieved complete remission, and the failure-free survival for the 28 patients was 64 per cent. There was no significant difference in failure-free survival among patients with large cell, lymphoblastic or undifferentiated (non-Burkitt's) lymphomas. However, relapses occurred during the first three years for lymphoblastic patients, but only during the first 8 months in the other two groups. Only 77 per cent of the 13 patients with large cell lymphoma of Murphy stage III achieved complete remission, while the predicted disease-free survival beyond three years for this subgroup was 65 per cent. Toxicity in this trial was severe with 77 per cent of all 107 patients experiencing severe or worse toxicity; 40 per cent exerienced life-threatening toxicity.

Differences in treatment between the POG and CCG trials were apparently minor, although radiation was used much more in the CCG study. Since patients in this study had, if anything, a worse outcome, this not only suggests that radiation may be of no benefit in the treatment of large cell lymphomas, but also raises the possibility that the dose intensity (i.e. mg drug administered/m^2) might have been adversely affected by treatment delays caused by radiation. However, the very small numbers of patients included in these trials precludes definitive conclusions.

All five patients with large cell lymphomas of the mediastinum treated with the LSA_2L_2 protocol achieved continuous complete remission,[28] while in a POG study (7905) 56 per cent of 22 patients with non-lymphoblastic lymphomas (other than Burkitt's) who received modified LSA$_2$L$_2$ therapy were disease-free at two years.[40]

Treatment of large cell lymphomas with regimens used for small non-cleaved cell lymphomas

It is difficult to determine the results of 'lymphoma-like' therapy of large cell lymphomas in children from the published literature since most publications have not evaluated this histological subgroup separately. Moreover, many treatment protocols have emphasized the treatment of B-cell tumours rather than specific histologies, and often do not attempt to break down the groups by histology. Although an attempt is made in these trials to confirm the phenotype of the tumours, this is not always possible, so that it is not even clear that the protocols are dealing excusively with B-cell tumours. This applies to the French LMB-02 study and the German BFM studies discussed in Chapter 17. Both of these studies, as well as the 77-04 protocol of NCI and the CCG randomized comparison of LSA$_2$L$_2$ and COMP, suffer from small numbers of patients. When stage and histology are taken into account, the number of patients in each of the final groups is so small as to render meaningful comparison impossible. Even in the CCG trial, in which 211 patients were evaluable at the time of the initial report, only 13 patients with large cell lymphoma (two localized) were treated with COMP. Subsequently, 16 patients with disseminated histiocytic lymphoma were reported to have a failure-free survival of 44 per cent at 3 years.

Bearing in mind the hazards of extrapolating from small numbers, it appears that the overall results of the protocols for B-cell lymphomas are very good, producing disease-free survival of between 65 and 80 per cent for patients with stage III disease (*see* Chapter 17). It would seem that these protocols provide very good therapy for at least the majority of large cell lymphomas of B-cell type. Further evidence that protocols designed for the treatment of lymphoma rather than leukaemia are effective in large cell lymphomas is provided by a retrospective analysis of 25 patients with non-lymphoblastic lymphomas of the mediastinum, 20 of which were immunoblastic and two large non-cleaved lymphomas. Eighteen were treated with a variety of 'lymphoma' regimens consisting predominantly of CHOP (cyclophosphamide, doxorubicin, adriamycin, vincristine Oncovin and prednisone). Twelve of these patients achieved continuous complete remission (median remission duration for the study was 42 months).[28] Similarly, in a POG trial in which patients with non-lymphoblastic lymphomas (except Burkitt's) were treated with the ACOP regimen (doxorubicin, cyclophosphamide, vincristine and prednisone), 76 per cent of patients were disease-free at two years.[42] There were no apparent differences in prognosis among the histological subtypes[2] (Fig. 18.7).

Although the prognostic significance of tumour cell phenotype in large cell lymphomas is largely unknown, a recent preliminary study in which patients with similar extents of disease were treated with similar chemotherapy protocols (COMP or D-COMP) suggested a survival advantage for patients with CD30 antigen expression.[43]

Optimal treatment

One potential advantage of the most recent protocols being used for B-cell lymphomas is their brevity (3–6 months total duration) and in spite of the fact that treatment protocols used for lymphoblastic lymphoma have been quite successful in small numbers of patients with large cell lymphomas, most paediatric oncologists would consider that large cell lymphomas, at least those of B-cell type, should be treated with protocols used for small non-cleaved cell lymphomas. There is no evidence that patients with large cell lymphomas have a worse prognosis than patients with other B-cell tumours (who enjoy overall a very good prognosis) when treated in this way. In fact the reverse may be true.

In the paediatric lymphomas radiation of regional disease has largely been abandoned as a component of primary therapy. In the few randomized studies of both localized and disseminated disease where its role has been evaluated, radiation appears to increase toxicity but provide no therapeutic benefit. In a series of six patients with CD30-positive lymphomas (initially misdiagnosed as histiocytoses, carcinoma or non-malignant disorder) relapse occurred frequently when radiation was used as the sole modality of treatment.[44] Thus, although it could be argued that its role in subtypes of large cell lymphomas is unknown, the weight of the evidence points away from it being of value.

Optimal therapy for other types of large cell lymphoma including those of T-cell type and CD30-positive lymphomas has not been defined, although a small number of such patients have been treated successfully with regimens used for other lymphomas. The most important aspect of devising appropriate therapy for these tumours is to recognize them. Only then can their response to the treatment regimens used in the larger trials be determined and rational strategies for their treatment developed. Since it is possible that CD30 lymphomas of B-type may differ in their response to treatment from those of T type, it is also important that, wherever possible, tumour is frozen so that detailed characterization,

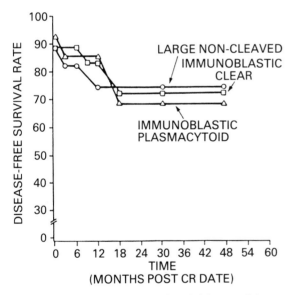

Fig. 18.7 Disease-free survival in children with large cell lymphomas. There were no significant differences in survival among the different morphological subtypes, although not all patients were treated according to the same treatment protocol. Reprinted[2] with permission from JB Lipincott & Co., Philadelphia.

including molecular studies can be carried out. There seems no cogent reason to explore in children the efficacy of the specific treatment regimens used in adult large cell lymphomas e.g. ProMACE-CytaBOM, M/m-BACOD, COP-BLAM and MACOB-B (*see* Chapter 21). Overall results are not as good as those that have been achieved in children with non-lymphoblastic lymphomas. In some of these protocols high-grade lymphomas (including immunoblastic lymphoma) tend to have a worse prognosis, although the basic strategies and drugs used are similar to those used in childhood B-cell lymphomas. Moreover, the majority of the large cell lymphomas in adults are of the follicular centre cell type. It is difficult to discern the relative effectiveness of treatment protocols used in adult diffuse aggressive lymphomas against immunoblastic lymphomas. This is because patient numbers tend to be small, prognosis in discrete histological groups is not always reported, the staging systems used differ and prognostic factors within histological groups are usually not provided. However, some patients do appear to achieve prolonged survival when treated with such protocols. In the French trial of the LNH-80 protocol, for example, 46 per cent or 23 patients with immunoblastic lymphomas were alive at five years. In this same trial, 74 per cent of diffuse large cell patients were alive at five years.[45]

Treatment of lymphomas arising in immunosuppressed patients

A particularly difficult problem is the management of patients with an underlying immunodeficiency syndrome in whom a lymphoma develops. Because the cause and degree of immunosuppression differs so markedly, the treatment of such patients must be individualized. Where immunosuppression is iatrogenic, cessation of the immunosuppressive drug or anti-T-cell monoclonal antibody therapy may permit tumour regression to occur. In patients with lymphoproliferative syndromes superimposed on an inherited immunosuppressive syndrome it is important to establish whether the proliferating cells have chromosomal abnormalities and whether they are monoclonal. These characteristics support the likelihood that the process is truly malignant. In such a situation the intensity of therapy will depend upon the propensity of the patient to infectious complications. Intensive chemotherapy in a severely immunosuppressed individual may simply hasten the occurrence of a fatal infectious process. It may be more appropriate to treat such immunosuppressed patients with localized disease by radiation, but if the process is disseminated there may be no way out of the dilemma, and a course of action must be taken upon which both family and physicians agree. Recent results with α-interferon in such patients show promise (*see* Chapter 8), and further exploration of the value of a wide range of lymphokines in severely immunosuppressed patients with lymphoma is appropriate in view of the gravely increased risks of conventional combination chemotherapy regimens. Patients without a history of repeated serious infections, however, should be treated with an intensive modern protocol as discussed above, since long-term survival is possible. In all of these patients, it must be borne in mind that the prognosis includes that of the underlying disease.

Follow-up

Appropriate intervals between follow-up studies for large cell lymphomas includes monthly examinations in the first six months after cessation of treatment and two-monthly assement of known disease sites for the first two years, after which relapse is unlikely. Thereafter the patient should be seen every six months to one year to ascertain that no long-term side-effects have developed and to ensure that accurate records are kept of survival duration.

References

1. Kjeldsberg CR, Wilson JF, Berard CW. *Human Pathogy*. 1983; **14**, 612.
2. Nathwani BN, Griffith RC, Kelly DR, *et al. Cancer.* 1987; **59**, 1138–42.
3. Koh S-J, Vargas GF, Cases JN *et al. American Journal of Clinical Pathology.* 1980; **74**, 417–26.
4. Thomas P, Said JW, Rosenfelt FP, *et al. American Journal of Clinical Pathology.* 1984; **81**, 243–8.
5. Van der Valk P, Meijer CJ, Willemze R, *et al. Histopathology.* 1984; **8**, 105–23.
6. Radzun HJ, Parwaresch MR, Kulenkampff CH, *et al. Blood.* 1980; **55**, 891–97.
7. Flavell DJ, Jones DB, Wright D. *Histochemistry and cytochemistry.* 1987; **35**, 1217–26.
8. Roholl PJM, Kleyne J, Pipers HW, *et al. Human Pathology.* 1985; **16**, 763.
9. Clearly ML, Trela M, Weiss LM, *et al. Laboratory Investigation.* 1985; **53**, 521.
10. Turner RR, Wood GS, Beckstead JH, *et al. American Journal of Surgical Pathology.* 1984; **8**, 485.
11. Gatter KC, Mason DY. In: Fer MF, Greco FA, Oldham RK, (eds). *Poorly Differentiated Neoplasms and Tumours of Unknown Origin.* Orlando, Florida: Grune and Stratton, 1986; 399–429.
12. Maclennan IC, Gray D. *Immunology Reviews.* 1986; **91**, 61–83.
13. Durnov LA, Ermakov ES, Molochkina AE. *Voprosi Onkologie.* 1975; **21**, 20–4.
14. Winberg CD, Nathwani BN, Rappaport H. *Laboratory Investigation.* 1979; **40**, 292 (abstract).
15. Frizzera G, Murphy SB. *Cancer.* 1979; **44**, 2218–35.
16. Isaacson PG, Norton AJ, Addis BJ. *Lancet.* 1987; **ii**, 1488–90.
17. Stein H, Mason DY, Gerdes J, *et al. Blood.* 1985; **66**, 848.
18. Agnarsson BA, Kadin ME. *American Journal of Surgical Pathology.* 1988; **12**, 264–74.
19. Stein H, Gerdes J, Tippelmann G, *et al. Third International Conference on Malignant Lymphoma.* June 10–13, 1987, Lugano, Switzerland. 0: 21.
20. Magrath IT. In: Sahlossberg D (ed). *Infectious Mononucleosis.* New York: Prader, 1983; 225–77.
21. 5th International workshop on chromosomes in leukemia-lymphoma. *Blood.* 1987; **70**, 1554–64.
22. Sigaux F, Berger R, Bernheim A, *et al. British Journal of Haematology.* 1984; **57**, 393–405.
23. Bloomfield CD, Arthur DC, Frizzera G, *et al. Cancer Research.* 1983; **43**, 2975.
24. Seibel N, Cossman J, Magrath IT. In: Pizzo PA, Poplack DG (eds). *Principles and Practice of Pediatric Onocology.* New York: Lippincott, 1988; 477–490.
25. Gonzalez-Crussi F, Mangkornkanok M, Hsueh W, *et al. American Journal of Surgical Pathology.* 1985; **11**, 59.
26. Cleary ML, Sklar J. *Proceedings of the National Academy of Sciences USA.* 1985; **82**, 7439.
27. Frizzera G, Hanto KJ, Gajl-Peczalska KJ, *et al. Cancer Research.* 1981; **41**, 4262–79.
28. Bunin NJ, Hvizdala E, Link M, *et al. Journal of Clinical Oncology.* 1986; **4**, 154–9.
29. Giovanella B, Nilsson K, Zech L, *et al. International*

Journal of Cancer. 1979; **24**,103–13.

30. Zaatari GS, Chan WC, Kim TH, *et al. Cancer.* 1987; **59**, 1040–5.

31. Porter BA, Shields AF, Olson DO. *Radiologic Clinics of North America.* 1986; **24**, 269–89.

32. Olson DO, Shields AF, Scheurich CJ, *et al. Investigative Radiology.* 1986; **21**, 540–6.

33. Porter BA, Shields AF, Olson DO. *Radiologic Clinics of North America.* 1986; **24**, 269–89.

34. Magrath I, Janus C, Edwards B, *et al. Blood.* 1984; **63**, 1102–11.

35. Wagner D, Kiwanuka J, Edwards BK, *et al. Journal of Clinical Oncology.* 1987; **5**, 1262–74.

36. Magrath IT, Lee YJ, Anderson T, *et al. Cancer.* 1980; **45**, 1507–15.

37. Pui C-H, Ip SH, Kung P, *et al. Blood.* 1987; **70**, 624–8.

38. Weinstein HJ, Lack EE, Cassady JR, *Blood.* 1984; **64**, 422–6.

39. Anderson JR, Wilson JF, Jenkin RD, *et al. New England Journal of Medicine.* 1983; **308**, 559–65.

40. Sullivan MP, Boyett J, Pullen J, *et al. Cancer.* 1985; **55**, 323–36.

41. Anderson JR, Jenkin RTD. *New England Journal of Medicine.* 1983; **309**, 311.

42. Hvizdala E, Berard C, Callihan T, *et al. Blood.* 1983; **62** (suppl. 1), 213a.

43. Kadin ME, Sposto R, Agnarsson BA, *et al. Blood.* 1989. (In press.)

44. Kadin ME, Sako E, Berliner N, *et al. Blood.* 1986; **68**, 1042–9.

45. Coiffier B, Bryon P-A, French M, *et al. Blood.* 1987; **70**, 1394–9.

CHAPTER 19

FOLLICULAR LYMPHOMAS

Dan L Longo and Wyndham Wilson

Definitions and general description

The follicular lymphomas comprise three of the 10 or so subtypes of lymphocytic lymphomas. They are linked by several features: their cell of origin is a follicular centre B lymphocyte; they grow in a nodular or follicular pattern; they predominantly originate in lymph nodes; they have a propensity to evolve into clinically more aggressive diffuse large cell lymphomas; and they share clonal cytogenetic abnormalities involving the same chromosomes in two-thirds to three-quarters of cases.[1] There are also several distinguishing features. Their natural histories are different from one another, a fact that has led to divergent approaches to the treatment of patients with follicular lymphomas. Their likelihood of being completely eradicated permanently by therapy being used today is different. They are distinguished from one another in an apparently arbitrary way.[2] The haematopathologist examines nodal tissue stained with haematoxylin and eosin and determines the pattern of growth. If the diagnosis of lymphoma is supported by the effacement of the lymph node architecture and the lymphoma is growing in an apparently nodular pattern, the pathologist counts the number of large cells in the centre of the nodules of the tumour.

All the follicular lymphomas are composed predominantly of two populations of morphologically atypical cells. The smaller of the two cells are larger than resting lymphocytes but smaller than normal lymphocytes responding to mitogenic stimuli, they contain sparse basophilic cytoplasm and a cleaved nucleus, and they are called small cleaved lymphocytes. The larger of the two cells has the morphology of a transformed lymphocyte and is the predominant cell in the most common lymphoma, diffuse large cell lymphoma. If there are up to five large cells per high power field, the lymphoma is categorized as follicular small cleaved cell (FSC) lymphoma. If there are five to 15 large cells, the lymphoma is called follicular mixed (FM) lymphoma. If there are 15 or more large cells per high power field in the centre of the nodules, the lymphoma is follicular large cell (FLC) lymphoma. It is quite clear that the three entities called follicular lymphomas lie on a continuous spectrum of disease, and it is remarkable that the arbitrary morphological distinctions provide an operational basis for dividing individuals with disease somewhere in the spectrum into subsets that are more or less clinically homogeneous and can be treated in a consistent way with a more or less predictable outcome.

The biology of the malignant follicular centre B-cell

In the normal lymph node, the follicular centre B-cell responds to antigen by proliferating and its progeny differentiate into memory B-cells and antibody-secreting cells. The proliferation and differentiation of the cell is at least partially influenced by other cell populations in the lymphoid follicle. When the follicular centre B-cell becomes malignant, the cell proliferates autonomously (or apparently so) and no longer responds to the normal stimuli that terminate a B-cell proliferative response. The aetiology of the malignant transformation is not known. The medical conditions known to predispose patients to the development of lymphoma have consistent features like chronic antigenic stimulation (e.g. coeliac disease), autoimmunity (e.g. Sjögren's syndrome), or immune deficiency (e.g. AIDS, iatrogenic immunodeficiency, X-linked immunodeficiency), but the lymphomas complicating these illnesses are generally diffuse, not follicular lymphomas. Follicular lymphomas do not appear to have particular predisposing factors. They are rare in developing countries, a finding that implicates environmental factors in their pathogenesis.

In some patients with follicular lymphomas, the host immune system appears to retain some control over the proliferation of the malignant cells, since up to 25 per cent of patients will have temporary spontaneous partial regressions (especially FSC histological subtype) and, rarely, patients have had complete regression of tumour.[3] The universal failure to generate lymphoma cell lines from patients with follicular lymphoma, the slow natural history of FSC subtype and the waxing and waning adenopathy seen in some patients had led some to suggest that follicular lymphomas in general, and FSC in particular may be benign lymphoid tumours.[4] However, the progression of disease in untreated follicular lymphoma patients, the tendency of the patients to develop diffuse large cell lymphoma and other more aggressive histological subtypes[5] and the clonal cytogenetic abnormalities found in these tumours[6] support the notion that they represent true malignant transformations of follicular centre B-cells.

The malignant cell of the follicular lymphomas was one of the first tumour cells to be recognized as B-cell derived and monoclonal on the basis of the detection of cell surface immunoglobulin of a single isotype.[7] With the development of a number of monoclonal antibodies that recognize B-cell specific antigens, it has become clear that the follicular lymphomas, and indeed all B-cell lymphomas, bear the cell surface phenotype of cells at discrete stages of normal B-cell differentiation.[8] The cell surface phenotype has suggested that tumours result from maturation arrest, and indeed, some laboratory evidence supports the idea that certain malignant B-cells may respond to signals that mimic normal differentiation signals.[9] However, since very little is known about the genetic events that characterize B-cells at different stages of development, the concept of maturation arrest does not offer much insight into the mechanism of lymphomagenesis or reveal vulnerabilities for potential therapeutic attack.

Most follicular lymphomas are B1, B2, B4, HLA-DR and surface immunoglobulin positive. Usually the isotype of the immunoglobulin is IgM. Rudders *et al.* have reported that a subset of their patients with FSC lymphomas had, in addition to IgM, a second immunoglobulin isotype, IgD on the surface, as well as complement receptors.[10] Those patients with IgM, IgD and complement receptors appeared to have significantly prolonged survival compared to the IgD-negative and complement receptor-negative FSC lymphoma patients. Unfortunately the patients were not managed in a consistent manner and it is not clear whether the conclusions reflect differences in natural history or differences in treatment outcome. There are no other reports in which identifying subsets of patients based on immunological phenotype provides prognostic information independent of histology. Rarely, patients with an unusual histological subtype of low-grade lymphoma called mantle zone lymphoma have tumours with a vaguely nodular appearance.[11] The mantle zone lymphoma is not derived from follicular centre cells but from small B-cells that surround the follicle. Immunological phenotype can assist in distinguishing mantle zone lymphoma from FSC (though this is virtually never necessary) as the mantle zone B-cell expresses the T65 antigen recognized by T101 and Leu-1 (CD5) antibodies.[12] Aside from identifying potential targets for therapeutic attack, immunological phenotyping plays no important role in the management of patients with follicular lymphoma.

The discovery of characteristic cytogenetic

abnormalities in up to 75 per cent of patients with follicular lymphoma of all histological types has stimulated an enthusiastic search for transforming genes that might be involved in the aetiology of follicular lymphoma. Yunis *et al.* found translocation between chromosomes 18 and 14 in 16 of 19 patients with follicular lymphoma.[6] The breakpoint of chromosome 18 was consistently at band q21;3 and its presence in untreated patients confirmed that the abnormality was not induced by exposure to mutagens during treatment. The gene on chromosome 18 that translocates to chromosome 14 was called *bcl*-2 but it has no homology to any known family of oncogenes.[13] *bcl*-2 translocates to band q32 of chromosome 14, the site of the immunoglobulin heavy chain joining segment genes (J_H), and more careful sequence analysis has demonstrated that the translocated gene is in proximity to the heavy-chain gene enhancer located between the joining region and IgM switch region. This suggests that the translocation occurred in the cell at a pre-B-cell stage during attempted heavy chain joining. It is not clear how this translocation might lead to transformation, but its mechanics are parallel to rearrangements of the c-*myc* gene in Burkitt's lymphoma.[14] *bcl*-2 does not transform 3T3 cells upon transfection and it is expressed by normal B-cells during mitogen-induced proliferation,[15] but its precise role in the development of follicular lymphoma awaits clarification.

Recently, Korsmeyer and his colleagues have demonstrated that the particular site of the t(14;18) can be used as a clonal signature, similar to the pattern of immunoglobulin gene rearrangements.[16] Since part of the job of a normal B-cell involves genetic instability that allows for the greatest possible diversity in the B-cell repertoire for antigen, it is not surprising that clonal malignancies could alter their genetic phenotype. Such phenotypic alteration has been observed in both the idiotype of the immunoglobulin molecule[17] and in the rearrangements of the immunoglobulin genes.[18] Such instability has mistakenly led some investigators to conclude that there is a high incidence of biclonal malignancy in the follicular lymphomas. Korsmeyer's data[16] clearly demonstrate that the subclones that have continued to rearrange their

immunoglobulin genes and thus appear to be derived from a different clone, are actually derived from the same clone, based on the precise site of t(14;18). In addition to possible insights into aetiology, the t(14;18) and other molecular probes appear capable of dramatically altering the criteria used to stage the extent of disease and/or the presence of residual disease in patients with follicular lymphoma since analysis of the genes is at least 100 times more sensitive than microscopic examination.[19] Although *bcl*-2 has not been clearly shown to be an oncogene, its behaviour suggests that a dissection of its effects on cell proliferation may provide an important clue to the aetiology of follicular lymphomas. This topic is more fully discussed in Chapter 6.

Although the specific aetiology of follicular lymphomas is not known, it is clear that the cell cycle kinetics of the individual histological subtypes is distinct.[20] Follicular small cleaved cell lymphomas have the lowest growth fraction and the lowest percentage of cells expressing the transferrin receptor, a rough immunological correlate to the growth fraction. Follicular mixed lymphomas have a higher growth fraction and more transferrin receptor positive cells than FSC lymphomas, and FLC lymphomas have the highest growth fraction.[20] It is a recurring theme in the study of the follicular lymphomas that the greater the fraction of large cells in the tumour, the higher the growth fraction of the tumour, the more rapid the clinical pace of disease and the more rapid the clinical pace of disease and the more susceptible to eradication by combination chemotherapy a tumour becomes. In many ways the follicular lymphomas behave analogously to bone marrow, another stem cell compartment with two stem cells. In this analogy, the tumour has two stem cell populations, the small cleaved lymphocytic stem cell that is not in cycle, is renewable and sensitive to inhibition (but not eradication) by combination chemotherapy, and a second stem cell that becomes more prominent as the fraction of large cells increases, is non-renewable, and sensitive to combination chemotherapy.[21] Thus, the more indolent growth and the more remote curability of FSC lymphoma relates to kinetics and the resistance of the stem cell of FSC lymphoma to chemotherapy.

The analogy to bone marrow seems apt. Although most chemotherapeutic agents at conventional tolerable doses can produce transient cytopenias and myelosuppression, the stem cell population almost always recovers and repopulates the marrow to the normal level. Follicular small cleaved cell lymphoma seems to be parallel to the marrow: the cells retain clinical sensitivity to conventional chemotherapy but continue to regrow and repopulate. A larger fraction of FM lymphoma patients are curable with combination chemotherapy, which correlates with the larger fraction of large cells and the kinetic advantage to treating a non-renewable stem cell population. This model is speculative at this point, but has the advantage of accurately describing the clinical course of disease. In addition, if the stem cell compartment of follicular lymphomas is analogous to that of the bone marrow, it is possible that treatment capable of ablating bone marrow might also ablate follicular lymphoma. Such a notion may provide theoretical support for high-dose therapy with autologous bone marrow support (*see* below).

Clinical features and staging

The follicular lymphomas account for 35–40 per cent of all lymphocytic lymphomas. Among follicular lymphomas, about two-thirds are FSC, one-quarter are FM and less than 10 per cent are FLC.[22] The natural histories of each of the histological subtypes were found to be significantly different before effective therapy was developed: median survival of FSC was 78 months, FM was 55 months and FLC was 29 months in one series.[23] When the large cell component is more prominent, the natural history is shorter.

The follicular pattern of growth is not uniform in patients with follicular lymphoma. The tendency of nodal sites of disease to have a diffuse pattern of growth of the same or different histological subtype also varies with the type of follicular lymphoma. About 25 per cent of patients with FSC, nearly 50 per cent of FM and virtually all FLC lymphomas will have areas of diffuse growth within predominantly follicular nodes. The impact of such areas of diffuse growth and histological discordance is not universally agreed upon.[23] However, when patients of a particular subgroup (e.g. FM) are examined for the presence of diffuse areas, it appears that patients whose nodes showed a 50 per cent, or greater, follicular pattern of growth had significantly better survival than those with less than 50 per cent follicular growth.[24] In addition, patients presenting with discordant histologies have been found to have a natural history that is intermediate between purely follicular and purely diffuse lymphomas of the same histological type.[25] Thus, the diffuse pattern of growth suggests more rapid or unregulated growth and the follicular pattern suggests slower progression perhaps with the retention of some responsiveness to normal regulatory control.

Follicular small cleaved cell lymphoma

These tumours arise primarily in the lymph nodes. Fewer than 10 per cent of patients have extranodal sites of presentation without nodal involvement. This lymphoma primarily affects adults over the age of 40 years (median age 55 years) and patients often give a history of prolonged asymptomatic lymphadenopathy. Systemic symptoms of fever, night sweats and unexplained weight loss are present in less than 15 per cent of cases. Despite the fact that patients may seek medical attention because they notice a single enlarged node, careful physical examination usually detects adenopathy in multiple sites. The disease may have been present for years and some patients will have had a lymph node biopsy in the past that failed to discern a cause for the adenopathy. Symmetrical adenopathy is common. Hilar nodes are often involved bilaterally, but mediastinal masses are rare. Abdominal lymph nodes, especially mesenteric nodes, are commonly involved and splenomegaly is found in about 40 per cent of patients. In about 5 per cent of cases, splenomegaly can cause hypersplenism or be associated with Coombs'-positive haemolytic anaemia. Splenectomy in such instances is therapeutic and has anecdotally been found to slow the progression of disease in some patients, similar to the findings in hairy cell leukaemia and prolymphocytic leukaemia, two other B-cell neoplasms with an indolent natural history. Bone marrow is involved in about 60–70 per cent of patients and the liver is involved in nearly half. Extranodal involvement of areas other than the bone marrow and liver is uncommon but ascites and pleural effusions may occur, particularly in late stages of the disease. Central nervous system involvement is uncommon, although peripheral nerve compression and epidural tumour masses causing cord compression may develop. Ureteral obstruction from enlarged pelvic nodes may require emergency surgical intervention to preserve renal function.

Routine examination of the peripheral blood at the onset of disease usually gives normal results, but may, on careful microscopic examination, reveal the typical cells with notched or cleaved nuclei ('buttock cells') characteristic of FSC lymphoma. Some patients (around 10 per cent) will present with, or will develop, markedly elevated white blood cell counts, up to 100 000/μl, consisting primarily of buttock cells. This was formerly called lymphosarcoma cell leukaemia. The presence of grossly detectable tumour cells in the peripheral blood does not apparently affect prognosis and may be predicted by detecting significant blast cell proliferation in the nodes.[26] More recently the presence of malignant cells in the peripheral blood of most patients with FSC lymphoma has been documented by sophisticated analysis of the presence of light chains on the cell surface. Normally, circulating B-cells have a 2:1 ratio of cells bearing κ light chains to cells bearing λ light chains. Any significant alteration from the 2:1 ratio implies a clonal excess of cells expressing one or the other light chain. The technique detects 1 per cent or fewer malignant cells in the peripheral blood and demonstrates that 70 per cent or more of lymphocytic lymphoma patients have circulating tumour cells.[27,28] It is unclear whether these circulating tumour cells are clonogenic and it is unknown what influence, if any, such cells should have on staging. One would imagine that circulating tumour cells at diagnosis would imply disseminated disease and after therapy would be the harbinger of short-lived remissions. Data on these points are being collected.

There are no characteristic laboratory abnormalities associated with FSC lymphoma, however, massive involvement of the liver can produce elevated liver enzymes, large nodes at the porta hepatis can produce a picture of extrahepatic obstruction, and marrow replacement can cause peripheral blood cytopenias. Unlike diffuse lymphomas, lactate dehydrogenase (LDH) level, bone marrow involvement, and anaemia do not appear to be prognostic factors for follicular lymphomas.

Follicular mixed lymphoma

Patients with FM lymphoma also present with diffuse adenopathy, but the disease involves the bone marrow less frequently and is more often associated with abdominal masses than FSC lymphoma. When the marrow is involved, it is often with the small cleaved cell component of FM lymphoma, which is thought to be the more migratory cell.

Follicular large cell lymphoma

Patients with FLC lymphoma are only about one tenth as common as those with the FSC type. The clinical presentations cannot distinguish one histological type from another very reliably. However, in patients with FLC lymphoma, biopsy of more than one site of disease at presentation nearly always demonstrates the synchronous presence of diffuse large cell (DLC) lymphoma. Patients with FLC lymphoma in the nodes have a high frequency of involvement of extranodal as well a nodal sites of disease. When the extranodal sites of disease are biopsied, they are virtually universally DLC lymphomas.

Staging evaluation of patients with follicular lymphoma

As discussed in Chapter 12, the Ann Arbor staging classification that was developed for use with Hodgkin's disease is routinely applied to patients with lymphocytic lymphoma; but the scheme does not suit the lymphocytic lymphomas. Unlike Hodgkin's disease, the lymphocytic lymphomas in general, and the follicular lymphomas in particular, spread both contiguously[29] and haematogenously. About 85 per cent of patients with FSC lymphoma will have stage III or IV disease at presentation. Furthermore, although there is some evidence that bulk disease may contribute to the outcome of follicular lymphoma, extranodal involvement of marrow and liver are certainly not such important prognostic factors as they are in diffuse lymphomas, but the presence of B symptoms does seem to exert an adverse effect on outcome.[21,23,26,30,31] The factor that appears to exert the greatest impact on outcome is histology. Thus, the most critical aspect of treatment planning is to be sure of the diagnosis. If organ involvement is not a major prognostic factor and if the vast majority of patients have advanced stage disease at presentation, what is the role of the staging work-up and how extensive does it need to be?

The evaluation begins with a careful history and physical examination with attention directed to epitrochlear, femoral and popliteal lymph node groups. Preauricular involvement is often associated with Waldeyer's ring involvement and Waldeyer's ring disease often heralds gastrointestinal tract disease. Posteroanterior and lateral chest radiographs are reliable at detecting intrathoracic disease. Lung tomography and chest computed tomographic (CT) scanning can add some additional information when plain radiographs are equivocal, but their use is optional. In our opinion, bipedal lymphangiography (LAG) is an essential and indispensible part of the staging evaluation. It is positive in the vast majority of patients with early stage disease on physical examination and gives the physician an additional site for following the response to treatment. In addition, the introduction of dye into the para-aortic nodes can be used to assess whether the ureters may be threatened by gross displacement or compression, this method gives a rapid result. Abdominal CT scanning and ultrasound may also be helpful, especially in the visualization of the upper abdomen, a site commonly involved by follicular lymphoma, but not easily assessed by LAG or other measures. Nuclear medicine tests have a small role in the

staging and management of patients with follicular lymphoma. Magnetic resonance imaging may play a role, but its strengths are still being ascertained.

What invasive tests need to be performed? Any patient whose clinical staging suggests stage I or II disease must have bilateral bone marrow biopsies and aspirates (which will be positive in up to 70 per cent of cases) and percutaneous liver biopsy (which will be positive in about 30 per cent of cases). In addition, despite the lack of influence of organ involvement on prognosis, we feel it is important to assess these sites of disease in any patient who is a candidate for potentially curative treatment (i.e. FM, FLC and many patients with FSC lymphomas). Treatment may well produce peripheral blood cytopenias; however the presence of bone marrow disease would certainly alter the interpretation of the cytopenias and the approach to dose modification. Similarly, the detection of liver involvement indicates that patients need re-evaluation of the liver at a time when they are thought to be in clinical complete remission before treatment can be safely stopped, if the aim of treatment is the complete eradication of disease. Patients are never taken to exploratory laparotomy purely for staging indications. Patients presenting with intra-abdominal disease not diagnosed in any other way may require diagnostic laparotomy, but this circumstance is rare (most commonly seen in FM lymphoma). When exploratory laparotomy was performed for experimental purposes at Stanford, it was found that 45 per cent of patients with FSC lymphoma who had clinical stage I or II disease had intra-abdominal disease, especially in the mesenteric nodes.[32] Therefore, it appears that nearly half of clinical stage I and II patients will have stage III disease.

At the completion of therapy, it is important to re-evaluate sites of disease that had been involved with lymphoma prior to treatment. Occasionally suspicious nodes or masses can be aspirated percutaneously with marker studies performed on the aspirate to evaluate the presence of clonal lymphocytes. Subsequent to achieving complete remission, patients are examined quarterly, re-evaluated with bilateral bone marrow biopsies on an annual basis and their retroperitoneal lymph nodes are kept opacified by repeat LAG for at least five years. It is possible that more sensitive detection methods for marrow and peripheral blood tumour cells[19,27,28] will alter criteria for complete remission.

Histological progression of follicular lymphoma

A common feature of all follicular lymphomas is their tendency to progress to a diffuse lymphoma.[5] When this transition occurs it is accompanied by a change to a more aggressive natural history similar to *de novo* diffuse large cell lymphoma (DLCL). In fact some have argued that the histological conversion may carry an even worse prognosis than *de novo* DLCL,[33] but aggressive postconversion treatment has produced long-term disease-free survival in around one-third of aggressively treated patients,[5,34] a level of success in keeping with the expected outcome if those particular treatment programmes were used in *de novo* DLCL. The progression from follicular to diffuse lymphoma occurs regardless of whether the follicular lymphoma is treated aggressively or conservatively,[35] and occurs at a rate of about 5–10 per cent per year depending on the degree of large cell component. The progression is such a constant feature of the disease that when patients who were initially diagnosed with follicular lymphoma are examined at autopsy, 95 per cent of the patients who died from lymphoma have progressed to diffuse lymphoma.[36] Examination of the molecular biology of the tumours during their follicular and diffuse stages of growth confirm that both tumour phases are derived from the same malignant clone.[16] Thus, the spectrum of follicular lymphomas must include the diffuse lymphomas of follicular centre cell origin.

Treatment and prognosis of patients with follicular lymphoma

The treatment of choice for patients with clinical stage I and II FSC and FM lymphoma is total nodal radiation therapy. Patients with stage I FLC lymphoma should be treated similarly to patients with localized DLCL, and should receive combination chemotherapy with CHOP (cyclophosphamide, doxorubicin, vincristine, prednisone) or modified ProMACE-MOPP (prednisone, methotrexate, doxorubicin, cyclophosphamide, etoposide, mechlorethamine, vincristine, procarbazine) with or without involved field radiation therapy. Patients with stage II, III, or IV FLC lymphoma should be treated with one of the newer second or third generation treatment programmes such as MACOP-B (methotrexate, doxorubicin, cyclophosphamide, vincristine, prednisone, bleomycin) or ProMACE-CytaBOM (prednisone, methotrexate, doxorubicin, cyclophosphamide, etoposide, cytosine arabinoside, bleomycin, vincristine) that have been used to induce complete remissions in over 80 per cent of patients with DLCL. The treatment of stage III and IV FM lymphoma should be combination chemotherapy with a programme at least as intensive as C-MOPP (cyclophosphamide, vincristine, procarbazine, prednisone), and preferably one of the newer second or third generation programmes used in DLCL.

The optimal treatment for stage III and IV FSC lymphoma is more uncertain. It is acceptable to withhold initial therapy or use drug or radiation treatment for symptomatic relief only. However, it would be preferable to use cyclic combination chemotherapy when therapy is needed, rather than chronic daily oral alkylating agent therapy, because of the marrow stem cell damage meted out by continuous exposure to alkylating agents. Although the conservative or palliative approach is acceptable, it is important to keep in mind ongoing research efforts that appear to demonstrate that improvements in primary treatment of stage III and IV FSC lymphoma may be associated with prolonged disease-free survival. Younger patients without intercurrent illnesses who wish to accommodate the short-term toxicities of the treatment for the potential long-term benefit of disease-free survival can be offered a more aggressive treatment option with one of the newer second or third generation lymphoma treatment regimens, perhaps followed by low-dose total lymphoid radiation therapy. Ongoing studies of biological treatment approaches may further improve the treatment outcome.

Treatment of stage I and II FSC and FM lymphomas

A number of studies have demonstrated the efficacy of radiation therapy in the treatment of clinically staged patients with localized disease. Perhaps the most impressive data were generated at Stanford.[37] Patients with stage I and II follicular lymphoma, determined by staging that stopped short of laparotomy in nearly 60 per cent of patients, were treated with involved field, extended field or total nodal radiation therapy. Overall, 54 per cent of the patients were free of disease after 10 years of follow-up. The freedom from relapse was significantly higher in the patients receiving total lymphoid radiation than in those receiving involved or extended field radiation. Only 10 per cent of the patients treated with total lymphoid radiation relapsed. Patients with FLC lymphoma had significantly poorer survival when treated with radiation therapy alone than did patients with FSC or FM lymphoma. If only patients with FSC and FM lymphoma undergoing clinical staging are considered, total lymphoid radiation should be able to cure over 75 per cent.

A retrospective analysis of results with radiation therapy in stage I and II follicular lymphoma at Yale demonstrated an 88 per cent five-year disease-free survival for stage I patients and a 61 per cent five-year disease-free survival for stage II patients.[38] At St. Bartholomew's Hospital, London, extended field radiation therapy obtained an 83 per cent relapse-free survival at 10 years in stage I and II follicular lymphoma patients.[39] Using involved field radiation for stage I patients and total lymphoid radiation for stage II patients, Gomez et al.[40] found an 83 per cent disease-free survival at 10

years. Thus, radiation therapy is effective therapy in early stage disease. The marginal and contiguous relapses seen in patients receiving limited field radiation in all the studies suggest that clinically staged patients should receive total nodal radiation.

The role of combination chemotherapy in the management of early stage follicular lymphoma is unclear. At least three randomized studies failed to demonstrate that the use of chemotherapy plus radiation therapy is superior to radiation therapy alone,[41–43] but the chemotherapy used in the studies was CVP (cyclophosphamide, vincristine, prednisone) or of similar efficacy. In a recent report from the M.D. Anderson Hospital, Houston, Texas, the relapse-free survival was significantly better for patients with stage I or II follicular lymphoma receiving chemotherapy with or without radiation (64 per cent at five years) than those treated with radiation alone (37 per cent at five years).[44] In this study the chemotherapy regime used was CHOP. Thus, it is possible that the use of more effective chemotherapy programmes might improve on the results obtained with involved field radiation therapy or might in fact be useful without added radiation therapy. However, at the moment, the data suggest that total lymphoid radiation therapy is the treatment of choice in stage I and II FSC and FM lymphoma.

Treatment of stage I FLC lymphoma

Stage I FLC lymphoma is clearly more aggressive in its natural history than either FSC or FM lymphoma and, when treated with radiation therapy alone, it has a significant early relapse rate. Since it is the small cleaved cell that is thought to be more migratory, the FLC lymphomas have a greater tendency to remain localized than the FSC type. However, as with localized diffuse large cell lymphoma, locally invasive bulky disease and haematogenous spread are important clinical problems. With the best radiation treatment technique, stage I FLC lymphoma patients may have nearly a 70 per cent chance of surviving five years free of disease.[45,46] Some groups have advocated the use of combined modality therapy in localized lymphomas of aggressive natural history, including FLC,[47] and a number of randomized trials have suggested that radiation plus chemotherapy is superior to radiation therapy alone in stage I disease.[41,42,48] Miller and Jones used CHOP followed by radiation therapy in only the 38 per cent of patients who either responded slowly to the chemotherapy or who required significant dose reductions due to myelotoxicity.[49] The disease-free survival was 84 per cent at 41 months. Cabanillas found that 100 per cent of his stage I patients obtained durable remissions in response to CHOP alone.[50] We have used a modified ProMACE-MOPP programme in which the doses of the myelotoxic drugs are reduced to about 75 per cent of the doses used in advanced stage DLCL.[51] Patients are given four cycles of chemotherapy followed by involved field radiation therapy. Thirty-nine of 41 patients have obtained long-term disease-free survival with this approach. There has been virtually no toxicity with this outpatient treatment programme. Thus, it appears that the treatment of choice for stage I FLC lymphoma is combination chemotherapy with either CHOP or modified ProMACE-MOPP with or without involved field radiation.

Treatment of stage III and IV FSC lymphoma

One of the most controversial areas in medical oncology is the treatment of patients with advanced stage FSC lymphoma. Over 20 years of painstaking clinical investigation has documented that advanced stage FSC lymphoma responds to single and multiple agent chemotherapy, radiation therapy and combined modality treatment approaches. However, the responses are not durable, lasting a median of around two years with 10 per cent or fewer patients remaining in remission for five years.[52] Follicular small cleaved cell lymphoma is an unusual advanced malignancy in that despite the absence of durable complete remissions, median survival is over eight years.[23] The capacity of patients to live so long with such short remissions implies that patients are living with their disease.

In the midst of the clamour that was generated in the effort to discern whether multiple agent chemotherapy was better than single agent chemotherapy or radiation therapy, Rosenberg, at Stanford, began managing a selected group of patients with no initial therapy.[53] His patients presented essentially without symptoms and often with a history of many months of gradually enlarging non-tender adenopathy. The patients selected for no initial therapy generally remained asymptomatic for 2 months following their initial evaluation. Some were of advanced age and had concurrent medical problems that made aggressive treatment somewhat more risky, or had an extended prior history of spontaneous waxing and waning in the nodes. Criteria for initiating therapy were rapid progression of disease, development of B symptoms or cytopenias related to marrow disease, or the development of a site of disease that threatened the function of an organ.

The median time to requiring treatment of patients with advanced stage FSC lymphoma was 4 years and the median survival period for the conservatively managed group was 11 years. The actual overall survival curves did not differ significantly from those of two prospective randomized studies being carried out at Stanford at the same time, one comparing single agent chemotherapy, combination chemotherapy, and total body radiation;[54] the other comparing the first two arms to combined modality therapy with chemotherapy plus total lymphoid radiation.[55] Thus, the data from the conservatively treated patients make it difficult to discern an effect from aggressive treatment. As a result, it is now routine to defer initial therapy in patients with advanced stage FSC lymphoma.

There are a number of findings that question the general applicability of the Stanford experience. First, many centres have found that their patients with FSC lymphoma do not fare as well as the group at Stanford. In fact, there may be subsets of patients who, based on histology or clinical features, should be treated aggressively at diagnosis because of a more accelerated natural history. Frizzera *et al.*[56] found a median survival of only 40 months in patients with neoplastic plasma cells as a component of their follicular lymphoma. Straus *et al.*[57] at Memorial Sloan-Kettering, found that patients with advanced stage disease had a median survival of less than five years with conservative treatment. At St. Bartholomew's Hospital, poor prognosis patients could be identified based on the presence of B symptoms, anaemia, abnormal liver function tests and hepatosplenomegaly.[39] Thus, there may be features associated with a more aggressive clinical course that would be poorly served by careful observation.

Furthermore, there are now a number of studies suggesting that improvements in therapy could well result in long-term disease-free survival. The Stanford experience with total nodal radiation in patients with laparotomy-documented stage III disease is instructive.[58,59] The 10-year relapse-free survival of stage III patients treated with radiation therapy was 40 per cent. For those with so-called limited stage III disease (no B symptoms, less than five sites of involvement, maximum size of disease < 10 cm), the 15-year freedom from relapse was 88 per cent.[59] The majority of patients relapsed in previously unirradiated lymph node groups suggesting that the addition of epitrochlear, mesenteric and Waldeyer's ring fields might have further improved the outcome. Studies by Cox *et al.*[60] and Flippen *et al.*[61] also suggest that 45–60 per cent of patients with stage III FSC lymphoma can achieve complete remissions lasting in excess of 5 years.

The use of combination chemotherapy in patients with advanced stage FSC lymphoma has rarely been more aggressive than CVP, a regimen designed in the mid-1960s. A feature of the response of FSC lymphoma to CVP is that 70 per cent of patients obtain a complete response (confirmed in numerous studies,[52] and patients relapse more or less continuously over time until by five years fewer than 10 per cent are in remission. The sites of relapse from chemotherapy-induced complete remission are nearly always previously involved nodal sites of disease,[62] unlike radiation relapses, which occur in previously uninvolved and unirradiated sites of disease. This observation forms the basis for the rationale for combined modality therapy. Radiation therapy appears to be extremely effective at eradicating disease within the beam field, and relapses occur because disease is disseminated. Combination chemotherapy appears extremely effective at eradicating disseminated sites of disease not detected clinically, but the bulk associated with involved nodes results in the persistence of disease even when the patient appears to be in complete remission.

With the dramatic advances in treatment of the more aggressive DLCL, the probability of long-term survival is higher with the more virulent tumour than in the indolent FSC lymphoma. However, the improvements in treatment obtained by the use of more aggressive treatment programmes have not been carefully sought in patients with FSC lymphoma, presumably because of the 5 per cent toxic death rates seen with most of the newer second and third generation chemotherpy programmes. Recently, somewhat more aggressive chemotherapy programmes have begun to be used in FSC lymphoma with early results suggesting that improvements in treatments might well produce prolonged disease-free survival. The group at the Dana-Farber Cancer Institute used M-BACOD (methotrexate, bleomycin, doxorubicin, cyclophosphamide, vincristine, dexamethasone) in patients with advanced stage FSC lymphoma and obtained five-year disease-free survival of around 40 per cent.[63] A programme called M-2, consisting of BCNU, cyclophosphamide, vincristine, melphalan and prednisone, gave data projecting an 83 per cent five-year disease-free survival for complete responders.[64] However, the short duration of follow-up makes it difficult to be certain of the durability of the remissions. The Eastern Cooperative Oncology Group demonstrated that COPP (cyclophosphamide, vincristine, procarbazine, prednisone) achieved a complete response in 56 per cent of patients with advanced FSC lymphoma and 57 per cent of the complete remissions lasted over five years.[65]

At the NCI, we have been engaged in a prospective randomized study comparing conservative treatment (no initial therapy) and aggressive combined modality therapy with ProMACE-MOPP flexitherapy followed by low-dose total lymphoid radiation therapy.[66] Among patients randomized to aggressive therapy, 76 per cent obtained a complete remission and 84 per cent of those remain in their initial complete remission with a median remission duration of over four years. Since the very best previous treatment results have resulted in median remissions lasting two years or less, it certainly appears that a substantial fraction of advanced stage patients may enjoy prolonged disease-free survival with this more aggressive treatment aproach. At this point in the study, there are no significant overall survival differences between patients treated with intent to cure versus those treated conservatively. However, patients initially randomized to conservative treatment whose symptoms progress to the point where treatment is indicated respond more poorly (complete remission rate 44 per cent) to the same therapy that induced 76 per cent remissions when used in patients at diagnosis. This demonstration that tumour bulk is a factor in response to therapy is also corroborated by retrospective data from the University of Chicago.[67] The complete response rate to initial aggressive therapy was 71 per cent, but the use of the same aggressive therapy after initial conservative management produced a complete response rate of only 25 per cent. Thus, it appears that the decision about treatment approach should be made at diagnosis. Once the palliative approach has been chosen, aggressive therapy should not be considered since its efficacy is markedly compromised by the delay.

In conclusion, no initial therapy is an acceptable management approach to patients with advanced stage FSC lymphoma. However, there is mounting evidence that aggressive treatment at diagnosis may permit a large fraction of patients to enjoy prolonged disease-free survival. Patients under the age of 50 years for whom a median survival of 10 years represents a significant foreshortening of life expectancy, patients without intercurrent illness, patients with B symptoms, abnormal liver function tests, effusions or other suggestions of more aggressive disease and patients initially treated conservatively who undergo histological conversion to DLCL or another aggressive lymphoma histology should probably receive aggressive treatment with a combination chemotherapy programme like ProMACE-MOPP with or without total nodal radiation for those who achieve a complete remission (not necessary in patients with converted histology). The decision about whether to treat aggressively should not be indefinitely delayed after diagnosis. Postponing the decision until symptoms demand treatment substantially reduces the efficacy of the treatment programme. Those who feel they must manage patients conservatively should consider the use of cyclical combination chemotherapy such as CVP to control the disease since, although the use of chronic oral alkylating agents like chlorambucil is well tolerated from the point of view of immediate side-effects, it is associated with irreversible damage to the bone marrow stem cells, the possible development of a myelodysplasia or secondary leukaemia, and a reduction in the capacity to delivery curative therapy should histological progression occur. CVP is not associated with such chronic marrow damage.

Treatment of stage III and IV FM lymphoma

It is no longer controversial that patients with stage III and IV FM lymphoma should be treated aggressively, with intent to cure, from diagnosis. In the first place, it is clear that the conservative approach is not associated with prolonged survival of FM lymphoma patients.[53] In addition, the benefits of the conservative approach in terms of the interval of freedom from therapy for patients with FM lymphoma are marginal (median time to treatment is only 16 months). Furthermore, the durability of chemotherapy-induced complete responses in patients with advanced stage FM lymphoma initially reported from the National Cancer Institute[68,69] has been confirmed in several other studies.[70–72] We obtained a complete remission in 72 per cent of stage III and IV patients with FM lymphoma treated with C-MOPP, with the median remission lasting over six years. At the M.D. Anderson Hospital, CHOP-bleomycin followed by involved field radiation therapy resulted in complete remissions in 74 per cent of stage III and 57 per cent of stage IV patients.[72] At four years, 64 per cent of the stage III complete responders and 48 per cent of the stage IV complete responders remained free of disease. No patient with an LDH under 250 relapsed more than two years after therapy. The NCI patients also demonstrated that high LDH, B symptoms and marrow involvement were poor prognostic factors. Even the application of the more sophisticated measures of complete remission, such as the presence of circulating clonal excess, confirms that complete remissions in FM lymphoma are durable and complete.[73] The circulating abnormal clone that is readily detectable in nearly 70 per cent of patients with advanced stage follicular lymphoma disappears with the achievement of clinical complete remission. In FSC lymphoma, clinical complete remission is not usually accompanied by clearing the malignant clone, and it now appears that this is the forerunner of relapse.[74]

There has been little experience with the more recently developed lymphoma treatment programmes in advanced stage FM lymphoma, but, extrapolating from the effects of C-MOPP in DLCL, it seems likely that the second and third generation combination chemotherapy programmes like MACOP-B, ProMACE-MOPP and ProMACE-CytaBOM would be excellent therapy for advanced stage FM lymphoma patients.

Treatment of stage II, III and IV FLC lymphoma

Follicular large cell lymphoma is one of the rarest forms of lymphocytic lymphoma, accounting for only about 3 per cent of cases at the National Cancer Institute.[22] Because FLC lymphoma represents a follicular lymphoma with an increasing fraction of kinetically active large cells, it seems likely that the low incidence is due to the fact that it represents a transition histology between FSC and FM lymphomas and the DLCL to which those follicular entities so commonly evolve.[5] However, if one examines the clinical course of FLC lymphoma, it is clear that conservative treatment is associated with a rapid downhill clinical course leading to death within a year, while aggressive combination chemotherapy is capable of achieving a complete remission in the majority of patients (eight out of 11; seven of the eight remissions were durable).[75] In every case in which a repeat biopsy was performed in patients with FLC lymphoma, the second biopsy revealed diffuse lymphoma. The Eastern Cooperative Oncology Group demonstrated similar results in a series of 25

patients with FLC lymphoma.[76] Since the natural history of FLC lymphoma is difficult to separate from DLCL, which it nearly always becomes, it is best to treat FLC lymphoma similarly to DLCL. The treatment approaches to DLCL are the subject of Chapter 21. Most investigators now include FLC lymphoma in the intermediate grade of malignant lymphomas together with DLCL and diffuse mixed lymphoma (DML).

Two of the most active new programmes are ProMACE-CytaBOM[77] and MACOP-B.[78] Both of the programmes are administered in the outpatient clinic, both utilize co-trimoxazole as infection prophylaxis and both have a toxic death rate under 4 per cent. Both achieve a complete response rate of 84 per cent. The projected plateau survival for ProMACE-MOPP is 70 per cent and for MACOP-B it is 69 per cent. These two programmes are not the only suitable programmes for patients with FLC lymphoma, but their ease of administration (ProMACE-CytaBOM is delivered two weeks out of three for 17 weeks, MACOP-B is delivered weekly for 12 weeks), acceptable toxicity and high incidence of durable complete responses make them among the most attractive.

Newer methods of treatment of follicular lymphoma

Several new biological treatment approaches to the follicular lymphomas have shown promise in early clinical testing. These include the interferons, monoclonal antibodies, adoptive cellular therapy with lymphokine activated killer cells plus interleukin-2 and bone marrow transplantation.

Among the biological response modifiers, interferons have been explored to the greatest extent. The direct antitumour and antiproliferative effects of interferons, as well as their immunomodulating effects, have made them very attractive to study.[79] The development of recombinant α-interferon has allowed adequate numbers of patients to be treated with nearly maximum tolerated doses and for prolonged periods. In an NCI study, 37 evaluable patients with malignant lymphoma were treated with 50 million units of recombinant α-interferon three times a week for at least three months.[80] The overall response of patients with follicular lymphoma was 54 per cent with a median duration of response of eight months. The responses lasted only while the patients were receiving interferon. As soon as the interferon was stopped the disease regrew, and the majority of patients who relapsed did so while receiving interferon. After a few weeks off treatment, retreatment of these patients who responded initially to interferon often produced second responses. Similar dose schedules in other studies have produced objective response rates of 25–35 per cent.[81,82]

Since the responses were seen near the maximum tolerated doses of interferon, it seems most likely that the effects of interferon are direct antitumour effects. If the mechanism of cytotoxicity of the interferons is distinct from that of conventional chemotherapy, steroids and radiation therapy, the interferons may have a role in combined modality regimens. A few pilot studies using interferon with combination chemotherapy and radiation therapy in a variety of doses and schedules are underway.

There are a large number of biologically active molecules in various phases of preclinical and clinical testing that may be useful in the management of patients with lymphoma. These include γ interferon, tumour necrosis factor and interleukin-1.

The first disease in which a monoclonal antibody was tested was a follicular lymphoma.[83] Ab89 produced a short-term minor reduction in the tumour burden in the first patient, but this did not qualify as a response, either in magnitude or duration. However, soon after, Levy and his colleagues used a monoclonal antibody directed at the idiotype of the immunoglobulin on the surface of the tumour and obtained a truly dramatic complete response that has lasted over five years without further therapy.[84] The tumour continued to regress even after the cessation of therapy, suggesting that the antibody might have induced an endogenous cellular host immune response against the tumour. Although extension of these results to 12 more patients has failed to reproduce the magnitude of response seen in the first patient,[85] other responses have been seen. In general these responses correlate with the degree of T-cell infiltration and Leu-7-positive NK-type cells present in the tumour-containing node. These observations certainly support the idea that in certain patients the anti-idiotypic antibody can recruit the host to reject the tumour.

Despite the theoretical appeal of anti-idiotype therapy, there are several serious problems that limit its widespread use: the antibodies are difficult to make; some patients have significant levels of circulating idiotype shed by the tumour that could prevent passive anti-idiotype from reaching the tumour; the host nearly always develops a human antimouse antibody response to the therapeutic antibody; the target immunoglobulin on the tumour cell may modulate; and finally, it is clear that there is substantial somatic mutation in B-cells and B-cell tumours that can result in the spontaneous loss of the idiotypic determinant on the tumour.[86,87] These drawbacks are serious, but there remain a number of strategies that are under active investigation to exploit the uniqueness of the tumour cell-associated immunoglobulin idiotype determinants in cancer treatment. One of these, the use of anti-idiotype conjugated to iodine-131 and supported by autologous bone marrow transplantation (because of the myelotoxicity of the radiation) has produced a complete remission in at least one lymphoma patient (F. Appelbaum, personal communication).

Other B-cell surface molecules may also be attacked by monoclonal antibodies. Press et al.[88] used IF5, an antibody specific for CD20, in four patients and obtained a brief partial response in one. It appears that naked murine antibodies are not very effective at killing the tumour cells to which they bind. It is expected that efficacy will be very greatly enhanced by coupling to antibodies any of a variety of toxic moieties that will be more efficient at tumour killing.

There has been tremendous excitement about the use of peripheral blood mononuclear cells activated *in vitro* and readministered to patients with cancer.[89] Although most of the patients treated to date have had renal cancer, melanoma, or colon cancer, there have also been eight patients with lymphoma who have received LAK cells plus IL-2. Four patients have had objective responses with the longest lasting for 10 months.

The use of bone marrow transplantation in support of patients receiving high dose chemotherapy plus or minus radiation therapy is the topic of Chapter 25. However, it is important to point out that this procedure has become extremely safe, with a mortality rate in experienced hands of 2 per cent. One of the diseases in which radiation and chemotherapy are most active and for which there is already evidence of a dose–response curve is follicular lymphoma. We propose that patients who achieve a complete remission with conventional combination chemotherapy programmes are highly likely to achieve durable complete remissions if they are treated with total body radiation and high-dose cyclophosphamide followed by marrow reconstitution with B-cell-purged bone marrow. Such a study needs to be performed first in the salvage setting and then as a component of primary remission induction. In our view, this aggressive approach is justifiable and likely to bring about the cure of the majority of patients.

References

1. Urba WJ, Longo DL. *Seminars in Oncology*. 1985; **12**, 250.
2. Braylan RC, Jaffe ES, Berard CW. In: Sommers SC (ed). *Pathology Annual*, vol. 10, 1975; New York: Appleton- Century-Crofts, 213.
3. Krikorian JG, Portlock CS, Cooney P, Rosenberg SA. *Cancer* 1980; **46**, 2093.
4. Jaffe ES. *Journal of the National Cancer Institute*. 1983; **70**, 401.
5. Hubbard SM, Chabner BA, DeVita VT Jr, *et al. Blood*. 1982; **59**, 258.
6. Yunis JJ, Oken MM, Kaplan ME, Ensrud KM, Howe RR, Theologides A. *New England Journal of Medicine*. 1982; **307**, 1213.
7. Jaffe ES, Shevach EM, Frank MM, Berard CW, Green I. *New England Journal of Medicine*. 1974; **280**, 813.
8. Freedman AS, Nadler LM. *Seminars in Oncology*. 1987; **14**, 293.
9. Kishimoto T. *Immunology Today*. 1983; **4**, 117.
10. Rudders RA, Ahl ET Jr, DeLellis RA, Bernstein S, Begg CB. *Cancer Research*. 1982; **42**, 349.
11. Weisenburger DD, Nathwani BN, Diamond LW, Winberg CD, Rappaport H. *Cancer*. 1982; **49**, 1429.
12. Cossman J, Neckers LM, Hsu SM, Longo DL, Jaffe ES. *American Journal of Pathology*. 1984; **115**, 117.
13. Tsujimoto Y, Finger LR, Yunis J, Nowell PC, Croce CM. *Science*. 1985; **226**, 1097.
14. Dalla-Favera R, Bregnim M, Erikson J, Patterson D, Gallo RC, Croce CM. *Proceedings of the National Academy of Sciences USA*. 1982; **79**, 7824.
15. Reed JC, Tsujimoto Y, Alpers JD, Croce CM, Nowell PC. *Science*. 1987; **236**, 1295.
16. Raffeld M, Wright JJ, Lipford E, *et al. Cancer Research*. 1987; **47**, 2537.
17. Raffeld M, Neckers L, Longo DL, Cossman J. *New England Journal of Medicine*. 1985; **312**, 1653.
18. Siegelman MH, Cleary ML, Warnke R, Sklar J. *Journal of Experimental Medicine*. 1985; **161**, 850.
19. Lee M-S, Chang K-S, Cabanillas F, Freireich EJ, Trujillo JM, Stass SA. *Science* 1987; **237**, 175.
20. Hansen H, Koziner B, Clarkson B. *American Journal of Medicine*. 1981; **71**, 107.
21. Longo DL, Young RC, Hubbard SM, *et al. Annals of Internal Medicine*. 1984; **100**, 651.
22. Anderson T, Chabner BA, Young RC, *et al. Cancer*. 1982; **50**, 2699.
23. Anderson T, DeVita VT Jr, Simon RM, *et al. Cancer*. 1982; **50**, 2708.
24. Hu E, Weiss LM, Hoppe RT, Horning SJ. *Journal of Clinical Oncology*. 1985; **3**, 1183.
25. Fisher RI, Jones RB, DeVita VT Jr, *et al. Cancer*. 1981; **47**, 2022.
26. Come SE, Jaffe ES, Andersen JC, *et al. American Journal of Medicine*. 1980; **69**, 667.
27. Smith BR, Weinberg DS, Robert NJ, *et al. New England Journal of Medicine*. 1984; **311**, 1476.
28. Ligler FS, Smith RG, Kettman JR, *et al. Blood*. 1980; **55**, 792.
29. Fuks Z, Glatstein E, Kaplan HS. *British Journal of Cancer*. 1975; **31**, 286.
30. Bennett JM, Cain KC, Glick JH, Johnson GJ, Ezdinli E, O'Connell MJ. *Journal of Clinical Oncology*. 1986; **4**, 1462.
31. Gospodarowicz MK, Bush RS, Brown TC, Chua T. *International Journal of Radiation, Oncology Biology and Physics*. 1984; **10**, 489.
32. Goffinet DR, Warnke R, Dunnick NR, *et al. Cancer Treatment Reports*; 1977; **61**, 981.
33. Armitage JO, Dick FR, Corder MP. *Cancer Treatment Reports*. 1981; **65**, 413.
34. Acker B, Hopper RT, Colby TV, Cox RS, Kaplan HS, Rosenberg SA. *Journal of Clinical Oncology*. 1983; **1**, 11.
35. Horning SJ, Rosenberg SA. *New England Journal*

of Medicine. 1984; **311**, 1471.

36. Garvin AJ, Simon RM, Osborne CK, Merrill J, Young RC, Berard CW. *Cancer.* 1983; **52**, 393.

37. Paryani SB, Hoppe RT, Cox RS, Colby TV, Rosenberg SA, Kaplan HS. *Cancer.* 1983; **52**, 2300.

38. Chen MG, Prosnitz LR, Gonzalez-Serva A, Fischer DB. *Cancer.* 1979; **43**, 1636.

39. Gallagher CJ, Gregory WM, Jones AI, *et al. Journal of Clinical Oncology.* 1986; **4**, 1470.

40. Gomez GA, Barcos M, Krishnamsetty RM, Pahahon AM, Han T, Henderson ES. *American Journal of Clinical Oncology.* 1986; **9**, 40.

41. Monfardini S, Banfi A, Bonadonna G, *et al. International Journal of Radiation, Oncology, Biology and Physics.* 1980; **6**, 125.

42. Landberg TG, Hakansson LG, Moller TR, *et al. Cancer.* 1979; **44**, 831.

43. Toonkel LM, Fuller LM, Gamble JF, Butler JJ, Martin RG, Schullenberger CC. *Cancer.* 1980; **45**, 249.

44. McLaughlin P, Fuller LM, Velasquez WS, Sullivan-Halley JA, Butler JJ, Cabanillas F. *Cancer.* 1986; **58**, 1596.

45. Kaminski MS, Coleman CN, Colby TV, Cox RS, Rosenberg SA. *Annals of Internal Medicine.* 1986; **104**, 747.

46. Leavitt SH, Lee CK, Bloomfield CD, Frizzera G. *Hematology and Oncology.* 1985; **3**, 33.

47. Mauch P, Leonard R, Skarin A, *et al. Journal of Clinical Oncology.* 1985; **3**, 1301.

48. Nissen NI, Ersboll J, Hansen HS. *Cancer.* 1983; **52**, 1.

49. Miller TP, Jones SE. *Blood.* 1984; **62**, 413.

50. Cabanillas F. *Hematology and Oncology.* 1985; **3**, 25.

51. Longo D, Glatstein E, DeVita V Jr. *et al. Proceedings of the American Association of Cancer Research.* 1987; **28**, 205.

52. Matis LA, Young RC, Longo DL. *CRC Critical Reviews in Haematology and Oncology.* 1986; **5**, 171.

53. Rosenberg SA. *Journal of Clinical Oncology.* 1985; **3**, 298.

54. Hoppe RT, Kushlan P, Kaplan HS, Rosenberg SA, Brown BW. *Blood.* 1981; **58**, 592.

55. Portlock CS, Rosenberg SA, Glatstein E, Kaplan HS. *Blood.* 1976; **47**, 747.

56. Frizzera G, Anaya JS, Banks PM. *Virchows Archives A.* 1986; **409**, 149.

57. Straus DJ, Gaynor JJ, Leiberman PH, Filippa DA, Koziner B, Clarkson BD. *American Journal of Medicine.* 1987; **82**, 247.

58. Glatstein E, Fuks Z, Goffinet DR, Kaplan HS. *Cancer.* 1976; **37**, 2806.

59. Paryani SB, Hoppe RT, Cox RS, Colby TV, Kaplan HS. *Journal of Clinical Oncology.* 1984; **2**, 841.

60. Cox JD, Komaki R, Kun LE, Wilson FJ, Greenberg M. *Cancer.* 1981; **47**, 2247.

61. Flippen T, McLaughlin P, Conrad FG, *et al. Cancer.* 1983; **51**, 987.

62. Schein PS, Chabner BA, Canellos GP, Young RC, DeVita VT Jr. *Cancer.* 1975; **35**, 354.

63. Anderson KC, Skarin AT, Rosenthal DS, *et al. Cancer Treatment Reports* 1984; **68**, 1343.

64. Case DC Jr. *Oncology.* 1984; **41**, 159.

65. Ezdinli EZ, Anderson JR, Melvin F, Glick JH, Davis TE, O'Connell MJ. *Journal of Clinical Oncology.* 1985; **3**, 769.

66. Young RC, Longo DL, Glatstein E, *et al. Proceedings of the American Society of Clinical Oncology.* 1987; **6**, 200.

67. Samuels B, Ultmann J, Pearson M, Barker C, Williams S, Watson S. *Proceedings of the American Society of Clinical Oncology.* 1987; **6**, 206.

68. Anderson T, Bender RA, Fisher RI, *et al. Cancer Treatment Reports.* 1977; **61**, 1057.

69. Longo DL, Young RC, Hubbard SM, *et al. Annals of Internal Medicine.* 1984; **100**, 651.

70. Lister TA, Cullen MH, Beard MEJ, *et al. British Medical Journal.* 1978; **1**, 533.

71. Ezdinli EZ, Costello WG, Icli F, *et al. Cancer.* 1980; **45**, 261.

72. Merchant N, McLaughlin P, Fuller L, *et al. Proceedings of the American Society of Clinical Oncology.* 1984; **3**, 249.

73. Sobel RE, Dillman RO, Collins H, Griffiths JC, Green MR, Royston I. *Cancer.* 1985; **56**, 2005.

74. Lindemalm C, Mellstedt H, Biberfeld P, *et al.* In: Cavalli F, Bonadonna G, Rozenczweig M (eds). *Malignant Lymphomas and Hodgkin's Disease.* 1985; Boston, Martinus Nijhoff: 225.

75. Osborne CK, Norton L, Young RC, *et al. Blood.* 1980; **56**, 98.

76. Glick JH, McFadden E, Costello W, Ezdinli E, Berard CW, Bennett JM. *Cancer.* 1982; **49**, 840.

77. Longo D, DeVita V Jr, Duffey P, *et al. Proceedings of the American Society of Clinical Oncology.* 1987; **6**, 206.

78. Klimo P, Connors JM. *Seminars in Hematology.* 1987; **24**, (suppl. 1), 26.

79. Clark JW, Longo DL. *Updates in Oncology.* 1987; **1**, 1.

80. Foon KA, Sherwin SA, Abrams PG, *et al. New England Journal of Medicine.* 1984; **311**, 1148.

81. O'Connell MJ, Colgan JP, Oken MM, Ritts RE, Kay NE, Itri LM. *Journal of Clinical Oncology.* 1986; **4**, 128.

82. Urba WJ, Longo DL. *Seminars in Oncology.* 1986; **13**, (suppl. 5), 40.

83. Nadler LM, Stashenko P, Hardy R, *et al. Cancer*

Research. 1980; **40**, 3147.

84. Miller RA, Maloney DG, Warnke R, Levy R. *New England Journal of Medicine*. 1982; **306**, 517.

85. Lowder JN, Meeker TC, Campbell M, *et al. Blood*. 1987; **69**, 199.

86. Raffeld M, Neckers L, Longo DL, Cossman J. *New England Journal of Medicine*. 1985; **312**, 1653.

87. Meeker T, Lowder J, Cleary ML, *et al. New England Journal of Medicine*. 1985; **312**, 1658.

88. Press OW, Appelbaum F, Ledbetter JA, *et al. Blood*. 1987; **69**, 584.

89. Rosenberg SA, Lotze MT, Muul LM, *et al. New England Journal of Medicine*. 1987; **316**, 889.

CHAPTER 20

DIFFUSE SMALL CELL LYMPHOMAS

Sandra J Horning

Definitions and general description

The Working Formulation of the Non-Hodgkin's Lymphoma (NHL) Classification Project, which groups NHL according to morphological criteria and survival data, includes a single histological subtype with diffuse architecture and small lymphocytic, cellular morphology under the rubric, 'low grade'.[1] While the Working Formulation categorizes another diffuse small cell lymphoma, diffuse small cleaved cell (DSC), as intermediate in grade due to somewhat less favourable survival data, the clinical behaviour of DSC often differs significantly from the large cell and high grade subtypes and will be included in this discussion. Also included herein is lymphocytic lymphoma, intermediate differentiation type, which is not considered

separately in the Working Formulation, but is thought to represent a distinct clinicopathological entity by some investigators.[2] The designations of these 'small cell' lymphomas according to several different classifications are shown in Table 20.1. In this chapter the clinical (Table 20.2) and pathological (Table 20.3) features of these lymphomas are reviewed together with the available data regarding their immunophenotypic and cytogenetic characteristics.

Small lymphocytic lymphoma

Small lymphocytic (SL) lymphoma consists of monomorphic small- to medium-sized round lymphocytes with few mitotic figures in a diffuse architectural pattern. Small lymphocytic lymphoma is morphologically indistinguishable

Table 20.1 Classification of diffuse small cell lymphomas

Name	Rappaport	Related terms Lukes–Collins	Kiel
Small lymphocytic (SL)	Diffuse, well-differentiated lymphocytic	Small lymphocytic	Lymphocytic lymphoplasmacytoid immunocytoma
Intermediate lymphocytic (IL)	–	–	–
Diffuse, small cleaved (DSC)	Diffuse, poorly-differentiated lymphocytic	Small cleaved follicular centre cell, diffuse	Small centrocytic

from chronic lymphocytic leukaemia (CLL); the clinical distinction between the two is based upon the presence of an absolute lymphocytosis in CLL (above 4000/mm^3).[3] Terms related to SL include diffuse, well-differentiated lymphocytic (Rappaport classification); lymphocytic, CLL (Kiel classification); and small lymphocytic (Lukes-Collins).[1] Small lymphocytic lymphoma may have plasmacytoid features with amphophilic or basophilic cytoplasm and intra-cytoplasmic (Russel bodies) or intranuclear (Dutcher bodies) inclusions of immunoglobulin. These may be accompanied by monoclonal gammopathy, usually of the IgM type. When significant quantities of IgM are secreted into the serum, the patients are usually referred to as having Waldenstrom's macroglobulinaemia. Although some advocate distinct categorization for SL lymphomas with plasmacytoid features (i.e. lymphoplasmacytoid immunocytoma in the Kiel classification), they are manifestations of a fundamentally similar process with similar natural histories and immunophenotypic and cytogenetic features as discussed below.

In the Working Formulation analyses of NHL, the SL subtype comprised 3.6 per cent of all NHL.[1] The median age at diagnosis was 61 years. The vast majority of SL lymphomas express B-cell markers including Ig – usually IgM with or without IgD – although in rather low intensity relative to follicular lymphomas. Other surface markers include complement receptors, receptors for the Fc portion of IgG, and the cells often express the CD5(T1/T101/Leu-1) pan-T-cell antigen. Clinical investigations have taken advantage of the latter in the treatment of patients with murine monoclonal antibodies directed against this T-cell antigen.[4,5] However, these have met with limited success due to a variety of factors including antigenic modulation and the development of antimurine antibodies.

A translocation involving chromosomes 11 and 14 has been observed in some cases of SL lymphoma and CLL. It has been proposed that a putative oncogene, *bcl*-1 (B-cell leukaemia/lymphoma 1), which is located on chromosome 11 at band q13, is deregulated or activated by its translocation to the rearranged immunoglobulin

Table 20.2 Clinical features of diffuse small cell lymphomas

	Median age	Male: female	Patients in stage IV (%)	Extranodal sites excluding marrow	Median survival (months)	Reference
Small lymphocytic	61	1.2:1	81	Uncommon	70	1
Intermediate lymphocytic	65	5:1	71	Uncommon	31	2
Diffuse, small cleaved	58	2:1	60	More common	41	1

Table 20.3 Pathological features of diffuse small cell lymphomas

	Cytology	Phenotype	Karotype
Small lymphocytic	Small round nuclei	B-cell	Trisomy 12, t(11;14)
Intermediate lymphocytic	Slightly irregular nuclei, mixed small round and indented nuclei	B-cell	Trisomy 12, t(11;14)
Diffuse, small cleaved	Small cleaved nuclei	B-cell (? T-cell)	Deletion chromosomes 8, 20

gene heavy chain locus on chromosome 14.[6] Trisomy 12 is also commonly seen in SL lymphoma and CLL.[7,8] It is speculated that neoplastic transformation or abnormal proliferation in these cases may be related to the cellular ki-*ras*-2 oncogene present on chromosome 12.[9]

Intermediate lymphocytic lymphoma

Lymphocytic lymphomas of intermediate differentiation (IL) have been described as a distinctive histological subtype with cytological features between those of SL and diffuse, small cleaved cell lymphoma. The architectural pattern of IL may be diffuse or may demonstrate a follicular, mantle-zone appearance. In IL, the predominant cell type has slightly irregular or indented nuclei and/or a mixture of cells, some with round nuclei like SL and others with indented, cleaved nuclei. Because of the combination of cell types, IL has been difficult to classify consistently. In the clinicopathological study of Weisenburger *et al*, the median age of patients was 65 years.[2] The male to female ratio was 5:1.

More recently, the immunophenotypic and cytogenetic features of IL have been described.[10] The immunophenotype was identical to that of SL lymphoma. Clonal cytogenetic abnormalities were identified in 10 of 12 cases, including structural or numerical abnormalities of chromosome 11 or 12 in nine cases. These data indicate a close relationship to SL.

Diffuse, small cleaved cell lymphoma

Diffuse, small cleaved cell (DSC) lymphoma is thought to represent the diffuse counterpart of follicular small cleaved cell (FSC) lymphoma; both are composed of small cells with indented or cleaved nuclei and scant cytoplasm. The frequency of mitotic figures is often higher in the diffuse subtype. Upon close inspection small foci of follicular lymphoma may be seen, particularly if enhanced by reticulin staining. Related terms are diffuse poorly-differentiated lymphocytic (Rappaport classification), small centrocytic (Kiel classification) and small cleaved follicular centre cell, diffuse (Lukes-Collins). Diffuse, small cleaved cell lymphoma comprised

a surprisingly large group (6.9 per cent of all NHL) in the Working Formulation.[1] The median age was 58 years and there was a 2:1 male predominance.

The classic phenotype of DSC lymphoma is of B-cell lineage with expression of monoclonal surface immunoglobulin. The DSC lymphomas are less likely to express common acute leukaemia associated antigen (CALLA) than their follicular counterparts. While it is often stated that DSC lymphomas are T1/T101/Leu-1 negative, in contrast to SL/CLL and IL, no difference in expression of this antigen among DSC, IL and SL/CLL was detected in a recent study.[11]

Only a few caes of DSC lymphomas have been submitted for cytogenetic analyses. Interestingly, the few published results do not demonstrate the 14;18 chromosomal translocation characteristic of FSC lymphoma. It is likely that some cases of DSC represent a progression from FSC lymphoma which express t14;18 but have not been reported due to small sample size, while other cases of DSC lymphoma are more akin to the SL/IL types and a few cases may be T-cell in origin. The cytogenetic abnormalities described for DSC include deletions and partial duplications.[8] Further studies, including those using 14;18 molecular probes and Southern blot analyses, may allow better classification of the DSC lymphomas and elucidate their aetiology.

Clinical features and staging

In the Working Formulation, the majority of cases (90 per cent) of SL lymphoma had advanced stage III or IV disease according to the Ann Arbor staging convention. Patients typically present with diffuse adenopathy and involvement of the bone marrow. In the majority of cases, patients are asymptomatic (without constitutional symptoms of weight loss, fevers or sweats) at diagnosis. Patients who present with an absolute lymphocytosis usually do not have a monoclonal gammopathy but, rather, have a relatively high incidence of hypogammaglobulinaemia and are the most likely to progress to a leukaemic phase.[3]

There is a relative paucity of literature

regarding the clinical features of IL lymphoma and much of the information that exists has been provided by pathologists rather than clinicians.[2] In contrast to SL lymphoma constitutional (B) symptoms are relatively common, and are present in 36 per cent of patients at diagnosis. Typical sites of involvement include diffuse adenopathy, spleen, liver and bone marrow. An absolute lymphcytosis is documented in 21 per cent of patients at diagnosis.

The majority of patients with DSC lymphoma in the Working Formulation had stage II or stage IV disease. Extranodal disease was not uncommon. However, the clinical characteristics of DSC lymphoma are actually quite heterogeneous. Some cases of DSC lymphoma present in middle age with diffuse adenopathy and marrow involvement and follow an indolent disease course. These clinical features, together with pathological features which often suggest a vague nodular pattern or a frank discordance in architecture that may be apparent when multiple tissues are available for review, suggest that many DSC lymphomas may have originated as follicular lymphomas. On the other hand, some DSC lymphomas have been reported in younger adults, presenting with a limited extent of disease, arising frequently in Waldeyer's ring, or in other extranodal sites and behaving as biologically aggressive neoplasms. The apparent heterogeneity of the reported clinical characteristics of DSC lymphomas may be partly due to the fact that historically the poorly differentiated lymphocytic category of Rappaport included some poor-prognosis, high grade lymphomas, including T-cell lymphoblastic lymphoma and quite possibly some diffuse, small non-cleaved lymphomas. Another explanation for these clinical differences is that many investigations were performed without the benefit of immunological studies and prior to the description of T-cell lymphomas. In an early study by Bloomfield *et al*, cell suspension analyses in 30 cases of diffuse poorly differentiated lymphocytic lymphoma resulted in the classification of five (17 per cent) as T-cell and nine (30 per cent) as surface immunoglobulin negative.[12]

As a group, the recommended staging procedures for the diffuse, lesser grade lymphomas include history and physical examination, complete blood count and chemistry panel, chest X-ray, computed tomography (CT) of the abdomen and pelvis, lymphogram and bone marrow biopsy. Additional studies that may prove helpful in management include serum protein electrophoresis in SL lymphoma/CLL and IL lymphoma and careful ear, nose and throat examination in DSC lymphoma.

Treatment and prognosis

Small lymphocytic lymphoma, like the follicular low-grade lymphomas, has an indolent natural history with median survivals in the six- to ten-year range. Also, as with the follicular low-grade lymphomas, SL lymphomas are responsive to a variety of therapeutic manoeuvres. These have included single alkylating agents, such as chlorambucil or cyclophosphamide; combination chemotherapy with CVP (cyclophosphamide, vincristine and prednisone); CVP and total lymphoid irradiation; and total body irradiation. Despite complete response rates as high as 75–80 per cent with each of these, SL lymphoma is characterized by a continuous pattern of relapse after remission, with a median remission duration of about 3–4 years.[13] Therapy in this group of patients is not infrequently complicated by concurrent medical problems in this older patient population as well as difficulty in the delivery of myelotoxic therapy due to infiltration of the bone marrow and hypersplenism.

Various prognostic factors have been reported which adversely affect survival in SL lymphoma including constitutional symptoms, age, anaemia, mitotic rate and stage.[14] In a recent analysis of 54 patients with SL lymphoma (excluding CLL) analysed at Stanford University, California, only constitutional symptoms and a diffuse rather than pseudofollicular nodal architecture predicted a significantly worse prognosis.[15]

Given that patients with advanced stage SL lymphoma have not been cured with conventional therapy, live a relatively long time with recurrent disease, are often elderly and are usually asymptomatic at diagnosis, it has become common practice to defer therapy until indicated by disease progression. In a group of patients managed at Stanford University with no initial treatment of their SL lymphoma, the median time to the institution of therapy was six years.[16] In an expanded group of selected SL lymphoma patients managed with no initial therapy, the survival at four years was 93 per cent.[15] Thus, the standard management for advanced stage SL lymphoma has become no initial treatment. Therapy, when indicated by disease progression, usually consists of alkylating agents such as chlorambucil or cyclophosphamide, alone or in combination with other agents, particularly steroids.

As a group, the DSC lymphomas had a median survival of 34 months in the Working Formulation Classification project, which was significantly shorter than FSC lymphoma and, therefore, DSC lymphoma is considered 'intermediate' in grade. In an interesting and important study being conducted at the National Cancer Institute, patients with low grade lymphomas, including SL and IL, are randomized to receive either no initial treatment or aggressive chemotherapy with ProMACE-MOPP (prednisone, methotrexate, doxorubicin, cyclophosphamide, etoposide, mechlorethamine, vincristine, procarbazine).[17] The study is designed to test whether an aggressive treatment approach can improve upon their natural history, particularly in younger patients.

For the subgroup of patients who have limited SL lymphoma, radiation therapy delivered with curative intent provides a prolonged freedom from relapse — 67 per cent at 10 years.[15,18] Thus irradiation should be offered for selected patients with stage I and II SL lymphoma, particularly those under the age of 50 in whom the planned treatment will be well-tolerated.

Whether treated or untreated, SL lymphomas may undergo histological transformation to a large cell lymphoma. This has been described in CLL and implies a poor prognosis with rapid disease progression, often refractory to intensive therapy (Richter's syndrome).[19] Immunological and molecular studies have been inconsistent; some have found the transformed lymphoma to

express identical markers and clonality as the original SL process and others indicate the development of a unique B-cell neoplasm.[19,20] Even with current, intensive, multiagent chemotherapy regimens, Richter's syndrome remains a major therapeutic challenge.

Two variants of SL/CLL should be considered separately. Benign monoclonal B-cell lymphocytosis is characterized by initial white blood counts from 10 000–44 000/mm^3, lack of disease progression, essentially normal humoral and cellular immunity and a normal karyotype.[21] T-cell CLL is a relatively rare form of CLL (about 2 per cent of all cases) and expresses a mature T-cell phenotype which may be subcategorized as helper/inducer (T4$^+$) or cytotoxic/suppressor (T8$^+$). Recent reviews indicate that T8$^+$ lymphocytosis may be a relatively indolent disease.[22] In contrast, T4$^+$ CLL has a poor prognosis (median survival 21 months) and is commonly accompanied by splenomegaly and cutaneous disease.[23] Serological testing for human T-cell lymphotrophic virus (HTLV-I) antibody has been negative in T-cell CLL.

In the report of Weisenburger et al.[2] the median survival among a group of IL lymphoma patients was only 31 months. Poor prognostic factors included systemic symptoms, advanced age, absolute lymphocytosis, significant anaemia, high mitotic rate and obliteration of the lymph node sinuses. Additional clinical data are needed to determine if IL lymphoma merits a separate category in the Working Formulation, especially since the early series may have included patients diagnosed late in their disease, given the difficulty in recognizing a new histological subtype. This may have been especially true in those cases with a 'mantle zone' histological appearance. Current treatment approaches should, in general, follow the recommendations stated above for SL lymphoma.

The approach to management of the DSC lymphomas should be guided by the clinical picture. Patients who are middle aged or older and who present with diffuse adenopathy, marrow involvement, typical cleaved nuclei and a B-cell phenotype may be managed in a fashion appropriate to FSC and SL lymphomas as discussed above. A small subgroup who received no initial therapy has been reported; their course was similar to the three histological subtypes considered to be low grade lymphomas.[24] Younger patients, particularly those presenting with limited and/or extranodal disease, bulky tumour, elevated lactic dehydrogenase and a greater degree of nuclear atypia are candidates for aggressive therapy with curative intent. Such therapy should include combination chemotherapy regimens such as ProMACE-CytaBOM, M-BACOD or CHOP (see Chapter 21 for details of these drug regimens). Central nervous system prophylaxis should be considered, as it is for the diffuse large cell lymphomas where prophylaxis is given for presentations in the paranasal sinuses, epidural space, testes and in the presence of circulating lymphoma cells. Of interest, the Vancouver group does *not* recommend MACOP-B for DSC lymphomas, based on poor outcome in three reported patients.[25]

The difficulties and confusion in the management of the diffuse small cell lymphomas result from our limited ability to predict their clinical behaviour. The prognostic significance of nuclear morphology alone in clinical studies has not been well established. Differences in outcome among the published studies may relate to difficulties in classification, as these neoplasms represent a morphological continuum. An additional contributing factor is the possible inclusion of T-cell neoplasms in the DSC lymphoma category.

The routine use of newer pathological techniques such as immunophenotyping, cytogenetics and the determination of a labelling index may prove superior in their ability to distinguish among prognostically significant subtypes. For instance, the cytogenetics of DSC lymphoma appear to be distinct from those of SL and IL lymphomas, which, cytogenetically, are essentially identical.

In a recent analysis of 64 B-lineage diffuse, small cell lymphomas (43 SL/CLL, 13 IL and 8 DSC) at Stanford University, there was no correlation between survival and histology (Fig. 20.1).[11] In this series a number of clinical and immunological features were studied including age, sex, stage, biopsy site, presence or absence of constitutional symptoms, lymphocytosis and

a variety of antigens. Of these, only three were significantly correlated with survival. Patients with biopsies containing 25 per cent or more proliferating cells as evidenced by expression of the Ki-67 nuclear proliferation antigen had a statistically significant reduction in survival ($P = 0.02$).

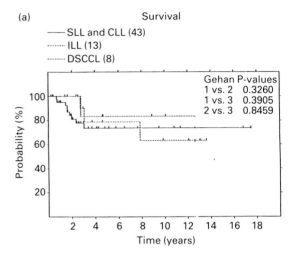

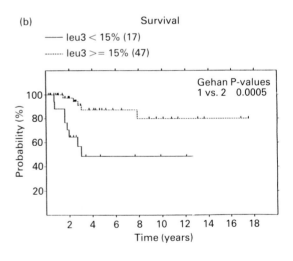

Fig. 20.1 (a) Survival data for 64 patients with diffuse, small cell lymphoma by histology. (*See* text for description). (b) Survival data according to expression of Leu-3[+] (helper T-cell) host infiltrate less than or greater than 15% of the total cell population.

Also, patients with lymphomas in which the host T-cell (Leu 4^+) or helper T-cells (Leu 3^+) were less than 25 per cent and 15 per cent of the total cell population, respectively, had a decreased survival ($P < 0.01$). More patients, particularly in the DSC group, are needed to establish the independent prognostic significance of immunophenotype in multivariate analyses of the diffuse, small cell neoplasms.

Given that many patients with IL and DSC lymphomas, and the majority of patients with SL lymphoma, may not be cured with conventional therapy, it is appropriate to consider investigational approaches for these patients. Treatment results with α-interferon have been disappointing in the SL lymphomas.[26] Trials employing anti-Leu-1 murine monoclonal antibody have shown only limited success due to the large circulating component of lymphoma cells, antigenic modulation and antimurine responses.[4,5] Further studies may possibly include drug-targeting with pan-B-cell antibodies including radiolabelled antibodies. Bone marrow transplantation has been employed with success in some cases of DSC lymphoma. This approach may be of particular benefit if young DSC lymphoma patients with a poor prognosis can be reliably identified with the aid of more sophisticated diagnostic tests as above. An additional problem relevant to the use of autologous bone marrow transplant in the diffuse small cell lymphomas is the presence of lymphoma in the marrow and therefore the need for adequate purging techniques or positive stem cell selection.

Follow-up

Once treatment is elected in the diffuse small cell lymphomas, it is important to maximize benefit in achieving as complete a response as possible. Even in the SL lymphomas, this approach renders the longest freedom from requiring further treatment. Therefore, it is recommended that patients be restaged by repeating initially abnormal studies during therapy. It must be recognized that some SL lymphoma patients may not be disease-free in the marrow after the resolution of all lymph node or splenic disease and it is not necessary to prolong treatment on this basis. Because of the propensity for these lymphomas to relapse continuously after treatment, it is important to examine patients, record blood counts and chemistries and monitor the abdomen and pelvis for occult disease on a regular basis. Patients who receive aggressive chemotherapy for DSC lymphoma are followed in a manner similar to those with diffuse large cell lymphoma.

References

1. The Non-Hodgkin's Lymphoma Pathologic Classification Project. *Cancer*. 1982; **49**, 2112.
2. Weisenburger DD, Nathwani BN, Diamond LW, *et al*. *Cancer*. 1981; **48**, 1415.
3. Pangalis GA, Nathwani BN, Rappaport H. *Cancer*. 1977; **39**, 999.
4. Dillman RO, Shawler DL, Sobol RE, *et al*. *Blood*. 1982; **59**, 1036.
5. Foon KA, Schroff RW, Bunn PA, *et al*. *Blood*. 1984; **64**, 1085.
6. Tsujimoto Y, Yunis J, Onorato-Showe L, *et al*. *Science*. 1984; **224**, 1433.
7. Yunis JJ, Oken MM, Kaplan ME, *et al*. *New England Journal of Medicine*. 1982; **307**, 1231.
8. Koduru PRK, Filippa DA, Richardson ME, *et al*. *Blood*. 1987; **69**, 97.
9. Jhanwar SC, Neel BG, Hayward WS, *et al*. 1983; *Proceedings of the National Academy of Sciences USA*. 1983; **80**, 4794.
10. Weisenburger DD, Sanger WG, Armitage JO, *et al*. *Blood*. 1987; **69**, 1617.
11. Medeiros LJ, Picker LJ, Gelb AB, *et al*. 1988;
12. Bloomfield CD, Kersey JH, Brunning RD, *et al*. *Cancer Treatment Reports*. 1977; **61**, 963.
13. Rosenberg SA. *Journal of Clinical Oncology*. 1985; **3**, 299.
14. Evans HL, Butler JJ, Youness EL. *Cancer*. 1978; **41**, 1440.
15. Morrison WH, Weiss LM, Picozzi VJ, *et al*. 1988;
16. Horning SJ, Rosenberg SA. *New England Journal of Medicine*. 1984; **311**, 1471.
17. Young RC, Longo DL, Glatstein E, *et al*. *Proceedings of the American Society of Clinical Oncology*. 1987; **6**, 200.
18. Paryani SB, Hoppe RT, Cox RS, *et al*. *Cancer*. 1983; **52**, 2300.
19. Harousseau JL, Flandrin G, Tricot G, *et al*. *Cancer*. 1981; **48**, 1302.

20. Van Dougen JJM, Hooijkan H, Michiels JJ, *et al. Blood*. 1984; **64**, 571.
21. Han T, Ozer H, Garigan M, *et al. Blood*. 1984; **64**, 244.
22. Phyliky RL, Li C–Y, Yam LT. *Mayo Clinic Proceedings*. 1983; **58**, 709.
23. Witzig TE, Phyliky RL, Li C–Y, *et al. American Journal of Hematology*. 1986; **21**, 139.
24. Portlock CS, Rosenberg SA. *Annals of Internal Medicine*. 1979; **90**, 10.
25. Connors JM, Klimo P. *Proceedings of the American Society of Clinical Oncology*. 1986; **5**, 192.
26. Horning SJ, Merigan TC, Krown WE, *et al. Cancer*. 1985; **56**, 1305.

CHAPTER 21

DIFFUSE AGGRESSIVE LYMPHOMAS IN ADULTS

Ellen R Gaynor and Richard I Fisher

Definitions and general description

The diffuse aggressive lymphomas of adults are a diverse group of diseases which have in common an aggressive clinical behaviour leading to rapid clinical deterioration of the patient and, at the same time, sensitivity to chemotherapeutic agents rendering them curable in a sizeable proportion of patients. Like all of the non-Hodgkin's lymphomas (NHLs), these diseases are malignant clonal expansions of lymphocytes arrested at a particular phase in the maturation sequence of normal lymphocytes. As can be seen in Table 21.1, these diseases are not neatly grouped by any of the current classification systems for the lymphomas. In the Rappaport classification system, the subtypes which comprise the diffuse aggressive lymphomas of adults include diffuse mixed cell lymphoma, diffuse histiocytic lymphoma and diffuse undifferentiated lymphoma. As classified by the Working Formulation, these lymphomas are included in the subgroups of diffuse mixed cell lymphoma and diffuse large cell lymphoma in the intermediate grade category and diffuse large cell immunoblastic lymphoma and diffuse small non-cleaved cell, non-Burkitt's lymphoma in the high grade category.

While lymphoblastic lymphoma and Burkitt's lymphoma are diffuse and aggressive they are more commonly seen in childhood than in adult patients. It is generally believed that the treatment of lymphoblastic and Burkitt's lymphoma should utilize different chemotherapy regimens than those commonly employed for the diffuse aggressive lymphomas of adults. Because they differ substantially in the age group affected and in the management

Table 21.1 Diffuse aggressive lymphoma of adults

Rappaport classification	*Working Formulation*
Intermediate grade malignancy	
Diffuse mixed, lymphocytic and histiocytic	Malignant lymphoma, diffuse mixed, small and large cell
Diffuse histiocytic	Malignant lymphoma, diffuse large cell
High grade malignancy	
Diffuse histiocytic	Malignant lymphoma, large cell, immunoblastic
Lymphoblastic	Malignant lymphoma, lymphoblastic
Diffuse undifferentiated	Malignant lymphoma, small non-cleaved cell

approach, further discussion of these lymphomas and of diffuse undifferentiated lymphoma can be found in Chapters 16 and 17.

Diffuse mixed cell lymphoma

This subtype accounts for approximately 7 per cent of all NHL. Slightly less than half of the patients present with stage I and II disease and extranodal involvement is common. In half of the cases of diffuse mixed cell lymphoma, the cells are cytologically similar to those of follicular mixed cell lymphoma and immunologically the cells mark as B-cells. It is likely that, in these instances, the disease represents histological evolution from a follicular growth pattern to diffuse involvement of the involved lymph node. The clinical course of this disease is more aggressive than that of follicular disease and while data are somewhat limited, it appears that with aggressive chemotherapy patients with diffuse mixed cell lymphoma can be cured of their disease.

In 50 per cent of cases, patients with diffuse mixed cell lymphoma have cells which are cytologically different from the cells seen in follicular mixed cell lymphoma. The cells in these cases are a pleomorphic mixture of atypical small and large cells. In the majority of cases studied, the malignant cells bear the immunological markers of mature or 'peripheral' T-cells (see Chapter 22). In some cases an epithelioid component is prominent and hence these lymphomas are referred to as lymphoepithelioid lymphoma or more commonly Lennert's lymphoma. The disease, which tends to occur in middle-aged people, is usually widely disseminated at diagnosis.

Diffuse large cell lymphoma

As a group, these lymphomas account for one-third of all cases of NHL. They are biologically diverse with respect to their cell of origin. It is now obvious that Rappaport's term 'diffuse histiocytic lymphoma' is a misnomer, since less than 5 per cent are of true histiocytic origin. The vast majority, greater than 95 per cent, are derived from lymphocytes of T- or B-cell origin. While the prognostic significance of T- or B-cell origin continues to be debated in the literature, it appears that with intensive chemotherapeutic regimens, the cell of origin impacts little, if at all, on potential curability.

Approximately one-third of patients present with stage I or II disease with the remainder having clinically disseminated disease at the time of diagnosis. Extralymphatic sites of involvement are common and the natural history of the disease is very aggressive with a median survival of less than one year in untreated patients.

Diffuse immunoblastic lymphoma

Using older chemotherapeutic regimens, it appeared that this subtype of lymphoma had a slightly worse prognosis and hence in the Working Formulation it is classified as a high-grade lymphoma. With newer treatment approaches, the prognostic difference compared to diffuse large cell lymphoma is less apparent. The Working Formulation further subdivides the immunoblastic lymphomas into three types: plasmacytoid, clear cell and polymorphous. While these names imply a particular cell of origin, immunological studies have demonstrated that T- or B-cell origin cannot be accurately predicted morphologically. Hence the subclassification has little clinical utility at the present time. Immunoblastic lymphomas of B-cell origin may be associated with circulating monoclonal immunoglobulins. Immunoblastic lymphomas are frequently found in the gastrointestinal tract and may occur in association with Sjögren's syndrome.

Like diffuse large cell lymphoma, this is an aggressive malignancy which is rapidly fatal if untreated. As with all of the diffuse aggressive lymphomas, it is frequently curable with intensive chemotherapy.

Summary

While the diffuse aggressive lymphomas can be classified into several morphological subtypes, it is important to appreciate the fact that the morphological distinction between diffuse mixed cell, diffuse large cell, or undifferentiated lymphoma does not provide significant information about prognosis. Statistically significant prognostic factors for these lymphomas relate to clinical presentation, e.g. stage of disease, sites of disease involvement and tumour burden. Furthermore, reproducibility of diagnosis among pathologists within this group of lymphomas is far from ideal.[1] Hence, while morphologically distinct, the diffuse aggressive lymphomas can be considered as a single entity from a clinical standpoint. The virulence of their behaviour, their tendency to early and widespread dissemination, and their potential curability warrant their being grouped together from a therapeutic perspective.

Clinical features and staging

As noted above, the diffuse aggressive lymphomas are, in general, diseases of middle-aged and older adults. Unlike their indolent counterparts which are almost always widely disseminated at the time of diagnosis, the diffuse aggressive lymphomas present as stage I or stage II disease in approximately 30 per cent of cases. Because they are potentially curable and because the best and frequently only chance of cure resides in the initial therapeutic choice, it is essential that the patient be completely and accurately staged at the time of diagnosis. It goes without saying that every patient deserves the expertise of a competent haematopathologist to establish the diagnosis and to ensure that the

patient's lymphoma is accurately classified.

The staging system used for the diffuse aggressive lymphomas is the Ann Arbor staging system (Table 21.2) which was originally proposed as a staging system for Hodgkin's disease. While it is used extensively, the four stage system has definite limitations when applied to the non-Hodgkin's lymphomas. For example, the distinction between stage III and stage IV in Hodgkin's disease has definite prognostic and therapeutic implications with the former being amenable to cure with radiation therapy in some cases, while the latter requires treatment with systemic chemotherapy. When dealing with NHL, stage III and stage IV both warrant systemic chemotherapy and the difference in prognosis between the two stages becomes less distinct with chemotherapy. Furthermore, while the Ann Arbor system clearly separates patients by extent of disease, it does not address the whole issue of bulk of disease. This has both prognostic and therapeutic importance in NHL. For example, patients with stage II disease which is non-bulky (< 10 cm tumour mass in one location) have a far better prognosis than a patient with bulky stage II disease (> 10 cm tumour mass in one location). While both patients, by definition, have stage II disease, the optimal therapy for each would be quite different.

A proposed staging evaluation is outlined in Table 21.3. As a minimum all patients should have (1) complete blood count and chemistry

Table 21.2 The Ann Arbor staging classification

Stage I	Involvement of a single lymph node region or of a single extranodal organ or site (I_E)
Stage II	Involvement of two or more lymph node regions on the same side of the diaphragm, or localized involvement of an extranodal site or organ (II_E) and of one or more lymph node regions on the same side of the diaphragm
Stage III	Involvement of lymph node regions on both sides of the diaphragm, which may also be accompanied by localized involvement of an extranodal organ or site (III_E) or spleen (III_S) or both (III_{SE})
Stage IV	Diffuse or disseminated involvement of one or more distant extranodal organs with or without associated lymph node involvement

Fever > 38 °C, night sweats, and/or weight loss >10 per cent of body weight in the six months preceding admission are defined as systemic symptoms, and denoted by the suffix B. Asymptomatic patients are denoted by the suffix A.

survey; (2) chest X-ray; (3) lymphangiogram; (4) computed tomographic (CT) scan of the abdomen to assess liver, spleen, and nodal areas not well visualized by the lymphangiogram; and (5) bilateral iliac crest bone marrow biopsies. Because bone marrow involvement increases the patient's likelihood of lymphomatous involvement of the meninges, a positive bone marrow biopsy is an indication for cytological and chemical studies on the cerebral spinal fluid. Patients who present with lymphomatous involvement of the meninges should receive a course of intrathecal methotrexate and cranial radiation therapy.

Table 21.3 Recommended staging work-up

A   *Required for all patients*
1. Complete history and physical examination with careful evaluation of all lymph node areas, liver, spleen, thyroid, testes and skin
2. Complete blood count and serum chemistries
3. Chest X-ray
4. Lymphangiogram
5. CT scan of the abdomen
6. Bilateral iliac crest bone marrow biopsies

B   *Required in certain circumstances*
1. CT scan of the thorax or whole lung tomograms
2. Gallium scan
3. Bone scan

In certain situations additional studies may be indicated. For example, if there is a question of nodal or parenchymal involvement on the chest X-ray, a CT scan of the thorax or whole lung tomograms should be obtained to assess this area further. Patients who are found to have an unexplained elevation of the alkaline phosphatase or who present with complaints of bone pain should be evaluated with a bone scan. Plain films of any abnormal area on the bone scan should be obtained to look for lymphomatous involvement of the skeleton. Gallium scanning is of limited use in the staging of lymphomas. While it is useful for detecting disease above the diaphragm, its utility in evaluating disease below the diaphragm is limited by the frequent intestinal faecal uptake of gallium.

While the staging procedures outlined very closely parallel those employed in the staging of a patient with Hodgkin's disease, there is one very important difference. Staging laparotomy is used routinely in patients with Hodgkin's disease who present with clinical stage I or II disease. Detection of disease in the abdomen not only upstages the disease but may also dictate a change in therapeutic strategy. Since the majority of patients with diffuse aggressive lymphoma are treated with systemic chemotherapy, staging laparotomy is reserved solely for those patients with diffuse large cell lymphoma who, after a complete staging work-up, are found to have clinical stage I disease. Such patients, who are shown by staging laparotomy to have pathological stage I disease, are potentially curable with radiation therapy. If one intends to use radiation therapy as the only treatment modality, staging laparotomy is justified in this select group of patients. Obviously, the procedure should be performed only in those institutions and by those surgeons who are highly experienced in the performance of a formal staging laparotomy. There is a general consensus of opinion that chemotherapy alone or in combination with radiation therapy is the treatment of choice for all patients with early stage disease. Staging laparotomy is thus rarely, if ever, indicated in the staging evaluation of these patients.

One further difference between the staging of Hodgkin's disease and the staging of NHL relates to the evaluation of the lymphoid tissue in Waldeyer's ring. This lymph node region is rarely involved in Hodgkin's disease but is often involved in NHL. Thus an examination of Waldeyer's ring is an essential part of the staging work-up of NHL. Because of a high correlation between gastrointestinal involvement and Waldeyer's ring involvement, the finding of disease in Waldeyer's ring necessitates barium studies of the gastrointestinal tract to document the presence or absence of disease.

Treatment and prognosis

Evolution of treatment approaches

While progress in the management of most solid malignancies has been painfully slow, tremendous advances have been made in the treatment of the diffuse aggressive lymphomas over the past 25 years. In order to understand the rationale for current treatment recommendations, one has to appreciate the evolution of management strategies from the 1960s to the present. For the sake of discussion, chemotherapy treatment can be divided into first, second, and third generation regimens (Table 21.4).

In the early 1960s, the diffuse aggressive lymphomas, of which diffuse large cell lymphoma is the most common, were almost universally fatal. Initial attempts at treatment used single chemotherapeutic agents. Although responses (including rare complete responses) were seen, the duration of remission was measured in months and the overwhelming majority of patients were dead within one year of diagnosis. Successful treatment of advanced stage Hodgkin's disease with combination chemotherapy prompted the use of a similar regimen C-MOPP (Table 21.5), in which cyclophosphamide was substituted for nitrogen mustard, in the treatment of diffuse aggressive lymphomas.[2] Of 24 patients treated, 46 per cent achieved a complete remission and 37 per cent of all treated patients remained in a complete unmaintained remission for five years. This study was the first to demonstrate the curability of diffuse large cell lymphoma. It also provided the insight that relapse after 18 months of attaining a complete remission was rare and that a disease-free survival of two years is equivalent to cure in the majority of these patients.

The introduction of the drug doxorubicin (Adriamycin) represented a major advance in cancer chemotherapeutics. The CHOP regimen (see Table 21.5) was one of the first chemotherapy programmes to incorporate this drug.[3] The CHOP combination has been used extensively in the treatment of large cell lymphoma and remains the most widely used regimen today in the treatment of this disease. Follow-up data of up to 12 years are now available from the Southwest Oncology Group for 418 patients treated in three consecutive studies employing the CHOP regimen. The

Table 21.4 Treatment programmes for diffuse aggressive lymphomas

Chemotherapy regimens	Patients	Complete remission (%)	Long-term survival (%)
First generation			
MOPP/C-MOPP	24	46	37
BACOP	32	48	34
CHOP (SWOG)	418	53	30
COMLA	48	40	32
Second generation			
COP/BLAM	33	72	61
M-BACOD	101	77	57
ProMACE-MOPP	79	73	65
Third generation			
m-BACOD	80	75	58
ProMACE d1/MOPP d8	54	76	60
ProMACE/CytaBOM	57	79	68
MACOP-B	61	84	75

For explanation of drug regimens *see* Table 21.5

complete remission rate was 53 per cent with 30 per cent of all treated patients achieving a sustained complete remission.[4]

The initial doxorubicin (Adriamycin) regimen devised at the National Cancer Institute (NCI) was the BACOP regimen (*see* Table 21.5).[5] This was the first of the chemotherapy regimens to use alternating myelosuppressive and non-myelosuppressive drug sequences. Of 32 patients treated, 48 per cent achieved a complete remission and about 34 per cent of all treated patients were apparently cured of their disease.

One of the initial regimens employing the antimetabolites cytosine arabinoside and methotrexate was the COMLA regimen (*see* Table 21.5) which was developed at Yale and subsequently used extensively at the University of Chicago. This regimen employed a treatment cycle of 11 weeks, with the drugs cytosine arabinoside and methotrexate being given on weeks 4–11. Forty-two patients were treated with a complete response rate of 55 per cent and 48 per cent long-term survivors. A subsequent update of this study with a 10-year follow-up period showed a decline in the complete response rate to 40 per cent with a 32 per cent long-term disease-free survival rate.[6]

Because the complete remission and cure rates were similar for the NCI C-MOPP and BACOP regimens, investigators analysed patients enrolled in these studies to ascertain if there were prognostic factors which might predict clinical outcome in similar studies. Of all parameters studied, those which adversely influenced prognosis were stage IV disease, a single tumour mass greater than 10 cm in diameter, elevated lactate dehydrogenase (LDH) > 250 u/ml, bone marrow involvement and large gastrointestinal masses.[7] It is of interest that while these clinical features were highly significant, the morphology of a given patient's lymphoma, i.e., diffuse mixed cell, diffuse large cell or diffuse undifferentiated, did not provide significant information about prognosis. Of greater interest is the fact that as treatment of the diffuse aggressive lymphomas has improved, the identified prognostic factors have become less important in predicting patient outcome. This probably simply reflects the fact that as treatment improves, those patients felt to be in poor prognostic subsets became more likely to achieve a complete remission.

While the first generation chemotherapy regimens represented a major advance in the treatment of the diffuse aggressive lymphomas, the fact remained that the majority of patients continued to die of their disease. The development of the second generation regimens in the 1970s and the third generation regimens of the 1980s were prompted by several observations. First and most obvious, there was a need to improve the complete remission and subsequent cure rate. Second, it was repeatedly observed clinically that patients' tumours would respond to treatment but would frequently regrow before initiation of a subsequent cycle of chemotherapy. Non-myelosuppressive drugs had been successfully used in an alternating fashion with myelosuppressive agents in the BACOP regimen. This approach would be extensively used in the second and third generation regimens. Third, the new drug, VP-16, which was shown to be active in the lymphomas, was introduced into some of the new treatment regimens. Finally, and perhaps most importantly, understanding of tumour-cell drug resistance matured. The Goldie–Coldman hypothesis proposed that, like bacteria, cancer cells have an inherent property of mutation toward drug resistance including drugs to which the tumour cells had not been previously exposed. The probability of mutant clones increases in direct proportion to tumour size and when cells become resistant to multiple drugs simultaneously, the efficacy of combination chemotherapy declines markedly.

The only approach which might overcome the propensity of tumour cells to drug resistance is to expose the tumour initially to a maximum number of drugs used in combination. Ideally these drugs should be shown to be non-cross-resistant. Several of the more recently introduced chemotherapy regimens are designed to test the Goldie–Coldman hypothesis, which predicts that the early introduction of all effective agents will overcome the problem of inherent drug resistance and will thereby increase the response rate and duration of response.

In an attempt to address the problem of

tumour growth during periods of myelosuppression, several chemotherapy regimens were designed which incorporated the use of non-myelotoxic drugs at times during the chemotherapy cycle when the patient's bone marrow was maximally suppressed. The COP/BLAM regimen (*see* Table 21.5), like the BACOP regimen, introduced the non-myelosuppressive drug bleomycin on day 15 of a 21 day cycle.[8] In addition to using a higher dose of bleomycin than that used in the BACOP regimen, the COP/BLAM regimen also employed a higher dose of doxorubicin. The drug procarbazine, which had demonstrated activity in the C-MOPP regimen, was also incorporated into the COP/BLAM programme. Of 33 patients treated, 72 per cent achieved a complete remission. Sixty-one per cent of all treated patients were disease-free at two years. The M-BACOD regimen (*see* Table 21.5) incorporated high dose methotrexate with leucovorin rescue at the midpoint of the treatment cycle to prevent the tumour growth which had been seen with the use of regimens given on a 21 or 28 day cycle.[9] Results were very encouraging, with a complete response rate of 77 per cent and long-term survival occurring in 57 per cent of patients. To decrease toxicity and to allow greater usage of this type of approach, the M-BACOD regimen was designed.[10] This regimen uses a much lower dose of methotrexate and can be given on an outpatient basis. With a shorter period of follow-up compared to the M-BACOD study, results are encouraging with 58 per cent of all treated patients remaining in complete remission.

While several regimens addressed the problem of mid-cycle tumour growth, investigators at the NCI devised a regimen, ProMACE-MOPP (*see* Table 21.5), which employed the simultaneous use of two non-cross-resistant regimens.[11] As originally devised, the treatment programme consisted of three phases. An induction phase using ProMACE was employed until the patient achieved a complete remission or until the rate of tumour responsiveness reached a plateau. Such a plateau was believed to represent either elimination of the drug-sensitive clone of cells or emergence of cells which were resistant to the ProMACE drugs. The second phase, following

ProMACE, utilized the MOPP regimen. The number of MOPP cycles given was equal to the number of ProMACE cycles used in the initial phase. Patients entering a complete remission received two cycles of intensification therapy using the ProMACE regimen. Seventy-three per cent of patients so treated achieved a complete remission, with 65 per cent of all treated patients experiencing long-term disease-free survival. Of particular significance is the fact that complete remissions were achieved using this regimen in 66 per cent of stage IV patients, 50 per cent of patients with bone marrow involvement and 64 per cent of patients with gastrointestinal involvement. These are subgroups of patients previously identified as being in poor prognostic categories. It appears that one of the most significant contributions of the ProMACE-MOPP treatment programme is that it affords the possibility of cure to those patients who previously responded poorly to therapy.

In an attempt to decrease toxicity and in order to expose the tumour cells to the maximum number of drugs early in the course of therapy, two subsequent treatment regimens were devised, ProMACE-CytaBOM and ProMACE d1/MOPP d8 (*see* Table 21.5). Within the first eight days of therapy these two regimens introduce multiple and maximum numbers of drugs known to be effective in the treatment of diffuse aggressive lymphomas. At the NCI a randomized study of these two treatment regimens showed a complete response rate of 76 per cent for ProMACE d1/MOPP d8 and 79 per cent for ProMACE-CytaBOM.[12] Disease-free survivals were 60 per cent and 68 per cent respectively. Toxic deaths were less than with the original ProMACE-MOPP regimen (4 versus 10 per cent) and both regimens were easily given in an outpatient setting. Hence these regimens appear to be equally effective but less toxic and less cumbersome than the original ProMACE-MOPP treatment regimen.

All of the regimens described above involve considerable cost to the patient in terms of treatment duration. Generally with these regimens, patients are treated for 6–10 months. The advantage of the MACOP-B regimen (*see* Table 21.5) is that the entire duration of therapy is 12 weeks.[13] Like the other third generation

Table 21.5   Chemotherapeutic regimens

	Regimen	Dose and route	Day	Frequency
1.	CVP			
	C – cyclophosphamide	400 mg/m² p.o.	1–5	Repeat every
	V – vincristine	1.4 mg/m² i.v.	1	21 days
	P – prednisone	100 mg/m² p.o.	1–5	
2.	C-MOPP			
	C – cyclophosphamide	650 mg/m² i.v.	1, 8	Repeat every
	O – vincristine (Oncovin)	1.4 mg/m² i.v.	1, 8	28 days
	P – procarbazine	100 mg/m² p.o.	1–14	
	P – prednisone	40 mg/m² p.o.	1–14	
3.	BACOP			
	B – bleomycin	5 u/m² i.v.	15, 22	Repeat every
	A – doxorubicin (Adriamycin)	25 mg/m² i.v.	1, 8	28 days
	C – cyclophosphamide	650 mg/m² i.v.	1, 8	
	O – vincristine (Oncovin)	1.4 mg/m² i.v.	1, 8	
	P – prednisone	60 mg/m² p.o.	15–28	
4.	CHOP			
	C – cyclophosphamide	750 mg/m² i.v.	1	Repeat every
	H – doxorubicin (Adriamycin)	50 mg/m² i.v.	1	21 days
	O – vincristine (Oncovin)	1.4 mg/m² i.v. (max 2.0 mg)	1	
	P – prednisone	100 mg p.o.	1–5	
5.	COMLA			
	C – cyclophosphamide	1500 mg/m² i.v.	1	Repeat every
	O – vincristine (Oncovin)	1.4 mg/m² i.v. (max 2.0 mg)	1, 8, 15	91 days
	M – methotrexate	120 mg/m² i.v. (bolus)	22, 29, 36, 43, 50, 57, 64, 71	
	L – leucovorin	25 mg/m² p.o. × 4	24 hours after methotrexate	
	A – cytarabine	300 mg/m²	Same as methotrexate	
6.	COP/BLAM			
	C – cyclophosphamide	400 mg/m² i.v.	1	Repeat every
	O – vincristine (Oncovin)	1 mg/m² i.v.	1	21 days
	P – prednisone	40 mg/m² p.o.	1–10	
	BL – bleomycin	15 u/m² i.v.	15	
	A – doxorubicin (Adriamycin)	40 mg/m² i.v.	1	
	M – procarbazine	100 mg/m² p.o.	1–10	
7.	M-BACOD			
	M – methotrexate*	3000 mg/m² i.v. (over 40–60 minutes)	14	Repeat every 21 days
	B – bleomycin	4 u/m² i.v.	1	
	A – doxorubicin (Adriamycin)	45 mg/m² i.v.	1	
	C – cyclophosphamide	600 mg/m² i.v.	1	
	O – vincristine (Oncovin)	1 mg/m² i.v.	1	
	D – dexamethasone (Decadron)	6 mg/m² p.o.	1–5	

Table 21.5 continued

8. **m-BACOD**

m	– methotrexate*	200 mg/m² i.v. (over 15 minutes)	8, 15	Repeat every 21 days
B	– bleomycin	4 u/m² i.v.	1	
A	– doxorubicin (Adriamycin)	45 mg/m² i.v.	1	
C	– cyclophosphamide	600 mg/m² i.v.	1	
O	– vincristine (Oncovin)	1.4 mg/m² i.v.	1	
D	– dexamethasone (Decadron)	6 mg/m² p.o.	1–5	

9. **ProMACE-MOPP**

Pro	– prednisone	60 mg/m² p.o.	1–14	Repeat every 28 days
M	– methotrexate*	1500 mg/m² i.v. (over 12 hours)	15	
A	– doxorubicin (Adriamycin)	25 mg/m² i.v.	1, 8	
C	– cyclophosphamide	650 mg/m² i.v.	1, 8	
E	– etoposide	120 mg/m² i.v.	1, 8	

Followed by MOPP after maximal response

M	– mechlorethamine	6 mg/m² i.v.	1, 8	Repeat every 28 days
O	– vincristine (Oncovin)	1.4 mg/m² i.v.	1, 8	
P	– procarbazine	100 mg/m² p.o.	1–14	
P	– prednisone	40 mg/m² p.o.	1–14	

10. **ProMACE-CytaBOM**

Pro	– prednisone	60 mg/m² p.o.	1–14	Repeat every 21 days
A	– doxorubicin (Adriamycin)	25 mg/m² i.v.	1	
C	– cyclophosphamide	650 mg/m² i.v.	1	
E	– etoposide	120 mg/m² i.v.	1	
Cyta	– cytarabine	300 mg/m² i.v.	8	
B	– bleomycin	5 u/m² i.v.	8	
O	– vincristine (Oncovin)	1.4 mg/m² i.v.	8	
M	– methotrexate*	120 mg/m² i.v. (bolus)	8	

11. **ProMACE d1/MOPP d8**

Pro	– prednisone	60 mg/m² p.o.	1–14	Repeat every 28 days
M	– methotrexate*	500 mg/m² i.v. (over 1 hour)	15	
A	– doxorubicin (Adriamycin)	25 mg/m² i.v.	1	
C	– cyclophosphamide	650 mg/m² i.v.	1	
E	– etoposide	120 mg/m² i.v.	1	
M	– mechlorethamine	6 mg/m² i.v.	8	
O	– vincristine (Oncovin)	1.4 mg/m² i.v.	8	
P	– procarbazine	100 mg/m² p.o.	d8-14	

12. **MACOP-B**

M	– methotrexate*	400 mg/m² i.v. (100 mg/m² i.v. bolus, then 300 mg/m² i.v. over 4 hours)	8, 36 64	Repeat every 84 days
A	– doxorubicin (Adriamycin)	50 mg/m² i.v.	1, 15, 29, 43, 57, 71	
C	– cyclophosphamide	350 mg/m² i.v.	1, 15, 29, 43, 57, 71	
O	– vincristine (Oncovin)	1.4 mg/m² i.v. (max. 2.0 mg)	8, 22, 36, 50, 64, 78	
P	– prednisone	75 mg/m² p.o.	1–84	
B	– bleomycin	10 u/m² i.v.	22, 50, 78	

*Leucovorin rescue is given 24 hours after each methotrexate dose.
i.v., intravenously; p.o., by mouth

regimens, MACOP-B introduces multiple drugs early in the course of treatment. Myelosuppressive therapy is given on alternate weeks relative to non-myelosuppressive therapy. As initially reported, the MACOP-B regimen yielded an 84 per cent complete remission rate with a relapse rate of only 10 per cent. In a recent update, the relapse rate is higher, at 16 per cent, with approximately 66 per cent of all treated patients achieving a durable complete remission.[14] Peculiar to this regimen is mucocutaneous toxicity which was seen in 40 per cent of patients. While myelosuppression was observed, the major dose-limiting toxicity of the regimen has been mucositis. Toxic deaths occurred in 3 per cent of patients similar to the rate seen with the other third generation regimens.

It appears that the second and third generation regimens for the diffuse aggressive lymphomas offer a considerable improvement over first generation regimens both with respect to complete remission rate and overall disease-free survival. This has been at the expense of increased toxicity as well as considerably increased cost. If, in fact, these regimens are superior, the increased cost and toxicity are certainly justified. A note of caution is warranted, however, in concluding that the results obtained are superior. Most of the second and third generation results have been obtained in single institution studies. In general, results from single institutions are better than those obtained in cooperative group trials. Furthermore, results obtained with the MACOP-B regimen at Memorial Sloan-Kettering[15] were significantly worse than the results reported by Klimo and Connor.[13] While there are many reasons why results are better at the institution where a regimen is designed and initially tested, the fact remains that most patients with diffuse aggressive lymphomas are not treated in the context of an academic institution. Hence it remains to be shown that in a cooperative group or a community setting, the second and third generation regimens are superior to the earlier regimens. As noted previously the CHOP regimen is probably the most widely used programme for the treatment of the diffuse aggressive lymphomas. As noted

above in a large group of patients, CHOP yielded a 53 per cent complete response rate with 30 per cent of all treated patients being cured. In a further analysis of the data, age proved to be a significant determinant of survival since 45 per cent of all patients who were less than 55 years old at the time of treatment were cured with this regimen. Older patients tended to be treated less aggressively with frequent dosage reductions; however, even the older patients who received full dosages had a worse prognosis. These facts must be taken into consideration when comparing the CHOP regimen with the more recently reported regimens.

Early stage disease (stage I and stage II (non-bulky))

With regard to stage, most investigators would agree that patients with stage I and stage II (non-bulky) disease should be approached differently from patients with stage II (bulky), stage III and stage IV disease.

The role of radiation therapy as the sole modality of treatment has now been clearly defined. Investigators at the University of Chicago staged 31 patients with exploratory laparotomy with 17 patients being staged as pathological stage I and 14 patients as pathological stage II.[16] All patients subsequently received extended field or total nodal radiation therapy with curative intent. Twenty-nine patients achieved a complete remission with radiation therapy alone. However, survival at 10 years was 70 per cent for patients with pathological stage I disease but only 46 per cent for patients who were pathological stage II disease. Hence it is clear that radiation therapy as the sole modality of treatment is appropriate for those few patients who, after meticulous staging including a formal staging laparotomy, are found to have stage I disease. In general, such extensive pathological staging is not undertaken and most investigators would now advise the use of systemic chemotherapy for patients with early stage disease since, in the majority of cases, the diffuse aggressive lymphomas are systemic diseases at diagnosis.

Issues which remain unanswered are whether

radiation therapy should be used in conjunction with chemotherapy and which combination chemotherapy regimen should be used in this setting. Ongoing studies at this time are attempting to answer these questions.

Investigators in Milan have recently reported the five-year results of treatment of 159 stage I and stage II patients with diffuse aggressive lymphomas.[17,18] Patients were randomized to receive CVP-radiation therapy-CVP (*see* Table 21.5), or BACOP-radiation therapy-BACOP (*see* Table 21.5). The design of the study was such that the relative merits of CVP and BACOP could be compared and, in addition, the advantage of a sandwich technique in avoiding or limiting disease progression as had been observed during radiation therapy could be evaluated. Relapse-free survival and overall survival were significantly superior in the group receiving the BACOP regimen suggesting that the drugs doxorubicin and bleomycin contributed to the improved results seen with the BACOP arm.

Miller and Jones in a non-randomized study have raised the issue of whether radiation therapy is needed in the setting of early stage disease.[19] A total of 41 patients with stage I and stage II diffuse large cell lymphoma were treated with the CHOP regimen. Seventeen of the 41 received involved field radiation therapy at the completion of chemotherapy. Ninety-eight per cent of patients entered complete remission and 84 per cent remained in remission with a median follow-up of 41 months. While there was a trend in disease-free and overall survival for the group which had received radiation therapy, the differences were not statistically significant.

Current cooperative group studies include randomized trials to determine whether radiation therapy is needed in addition to chemotherapy and what the optimal number of cycles of chemotherapy is. At present the CHOP regimen is being used, since it has been shown to produce excellent results in early stage disease. Whether second and third generation regimens will offer any advantage over the CHOP regimen remains to be tested in randomized studies.

Advanced stage disease stage II (bulky), stages III and IV

For patients with stage II (bulky), III and IV disease, it is clear that an aggressive chemotherapy approach is mandatory if the patient is to be cured. While it would appear that second and third generation regimens give significantly better results than those achieved with the CHOP regimen, it is important to appreciate that each of these regimens has been reported as a single institution study and one cannot compare these newer regimens with the CHOP regimen, as given by the Southwest Oncology Group (SWOG) in a retrospective manner. Of note, SWOG recently completed a series of phase II studies in which the m-BACOD, ProMACE-CytaBOM and MACOP-B regimens were tested in a cooperative group setting.[20] These pilot studies showed that the aggressive regimens can be safely used in multi-institutional trials. As expected, the complete remission rates of 58–65 per cent which were observed were less than those reported in single institution studies. It is also of interest that these response rates are not markedly different from the complete response rates seen with the CHOP regimen in cooperative group studies. The expense and increased toxicity of the newer regimens are acceptable if response rates and cure rates are improved. However, if there is no difference as compared with the CHOP regimen, such increased risk to the patient is not warranted.

A randomized trial comparing the four regimens, CHOP, M-BACOD, ProMACE-CytaBOM and MACOP-B is currently being conducted. The study, which will involve several hundred patients, will hopefully provide the answer as to whether any of these regimens is superior to the others. It is anticipated that the results of this study will have a major impact on the treatment of the diffuse aggressive lymphomas.

Until this study is completed, there is no correct answer regarding the most appropriate regimen to use in the treatment of these lymphomas. We believe that if patients are not participating in a clinical trial, then the choice of regimen should be dictated by which regimen the treating physician is familiar with and by the sophistication of the support facilities available to the treating physician. The more aggressive regimens are associated with significant morbidity and a toxic death rate of approximately 4–5 per cent. Such treatment should be undertaken only in situations where the patient can be supported through the complications of therapy. Because of our familiarity with the ProMACE-based regimens and because we believe these are effective, our choice would be to use one of these in treating a patient who is not participating in a research protocol. For patients who are not able to tolerate the drug doxorubicin, we believe that the COMLA or C-MOPP regimens are reasonable alternatives.

Salvage therapy

Patients who do not achieve a complete remission with initial therapy present difficult management problems. A rare patient may enter a short complete remission with another first line regimen. The vast majority of patients, however, will not achieve a meaningful response with this approach. There are at present no truly useful salvage regimens for patients who fail to achieve complete remission with initial therapy. The drugs cisplatin, amsacrine, etoposide and ifosfamide used either alone or in combination in single institution studies have yielded responses in some patients failing conventional therapy.[21] Unfortunately durations of remissions have been short in most instances.

The role of biological response modifiers (BRM) in the treatment of the diffuse aggressive lymphomas remains to be defined. From preliminary studies, it appears that α-interferon contributes very little to the management of refractory diseases. Currently the role of interleukin-2 in combination with lymphocyte activated killer cells (LAK) as a salvage approach is being evaluated in clinical trials conducted under the auspices of the National Cancer Institute. While BRM may play a role in salvage therapy, it appears more likely that immunological approaches will be more successful in those situations where the tumour burden is low.

The most encouraging results of salvage therapy have been achieved with high dose chemotherapy in conjunction with autologous bone marrow transplantation. Approximately 20 per cent of all patients have achieved long-term unmaintained complete remissions with autologous bone marrow transplant. This topic is discussed in detail in Chapter 25.

Patient follow-up

Patients with diffuse aggressive lymphoma require follow-up for the remainder of their lives. The period of greatest risk of relapse is in the 24 months following completion of therapy. Approximately one month after completion of therapy, patients should undergo a restaging evaluation. This involves the repetition of all tests which were abnormal prior to the initiation of therapy. Patients who have achieved a complete remission should be examined at one-month intervals during the first year and two-month intervals during the second year following completion of therapy. Following a two-year disease-free interval, patients should be evaluated every three months thereafter.

Conclusion

The diffuse aggressive lymphomas, while fatal if untreated, can be cured in a significant number of patients. Because the patient's only significant chance of cure rests with initial therapy, we recommend that the physician choose therapy wisely, treat aggressively and modify drug dosages only as specified for each regimen. To do otherwise may unnecessarily deny the patient the possibility of cure.

References

1. Cossman J, Jaffe ES, Fisher RI. *Cancer*. 1984; **54**, 1310.
2. DeVita VT, Canellos GP, Chabner BA, *et al. Lancet*. 1975; **i**, 248.
3. Jones SE, Grozea PN, Metz EN, *et al. Cancer*. 1979; **43**, 417.
4. Coltman CA, Dahlberg S, Jones SE, *et al. Advances in Cancer Chemotherapy*. 1986; 71–8.

5. Schein P, DeVita VT, Hubbard S, *et al. American Journal of Medicine.* 1976; **85**, 417.

6. Gaynor ER, Ultmann JE, Golomb HM, *et al. Journal of Clinical Oncology.* 1985; **3**, 1596.

7. Fisher R, Hubbard SM, DeVita VT, *et al. Blood.* 1981; **58**, 45.

8. Lawrence J, Coleman M, Allen SL, *et al. Annals of Internal Medicine.* 1982; **97**, 190.

9. Skarin AT, Canellos GR, Rosenthal DS, *et al. Journal of Clinical Oncology.* 1983; **1**, 91.

10. Skarin AT, Canellos GP, Rosenthal DS, *et al.* In: Cavalli F, Bonadonna G, Rosenczweig M (eds). *Proceedings of the Second International Conference on Malignant Lymphoma* 1984; Boston: Martinus Nijhoff. 59.

11. Fisher RI, DeVita VT, Hubbard SM, *et al. Annals of Internal Medicine.* 1983; **98**, 304.

12. Longo D, DeVita VT, Duffey P, *et al. Proceedings of the American Society of Clinical Oncology.* 1987; **6**, 811. (Abstract)

13. Klimo P, Conner JM. *Annals of Internal Medicine.* 1985; **102**, 596.

14. Conners JM. *Issues in Oncology.* 1986; **3**, 1.

15. Lowenthal DA, White A, Koziner B, *et al. Proceedings of the American Society of Clinical Oncology.* 1987; **6**, 201.

16. Voves EE, Ultmann JE, Golomb HM, *et al. Journal of Clinical Oncology.* 1985; **3**, 1309.

17. Monfardini S, Banfi A, Bonnadonna G, *et al. International Journal of Radiation, Oncology, Biology and Physics.* 1980; **6**, 125.

18. Bonaddona G. *Seminars in Oncology.* 1985; **12** (supplement 6), 1.

19. Miller T, Jones SE. *Blood.* 1983; **62**, 413.

20. Fisher RI, Miller TP, Dana BW. *Seminars in Hematology,* 1987; **24**, (supplement 1), 21.

21. Cabanillas F, Hagemeister FB, Bodey GP, *et al. Blood.* 1982; **60**, 693.

CHAPTER 22

T-CELL LYMPHORETICULAR MALIGNANCIES IN ADULTS

Ray Lamb and Paul A Bunn Jr

With the advent of phenotypic cell surface marker analysis, using immunohistological stains, flow cytometry and genotypic analysis with immunoglobulin and T-cell receptor gene probes, we can classify lymphomas more specifically. Prior to the availability of these tools the non-Hodgkin's lymphomas (NHLs) were classified by morphological analysis. Now, using new technology we can classify the NHLs not only into B-cell or T-cell subsets but can also subclassify the T-cell diseases into helper, suppressor, immature, intermediate or mature groups.[1–5] This new technology has allowed recently identified diseases of T-cell origin to be classified and has led to the first direct evidence of viral induction of human malignances.[6–9]

In the USA, T-cell lymphomas are not as common as B-cell lymphomas, but in other parts of the world, such as Japan, the reverse is true. In the USA, lymphomas of T-cell origin comprise less than 1 per cent of the low-grade lymphomas; whereas 15–40 per cent of high grade malignancies are of T-cell origin.[4] Acute lymphoblastic leukaemia (ALL) of T-cell origin is the second most common type of ALL and can be considered as the haematological phase of the T-cell lymphoblastic lymphoma.[10] This chapter deals with diseases of T-cell origin not covered in Chapter 16 (lymphoblastic lymphoma) or Chapter 19 (high grade lymphomas including T-cell). Table 22.1 gives an overview of the classification of T-cell neoplasms.

Cutaneous T-cell lymphoma (mycosis fungoides and the Sézary syndrome)

Definition and general description

Descriptions of the cutaneous and clinical manifestations of the cutaneous T-cell lymphomas (CTCLs) have evolved over 50 years, but the pathophysiological understanding of these diseases has developed over the past 15 years.[11,12] Cutaneous T-cell lymphoma was first described by Alibert in 1806 with the name mycosis fungoides (MF) being based on the mushroom-like nature of the tumours.[13] In 1870, Bazin described the classical cutaneous stages of the disease with the usual progression from a premycotic phase, infiltrated plaques and finally to cutaneous tumours.[11] The *d'emblee* variant, characterized by the *de novo* appearance of tumours without prior skin involvement, was described in 1885. Pathologically, Pautrier described the characteristic finding of intraepidermal microabscesses of tumour cells in the early twentieth century.[11] This led to the theory of the epidermotropic nature of the malignant cells and the concept of skin-associated lymphoid tissue (SALT).[14] While an erythrodermic variant of MF was described as early as 1892, it was Sézary who, in 1938, recognized the classic syndrome which now bears his name, consisting of generalized erythroderma and malignant cells in the peripheral blood.[15] Lutzner and Jordan in 1968 described the ultrastructural appearance of the Sézary and mycosis cell with a convoluted or cerebriform nucleus with condensed heterochromatin.[16] In 1970, Crossen *et al.* described the lymphocytic properties of the abnormal cell, first establishing these disorders as malignant lymphomas.[17] The work of Broder *et al.*[18] and Haynes *et al.*[19] characterized the malignant cell as having phenotypic and functional characteristics of helper T-cell subset. Subsequently Bunn and co-workers[20] showed that these cells always have the genotype of T-cells with monoclonal T-cell receptor gene rearrangements. Recently, evidence has been accrued which indicates a role for a retrovirus related to, but possibly distinct from, human T-cell lymphotrophic virus (HTLV-1) in the pathogenesis of some cutaneous T-cell lymphomas.[8,9]

The malignant cells almost always have identifiable cytogenetic abnormalities although no single abnormality has been universally found.[21] A variety of clonal abnormalities has been reported; none are specific for CTCL.

Clinical features/staging

Natural history

Early estimates had similar numbers of new cases of CTCL with that of Hodgkin's disease but it is now estimated that about 400 new cases of CTCL occur each year with 100–200 deaths per year. While CTCL occurs more frequently in middle-aged individuals it has been shown to occur below the age of 20 and above age 70. It can affect all racial groups and has a slight male predominance of 1.8:1.[22]

The mean interval between onset of skin lesions and histological diagnosis is six years with a range between one month and 48 years. Because of the non-specific nature of the pathological findings it is often difficult to establish a diagnosis during this period. Repeat biopsies are always required and modern immunological and molecular probes should be used. The classic case follows an indolent course

Table 22.1 T-cell lymphoreticular malignancies in adults

		Chemical characteristics	*Surface phenotype*
I.	Diseases with immature phenotypes 1. T-cell acute lymphoblastic leukaemia 2. Lymphoblastic lymphoma	TdT+; aggressive children/adolescents mediastinal masses common	Early thymic or primitive T-cell antigens (3A1, Leu-9, T10, T9)
II. A.	Diseases with mature phenotypes Diseases with aggressive courses 3. Peripheral T-cell lymphomas T-diffuse histiocytic lymphoma T-immunoblastic lymphoma T-diffuse mixed lymphoma	TdT – adults	Post-thymic usually T11+, T4+, T8–, Tac– occasionally T11+, T4+, T8+, Tac–
	4. Adult T-cell leukaemia/lymphoma	Function as T-suppressor cells HTLV-I-positive	T11+, T4+, T8–, Tac+
B.	Diseases with indolent courses 5. Mycosis fungoides and Sézary's syndrome (cutaneous lymphomas)	Function as T- helper cells	T11+, T4+, T8–, Tac–
	6. T-chronic lymphocytic leukaemia		T11+, either T4+ or T8+
	7. T-gamma lymphocytosis with neutropenia		T11+, usually T4–, T8+, T gamma+

with variable duration of the individual phases. The premycotic, erythematous or eczematoid phase progresses from patches to infiltrated, indurated plaques, nodules and tumours which can ulcerate. Erythrodema may be a presenting feature or, less commonly, can evolve from later disease stages. While circulating Sézary cells are mostly associated with erythroderma, up to 25 per cent of patients with MF in plaque and tumour stages have circulating Sézary cells. Several types of clinical lesions may coexist at the same time. Other, less common, presentations of CTCL include lymphomatoid papulosis, alopecia mucinosa, and granulomatous, pustular, bullous or verrucous variants. It is difficult to predict which of these cases will evolve into frank malignant lymphomas and when. These patients should thus be followed carefully with serial biopsies in an identical fashion to those with suspicious patch lesions. Cutaneous T-cell lymphoma can be confused with benign chronic dermatitis with differentiation being made through clinical, immunological, and genotypic studies. The malignant cells, as do normal lymphocytes, migrate through different body compartments. Although cutaneous T-cell lymphoma cells are epidermotropic, kinetic and cell labelling studies indicate the major region of cell replication is in the skin and in the lymph nodes.[23] The question of whether the initial site of oncogenesis in cutaneous T-cell lymphoma is cutaneous or whether the skin acts as a homing organ for these neoplastic T-cell remains unresolved.

In various series the median survival after biopsy diagnosis ranges from three to 10 years; earlier series report post-diagnosis survival of three to five years, but more recent studies show median survival of 9–10 years after diagnosis.[11,12,24] It is not known if this difference is due to earlier diagnosis, improved survival with newer modalities of treatment or both. Cytological transformation to more aggressive histological types of lymphoma in CTCL patients has recently been shown to be associated with a poor outcome in analogy to similar conversion with low-grade B-cell lymphomas.[25]

The most frequent cause of death is infection, accounting for 50 per cent of all deaths.[24,26] The skin is the most common site of infection with the lungs as the second most frequent. Progressive, disseminated cutaneous T-cell lymphoma with widespread visceral involvement is the second most common cause of death after infection.

Cutaneous T-cell lymphoma has been associated with other malignant diseases, especially Hodgkin's disease. The reasons for the higher than expected concurrence of these two malignancies is unclear. Associated acute myeloblastic leukaemia, sideroblastic anaemia or refractory anaemia with excess myeloblasts have been reported.[27] Epithelial skin cancers, basal cell or squamous cell, have also been reported in approximately 10 per cent of cases. These neoplasms developed prior to treatment in 4 per cent of patients and after topical nitrogen mustard in 6.5 per cent. Second skin cancers have also been reported after PUVA and electron beam therapy.[28–30].

Aetiology

The aetiology is unknown, but various environmental, genetic, and infectious factors have been implicated. There is a frequent history of exposure to toxic chemicals, physical agents, and drugs, and a higher-than-expected employment in plants manufacturing textiles, petrochemicals, metals, and machinery.[22,31,32] These observations are consistent with chronic immunological stimulation leading to malignant transformation. There are reports of at least four families with more than one member having mycosis fungoides in addition to other lymphomas and leukaemias.[22]

Virus-like particles have been reported in biopsies of patients with cutaneous T-cell lymphoma.[33] The human T-cell lymphotrophic virus (HTLV-I), a type C retrovirus known to be the causative agent for adult T-cell leukaemia/lymphoma (ATLL, *see* below), has been implicated in CTCL.[8,33–35] In a European study of patients with early or suspected disease, a higher than expected frequency of anti-HTLV-I antibody was found.[35] However, most serological surveys of CTCL patients have shown a very low presence of antibodies to this virus.[36] The absence of epidemiological evidence for clustering of cases argues against a common retroviral aetiology. Recently a putative aetiological retrovirus, HTLV-V, was isolated from a cell line derived from a CTCL patient.[9] However, the absence of epidemiological evidence for clustering of cases argues against a retroviral aetiology.

Clinical and pathological staging

Age, absolute lymphocyte count, extent of disease and symtomatology have been reported to have prognostic significance. However the only consistent factor is extent of disease.[11,12,24,37–39] As shown in Fig. 22.1(a-d) survival is dependent upon extent of disease at time of diagnosis. The extent of disease is determined by the type and extent of skin lesions (T-stage), the presence or absence of peripheral blood involvement (B-stage), whether or not peripheral nodes are positive or effaced (N-stage), and the presence or absence of extracutaneous disease (M-stage).

This TNM system was devised by the Mycosis Fungoides Cooperative Study Group and modified by the cutaneous T-cell lymphoma workshop[40] (Table 22.2). Cutaneous forms of the disease in which erythematous patches and plaques cover less than 10 per cent of the skin surface are called T1 (limited plaque stage). When plaques cover 10 per cent or more of the skin surface, the designation is T2. When one or more cutaneous tumours are present the designation is T3, and generalized erythroderma is classified as T4. The frequency of each of these types in recent large series is: limited plaque (38 per cent), generalized plaque (28 per cent), cutaneous tumour (17 per cent) and generalized erythroderma (17 per cent).

The lymph nodes are classified as N0 if there are no clinically or pathologically abnormal lymph nodes; N1 is the designation for clinically abnormal lymph nodes with pathology negative for CTCL (pathological stage LN1 or 2); N2 represents no clinical abnormal lymph nodes but pathology is positive (LN3 or 4); and N3 represents lymph nodes which are clinically abnormal and pathologically positive (LN3 or 4). Peripheral blood involvement is called B0 if less than 15 per cent atypical circulating cells are found or B1 if more than 15 per cent typical circulating cells are present. M0 is reserved for no clinical evidence of visceral organ involvement and M1 is for positive visceral involvement, as proven by pathological specimens.

The TNM system is used to stage CTCL; however, the presence or absence of peripheral blood involvement should always be noted. Stage I is where skin lesions are limited to the plaque stage (T1 or 2) without any lymph node or visceral involvement. Stage II is plaque stage (T1 or 2) with clinically abnormal but pathologically uninvolved lymph nodes (LN1 or 2) or tumour stage T3 with normal or clinical involvement of nodes. Stage III is similar to stage II in terms of node status and visceral involvement but with generalized erythroderma. Stage IV can be any skin stage but has pathologically involved lymph nodes (LN3 or 4; stage IVA) or visceral involvement (stage IVB).

The cutaneous manifestations of cutaneous T-cell lymphomas vary widely. They are typically non-specific, being diagnosed as eczema, psoriasis, neurodermatitis, erythema, parapsoriasis-en plaque, poikiloderma, tinea corporis, contact dermatitis, and even secondary syphilis.[11,12,24] These lesions of the 'premycotic or erythematous stage' may be transitory in nature over a period of months to years and may be associated or even preceded by severe pruritus.

The patch/plaque stage represents the earliest stage where the clinical lesions show definitive histological features of cutaneous T-cell lymphoma (Fig. 22.2a). The plaques can occur anywhere on the body but have a predilection for buttocks, thighs, abdomen and the breast area of women. The random distribution of lesions is a distinguishing feature that contrasts with the symmetry of psoriasis and the flexural involvement in atopic dermatitis. Lesions tend to persist with little spontaneous resolution, although temporary improvement can occur with non-specific treatment. With progression of disease, new lesions may appear and/or gradual thickening of the patches can occur to evolve into plaques. Pruritus is a prominent but variable feature. The plaques gradually increase in size and can coalesce so that extensive lesions

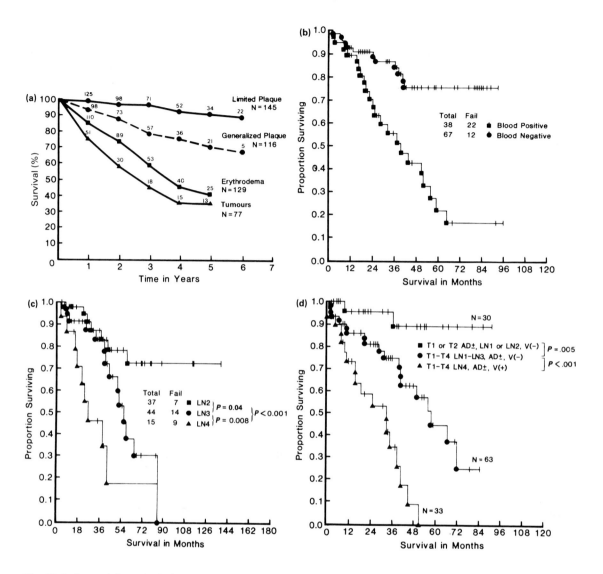

Fig. 22.1 Actuarial survival of patients by skin stage, peripheral blood, lymph node, and visceral involvement.
(a) Survival of patients by skin stage. Patients with tumours or generalized erythroderma have a shorter
survival time than do patients with only limited or generalized plaques.[11] (b) Patients with peripheral blood
involvement have a significantly shorter survival than those patients whose blood is not clinically involved.[31]
(c) Patients with dermatopathic lymphadenopathy and only a small number of MF cells (LN2) had superior
survival to those with dermatopathic changes and large clusters of paracortical MF cells (LN3), who in turn had
a superior survival to those with partially or completely effaced node architecture (LN4).[30] (d) This graph shows
survival in patients can be divided into three prognostic groups based on skin, node and visceral findings.
Patients with plaque disease (T1-2) with minimal node involvement (LN1-2) and no visceral involvement V(−)
have an excellent prognosis with 90% predicted survival at 7+ years as shown in the upper curve. Patients with
tumours or erythroderma (T3-4) without effaced nodes (LN2) or visceral involvement V(−) and patients with
plaques (T1-2) with moderate node involvement (LN3) and no visceral involvement V(−) have an intermediate
prognosis as shown by the middle curve. Patients with effaced lymph nodes (LN4) or visceral involvement V(+)
have the worst prognosis as shown in the lower curve. (AD± means with or without palpable adenopathy). The
data in (d) are from unpublished results from the NCI series.

are formed. Healing in the centre can give rise to annular figures; they may be thin and only slightly elevated or may show marked induration. Lesions of the scalp may be associated with alopecia, while lesions on palms and soles show either localized plaques or diffuse hyperkeratosis.

In the tumour stage, masses may appear in previously normal skin, in premycotic lesions or in infiltrated plaques (Fig. 22.2b). They tend to occur on the face or in the body folds, e.g. axillae, groin, antecubital folds, neck and breasts, but can occur anywhere. The rate of growth of the tumours can vary from very slow to a rapid growth rate. Tumours may regress spontaneously but the majority persist and

Table 22.2 Staging of cutaneous T-cell lymphoma

Classification		Description
T:	Skin	
	T0	Clinically and/or histopathologically suspicious lesions
	T1	Limited plaques, papules, or eczematous patches covering <10% of skin
	T2	Generalized plaques, papules, or erythematous patches covering >10% of skin surface
	T3	Tumours, one or more
	T4	Generalized erythroderma
N:	Lymph nodes	
	N0	No clinically abnormal peripheral lymph nodes, pathology negative for CTCL
	N1	Clinically abnormal peripheral lymph nodes, pathology negative for CTCL
	N2	No clinically abnormal peripheral lymph nodes, pathology positive for CTCL
	N3	Clinically abnormal peripheral lymph nodes, pathology positive for CTCL
B:	Peripheral blood	
	B0	<15% atypical circulating cells
	B1	>15% atypical circulating cells: total WBC, total lymphocyte count and number of atypical cells/100 lymphocytes recorded
M:	Visceral organs	
	M0	No involvement of visceral organs
	M1	Visceral involvement (must have confirmation of pathology and organ involved should be specified)

Stage	T	N	M
IA	1	0	0
IB	2	0	0
IIA	1–2	1	0
IIB	3	0,1	0
III	4	0,1	0
IVA	1–4	2,3	0
IVB	1–4	0–3	1

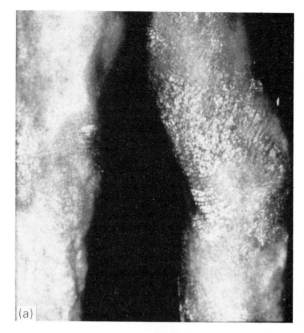

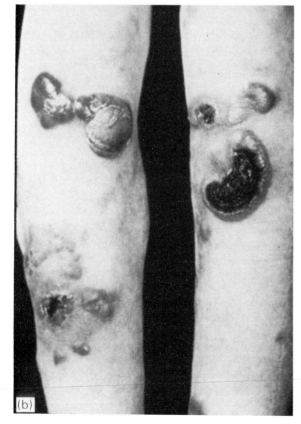

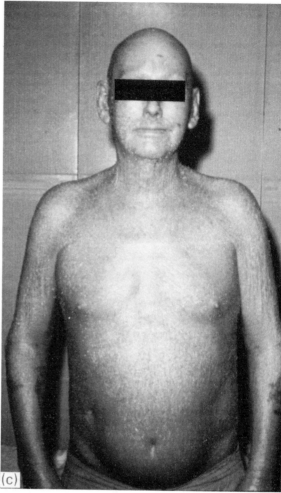

Fig. 22.2 (a) An example of the generalized plaque (T2) stage of CTCL; (b) An example of the tumour stage (T3) of CTCL; (c) An example of generalized erythroderma (T4) stage of CTCL.[11]

continue to grow; many will eventually ulcerate. They are usually painless but have a tendency to become secondarily infected, especially if ulcerated. Pruritus tends to decrease in the tumour stage. Occasionally cutaneous T-cell lymphoma may result in a leonine facies suggestive of leprosy.

A variant of the tumour stage that tends to develop within clinically normal skin instead of pre-existing plaques or patches has been termed *d'emblee*. Patients with the *d'emblee* form of CTCL tend to have a more rapid progression of their disease than patients with the classic forms.

Generalized erythroderma may be the presenting sign of cutaneous T-cell lymphoma or, less commonly, may develop from pre-existing premycotic, plaque, or patch stages of disease (Fig. 22.2c). Erythroderma usually involves most of the skin surface, although areas of normal skin can persist. Pruritus leading to excoriation and secondary infections is extremely common. The Sézary syndrome represents the leukaemic phase of CTCL, with clinical features of pruritus, generalized exfoliative erythroderma and abnormal hyperchromatic and hyperconvoluted mononuclear cells in the peripheral blood. Since most patients with generalized erythroderma have circulating Sézary cells there is no clear distinction between the erythrodermic form of mycosis fungoides and the Sézary syndrome. There debate as to the level of circulating Sézary cells that is necessary to make the diagnosis; more than 15 per cent of circulating lymphocytes is generally accepted.[39] Other features associated with the Sézary syndrome include ocular ectropion, dystrophic nails, hyperkeratosis of the palms and soles with painful fissuring, partial alopecia and generalized hyperpigmentation.

At the time of diagnosis and in autopsy series, extracutaneous disease is most common in lymph nodes or in the peripheral blood.[11,37–39] The presence or absence of and extent of disease in these sites provides important prognostic information.[37–39] Lymphadenopathy is present in about 47 per cent of patients at diagnosis. The frequency of adenopathy is related to cutaneous findings. It is present in 17 per cent of those with limited plaque lesions; 44 per cent with generalized plaques; 56 per cent with tumours; and 85 per cent with generalized ery-

throderma.[37,38] Histological classification of nodal involvement improves the prognostic information provided by the physical examination of nodal areas. The classification of Matthews is recommended in which nodal histology is divided into the presence of dermatopathic changes alone, dermatopathic changes with small clusters of mycosis cells, dermatopathic changes with large clusters of mycosis cells, or effacement of nodal architecture.[38] Prognosis is related to the degree of nodal involvement. Lymph node biopsies should be performed on all patients with adenopathy and blind lymph node biopsies should be considered in early stage patients without adenopathy. Lymphangiograms do not appear to provide prognostic information not provided by physical examination and node biopsy.[38] Therefore the routine use of this procedure is not recommended.

Evaluation of peripheral blood should be performed in all patients as it also provides prognostic information.[39,41] The complete blood count may show lymphocytosis with Sézary cells in patients with any stage; lymphopenia is also frequently found. Patients with generalized erythroderma invariably have circulating Sézary cells. The reporting should include the total white blood cell count, the total lymphocyte count, and the number of Sézary cells, because studies show that the absolute number of Sézary cells as well as their presence or absence provides prognostic information.[39,41]

While visceral spread is found in the vast majority of patients at autopsy, it is identified in a minority of patients at the time of diagnosis. Cutaneous T-cell lymphoma can involve any organ system, with autopsy series showing 72 per cent having some form of extracutaneous involvement. Since most tests of organ systems have no pathognomonic findings for CTCL any true involvement must be diagnosed by a high index of suspicion and have histological confirmation.[37–39] The most frequently involved organs, in descending order include spleen (52 per cent); liver (42 per cent); bone marrow (32 per cent); gastrointestinal tract (31 per cent); kidneys (28 per cent); heart (21 per cent); and central nervous system (18 per cent).[11]

Clinical manifestations of pulmonary lesions include parenchymal nodules, infiltrates, effusions and adenopathy of the mediastinum and/or hilum. Bone marrow involvement is uncommon at diagnosis; circulating cells may originate in skin or lymph nodes. Bone lesions are rare and the presence of osteolytic lesions should lead to a search for HTLV-I. Involvement of the oral–gastrointestinal tract including lips, buccal mucosa, tongue and lower gastrointestinal tract is rare. When involved, these may present with diarrhoea, ascites and gastrointestinal bleeding.[11] Central nervous system involvement is usually manifested as lymphomatous leptomeningitis. Work-up for other organ involvement should only be undertaken when directed by clinical signs and symptoms because asymptomatic organ infiltration is uncommon.

Baseline radiological studies should include a chest film to detect pulmonary involvement; findings of parenchymal disease are usually seen only in advanced disease, but a baseline film may prove useful when symptoms appear and one wishes to know if the X-ray findings are old or new. Consideration of abdominal computed tomographic (CT) scans may be entertained as a staging procedure to reveal hepatosplenomegaly or other signs of visceral involvement, but the benefits gained may not be worth the expense. Additional radiological studies are not necessary in the staging work-up unless clinically indicated by specific signs or symptoms. Routine chemical screening is generally unremarkable until late-stage disseminated disease. While elevated levels of serum lactic acid dehydrogenase, serum IgE, and eosinophils are frequently found, the utility of following these parameters has never been determined. The use of bone marrow biopsy is reasonable, especially in patients with erythroderma or who have positive lymph nodes. A liver biopsy is recommended in patients who have a positive bone marrow, lymph nodes or peripheral blood. Evaluation of the immune system is not warranted in all patients since clinical evidence of alterations in immune function is not seen until advanced stages of the disease. Delayed hypersensitivity reactions to skin test antigens are normal in early stages but become depressed in later stages of disease. Mitogenic responses of the malignant cells are usually depressed compared to normal lymphocytes.

Immunohistological and molecular studies can be very helpful in differentiating between chronic benign dermatitic lesions and cutaneous T-cell lymphoma.[42,43] A complete drug history should be obtained since the use of certain antihypertensive agents may produce a cutaneous histopathology similar to that of cutaneous T-cell lymphoma.[44] The typical histological features of CTCL in skin biopsies include the presence of a band-like polymorphic infiltrate of mononuclear cells in the upper dermis, hugging the epidermis.[11,12] Epidermotropism with single cell or clusters of cells invading the epidermis is always present. The presence of such intraepidermal clusters of cells, termed Pautrier's microabscesses (Fig. 22.3), is nearly pathognomonic of CTCL. The infiltrate may extend deeper into the dermis as the disease progresses. Involvement of the deep dermis with sparing of the upper dermis suggests the presence of a different form of lymphoma.

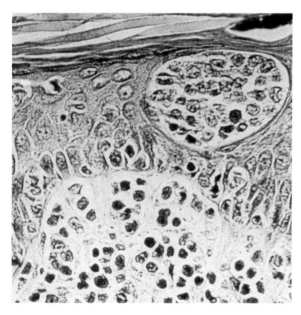

Fig. 22.3 Skin biopsy showing an infiltrate containing atypical convoluted lymphocytes in the upper dermis and intraepidermal Pautrier abscesses.

Treatment

There are four standard therapeutic modalities for treatment of CTCL: topical chemotherapy, particularly with topical application of mechlorethamine (nitrogen mustard, HN2); radiation therapy, including whole body electron-beam irradiation; photochemotherapy with oral methoxsalen and ultraviolet A light (PUVA); and systemic chemotherapy.[28–30,45] These modalities give remission rates of 90 per cent, but duration of remission is quite short. Much recent work has been undertaken using investigational therapeutic modalities including interferon, monoclonal antibodies, leucopheresis, antithymocyte globulin (ATG), retinoids, acyclovir, cyclosporin, and extracorporeal photochemotherapy.[45–52]

Topical chemotherapy

The clinical use of topical HN2 for CTCL has been known for over 25 years. The use of dilute aqueous solutions (10 mg/50 ml) of HN2 applied to the entire cutaneous surface of patients on a daily basis has led to remission rates ranging from 59 to 94 per cent, depending on the skin stage at time of treatment.[45] In 243 patients treated with HN2 the remission rate was 94 per cent of T1 patients versus 59 per cent of T4. Topical HN2 is available throughout the country, is inexpensive and is free of systemic side-effects; all attributes which have led to it becoming a standard approach in CTCL treatment. However, the limitations include 40 per cent of patients developing hypersensitivity reactions, the inconvenience of daily application, the recurrence of hypersensitivity reactions, the recurrence of disease after cessation of therapy in a majority of patients, xerosis, hyperpigmentation and an increased frequency of epithelial neoplasms. In some cases hypersensitivity can be overcome by topical desensitization procedures. The Stanford series[61], using HN2 in polyethyleneglycol (PEG) or in aquaphor, shows excellent results with markedly decreased rates of hypersensitivity reactions.

Other topical agents include the nitrosourea, BCNU, and bleomycin.[28] Similar to HN2, BCNU can be applied to the skin in aqueous solutions or ointment-based preparations. However, BCNU must be used intermittently, as opposed to daily HN2, due to its myelosuppressive ability. In addition, other adverse side-effects include cutaneous irritation, telangiectasia, hyperpigmentation and potential for secondary epithelial neoplasms. The main use of BCNU is therefore for patients unable to use HN2 because of cutaneous allergies or progression limited to the skin.

Radiation therapy

The lesions of CTCL are very sensitive to ionizing radiation and tend to regress with relatively small doses of superficial X-rays, electron-beam or photon radiation. The total dose of radiation is very important with doses of 3000 cGy, or more, having a higher complete remission rate and better disease-free survival rates than lower doses.[28,29] The Stanford group has reported long-term follow-up on a large number of patients given total skin electron-beam therapy.[29] Complete remissions were obtained in 84 per cent of patients with five-year survival of 65 per cent. Of interest, only 20 per cent of the patients were still disease free at three years, but late relapses after three years were not reported in the Stanford experience as opposed to the continued late relapse rates seen with topical HN2. Similar to topical chemotherapy, the complete responses were associated with the cutaneous stage of disease; rates were highest for T1 lesions and lowest for T3 and T4 lesions. The best fractionation schedule has yet to be determined, but most groups employ the four times weekly schedule developed at Stanford. This provides results which appear superior to a once weekly schedule.[29,53] However, it is felt that this modality of therapy is quite toxic and rarely curative. Thus, it is being used less often as an initial therapy. It is not clear whether the early use of this modality is superior to topical HN2 or PUVA which are, perhaps, less toxic.

The use of local-field radiation is felt to be useful to clear deep-seated cutaneous lesions or lesions located in difficult to treat areas in patients treated primarily with other topical modalities. Some patients with indolent disease may enjoy extended disease-free periods with the use of local-field radiation alone.[28]

Difficulties in the use of radiation include unequal exposure to all parts of the skin, especially the scalp, perineal area, and soles of the feet. Attempts to overcome this problem include the use of multiple overlapping fields. Adverse effects of total skin electron-beam therapy are dose dependent; they include erythema, blistering, temporary or permanent hair loss, nail loss, arthralgias, gynaecomastia, skin atrophy, telangiectasias, xerosis, hyperpigmentation, and loss of eccrine gland function. Skin cancers occurring after radiation therapy occur but are no more common than compared to the chronic use of topical HN2 or PUVA therapy.

The utility of combining total-skin electron-beam irradiation with total nodal irradiation has been evaluated preliminarily.[54] Complete responses were seen in the majority of cases. Patients with all known disease limited to the skin had a longer duration of remission compared to patients with known adenopathy. Further controlled trials to ascertain the clinical value of this expensive and potentially toxic approach are needed prior to recommending it for routine therapy. Similarly, the use of total body photon irradiation has been tried with only limited success and should not be used outside a research setting.[50]

PUVA

Methoxsalen (8-methoxypsoralen) is a phototoxic furocoumarin compound which is activated by ultraviolet light, usually in the A range. When used at 0.6 mg/kg followed two hours later by exposure to long-wave ultraviolet light (PUVA), it results in the binding of the photon excited psoralens to pyrimidine bases in DNA.[30] Since ultraviolet light A penetrates through the upper part of the dermis but only 1 per cent penetrates further into the subcutaneous fat, the activated psoralens affect cells primarily in the epidermis and papillary dermis. Thus, patients with tumours have lower response rates than patients with the plaque or patch stage of disease. Complete remission rates are below that seen with electron-beam but

comparable to those found using topical HN2, averaging 62 per cent. Again, in early stage disease a higher complete remission rate will be seen – up to 90 per cent – but like the aforementioned topical modalities, the curative potential is low.

Adverse reactions to PUVA are primarily cutaneous and are seen as acceleration of pre-existing actinic damage and photocarcinogenesis. Atrophy and dryness of skin is common. Other complications including acute phototoxicity (erythema, pruritus), hyperpigmentation, xerosis, potential cataracts of eyes, and activation of herpes simplex infections.

The exposure of patch or early plaque stage disease to sunlight or ultraviolet light B range can clear a number of the lesions, the mechanism being felt to be direct lymphocytotoxicity. Due to the greater risk of photocarcinogenesis of the B range of ultraviolet light, this practice is not to be recommended as a standard form of therapy.

Systemic chemotherapy

A number of authors have evaluated systemic chemotherapy in the treatment of CTCL with either single agent or combination therapy.[28] Single agents have a reported response rate, (complete response + partial) of 60–70 per cent. The most active agents are methotrexate, alkylating agents, VP-16, and cisplatin. Complete responses are generally in the 20–25 per cent range for the more commonly used single agents but have been reported as more than 60 per cent in patients treated with moderate dose methotrexate (60–240 mg/m^2) with citrovorum rescue.[55]

The use of a combination of active agents has resulted in higher complete remission rates and longer duration of remission.[28,56] Combination chemotherapy has generally been evaluated in patients with advanced stages. Although response rates are quite high, these regimens are *not* curative.[28] And, it has never been proven that combinations improve survival when compared to single agent therapy. Thus, results are similar to those with low grade B-cell lymphomas. It also appears that regimens used in B-cell lymphomas have similar response rates in T-cell lymphomas. The chlorambucil and prednisone, cytoxan plus vincristine plus prednisone (CVP), and CVP plus bleomycin or doxorubicin regimens have been utilized most often.[28,56–59] Increasingly, combination regimens have been used with cutaneous therapies since the skin is the site of 'bulk' disease and the most frequent site of progressive disease.

Combined modality therapy

The systemic nature of CTCL, the presence of bulk disease within the skin, and the failure of single modality therapy to cure the disease led to development of combined treatment approaches. The most heavily studied combinations have included: electron-beam radiation therapy (EBRT) plus chemotherapy; EBRT plus topical HN2; and topical HN2 plus chemotherapy. Trials of PUVA plus chemotherapy or biological response modifiers, and combinations of biological agents are in progress.

Total skin electron irradiation plus chemotherapy was evaluated at the University of Chicago,[57] the National Cancer Institute (NCI),[58,59] and at Yale University.[60] The University of Chicago series employed total skin electron-beam (TSEB) irradiation according to the Stanford technique and combination chemotherapy with MOPP or COPP. In this non-randomized study, survival of patients with advanced stages (about 80 per cent at three years) was felt to be superior to their experience with single modality therapy. The results in patients with cutaneous tumours were felt to be especially gratifying. Results from Yale were similar.[60] A preliminary study at the NCI[58] combined TSEB irradiation with single agent HN2 or with two alternating three drug regimens. The trial showed that the agents could be safely combined, were associated with high complete response rates and produced long disease-free periods in some early stage patients.

Currently the NCI is actively conducting a randomized trial comparing conservative treatment with topical HN2 to combined modality therapy with TSEB irradiation (given by the Stanford technique) plus systemic chemotherapy consisting of cyclophosphamide,

doxorubicin, VP-16, and vincristine (CAPO). This trial has been reported, in abstract form, showing a survival advantage to stage I and II patients treated with combination therapy but no advantage for advanced stage III and IV patients.[59] Final conclusions from this trial await longer follow-up.

At Stanford University the combination of topical HN2 with TSEB irradiation has prolonged remission compared to TSEB irradiation alone.[61] In the Yale experience with TSEB irradiation plus chemotherapy, topical HN2 was often used to prolong remission duration as well.[60] A single institution trial combining topical HN2 with combination chemotherapy (bleomycin + doxorubicin + methotrexate) reported a 70 per cent complete response rate in 10 patients with some responses lasting in excess of 100 months.[62] Thus, it does appear reasonable to combine topical HN2 with either TSEB irradiation or chemotherapy in an attempt to prolong remission duration.

Biological response modifiers

Several biological response modifiers including interferons, polyclonal antibodies, monoclonal antibodies, and antibody conjugates have been evaluated recently and other agents (tumour necrosis factor, interleukin) are likely to be studied in the next few years. The recombinant interferons have a definite role in the therapy of CTCL. Initial studies at the NCI[46] revealed that recombinant interferon is an active single agent in advanced CTCL. In these patients who had failed prior chemotherapy, a response rate of 45 per cent was obtained. Of the 20 original patients, the two who achieved a complete response have both been disease free for more than four years. More recent studies performed at other institutions with earlier stage patients show even more impressive results. In an Italian study, 12 previously untreated patients achieved a response rate of 92 per cent; there were five complete responses, six partial responses, and only one progression.[63] In a US multicentre study there was a mixed patient population of four untreated patients, 10 with prior single agent therapy, and six patients who had received multiagent therapy.[64] Patients received either low dose α-interferon or an escalated dose schedule over a 10-week induction period. Seventy per cent of patients achieved objective antitumour response with three patients (15 per cent) achieving a complete response. A greater percentage of patients treated with the higher dose achieved an objective response. These studies show that human interferon is an effective single-agent therapy for early as well as advanced CTCL. The major dose-limiting toxicity of interferon is a 'flu-like syndrome which is generally transient in nature; other toxicities include liver damage, diarrhoea, and depression. Long-term follow-up will be necessary to determine the durability of the complete responses in these patients.

With the recognition that mycosis fungoides and the Sézary syndrome were malignancies of T-cells, trials of antithymocyte globulin and anti-T-cell antibodies ensued.[28,48] Trials from several centres demonstrated that ATG could produce objective remissions. However, these remissions were of short duration and the ATG was extremely expensive and toxic. This led to monoclonal antibody trials. T65 is a 67 000 dalton antigen present on mature T-cells and nearly all CTCL cells and is recognized by the Leu-1 and T101 (CD5) antibodies. Levy and Miller documented transient decreases in circulating malignant T-cells and an objective remission of cutaneous lesions following the intravenous use of Leu-1.[65,66] Larger follow-up studies at the NCI, the University of California-San Diego, and the University of Southern California[47,67,68] showed that objective remissions were uncommon. This was attributed to antigen modulation and the development of human antimurine antibodies neutralizing the effect of the antibody.

The use of radiolabelled T101 has been investigated for both imaging and therapeutic uses. Indium-111-labelled T101 can be used to image CTCL in cutaneous and nodal sites.[69,70] Objective responses to iodine-133-labelled-T101 were observed in five of six patients treated by Rosen *et al.*; however, ^{131}I-labelled T101 is less stable than the chelated indium conjugate.[71] This therapy produced considerable toxicity and short remissions due in part to dehalogenation *in vivo*. Studies with improved conjugates can be expected in the future.

Miscellaneous

Other treatments of interest include 2'-deoxycoformycin (2'DCF) acyclovir, cyclosporin, and extracorporeal photo-chemotherapy using methoxypsoralen. In general, initial reports of activity for most of these therapies have not yet been confirmed in larger trials. Thus, these therapies must be considered experimental until their role is defined by prospective randomized trials or large multicentre trials. Deoxycoformycin is a potent inhibitor of the enzyme adenosine deaminase. It has been shown to be active in a number of lymphoid malignancies including those of T-cell origin.[72] The drug has considerable toxicities including severe immune depression, anaemia and infections. It is being evaluated in combination with interferon in patients with hairy cell leukaemia. Its use in CTCL patients remains experimental at present.

Acyclovir used in an MF patient with herpes simplex infection was observed to give a temporary complete regression of tumour lesions following intravenous administration of 5 mg/kg every 8 hours for 12–18 days.[50] The patient was maintained on oral acyclovir which kept the disease under partial control. Additional patients are being studied to help ascertain the response rate and toxicity profile of the drug. Some authors have argued that responsiveness to acyclovir is suggestive evidence for a viral aetiology of CTCL.

Meyskens and co-workers have shown short-term benefits in the use of retinoids in CTCL.[49,50] Response rates are lower than those seen with combination systemic and topical therapy but comparable to other single agent therapies. The advantage in the use of retinoids lies in their low toxicity compared to cytotoxic drugs. Trials using retinoids in conjunction with photo-chemotherapy, interferon, or combined chemotherapeutic drug regimens have yet to be reported.

Anecdotal reports of activity of cyclosporin A have also appeared.[51,73] Cyclosporin is a potent inhibitor of T-cell function and proliferation. Thus it is highly toxic and can result in death due to immunosuppression, increased capillary permeability, and renal failure. Patients treated with cyclosporin A have been reported to have their disease rebound when the drug is discontinued, resulting in a worse state than that prior to treatment. Thus, it must be regarded as highly investigational until large trials are complete.

The use of leucopheresis in Sézary syndrome was shown to provide clinical palliation in some CTCL patients especially those with high circulating Sézary cell counts.[74] With the appreciation of PUVA effectiveness, Edelsen *et al.* evaluated extracorporeal photochemotherapy using oral methoxsalen two hours before leucopheresis.[52] The patients had 30–50 per cent of their circulating leucocytes removed and exposed to ultraviolet A (UVA) light. Of 37 evaluable patients, 64 per cent showed a decrease in cutaneous involvement, including 28 patients whose disease was resistant to systemic chemotherapy (the combination of drugs and schedule was not identified). Complications included thrombophlebitis, transient transaminase elevation, fever, hepatitis, herpes zoster, pneumonia and sepsis, each occurring in one patient. The mechanism of action is not known but an immune reaction to the infused damaged cells is felt to be the mode of action. As with other promising modalities, further trials will be necessary to determine the ultimate role of this modality in the treatment of CTCL.

Recommendations for treatment

The treatments listed in the previous sections produce frequent remissions but few cures. Therefore, treatment modalities are considered palliative for most patients; symptomatic improvement can be achieved in a majority of patients with median survival in excess of eight years being common. Optimal stage specific treatment is not known thus it is difficult to make definitive treatment recommendations. For this reason all patients are candidates for investigational protocols evaluating new approaches to therapy. Before treatment begins in any patient with CTCL the decision must be made if the goal of therapy is to be palliative or curative. Currently it is thought that only early stage patients have the potential for cure. The use of monoclonal antibodies and interferon in patients with CTCL has shown encouraging results in clinical trials and should be considered in protocol settings.

Adult T-cell leukaemia/ lymphoma

Definition and general description

The disease process known as adult T-cell leukaemia/lymphoma (ATLL) is the first human malignancy shown to be caused by a type C retrovirus, HTLV-I.[7,34,75] It is classified as a mature T-cell malignancy of aggressive nature with a clinical syndrome of lymphadenopathy, splenomegaly, skin lesions, pulmonary infiltrates and lymphocytosis of multilobed T lymphocytes.[34] When first described in Japan, the disease was noted to have an increased incidence in certain geographical regions leading to the hypothesis that it was either genetically derived or transmitted by an infectious agent.[76] Subsequent studies from the NCI showed that the malignant cells were infected by a C-type human retrovirus known as human T-cell lymphotrophic virus type I (HTLV-I).[7,75] The HTLV-I retrovirus possesses an RNA genome and the enzyme reverse transcriptase. This virus and related retroviruses, which bind specifically to helper T-cells, have been associated with a number of illnesses, including the acquired immunodeficiency syndrome (AIDS) caused by human immunodeficiency virus (HIV-1); HTLV-II is the least common of the type C retrovirus infections in terms of incidence. It has been found in intravenous drug abusers and in certain patients who have an atypical form of hairy cell leukaemia, but to date, no specific disease, malignancy or syndrome has been caused by the HTLV-II virus.[75,77]

Human T-cell lymphotrophic virus was discovered during investigations of the properties of T-cell growth factor (now called interleukin-2 or IL-2).[6] A cell line established from a patient with ATLL grew in the absence of IL-2. This cell line, Hut 102, was shown to produce IL-2 and to have a high constitutive expression of IL-2 receptors. Thus, an autocrine mechanism of tumour growth was postulated. Subsequent studies have shown that malignant cells from most ATLL patients express IL-2 receptors but do not produce IL-2. The Hut 102 cell line was shown to contain virus particles and reverse transcriptase.[7] The HTLV-I virus genome, isolated from this and other cell lines, has subsequently been sequenced completely.[78] The long terminal repeats (LTRs) are positioned at the 5′ and 3′ ends of the proviral RNA and regulate transcription by providing sites for RNA polymerase attachment. The *gag* region encodes the internal core proteins of the virus of which three have so far been demonstrated: they are called p24, p19 and p15, on the basis of molecular weight (e.g. p24 is a 24 000 dalton protein). The *pol* region codes for the enzyme reverse transcriptase with the *env* region carrying the code for the viral envelope. The region known as pX is felt to direct translation of a protein which acts as a transcriptional activator of the LTR regions (see Chapter 11).

Evidence suggesting causation of ATLL by HTLV-I includes: the virus has consistently been demonstrated in patients with ATLL; areas endemic for ATLL are also areas of high prevalence for asymptomatic carriers of HTLV-I; the HTLV-I proviral genome is monoclonally integrated into DNA of ATLL leukaemic cells. *In vitro*, HTLV-I can infect T-cell cultures, most readily OKT4 positive T-cells which is the subset of T-cells most often affected *in vivo*. After infection, the T-cell cultures show changes in cell morphology, expression of certain cell surface antigens and changes in growth properties. As a result, the *in vitro* cells closely resemble the *in vivo* leukaemic cells. The fact that the proviral DNA segments are monoclonally integrated indicates that all leukaemic cells are clonal in origin and are descendants of a single infected cell. The actual site of proviral insertion varies from one individual to another, but is always the same within cells of a single tumour. This fact precludes the possibility that an oncogene is activated by adjacent insertion of HTLV-I. The fact that numerous cells are infected by HTLV-I, but the tumour is monoclonal suggests that virus *alone* may be necessary but not sufficient to induce ATLL. Additional genetic changes presumably occur in a single cell to give rise to the tumour. The viral infection may trigger initial polyclonal proliferation with a subsequent second genetic change.

Clinical manifestations of adult T-cell leukaemia/lymphoma

The clinical features of ATLL are contrasted with those of CTCL in Table 22.3.[34,75] Adult T-cell leukaemia/lymphoma patients are younger, on average, with a median age of 35–58 years. The disease is most often rapid in progression with an interval from symptoms to diagnosis averaging only two months. Patients usually present with hypercalcaemia, skin lesions or both. Opportunistic infections are common and may develop at any time. The types of infections range from Gram-negative bacteria to *Mycobacterium*, *Pneumocystis carinii*, *Cryptococcus*, cylomegalovirus, herpes zoster, and *Candida* infections. Although immunosuppression from chemotherapy or glucocorticords may be a factor involved in the acquisition of these opportunistic infections, the underlying malignancy is felt to be the chief protagonist, due to its suppression of normal helper T-cells. Lymphadenopathy is invariably present though massive mediastinal lymphadenopathy is less common than in peripheral T-cell lymphomas, lymphoblastic lymphoma or T-cell ALL. Almost all patients are stage IV (Ann Arbor or Rye classification) at diagnosis with involvement of one or more organs.

Hypercalcaemia is present in most patients and its absence may imply a good prognosis. The hypercalcaemia is refractory to many standard forms of therapy. It is best controlled by achieving an antitumour response to chemotherapy. Most patients have evidence of metabolic bone disease evidenced by abnormal bone scans with diffuse uptake ('superscans') and elevated alkaline phosphatase. Osteolytic bone lesions with evidence of osteoclast activation are often seen on X-ray. The mechanism of bone lesions and hypercalcaemia is felt to be the secretion of a bone-resorbing, osteoclast-activating substance by the ATLL cells. Such a protein has not yet been isolated, however. Vitamin D and parathormone levels are usually normal.

Involvement of the skin is frequent and often a presenting problem. Skin lesions are quite variable; cutaneous nodules are most frequent, but plaques and erythroderma have been described. These lesions are less pruritic than

CTCL lesions. Involvement of the CNS (lymphomatous leptomeningitis), the pulmonary system and the gastrointestinal tract (including the liver) are most common after skin involvement. Invasion of these organs is usually symptomatic as the cells are quite invasive. Bone marrow involvement is frequent. A leukaemic phase is present in many but not all patients. The leukaemic cells have a characteristic appearance (*see* below). Involvement of nearly every organ has been described, albeit in lesser frequency.

The majority of ATLL patients have a rapidly progressive, rapidly fatal illness. However, subacute and smouldering forms of the disease have been described. These patients generally have an indolent course which lasts up to several years. Progression to an acute disease often occurs as the terminal event though patients may also die of opportunistic infections.

Differential diagnosis

The diagnosis of ATLL is established by histological and immunological evaluation of the malignant cells and by proof of HTLV-I infection. Patients must have histological evidence of a malignant lymphoma. These malignant lymphomas always have T-cell receptor gene rearrangements and a surface phenotype of mature helper T-cells (T4$^+$, T8$^-$). Terminal deoxyribonucleotidal transferase (Tdt) is negative. In addition the cells express the IL-2 receptor. This latter feature is unusual in any of the other T-cell malignancies.

Evidence of HTLV-I infection in patients with

Table 22.3 Comparison of disease features

Features	ATLL	CTCL	PTCL	TCLL
Median age (years)	34–58*	52	63.5	>60
Sex (M:F)	1:1	M>F	2.8:1	2:1
Race	Japanese or Black	Variable	Variable	Variable
Endemic area	Yes	No	No	No
Aggressive behaviour	Usually	No	Yes	No
Median survival (months)	11	102	<20	100
Site of disease				
visceral	++++	+	+++	0
bone marrow	++++	+−	++	++++
skin	+++	++++	+	++
CNS	++++	++	+	+
bone	++	0	0	0
mediastinal mass	0	0	+	0
Immunological features				
opportunistic infections	++++	0	+	++
pre-existing immune defect	0	0	++	++
Laboratory features				
hypercalcaemia	++++	0	+	0
T4$^+$	++++	++++	+++	++
Tac+	++++	0	0	0
anti-HTLV-I antibody	++++	0	0	0
HTLV-I provirus	++++	0	0	0

* = Age varies with endemic age studied

lymphoid malignancy generally begins with serological tests for HTLV-I antibodies. Unfortunately, there are 10 per cent false-positive and false-negative rates associated with these antibody tests. More direct evidence is obtained by finding viral antigens or the viral genome in the malignant cells. Radiolabelled probes are now available for these analyses.

Histopathology

There are a number of common histopathological characteristics of ATLL, although none are sufficiently specific to be pathognomonic. A characteristic irregular nuclear contour (multilobed, convoluted or pleomorphic in shape) leukaemic cell has been described (*see* Fig. 22.4). This cell can be differentiated from the circulating Sézary cells of CTCL by use of either light microscopy or, if needed, electron microscopy. It is not present in all ATLL patients and other less characteristic variants may be seen in 20 per cent of patients. The nodal pathology is never pathognomonic for the diagnosis of ATLL since there is no characteristic feature. Nodal involvement reveals a diffuse

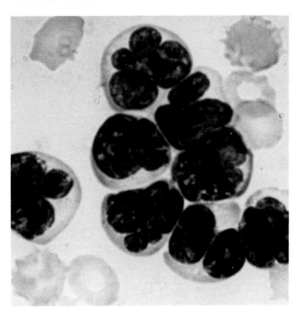

Fig. 22.4 Histopathology, by light microscopy, of a patient with ATL showing the multilobed leukaemic cells.

pattern of cellular involvement but preservation of the underlying architecture can be observed. The infiltrating cells are of a variety of sizes and shapes with the multilobed tissue variant of the leukaemic cell being a minor constituent of the total cell population. The multilobed cell is seen most frequently in the subcortical areas of the node. In addition, no correlation has been shown between the nodal histopathology and the patients' clinical course. Nodal histopathological descriptions may fit into several categories of the Rappaport and NCI Working Formulations.

Histopathological findings in visceral organs are also variable. There is generally a higher degree of pleomorphism and the final diagnosis may be one of several categories of NHL. The histopathology does not appear to correlate with survival. Histological sectioning of skin lesions shows that ATLL dermal infiltrates are typically dense nodules of malignant cells where CTCL shows a more band-like infiltration with less dense infiltration of malignant cells. Both ATLL and CTCL may show epidermal Pautrier's microabscesses.

Cytogenetics

Karyotypic abnormalities in ATLL have involved almost all chromosomes, however, only four of these aberrations were observed in more than one series. These four abnormalities are: trisomy of chromosome 3; deletion of part of the long arm of chromosome 6 ($6q^-$); trisomy of chromosome 7; and elongation of the long arm of chromosome 14 with breaks at bands q11 and q32.[79,80] The chromosome 14 break at q11 is at the locus for the α-chain of the T-cell receptor. These four chromosome abnormalities have also been reported in B-cell malignancies. It is notable that none of these karyotypic defects has been shown to involve the reproducible separation of an oncogene from its regulator, or relocation to a site where its expression could be enhanced. More specific cytogenetic abnormalities are reviewed in Chapter 5.

Treatment and prognosis

To date the treatment modalities employed as therapy for ATLL have not resulted in any long-term survivors. Use of aggressive combination chemotherapy is made most often. Clinical complete remission can be obtained in approximately 70 per cent of patients; unfortunately, these patients tend to relapse after a median time of 13 months (in the NCI series the range was 6–26 months). Second remissions have been difficult to achieve with median actuarial survival of all American series patients being only 11 months. In patients with smouldering disease the option of therapy can be held until the disease process transforms into an acute process. Thus far, no benefit to early therapy in this subpopulation has been demonstrated.

Since standard therapy has shown such a poor response, experimental therapy is now actively being investigated. At the NCI the use of monoclonal antibodies specific for the the IL-2 receptor has been evaluated since the malignant cells have an abnormally high expression of this receptor. A few transient responses were observed with unlabelled antibody. *In vitro* studies show a greater degree of cytotoxicity with toxin labelled antibody. Clinical trials with these toxin conjugates are in progress at the NCI. Other investigational therapies need to be evaluated. The use of radiolabelled monoclonal antibodies and autologous bone marrow transplantation warrant investigation.

It is not known whether any antiviral agents including azidothymidine (AZT; Retrovir) have a beneficial role in ATLL patients. This also warrants investigation. Interferon is being considered after standard chemotherapy, to reduce tumour bulk; or without chemotherapy in the subacute patients, who do not need acute intervention. The use of any of these modalities or combinations thereof has yet to be proved effective in clinical trials. Since the number of cases of ATLL is still low, it is hoped that all cases can be referred to appropriate research institutions so that more successful therapy can be developed.

Peripheral T-cell lymphomas; diffuse intermediate and high grade lymphomas

T-cell non-Hodgkin's lymphomas comprise approximately 20 per cent of the diffuse intermediate and high grade non-Hodgkin's lymphomas with a range of 15–40 per cent.[4,81] The classification of intermediate and high grade T-cell lymphomas has been muddled by changes in the overall lymphoma classifications and the lack of systematic immunological analyses. Thus, the terms T-immunoblastic lymphoma (or sarcoma), T-large cleaved, Lennerts T-zone, T-large non-cleaved and peripheral T-cell lymphoma appear in the literature. At present, these disorders should probably be considered as one entity. They generally have a mature helper T-cell phenotype. In the Rappaport classification these are usually classified as diffuse mixed or diffuse histiocytic lymphomas.

The clinical manifestations are summarized in Table 22.3. The median age is 63 years with a 2.8:1 male predominance. There is no evidence for a viral causation at present. A large percentage of cases have pre-existing illness including angioblastic lymphadenopathy,[81,82] lymphomatoid granulomatosis, Sjögren's syndrome and other 'autoimmune' disorders.

Most patients present with advanced stages and B symptoms are relatively common. In a series of 42 cases from Vanderbilt it is noteworthy that at presentation 79 per cent had stage III/IV disease, 67 per cent had B symptoms, 69 per cent had lymphadenopathy, 37 per cent had bone marrow involvement, 21 per cent had pleural or lung involvement, 29 per cent had hepatomegaly and 43 per cent had splenomegaly. During their illness 19 per cent experienced hypercalcaemia and 29 per cent had eosinophilia.[82]

The optimal therapy for peripheral T-cell lymphoma (PTCL) is unknown. Many series have reported that these patients have a worse prognosis than other patients with intermediate and high grade lymphomas. In contrast, the NCI has reported equivalent complete response rates and long-term survival rates in high grade B-cell versus T-cell lymphomas. It is possible that these differences reflect the more aggressive regimens employed at the NCI such as ProMACE (prednisone, methotrexate, Adriamycin (doxorubicin), cyclophosphamide, etoposide)-MOPP (mechlorethamine, Oncovin, procarbazine, prednisone) or ProMACE-CytaBOM (cytosine, arabinoside, bleomycin, Oncovin, methotrexate), or that these differences reflect patient selection. Patients with underlying diseases (Sjögren's) and prior therapies for these disorders may have a worse prognosis. The use of autologous bone marrow transplantation, monoclonal antibodies, etc. is largely unexplored.

Histologically, all cases of PTCL have been diagnosed as diffuse histocytic, diffuse mixed, or diffuse poorly differentiated lymphocytic lymphomas, in the Rappaport classification with none having the appearance of a nodular lymphoma.

Since the experience of investigators using earlier combinations of chemotherapy did not show as good complete response rates and duration of response when compared to the use of ProMACE-MOPP at the NCI, one must assume the need for an aggressive modality of therapy until the time comes when clinical trials demonstrate optimal therapy.[81] Additional information concerning T-cell lymphomas can be found in Chapter 16 (lymphoblastic lymphoma) and Chapter 21 (diffuse aggressive lymphomas).

T-cell chronic lymphocytic leukaemia

The vast majority of chronic lymphocytic leukaemias (CLL) are of B-cell origin, by some estimates up to 98 per cent.[4,81–87] In B-cell CLL the T-cell concentration is at a normal or low level.[88] Those CLLs which are of T-cell origin have a slightly different presentation from the B-cell variety. Prominent features include the absence of lymphadenopathy in the majority of cases; and prominent splenomegaly, anaemia, lymphocytosis and skin involvement. The skin involvement includes erythroderma not unlike the erythroderma of CTCL.

T-cell CLL cells form sheep erythrocyte rosettes but do not have surface immunoglobulins. The cases are equally divided into helper (T4+, T8−) or suppressor (T8+, T4−) phenotypes. No prognostic or clinical significance is attributed to the phenotype. A number of chromosome abnormalities have been detected, with chromosome 14 showing the most consistent abnormality.[89–93] A number of studies have attempted to compare the phenotype, morphology and function of T chronic lymphocytic leukaemic cells with results showing decreased function of some cells but preservation of function in others.[94–97] While T-CLL cells can retain some of the functional activity of their normal T subpopulations, it requires combinations of several tests to characterize this activity which is of little clinical use.

The therapy and problems of T-cell CLL, are similar to B-cell CLL. The appropriate use of alkylating agents and steroids are still the initial regimen of choice for patients who require treatment. It has been assumed that patients with T-cell CLL have a more aggressive clinical course, but no trials have been performed to document this assumption. The use of recombinant interferons or deoxycofomycin have not been fully assessed in this malignancy. It should be noted that a new aggressive variant of suppressor cytotoxic T-CLL has been noted.[98] The three patients indexed in this study were all young, mean age 24, and all died within 20 months of presentation. The possibility of subsets of patients in T-CLL with a more progressive clinical course exists and appropriate evaluation of all patients who appear resistant to initial treatment may be warranted.

T-gamma lymphocytosis with neutropenia (large granular lymphocytic leukaemia)

Originally considered not to be a neoplastic condition, the entity known as T-gamma lymphocytosis with neutropenia is becoming recognized as a variant of T-cell CLL with a more indolent, protracted course.[81,99–101] First thought to involve only males this process showed 36 per cent female involvement in one series.[102] Most patients present with an absolute lymphocytosis and granulocytopenia, less than 500 granulocytes/μl in 50 per cent of patients and associated with a mild to moderate anaemia. Lymphadenopathy is not prominent but splenomegaly is common as is skin involvement with abnormal lymphocytes, and other autoimmune disorders. Rare cases of conversion to more aggressive disease have been reported.[103] The major morbidity lies in granulocytopenic-induced infections.

The abnormal cell in this disorder is a large granular lymphocyte which has been reported to have receptors for the Fc portion of the IgG molecule as well as T-cell markers. The majority of the cells show OKT8 positivity compatible with cytotoxic/suppressor phenotype. They show high levels of antibody-dependent cytoxicity but low to absent levels of natural killer activity.[104–106] Cytological studies reveal distinctive azurophilic granules in the cells which possess acid phosphatase activity.[106] Ultrastructural analysis reveals cytoplasmic inclusion bodies consisting of parallel tubular arrays; these arrays correspond to the azurophilic granules seen on light microscopy.[101] Less than 1 per cent of B-chronic lymphocytic leukaemic cells contained similar granules.

In a review of the literature of T cytotoxic/suppressor cell CLL, 25 cases which fulfilled the criteria for this process were found.[102] Of the 25 cases found only four had died at the time of the report with one of the four deaths secondary to an accident. The other three patients died as a result of complications of their disease. Follow-up time on the living patients ranges from 3 months to over 20 years.

Therapy in this disorder is mostly symptomatic with patients who have decreased erythrocyte production sometimes requiring erythrocyte transfusion. Other considerations of treatment include the use of the recombinant colony stimulating factors (CSFs), recombinant erythropoietin, or interferons. The major morbidity lies in the recurrent infections experienced by these patients which may preclude the use of chemotherapy as a treatment modality.

References

1. Rappaport H. In: *Atlas of Tumor Pathology*, Sec. III, Fasc. 8. Washington, DC: Armed Forces Institute of Pathology. 1966.
2. Dorfman RF. *Lancet*. 1974; **i**, 1295.
3. Rosenberg S, and members of the Non-Hodgkin's Lymphoma Pathologic Classification Project. *Cancer*. 1982; **49**, 2112.
4. Jaffe ES. *Seminars in Oncology*. 1986; **13** (suppl. 5), 4.
5. van Vloten WA, Willemze R. *Dermatologic Clinics*. 1985; **3**, 665.
6. Gazdar AF, Carney DN, Bunn PA Jr. *Blood*. 1980; **55**, 409.
7. Poiesz NJ, Ruscetti FM, Gazdar AF, *et al*. *Proceedings of the National Academy of Sciences USA*. 1980; **77**, 7415.
8. Soloman AR. *Dermatologic Clinics*. 1985; **3**, 615.
9. Manzari V, Gismandi A, Barillori G *et al*. *Science*. 1987; **238**, 1581.
10. Nathwani BN, Kim H, Rappaport H. *Cancer*. 1976; **38**, 964.
11. Carney DN, Bunn PA Jr. *Journal of Dermatology, Surgery and Oncology*. 1980; **6**, 369.
12. Carney DN, Bunn PA Jr. *Journal of Dermatology, Surgery and Oncology*. 1980; **6**, 369.
13. Alibert JLM. *Tableau du plan fungoide: Description des maladies de la peau observées à l'hôpital St. Louis, et exposition des meilleures méthodes suivies pour leur traitement*. Paris: Barrois l'Ainé et Fils. 1806.
14. Toback AC, Edelson RL. *Dermatologic Clinics*. 1985; **3**, 605.
15. Sézary A, Bouvrain Y. *Bulletin de la Société Française de la Dermatologie et la Syphiligraphie*. 1938; **45**, 254.
16. Lutzner MA, Jordan HW. *Blood*. 1968; **31**, 719.
17. Crossen PE, Mellor JEL, Finley AG, *et al*. *American Journal of Medicine*. 1970; **50**, 25.
18. Broder S, Edelson RL, Lutzner M, *et al*. *Journal of Clinical Investigation*. 1976; **58**, 1297.
19. Haynes BR, Metzger RS, Minna JD, Bunn PA Jr. *New England Journal of Medicine*. 1981; **304**, 1319.
20. Bertness V, Kirsch I, Gollis G, Johnson B, Bunn PA Jr. *New England Journal of Medicine*. 1985; **313**, 534.
21. Whang-Peng J, Bunn PA Jr., Knutsen T, *et al*. *Cancer*. 1982; **50**, 1539.
22. Greene MH, Dalager NA, Lamberg SI, *et al*. *Cancer Treatment Reports*. 1979; **63**, 597.
23. Bunn PA Jr, Edelson RL, Ford SS, Shackney SE. *Blood*. 1981; **57**, 452.
24. Epstein EH, Levin DL, Craft JD, *et al*. *Medicine*. 1972; **51**, 61.
25. Dmitrovsky E, Matthews MJ, Bunn PA, *et al*.

Journal of Clinical Oncology. 1987; **5**, 208.

26. Posner LE, Fossieck BE Jr, Eddy JL, Bunn PA Jr. *American Journal of Medicine.* 1981; **71**, 210.

27. Rastaker G, Raphael M, Boisnic S, Charron D. *Journal of the American Academy of Dermatology.* 1986; **15**, 1296.

28. Winkler CF, Bunn PA Jr. *Conn's Current Therapy.* 1985; 317.

29. Hoppe RT, Cox RS, Ruks Z, *et al. Cancer Treatment Reports.* 1979; **63**, 691.

30. Roenigk HH Jr. *Cancer Treatment Reports.* 1979; **63**, 669.

31. Tuyp E, Burgoyne A, Aitchison T, MacKie R. *Archives of Dermatology.* 1987; **123**, 196.

32. Fischmann AB, Bunn PA, Guccion JG, *et al. Cancer Treatment Reports.* 1979; **63**, 591.

33. Van der Loo EM, van Muijen GNP, van Vloten WA, *et al. Virchows Archives B-Cell Pathology.* 1979; **31**, 193.

34. Bunn PA Jr, Schechter GP, Blayney D, *et al. New England Journal of Medicine.* 1983; **309**, 257.

35. Wantzin GL, Thomsen K, Nissen NI, Saxinger C, Gallo RC. *Journal of the American Academy of Dermatology.* 1986; **15**, 598.

36. Gallo RC, Kalyanaraman VS, Sarngadharan MG, *et al. Cancer Research.* 1983; **43**, 3892.

37. Bunn PA, Huberman MS, Wang-Peng J, *et al. Annals of Internal Medicine.* 1980; **93**, 223.

38. Sausville EA, Worsham GF, Matthews MJ, *et al. Human Pathology.* 1985; **16**, 1098.

39. Schechter GP, Sausville E, Fischmann BA, *et al. Blood.* 1987; **69**, 841.

40. Bunn PA Jr, Lamberg SI. *Cancer Treatment Reports.* 1979; **63**, 275.

41. Vonderheid EC, Sobel EL, Nowell PC, *et al. Blood.* 1985; **66**, 358.

42. Sentis HJ, Willemze R, Scheffer EL. *Journal of the American Academy of Dermatology.* 1986; **15**, 1217.

43. Chu AC, Robinson D, Hawk JLM, *et al. Journal of Investigative Dermatology.* 1986; **86**, 134.

44. Furness PN, Goodfield MJ, Maclennan KA, *et al. Journal of Clinical Pathology.* 1986; **39**, 902.

45. Vonderheid EC, Van Scott EJ, Wallner PE, Johnson WC. *Cancer Treatment Reports.* 1979; **63**, 681.

46. Bunn PA Jr, Foon KA, Ihde DC, *et al. Annals of Internal Medicine.* 1984; **101**, 484.

47. Foon KA, Schroff RW, Bunn PA Jr. In: Foon KA, Morgan AC Jr (eds). *Monoclonal Antibody Therapy of Human Cancer.* Boston: Martinus Nijhoff Publ. Co. 1984: 85–101.

48. Edelson RL, Raafat J, Berger CL, *et al. Cancer Treatment Reports.* 1979; **63**, 675.

49. Kessler JF, Meyskens FL, Levine N, *et al. Lancet.* 1983; **i**, 1345.

50. Vonderheid EC, Micaily B. *Dermatology Clinics.*

1985; **3**, 673.

51. Jensen JR, Thestrup-Pedersen K, Zachariae H, Sogaard H. *Archives of Dermatology.* 1987; **123**, 160.

52. Edelson R, Berger C, Gasparro F, *et al. New England Journal of Medicine.* 1987; **316**, 297.

53. Nisce LZ, Safai B, Kim JH. *Cancer.* 1981; **47**, 870.

54. Micaily B, Vonderheid EC, Brady L, *et al. International Journal of Radiation, Oncology, Biology and Physics.* 1985; **11**, 111.

55. McDonald CJ, Bertino JR. *Cancer Treatment Reports.* 1978; **62**, 1009.

56. Grozea PN, Jones SE, McKelvey EM, *et al. Cancer Treatment Reports.* 1979; **63**, 647.

57. Griem ML, Tokars RP, Petras V, *et al. Cancer Treatment Reports.* 1979; **63**, 655.

58. Winkler CF, Sausville EA, Ihde DC, *et al. Journal of Clinical Oncology.* 1986; **4**, 1094.

59. Kaye F, Ihde D, Fischmann A, *et al. Proceedings of the American Society of Clinical Oncology.* 1986; **5**, 195.

60. Braverman IM, Yager NB, Chen M, *et al. Journal of the American Academy of Dermatology.* 1987; **16**, 45.

61. Hoppe RT, Abel EA, Deneau DG, Price NM. *Journal of Clinical Oncology.* 1987; **5**, 1796.

62. Zakem MH, Davis BR, Adelstein DJ, Hines JD. *Cancer.* 1986; **58**, 2611.

63. Covelli A, Cavalieri R, Coppola G, *et al. Proceedings of the American Society of Clinical Oncology.* 1987; **6**, A745.

64. Olsen E, Rosen S, Villmer R, *et al. Proceedings of the American Society of Clinical Oncology.* 1987; **6**, A746.

65. Miller RA, Levy R. *Lancet.* 1981; **i**, 226.

66. Miller RA, Maloney DG, McKillop J, Levy R. *Blood.* 1981; **58**, 78.

67. Dillman RO, Shawler DL, Dillman JB, Royston I. *Journal of Clinical Oncology.* 1984; **2**, 881.

68. Bertram JH, Gill PS, Levine AM, *et al. Blood.* **68**, 752.

69. Bunn PA Jr, Carrasquillo JA, Keenan AM, *et al. Lancet.* 1984; **ii**, 1219.

70. Carrasquillo JA, Bunn PA Jr, Keenan AM, *et al. New England Journal of Medicine.* 1986; **315**, 673.

71. Rosen ST, Zimmer M, Goldman-Leikin R, *et al. Journal of Clinical Oncology.* 1987; **5**, 562.

72. Grever MR, Leiby JM, Kraut EH, *et al. Journal of Clinical Oncology.* 1985; **3**, 1196.

73. Puttick L, Pollock A, Fairburn E. *Journal of the Royal Society of Medicine.* 1983; **76**, 1063.

74. Edelson RL, Facktor M, Andrews A, *et al. New England Journal of Medicine.* 1974; **291**, 293.

75. Broder S, Bunn PA Jr, Jaffe ES, *et al. Annals of Internal Medicine.* 1984; **100**, 543.

76. Matsumoto M, Nomura K, Matsumoto T, *et al.*

Japanese Journal of Clinical Oncology. 1979; **9**, 325.

77. Weiss SH, Beggar RJ. *Mount Sinai Journal of Medicine.* 1986; **53**, 579.

78. Wong-Staal F, Grallo RC. *Blood.* 1985; **65**, 253.

79. Fifth International Workshop on Chromosomes in Leukemia-Lymphoma. *Blood.* 1987; **70**, 1554.

80. Marx J. *Nature.* 1984; **224**, 859.

81. Sausville EA, Bunn PA Jr. In: Braunwald E, Isselbacher K, Petersdorf R, Wilson J, Martin J, Fanci A (eds). *Harrison's Principles of Internal Medicine, Update VII Oncology.* New York: McGraw-Hill, 1986; 159.

82. Greer JP, York JC, Cousar JB, *et al. Journal of Clinical Oncology.* 1984; **2**, 788.

83. Aisenberg AC, Wildes BM, Harris NL, Koh HK. *American Journal of Medicine.* 1982; **72**, 695.

84. Huhn D, Thiel E, Rodt H, Schlimok G, Theml H, Rieber P. *Cancer.* 1983; **51**, 1434.

85. Sullivan AK, Vera JC, Jerry M, *et al. Cancer.* 1978; **42**, 2920.

86. Rudders RA, Howard JP. *Blood.* 1978; **52**, 25.

87. Brouet JC, Flandrin G, Sasportes M, *et al. Lancet.* 1975; **ii**, 890.

88. Rowlands DT, Daniele RP, Nowell PC, Wurzel HA. *Cancer.* 1974; **34**, 1962.

89. Ueshima T, Rowley JD, Variakojis D, *et al. Blood.* 1984; **63**, 1028.

90. Pittman S, Morilla R, Catovsky D. *Leukemia Research.* 1982; **6**, 33.

91. Gramatzki M, Pandolfi F, Maples J, *et al. Immunobiology.* 1985; **169**, 186.

92. Erikson J, Croce CM. *Current Topics in Microbiology and Immunology.* 1986; **132**, 175.

93. Hecht F, Morgan R, Hecht DKM, Smith SD. *Science.* 1984; **226**, 1445.

94. Pandolfi F, De Rossi G, Semenzato G, *et al. Blood.* 1982; **59**, 688.

95. Reinherz EL, Nadler LM, Rosenthal DS, *et al. Blood.* 1979; **53**, 1066.

96. Marks SM, Yanovich S, Rosenthal DS, *et al. Blood.* 1978; **51**, 435.

97. Spiers ASD, Lawrence DA, Levine M, Weitzman H. *Scandinavian Journal of Haematology.* 1986; **37**, 421.

98. Hui PK, Feller AC, Pileri S, Gobbi M, Lennert K. *American Journal of Clinical Pathology.* 1987; **87**, 55.

99. Hooks JJ, Haynes BF, Detrick-Hooks B, *et al. Blood.* 1982; **59**, 198.

100. Rumke HC, Miedema F, Ten Berge IJM, *et al. Journal of Immunology.* 1982; **129**, 419.

101. McKenna RW, Parkin J, Kersey JH, Gajl-Peczalska KJ, *et al. American Journal of Medicine.* 1977; **62**, 588.

102. Phyliky RL, Li CY, Yam LT. *Mayo Clinic Proceedings.* 1983; **58**, 709.

103. Kruskall MS, Weitzman SA, Stossel TP, *et al. Annals of Internal Medicine.* 1982; **97**, 202.

104. Bakri K, Ezdinli EZ, Wasser LP, Han T, *et al. Cancer.* 1984; **54**, 284.

105. Aisenberg AC, Wilkes BM, Harris N, *et al. Blood.* 1981; **58**, 818.

106. Chan LWC, Check I, Schick C, *et al. Blood.* 1984; **63**, 1133.

CHAPTER 23

PRIMARY INTESTINAL LYMPHOMA AND ALPHA HEAVY CHAIN DISEASE

B Ramot and G Rechavi

Definitions and general description

The association between intestinal malabsorption and small bowel lymphoma has been described by Fairley and Mackie,[1] but this syndrome has remained a rare condition in the Western world.[2,3] In 1965 we described a clinical entity affecting young adult Arabs and non-European Jews, characterized by severe malabsorption that terminated in malignant lymphoma.[4] In 1966 Eidelman et al.[5] reported detailed clinical information and the results of intestinal biopsy studies on nine such patients. In 1968 Seligman's group reported a new immunoglobulin abnormality in a patient with malabsorption associated with plasma cell infiltration of the gut, and called it α heavy chain disease.[6] It soon became apparent that these two clinical entities were part of a spectrum of small intestinal lymphoproliferation observed in the Mediterranean region.[7,8] The disease is not restricted to this area but has a wider distribution in many developing countries. Up to now the disease has been reported mainly in Algiers, Tunis, Morocco, Lebanon, Israel, South Africa and Iran, with sporadic cases from other parts of the world.[8–14]

The term immunoproliferative small intestinal disease (IPSID), introduced during the WHO workshop in 1976,[8] is an appropriate term for the premalignant phase of this clinical entity which covers a spectrum of clinical and pathological disorders. α-heavy chain disease and IPSID are most probably both manifestations of the same condition, with malabsorption as a dominant clinical feature. Although intestinal lymphoma appears to be an important cause of malabsorption in developing countries, there are no reported incidence rates, except for Israel, where the mean annual incidence of primary intestinal lymphomas was 4.8 per million during the years 1960–1967, differing in the various ethnic groups.[15] This rate had dropped to 3.6 per million between 1968 and 1975.[16] The decrease was due to a marked fall in the rates in children and young adults with a concomitant rise in older age groups, resulting in a pattern of bowel involvement which more closely approximates that observed in developed countries.[14,17]

This trend is persisting and has resulted in almost complete disappearance of diffuse small intestinal lymphoma in Israel, although no recent systematic study has been performed.

Pathological findings

The disease can be divided into two phases. Phase 1a: a reactive lymphoplasmocytic infiltration (IPSID) of the intestinal mucosa of the upper gastrointestinal tract causing wide separation of the crypts of Lieberkühn and obliteration of the villous architecture without significant impairment in the surface epithelium. This infiltrate can also be found in the mesenteric lymph nodes. The lymphoplasmacytic infiltration is detectable only on intestinal biopsy since, on macroscopic examination the gut appears normal. This phase is probably reversible by antibiotic therapy. Phase 1b: the infiltrate is composed of abnormal lymphoplasmacytic cells. Macroscopically there is a diffuse thickening of mucosal folds which is sometimes associated with a nodular mucosal pattern. This is probably a transitional phase and is not reversible. Phase 2: lymphoma with diffuse infiltration of the gut: the disease extends from the gut to the mesenteric and retroperitoneal lymph nodes. Extra-abdominal involvement is rare. Of interest is the finding that the spleen is frequently small and fibrotic.

Histologically, the malignant phase is characterized by an abnormal plasmacytoid, centroblastic and/or centrocytic infiltrate and the appearance of large immunoblasts, sometimes resembling Reed–Sternberg cells. These cells can predominate in the infiltrate. More frequently, occasional large pleomorphic immunoblasts are seen among the predominating lymphoplasmacytic cellular infiltrate of the bowel (Fig. 23.1). It has been suggested that these large immunoblasts result from de-differentiation of the monoclonal plasma cell infiltrate,[18–21] but they could also arise from immature precursors of the plasma cells situated in Peyer's patches.[19–21]

The detailed histopathological description of this entity has been reported by Rappaport *et al.*,[22] Nassar *et al.*[23] and has been extensively reviewed by Haghighi and Wolf.[14]

These observations have led to the following hypothesis concerning the evolution of the disease. In underprivileged populations repeated gastrointestinal tract infections in a host with an appropriate genetic background result in a local lymphoplasmacytic response. The abnormal gut is the portal of entrance for additional 'noxious' agents and antigens that further stimulate the lymphatic tissue. Spontaneous or environmentally induced mutations in the proliferating pool result in chromosomal translocations, oncogene rearrangement and activation that can result in a malignant transformation. Although cytogenetic abnormalities have been reported in a number of cases, a specific consistent chromosomal abnormality has not yet been described.[24] The predominant stage of cell differentiation in the

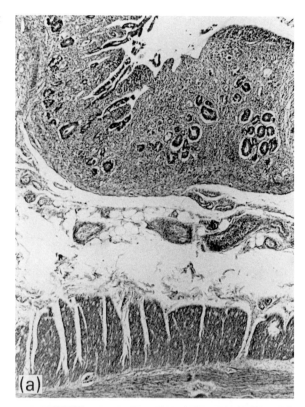

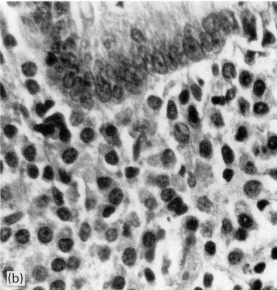

Fig. 23.1 Diffuse lymphoplasmacytic infiltration of the intestinal mucosa (intestinal biopsy) in the presence of α heavy chain in the serum.

proliferating pools at the time of the transforming event will influence the cytological pattern, and hence the cytological heterogeneity; lymphoplasmacytic, centrocytic (small cleaved cell), centroblastic (large cleaved or non-cleaved cell), mixed or immunoblastic lymphoma will result. Histological evolution has been proved.[14] This is the authors' interpretation of the histological findings. Whether de-differentiation of the infiltrating cells, and whether transforming events occur in cells at different maturation stages of the proliferating cell pool remains to be determined.

Clinical features and staging

The age distribution and clinical manifestations do not vary in different geographical regions.[4–14] Abdominal pain, chronic severe intermittent diarrhoea and weight loss in young adults of both sexes are features in all series. The diarrhoea is mainly due to steatorrhoea, and a protein-losing enteropathy has been reported.[14] Peripheral oedema, tetany and clubbing have been observed in about 50 per cent of patients. Peripheral lymphadenopathy and hepato-splenomegaly are very rare and in their presence intestinal lymphoma is an unlikely diagnosis.[8]

At presentation, abdominal masses occur in 30–50 per cent of the patients. This finding is a late manifestation of the disease and its frequency will depend in part on the quality of the medical services in the region and on the time taken to diagnose the disease. The clinical course is frequently indolent with spontaneous remissions. Some patients have been diagnosed 1–4 years after the onset of symptoms.

Unfortunately, routine laboratory tests are not diagnostic. The abnormalities result from malabsorption as evident by steatorrhoea and hypoproteinaemia; less frequently hypocalcaemia, hypomagnesaemia and hypokalaemia are seen. The cholesterol levels are frequently very low; hypochromic anaemia is usually present and elevated alkaline phosphatase, often of intestinal origin, is a common finding.[8] The presence of alpha heavy chain in the serum, urine, saliva and intestinal fluids is diagnostic but not essential to the diagnosis, since it has

been detected in the serum in only 25–60 per cent of patients with primary intestinal lymphoma in developing countries. Therefore, the question of whether this protein abnormality is an integral part of the clinical syndrome of intestinal lymphoma with malabsorption remains unresolved.

Cases with these clinical syndromes, but also with unusual immunoglobulin abnormalities, have been reviewed by Haghighi and Wolf.[14] Doe *et al.*[18] developed an immunoselection method by immunoelectrophoresis in a gel containing a specially developed anti-Fab α antiserum which provides a very sensitive screening method for detecting α heavy chain disease. This method, however, has not been applied to systematic screening of intestinal lymphoma patients, and therefore present estimates of the prevalence of α heavy chain in the serum of patients with this clinical entity may be underestimated.

X-rays of the gastrointestinal tract can be helpful, although the pattern is not specific. Barium studies in IPSID patients frequently show a malabsorption pattern which is more prominent in the upper small intestine. A coarse pseudopolypoid mucosal pattern, strictures and segmentation, and pressure by extrinsic masses are usually observed in patients with intestinal lymphoma.[4,8]

Staging

Clinical staging is important for the understanding of the course of the disease and for better evaluation of the response to therapy. The WHO workshop committee has recommended that pathological staging be performed in most cases.[8] The following staging classification was reported by Salem *et al.*[25] and it is recommended that it be adopted.

Stage 0 – diffuse benign-appearing mucosal cellular infiltrate with α heavy chain, without evidence of lymphoma on staging laparotomy

    I – malignant lymphoma either in intestine (Ii) or in mesenteric nodes (In) but not in both

    II – malignant lymphoma in both intestine and mesenteric nodes

III– involvement of retroperitoneal and extra-abdominal nodes

IV– involvement of non-contiguous extranodal tissues.

Pathological staging (i.e. laparotomy) should probably be avoided as a routine procedure in developing countries if per oral intestinal biopsies, ultrasound or computed tomography (CT) are available. Pathological staging is, however, important for the understanding of the biology of this disease.

Treatment and prognosis

There is no generally accepted mode of therapy. Undoubtedly patients in stage 0, which is probably the premalignant phase, should be treated with antibiotics. We have used tetracyclines extensively – 1–2g/day for prolonged periods of time, as the steatorrhoea is related to bacterial overgrowth. The routine addition of steroids is debatable,[8] but in our experience patients improve much faster when steroids are added.

This premalignant phase can be reversible; the steatorrhoea and α heavy chain in the serum may disappear, the patients gain weight and appear clinically normal. The pathological intestinal changes are also, in part, reversible. Flattening of the villi, commonly observed in intestinal biopsies, is a 'normal' finding in developing countries and should be taken into account when making comparisons with intestinal biopsies obtained in western countries.

Patients in stage I should be treated with antibiotics, steroids and alkylating agents. Cyclophosphamide or melphalan are the drugs which have been most commonly used. Such therapy results in clinical remissions but recurrence occurs in essentially all cases after varying periods of time. We observed a patient with α heavy chain disease for 10 years. He was treated with antibiotics, steroids and alkylating agents for short periods of time and finally died from pneumococcal meningitis. His course demonstrates again that the biological behaviour of the disease is similar to that of low grade malignant lymphoma.

Treatment of patients in stages II, III and IV will depend not only on the stage but on the type of proliferating cell. The immunoblastic lymphomas usually have a more acute, aggressive course. Patients have been treated with COP (cyclophosphamide, vincristine, prednisone), CHOP (cyclophosphamide, doxorubicin, vincristine, prednisone) and C-MOPP (cyclophosphamide, vincristine, procarbazine, prednisone). Unfortunately, there are no clinical studies to prove the superiority of any of these protocols, as most patients eventually succumb. Chemotherapy has been complicated in some cases by perforation of the gut or intussusception. Radiotherapy to the abdomen has been employed in a number of patients, with the induction of temporary remissions. It is clear, however, that the present day protocols are not effective enough in the late stages of this disease, and have not been explored sufficiently in early disease.

In the future, if randomized studies are performed, it will be important to randomize the patients with advanced disease according to the histological classification. Whether such patients should be treated by aggressive chemotherapy with autologous bone marrow transplantation remains an open question. Since this approach is probably not applicable to patients in developing countries, efforts should be made to prevent the disease, which is undoubtedly related to environmental factors. Until this is achieved, early diagnosis should be the goal.

Speculation concerning pathogenesis

Analyses of some B-cell tumour models indicate a multistep process, the first event being a polyclonal proliferation. In the case of African Burkitt's lymphoma and in Burkitt's lymphoma in immunodeficient patients, the first stage is presumed by many to be Epstein–Barr virus (EBV) induced proliferation and immortalization of B-cells. Malignant transformation will take place if another genetic event, such as activation of the c-*myc* oncogene, occurs. A similar two-step model for malignant transformation has also been suggested for mouse plasmacytomas where a preneoplastic stage is induced by chronic stimulation from intraperitoneal injection of mineral oil, followed by a malignant transformation due to c-*myc* activation.[26]

The evolution of α heavy chain disease suggests an analogous two-step model (Fig. 23.2). The first step results in a lymphoplasmacytic proliferation with synthesis of a defective α heavy chain protein. This stage may be attributed to a combination of environmental factors, such as enteric pathogens and/or dietary factors acting in the context of an, as yet poorly defined, appropriate host milieu. This potentially reversible stage is followed by malignant transformation resulting in a high grade immunoblastic lymphoma. The molecular events responsible for the transformation remain unknown.

Information on the structure of the abnormal α heavy chain protein is limited. Because of amino-terminal sequence heterogeneity, protein sequence data are scarce. Structural analysis of the proteins has revealed an internal deletion.[27] It is important to stress that the deletions in the

α heavy chain proteins, like the deletions in γ and μ heavy chain proteins (in γ and μ heavy chain diseases) terminate at exon boundaries and not at random. They involve one, two or three heavy chain domains, i.e. the deletion of entire exons. Based on very limited studies of the genomic structure of heavy chain genes in murine myeloma mutants, several genetic mechanisms can be suggested to explain these findings[28-32] (Fig. 23.3).

Heavy chain disease proteins, for example, can result from a genomic deletion (i.e. in the

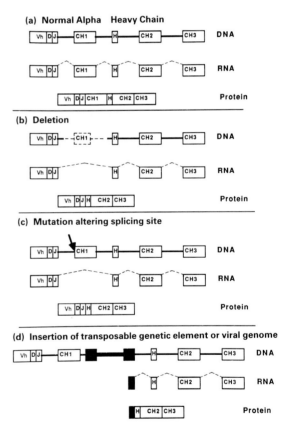

Fig. 23.3 Possible genetic mechanisms that can result in an abnormal α heavy chain protein. Vh, variable region of Ig heavy chain; D, diversity segment; J, joining segment; CH1, CH2, CH3, exons 1, 2, 3 of the constant region of the Ig α chain; H, hinge segment.

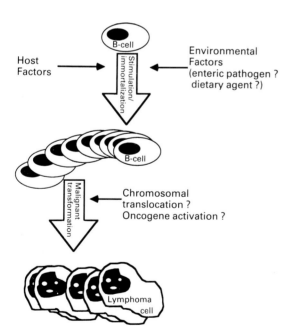

Fig. 23.2 Schematic representation of the hypothetical two-step evolution of primary intestinal lymphoma.

gene itself). Such large deletions were identified in murine myeloma IF2 that produces an abnormal γ 1 heavy chain protein, and in the murine α heavy chain-producing mutants of the myeloma W3129. A deleted immunoglobulin κ light chain gene was also described in the mutant MPC11 plasmacytoma. The above mentioned examples suggest that some of the internal deletions that result in the synthesis of abnormal Ig chain proteins involve aberrant V-J joining or heavy chain switching signals.[29,31] Another mechanism that could give rise to abnormal proteins is a localized mutation changing the splice consensus sequence, resulting in aberrant splicing events. Some heavy chain proteins that have a non-immunoglobulin amino-terminal sequence have been identified. For example, a μ heavy chain disease protein was recently identified that has 40 amino-terminal residues of unknown origin.[27] It is tempting to speculate that such non-immunoglobulin sequences were derived from unusual events such as the insertion of a viral or repetitive transposable element genome in the vicinity of the Ig genes. Such events have been described in mouse and rat Ig-producing tumours.[31,32] Chromosomal translocations that bring the Ig genes to the vicinity of sequences derived from another chromosome are known to occur in B-cell tumours. Chromosomal translocations involving chromosome 14 (the location of the heavy chain genes) have been described in some cases of α heavy chain disease,[22,23] but no band localization has been reported. It should be mentioned, however, that in tumours involving such translocations, (e.g. Burkitt's lymphomas and mouse plasmacytomas) the translocations occur in the non-expressed allele.

The high prevalence of α heavy chain proteins in primary intestinal lymphoma in developing countries suggests that there is a selective advantage favouring the proliferation of α heavy chain producing cells during the evolution of the disease. It might be that the heavy chain protein confers a selective advantage upon these cells which is unrelated to the malignant transformation. A possible mechanism leading to an external selective pressure is provided by the observation that all α heavy chain proteins described so far have been α 1 and not α 2

proteins,[20] suggesting that an external selective pressure must operate specifically on IgA1-producing cells. Figure 23.4 illustrates the main difference between IgA1 and IgA2 protein. The hinge domain of IgA1 is 13 amino acids longer than that of IgA2. Many bacteria have been shown to possess active IgA1 proteases. The cleavage sites for these enzymes are clustered in the short segment of the IgA1 hinge domain.[34] Enteric growth of IgA1 protease-producing bacteria could suppress the proliferation of IgA1-producing cells and so only cells that synthesize the aberrant α 1 heavy chain proteins would be resistant to the proteolytic activity, because of the deletions involving the hinge or neighbouring sequences. Antibiotic treatment would be expected to eliminate this selective pressure and could thus explain the reversibility of this process.

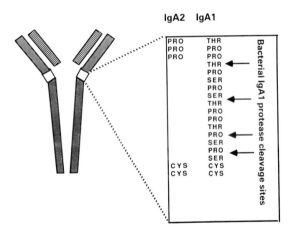

Fig. 23.4 Hinge region sequence comparison of normal IgA2 and IgA1 α heavy chain. IgA1 has a 13 amino acid sequence that is the site for several bacterial IgA1 proteases.

Another possibility to account for the selection process is that the membrane-bound abnormal immunoglobulin confers a growth advantage and contributes to the uncontrolled proliferation. Surface immunoglobulin functions as a membrane receptor and it has been shown that aberrant expression of membrane receptors can result in cellular transformation. For example, the *erbB* oncogene was found to be homologous to the epidermal growth factor receptor and the *fms* oncogene to the macrophage-colony-stimulating factor receptor. Alterations in the structure of these membrane receptors confer the ability to transform.[35,36]

During B-cell maturation, a programmed differentation takes place. There is a hierarchy of immunoglobulin gene rearrangements that occurs during cellular maturation of B-cells,[37] although the factors controlling the step-by-step differentiation are poorly defined. It might be suggested that the genetic defects in heavy chain genes disrupt the programmed differentiation, resulting in uncontrolled proliferation. All of the above mentioned hypotheses can be proved or disproved by current techniques.

References

1. Fairley NH, Mackie FP. *British Medical Journal*. 1937; **1**, 375–80.
2. Gary GM, Roseberg SA, Cooper AD, Gregory PB, Stein DT, Herzenberg H. *Gastroenterology*. 1982; **82**, 143–52.
3. Ramot B. *Annual Review of Medicine*. 1971; **22**, 19–24.
4. Ramot B, Shahin N, Bubis JJ. *Israeli Journal of Medical Science*. 1965; **1**, 221–6.
5. Eidelman S, Parkins RA, Rubin CE. *Medicine*. 1966; **45**, 111–37.
6. Rambaud JC, Bognel C, Prost A, *et al*. *Digestion*. 1968; **1**, 321–36.
7. Ramot B, Hulu N. *British Journal of Cancer*. 1975; **31**, 343–9.
8. *Bulletin of the World Health Organization*. 1976; **54**, 615–24.
9. Nassar K, Haghighi P, Bakshandeh K, Haghshenas M. *Gut*. 1970; **11**, 673–8.
10. Novis BH, Bank S, Marks IN, Selzer G. *Quarterly Journal of Medicine*. 1971; **161**, 521–40.
11. Khojasteh A, Haghshenass M, Haghighi P. *New England Journal of Medicine*. 1983; **308**, 1401–5.
12. Shahid NJ, Alami SY, Nassar VH, Balikian JB, Salem AA. *Cancer*. 1975; **35**, 848–58.
13. Haghshenas M, Haghighi P, Abadi P, Kharazmi A, Gerami C, Nasr K. *American Journal of Digestive Diseases*. 1977; **22**, 866–73.
14. Haghighi P, Wolf PL. *Clinical and Laboratory Medicine*. 1986; **6**, 477–89.
15. Shani M, Modan B, Goldman B, Brandstaeter S, Ramot B. *Israeli Journal of Medical Science*. 1969; **5**, 1173–7.
16. Selzer G, Sacks M, Sherman G, Naggan L. *Israeli Journal of Medical Science*. 1979; **15**, 390–6.
17. Seligmann M, Rambaud JC. *Israeli Journal of Medical Science*. 1969; **5**, 151–7.
18. Doe WF, Danon F, Seligmann M. *Clinical and Experimental Immunology*. 1979; **39**, 189–97.
19. Ramot B, Levanon M, Hahn Y, Lahat N, Moroz C. *Clinical and Experimental Immunology*. 1977; **27**, 440–5.
20. Seligmann M, Mihaesco E, Preud'homme JL, Danon F, Brouet JC. *Immunologic Reviews*. 1979; **48**, 145–67.
21. Asselah F, Slavin G, Fimls GS, Asselah H. *Cancer*. 1983; **52**, 227–37.
22. Rappaport H, Ramot B, Hulu N, Park JK. *Cancer*. 1972; **29**, 1502–11.
23. Nassar VH, Salem PA, Shahid MJ, *et al*. *Cancer*. 1978; **41**, 1340–54.
24. Gafter U, Kessler E, Shabtay F, Shaked P, Djaldettim. *Journal of Clinical Pathology*. 1980; **33**, 136–44.
25. Salem P, El-Hashimi L, Anaissie E, *et al*. *Cancer*. 1987; **50**, 1670–6.
26. Klein G, Klein E. *Nature*. 1985; **315**, 190–5.
27. Seligmann M, Rambaud JC. *Annals of the New York Academy of Science*. 1983; **409**, 478–85.
28. Dunnick W, Rabbits TH, Milstein C. *Nature*. 1980; **286**, 669–75.
29. Dackowski W, Morrison SL. *Proceedings of the National Academy of Sciences USA*. 1981; **78**, 7091–5.
30. Seidman JG, Leder P. *Nature*. 1980; **286**, 779–83.
31. Hawley RG, Shulman MJ, Murialdo H, Gibson DM, Hozumi N. *Proceedings of the National Academy of Sciences USA*. 1982; **79**, 7425–9.
32. Economou-Pachins A, Lohse MA, Furano AV, Tsichlis PN. *Proceedings of the National Academy of Sciences USA*. 1985; **82**, 2857–61.
33. Berger R, Bernheim A, Tapis A, Brout J–C, Seligmann M. *Cancer Genetics and Cytogenetics*. 1986; **22**, 219–23.
34. Killian M, Thomsen B, Petersen TE, Bleeg HS. *Annals of the New York Academy of Science*. 1963; **409**, 612–24.
35. Downward J, Yarden Y, Mayes E, *et al*. *Nature*. 1984; **307**, 521–7.
36. Sherr CJ, Rettenmeir CW, Sacca R, Roussel MF, Look AT, Stanley ER. *Cell*. 1985; **41**, 665–76.
37. Krosmeyer SJ, Hieter PA, Ravetch JV, Poplack DG, Waldmann TA, Leder P. *Proceedings of the National Academy of Sciences USA*. 1981; **78**, 7096–100.

CHAPTER 24

MANAGEMENT OF RECURRENT OR REFRACTORY DISEASE

Fernando Cabanillas, Sundar Jagannath and Thierry Philip

Even though the malignant lymphomas can be considered among the disorders which are most sensitive to chemotherapy and radiation therapy, there still exists a significant fraction of adult patients who fail to achieve complete remission on 'frontline' chemotherapy regimens. Similarly, a small fraction of the complete responders will eventually relapse. The prognosis for such patients is extremely poor if the diagnosis is that of an intermediate or high grade lymphoma and particularly if subsequent salvage attempts fail to result in a complete remission. Patients with low grade lymphomas, in contrast, can survive for longer periods of time, even with recurrent disease. Until recently, there existed few drugs or combinations that were capable of inducing second complete remissions in these patients. Recent combination regimens, however, are able to induce a major response in the majority of adult patients with relapsed lymphoma and complete responses in a significant fraction.[1,2] In fact, a modest fraction of the complete responders have achieved long-term disease-free survival and can probably be considered cured. Advances in the area of bone marrow transplantation have also resulted in high response rates and cures in a small proportion of adult patients[3] and even better results in paediatric Burkitt's lymphoma.

The purpose of this chapter is to review the status of both single agent and combination chemotherapy studies as well as autologous bone marrow transplantation with very high dose chemotherapy in recurrent or refractory lymphomas in both children and adults.

What is refractory lymphoma?

Not every patient with recurrent lymphoma has refractory disease. The term refractory lymphoma has frequently been used in an ambiguous context and thus needs to be better defined. In describing the results of salvage studies, the frequently used statement 'patients who have failed front line regimens' is not appropriate. The setting in which these patients 'failed' is much more important than the fact that they failed. Those patients who achieve less than a partial response to frontline chemotherapy regimens are without doubt the best example of refractory disease. Those who respond to front-line regimens but who develop progressive disease while still undergoing treatment can also be considered as having refractory lymphoma, in this instance 'acquired resistance'.

Patients who only achieve partial response to frontline therapy can also be considered to be refractory because, undoubtedly, they will soon develop progressive disease and die from their malignancy. It is important to recognize such patients, who have partial sensitivity to chemotherapy, prior to the onset of disease progression. If they are properly identified at the time of the plateau of their response to therapy, a change in chemotherapy to a non-cross-resistant regimen can result in a complete response in most cases. Another situation which can be considered as acquired refractoriness is that of the patient who achieves a complete remission on frontline therapy and then develops progressive disease within six months of the treatment being discontinued.

Establishing the presence of recurrent or residual lymphoma

Before undertaking treatment for recurrent or refractory lymphoma, it is mandatory to establish the existence of such a problem. Several situations can mimic the presence of lymphoma. Bulky abdominal or mediastinal masses at presentation in particular can cause problems. After therapy, these masses can shrink without completely disappearing. Re-biopsy has shown that very frequently such residual masses consist only of fibrotic tissue and fatty changes without any viable tumour. This phenomenon appears to be more frequent in patients with nodular lymphomas where the collagen matrix is not affected by the treatment. Radiation therapy when applied to these areas of residual abnormalities can make the situation even more confusing by virtue of the fibrosis it produces, particularly in lung tissue adjacent to the mediastinum.

Another source of problems can be pleural effusions. An exhaustive investigation of the pleural fluid should be carried out in patients whose effusion does not reveal cytological evidence of malignancy. Surface markers, flow cytometry and even cytogenetics should be performed in these circumstances. Second malignancies such as carcinoma of the lung can complicate the picture and need to be considered in the differential diagnosis. Benign processes such as constrictive pericarditis secondary to radiotherapy can also closely mimic malignancy by presenting with recurrent pleural effusions; in these cases, most of the time the fluid will show the characteristics of a transudate which should alert the physician to this possibility.

An effort to obtain tissue to establish the presence of tumour should be a requisite. This can be done via an excisional biopsy, or in cases of deep seated abdominal masses, by means of

a fine needle aspirate. Re-biopsy is also mandatory in cases of recurrent low grade lymphoma to rule out transformation to a large cell lymphoma.

Management of recurrent or refractory lymphoma in adults

Clinical problems of the adult patient with recurrent lymphoma

The patient with recurrent lymphoma usually tolerates salvage chemotherapy less well than the patient who presents with lymphoma *de novo*. This is largely due to the fact that most of these patients have had a considerable amount of prior chemotherapy and many of them might also have received radiotherapy to abdominal or pelvic fields. Also, bone marrow invasion by lymphoma occurs more frequently in patients with recurrent lymphoma than at the time of initial presentation. Nevertheless, administration of maximum tolerated doses is necessary in order to achieve the maximum response. Many of these patients develop infections or febrile neutropenic episodes and consequently adequate supportive care facilities are necessary for optimal management.

In addition to the potential problems of myelosuppression, these patients frequently have underlying metabolic abnormalities. Biliary and ureteral obstruction are common in the presence of intra-abdominal lymphoma. Renal failure and hyperbilirubinaemia complicate the use of some drugs which are metabolized by the liver and kidneys. In such cases, it might be necessary to use biliary or ureteral decompression by means of a percutaneous catheter until an antitumour response is obtained.

Clinical features associated with survival after relapse of adult lymphoma

A prognostic factor study conducted on all patients with all histological types entered on the MIME salvage regimens revealed that seven factors were important when analysed with univariate technique (Table 24.1).[4] The complete response to salvage therapy correlates well with the quality of response to frontline therapy. Patients who achieve a complete response on frontline therapy tend to respond better to salvage therapy than those who fail to respond or who only achieve a partial response on front line therapy. Another important variable associated with a favourable prognosis is the serum lactic dehydrogenase (LDH) level; the higher the LDH the worse the response to salvage treatment and the shorter the survival.[4] In general, the higher the number of relapses the patient has experienced in the past, the more unfavourable the outcome in terms of both response to salvage treatment and survival.[4]

On the other hand, patients with indolent (low grade) lymphomas will frequently survive for several years even after having experienced multiple relapses. In a recent study, we showed that the median survival of low grade follicular lymphomas after the first or second relapse is 36 months, and after the third relapse, it is 14 months.[5] Prognostic features associated with

Table 24.1 Complete response rates according to statistically significant pretreatment variables

Characteristic	No. of patients	CR (%)	P value
Response to first-line therapy			
CR	89	33(37)	
PR	59	11(19)	<0.01
failure	43	4(9)	
LDH (100–225 μg/ml)			
<250	72	30(42)	
250–399	58	15(26)	
400–599	35	2(6)	<0.01
>600	43	2(5)	
No. previous relapses			
0	3	3(100)	
1	90	35(37)	
2	63	8(13)	<0.01
3	27	4(15)	
≥4	25	1(4)	
Bulky disease			
no	127	42(33)	
yes	81	7(9)	<0.01
No. sites involved			
1	56	24(43)	
2	59	13(22)	
3	50	10(20)	<0.01
≥4	43	2(5)	
Diagnosis			
aggressive	123	39(32)	
indolent	85	10(12)	<0.01
Marrow involvement			
no	119	35(29)	
yes	77	9(12)	0.01

CR: complete response; PR: partial response; LDH: lactic dehydrogenase short median survival after relapse were the presence of B symptoms, bulky tumour mass, more than two relapses, LDH > 400 μg/ml, and a haemoglobin < 1.55 mmol/l (10 g/dl). Whenever one of these variables was present, the median survival was 28 months and when two or more were present, it was 8.5 months. On the other hand, when none of these adverse features was present, the median survival was not reached at six years. Another feature associated with a very short median survival is the transformation from low grade follicular lymphoma into an intermediate grade type. This happened in 38 per cent of the relapsed cases and was associated with a median survival of 14 months from the time of transformation.

As a strategy, it seems reasonable to select patients with low grade lymphomas who have adverse prognostic features to investigate the role of intensive regimens such as megadose chemotherapy with bone marrow transplant. This will avoid jeopardizing those who have a favourable life expectancy and also allows investigators to reach conclusions about therapeutic effectiveness faster.

Results of chemotherapy with single agents for recurrent or refractory adult lymphoma (Table 24.2)

Even though responses can be obtained with several available single agents, most of the time these remissions are only partial and usually of very short duration resulting only in palliation.

Etoposide (VP-16)

This is among the most active agents in the treatment of recurrent lymphoma. Response rates have varied anywhere from 5 per cent in a study performed by the Southwest Oncology Group (SWOG)[6] to 60 per cent in a study conducted in South Africa.[7] In a total of 116 patients treated in four different series using VP-16 as a single agent, the total response rate was 22 per cent.[6–9] The reason for the broad range of responses is the fact that the prognostic features in the different series varied greatly. Some patients, like those in the SWOG series were very heavily pretreated and, in addition, the

dose used in that particular study was half of what is considered optimal. If that series was excluded, then the response rate in the remaining 60 patients in other three series was 37 per cent.

Mitoxantrone

Mitoxantrone is one of the most recently identified drugs active against lymphoma. In a collaborative multi-institutional trial using a dose of 14 mg/m^2 every three weeks, a response rate of 40 per cent was obtained in a total of 122 patients.[10] Of these, 32 per cent were partial responses and 8 per cent complete. Activity was greater in the follicular lymphomas where the overall response rate was 56 per cent, while in the large cell lymphomas it was 25 per cent. A median duration of eight months was observed in responding patients with low grade follicular lymphoma, while in the large cell group it was six months. For a single agent, this median duration of response is considered very satisfactory. It appears that the schedule of administration of mitoxantrone has an important effect on the response rate. When a weekly schedule using 5 mg/m^2 for six weeks was utilized in a SEG (Southeastern group) study, the response rate was only three out of 29 (10 per cent).[10]

Ifosfamide

This drug has been widely used in Europe where it is commercially available. Four independent studies carried out in the USA and Europe, in which a total of 41 patients were treated, achieved a combined response rate of 68 per cent.[11] Most of these responses were partial but some of the patients were resistant to cyclophosphamide and yet were still able to respond to ifosfamide. The major dose-limiting toxicity of ifosfamide is haemorrhagic cystitis. With the use of the antidote, mesna, this complication has practically disappeared.

Platinum

In early phase I studies, platinum was found to have some activity in the lymphomas, but the doses used in those studies were highly variable.

A phase II trial in the lymphomas carried out by the Cancer and Leukaemia Group B (CALGB) accrued 27 patients, 19 of which were lymphoma and eight Hodgkin's disease.[12] A 26 per cent response rate was observed in lymphoma and 25 per cent in Hodgkin's disease. All of the responses were partial and the median duration of response was only six weeks. The dose used in this study was 70 mg/m² once every three weeks.

High dose methotrexate

As a single agent, high dose methotrexate with leucovorin rescue has been associated with a high response rate but usually a short duration of response. In a study in which the dose ranged from 3 g to 7 g/m², 26 patients with lymphoma were entered; responses were seen in 13, giving an overall response rate of 50 per cent.[13] Of these responses, five, or 19 per cent, were complete.

High dose cytosine arabinoside

In one study in which cytosine arabinoside (ara-C) was administered as a single agent at a dose of 2 g/m² over three hours every 12 hours for a total of 4–8 g/m² per course, the response rate

Table 24.2 Single agent activity in lymphomas

Drug	No.	CR (%)	CR + PR (%)	Comments	Reference
Etoposide	116	?	22	When SWOG series excluded (which used 50% of optimal dose), response rate = 37%	6–9
Mitoxantrone	122	8	40	Response higher in follicular low grade lymphoma	10
Ifosfamide	41	?	68	Some responses in cyclophosphamide-resistant patients	11
Platinum	19	?	26	Short response duration	12
High dose methotrexate	26	19	50	No mention of response duration	13
High dose Ara-C	28	–	29	Median response duration = 10 weeks	14
Bleomycin (intermittent)	190	14	41	Response duration = 10 weeks	15–17
Bleomycin (continuous infusion)	21	5	38	14 patients had received prior bleomycin; median response duration = 8 weeks	18
5-FU	21	?	26		19–24
L-Asp	20	–	10		25,26

CR: complete response; PR: partial response: Ara-C: cytosine arabinoside; 5-FU: 5-fluorouracil; L-Asp: L-asparaginase; SWOG: Southwestern Oncology Group in malignant lymphoma was 29 per cent of 28 evaluable patients or 25 per cent of the 32 patients entered.[14] The median response duration, however, was relatively short (10 weeks) with a range of 6–33 weeks. None of the responses were complete in this study.

Bleomycin

This drug has been extensively studied as a single agent in lymphomas where it was found to be active early during the initial clinical trials. Several doses and schedules have been used which have resulted in some confusion. It is important to bear in mind that most single agent trials conducted in lymphoma have used doses higher than those utilized in combination regimens.[15–17] The study conducted by Terjanian *et al.* in which relatively high doses were used (5 u/m² daily × 5 as continuous infusion) revealed a response rate of 38 per cent which, when interpreted in the context that most patients had been exposed to bleomycin in the past, is rather impressive.[18]

5-Fluorouracil (5-FU)

Experience with this drug in lymphomas is fragmented and limited. Traditionally, it has been considered as a drug effective against carcinomas but not against haematological neoplasms. The overall response rate of 28 per cent is, however, interesting.[19–24] A combination trial with drugs such as platinum with which 5-FU is known to synergize would be of interest.

L-Asparaginase

This agent is known to be active against acute lymphoblastic leukaemia. Its poor activity in lymphoma is thus difficult to understand.[25,26] However, there are not many data in this regard to make a definitive statement.

Results of combination chemotherapy

The complete remission rates obtained with single agents are low. For this reason, many investigators have been examining combinations of drugs with the goal of improving both the complete response rate and survival. One of the most extensively used drugs in patients who have been exposed to doxorubicin (Adriamycin) in the past has been VP-16. VM-26 which is closely related to VP-16 has also shown some activity in recurrent lymphoma, but as of this time, it is not clear whether one of these agents is superior to the other.[27] Most of the salvage combination regimens in use today contain one of these two drugs. VM-26, for reasons which are unclear, has been used more widely in paediatric patients.

A recent clinical trial in 29 patients with recurrent lymphoma carried out by Lachant and coworkers from the Cancer and Leukemia Group B examined the response of a combination of methotrexate at intermediate doses, VM-26, procarbazine and prednisone.[28] Nearly one-half of the patients had diffuse large cell 'histiocytic lymphoma'. The overall response rate obtained was 41 per cent with a complete response rate of 7 per cent. These results, particularly in view of the low complete remission rate, are considered suboptimal especially when compared to recent results obtained with other combinations.

At M.D. Anderson Hospital, we have conducted a series of clinical trials using combinations containing VP-16 and ifosfamide.[1] The first study, IMVP-16, included ifosfamide, methotrexate and VP-16[29] (Table 24.3). In the second trial, methotrexate was substituted by AMSA (AIVP-16).[30] More recently, a large study in which 208 patients with lymphoma were treated utilized the MIME combination of methyl Gag, ifosfamide, methotrexate, and etoposide (VP-16)[4] (Table 24.3). The AIVP-16 combination has shown inferior results when compared to IMVP-16 and MIME. This difference in results could not be explained by any disparity in the distribution of prognostic features in these three series. The VP-16 dose in the AIVP-16 trial was 30 per cent lower than in the IMVP-16 and MIME studies. Furthermore, the dose of AMSA was only 75 per cent of the full single agent dose in phase II trials. We feel that this possibly explains the lower response rate in the AIVP-16 study. The response rate of MIME has been similar to IMVP-16, but the addition of methyl Gag appears to have contributed to a higher response rate in the low grade follicular lymphomas. However, in the large cell lymphomas, the activity of MIME was very similar to IMVP-16 and methyl Gag did not appear to contribute anything.

Numerous ifosfamide-VP-16 trials have been recently conducted in Europe. The number of patients in each of these studies has ranged from 10 to 30. These are summarized in Table 24.4.[31] When the 127 cases treated in these European series which used ifosfamide-VP-16 combinations are compared to the 324 cases treated in the USA, the results are remarkably similar both with regards to the complete response rate as well as the overall response rate. The European results were particularly close to those reported in the MIME study.

An analysis of the various clinical trials conducted using ifosfamide-VP-16 combinations shows that in practically all series which included more than 10 patients a lower response

rate was observed whenever the total dose of ifosfamide or VP-16 was reduced to less than 5 g/m^2 or 300 mg/m^2, respectively. An example of this is the ifosfamide-VP-16 combination study reported by Segal where the dose of VP-16 was 40 mg/m^2 daily $\times$ 3 which is 40 per cent of the optimal dose[32] (*see* Table 24.3). Similarly, the BMV-VIP study[31] from Westminster Hospital, London (*see* Table 24.4) used one-half of the standard dose of ifosfamide and the AIVP-16 trial (*see* Table 24.3) from M.D. Anderson Hospital used 70 per cent of the optimal dose of VP-16.[30] Also, the low dose single agent phase II study of VP-16 conducted by the Southwest Oncology Group was associated with a low response rate of 5 per cent.[6] All these observations support the fact that the dose of VP-16 as well as that of ifosfamide seems to be of critical importance in obtaining an optimal response rate.

Table 24.3 Summary of studies conducted in USA with ifosfamide-VP-16 combinations

	No. patients	CR (%)	CR + PR (%)	Comments	Reference
Ifosfamide, MTX, VP-16 (IMVP-16)	52	19(37)	32(62)	Response rate higher in LCL. Median duration response 12 months	29
AMSA, Ifosfamide, VP-16 (AIVP-16)	45	12(26)	17(37)	Dose of VP-16 70% of dose in IMVP-16	30
Ifosfamide, VP-16	19	2(11)	5(26)	Ifosfamide and VP-16 doses much lower than in IMVP-16 study	32
MeGag, Ifosfamide, MTX, VP-16 (MIME)	208	50(24)	125(60)	Best response in LCL. Median relapse-free survival of CRs = 18 months	4
Total	324	83(26)	179(55)		

CR: complete response; PR: partial response; MTX: methotrexate; LCL: lymphoblastic cell leukaemia

Platinum-based combinations

Based on the synergism *in vitro* of platinum and high dose cytosine arabinoside (ara-C), we have recently completed a study utilizing these drugs in addition to dexamethasone. Both platinum and high dose ara-C have only marginal activity as single agents for recurrent lymphoma. However, when these drugs are combined in the regimen we have named DHAP, a high response rate has been observed. The overall response rate of 60 per cent with a 24 per cent complete response rate is very similar to that obtained with MIME.[33] However, in the low grade lymphomas, the complete response rate obtained with DHAP was 36 per cent which contrasts with 12 per cent with MIME. This DHAP regimen can be very useful, particularly since VP-16 is frequently used as part of front line treatment and VP-16 salvage regimens might not be as active in these patients if their tumour has become resistant to this drug.

Autologous bone marrow transplant in relapsed lymphoma

There are sufficient experimental and clinical data supporting the existence of a steep dose–response curve in chemotherapy sensitive tumours.[34] Some drugs, however, will show a steeper curve than others. This type of dose–response curve would imply a better therapeutic effect if higher doses could be given. However, dose is generally limited by anticipated toxicity to normal organs, as well as to haematopoietic tissue. The use of autologous bone marrow transplant (ABMT) provides a means of support

Table 24.4 Ifosfamide (IFX) combinations as salvage therapy for lymphoma

Acronym/Centre	Drugs	No.	CR (%)	PR (%)	Overall (%)
VIM(B)/U.Essen, W. Germany	VP-16,IFX,MTX bleomycin	30	9(30)	16(53)	83
VIM-Bleo/U. Freiburg, W. Germany	VP-16,IFX,MTX, bleomycin	18	8(44)	3(17)	61
IMP-M/Ben Gurion U., N. Israel	IFX,MTX,VP-16, mesna	10	1(10)	1(10)	20
IBEP/Augusta Hosp., Bochum, W. Germany	IFX,bleomycin, VP-16, procarbazine	10	3(33)	4(40)	73
VIM/Vienna Lymphoma Study Group	VP-16,IFX, mitoxantrone, prednisone, bleomycin	30	5(17)	10(33)	50
BMV-VIP/ Westminster, London	Bleomycin, methylprednisone, vindesine, VP-16, IFX*	29	8(28)	–	28
Overall total		127	34(27)	34(27)	54

CR: complete response; PR: partial response; IFX: ifosfamide; MTX: methotrexate. *Ifosfamide dose ½ of standard by which the duration of myelosuppression resulting from massive doses of chemotherapy can be shortened. Currently, the basic requirements for a successful ABMT programme using high dose chemotherapy are as follows:

1. tumour cells should still express sensitivity to chemotherapy at standard dose levels
2. the tumour burden should ideally be minimized prior to ABMT because cumulative organ toxicities usually do not allow repetition of high dose chemotherapy
3. the drug or drugs used should be known to be active against the tumour involved
4. transplanted marrow must be free of viable tumour cell contamination.

Encouraged by the initial reports of Appelbaum et al.[35] using ABMT in lymphoma, a large number of investigators have applied high dose chemotherapy and ABMT as salvage therapy for resistant or recurrent intermediate and high grade lymphoma. Several reviews of the state of the art of ABMT have recently been published on this subject.[36–38]

The experience of major centres, both in Europe and America, was reviewed by Philip *et al.*[39] There were 100 patients with relapsed intermediate and high grade lymphoma (with the exception of Burkitt's lymphoma) in this retrospective study. The two-year disease-free survival for the entire group was 20 per cent, with the latest death occurring at 31 months. This study revealed that, similar to the experience with conventional salvage chemotherapy, the quality of previous response to chemotherapy had an important impact on outcome after ABMT. Patients with primary refractory disease (those who either failed to respond or who had transient partial responses on frontline chemotherapy) were all either dead or had recurred within two years of the ABMT. Those who had achieved a complete remission with frontline chemotherapy had, in general, a much more favourable outcome after ABMT.

This latter group could in turn be further subdivided into two groups: those who had responded to conventional salvage chemotherapy preceding ABMT and those who had failed to respond. Those who failed to respond ('resistant relapses') had a two-year disease-free survival of 14 per cent, while those who did respond ('sensitive relapses') had a 38 per cent disease-free survival at two years. The latter was clearly the group who most benefited from megadose chemotherapy and ABMT. It remains to be seen whether the use of ABMT in this group of sensitive relapses is associated with a significantly longer survival than continuing conventional dose salvage chemotherapy. A large collaborative randomized study has been designed to test this point.

In conclusion, prior response, both to front line as well as salvage chemotherapy, is an important prognostic variable which predicts for clinical outcome in patients with intermediate or high grade lymphoma undergoing ABMT. Most investigators nowadays prefer to use ABMT only in those patients who have achieved a complete response to front line treatment and who have shown response to conventional salvage chemotherapy at the time of relapse.

In vitro manipulation of autologous bone marrow

Autologous bone marrow transplant carries with it the risk of marrow contamination. It is impossible to distinguish relapses due to failure to eradicate established tumour from those due to infused tumour cells at the time of transplantation. In a review of 100 patients treated with unpurged ABMT, the most frequent site of failure (85 per cent) was the area of bulk disease at the time of transplantation. Similar experience with syngeneic and allogeneic transplantation points to the inadequacy of current cytoreductive programmes as a major cause of failure.

Several investigators have tried to accomplish removal of residual bone marrow lymphoma cells by immunological methods or by incubating the marrow with drugs such as hydroperoxycyclophosphamide (4HC) or maphosphamide. Takvorian *et al.* have treated 33 patients with recurrent lymphoma using high dose cyclophosphamide, total body irradiation and immunologically treated ('purged') autologous bone marrow.[40] These patients' tumour cells expressed B1 surface antigen and their bone marrow was treated with a monoclonal antibody against this antigen. They were selected for ABMT only if they responded to conventional salvage chemotherapy, defined as a decrease of the disease to less than 2 cm in diameter and bone marrow involvement less than 5 per cent. Twenty patients remain in an unmaintained remission with a median follow-up of one year.

Yeager *et al.*[41] and Santos *et al*[42] have used Leu-1 and Leu-9 as well as complement to purge the marrows of patients with T-cell lymphoma. Of the seven patients reported, four have relapsed. These results are not significantly different to those obtained with the use of unpurged bone marrow in patients with sensitive relapse, although small numbers preclude definitive statements.

The results of transplant using marrow incubated with one of the cyclophosphamide analogues mentioned above are also not clearly different from those when the unpurged ABMT is used in similar patient groups.

Conclusions

Although the response rates obtained with salvage regimens are still suboptimal when compared to the results of front line treatment, a response can be obtained in the majority of patients with refractory or recurrent lymphoma and a modest fraction of these patients can be cured. The strategy of conventional salvage chemotherapy followed by consolidation with autologous bone marrow transplant using megadoses of chemotherapy is likely to result in further improvement of these results in the future and appears to be the most logical approach at the present time. The conventional salvage regimen should, if possible, include drugs not used before as part of the patient's management. A regimen which usually meets this specification is the DHAP regimen.[33]

Management of recurrent or refractory lymphoma in children

For many years, lymphoid malignancies in children were divided into two different entities, namely the chemosensitive leukaemias and the chemoresistant 'lymphosarcomas' and 're-ticulosarcomas'.[43] Recently, serious doubts have arisen as to the validity of this distinction since several reports have shown that similar treatment results to those in leukaemia can be obtained in B- and T-cell derived lymphomas.[44,45] Therefore, the leukaemia versus lymphoma question appears to be, at least in this respect, a worthless one as extensively reviewed by Bernard.[43] T-cell and B-cell malignancies with a lymphomatous presentation are considered as lymphoma regardless of the degree of bone marrow involvement. However, B-cell lymphomas are treated with a sequential protocol,[46] whereas T-cell lymphomas are treated with leukaemia-type protocols.[47] Interest in the management of childhood lymphoma has grown rapidly during the past decade and the current situation is quite clear and is summarized in Chapters 16, 17 and 18.

Despite the acute sensitivity of Burkitt's lymphoma to both chemotherapy and radiotherapy, the outcome in relapsed patients was until recently very poor and long-term survival was almost unknown. Salvage therapy in this disease has been successful only when high dose therapy has been employed with the exception of one report from Villejuif.[48] Encouraging results with allogeneic transplantation in high risk and relapsed leukaemias, and the likelihood that Burkitt's lymphoma would demonstrate a dose–response effect with intensive chemotherapy, made this tumour an obvious candidate for the assessment of massive chemotherapy and autologous bone marrow transplantation (ABMT).

The first studies by Appelbaum *et al.* showed clearly that a dose–response relationship existed[35] and this was subsequently confirmed by a number of groups with a variety of chemotherapeutic regimens.[49,50] A remarkably high response rate was observed in patients who had relapsed after conventional regimens and were resistant to reinduction at standard doses.[50] The long-term survival and probable cure of a small number of patients from the early series, and the subsequent demonstration of cure rates in selected cases leaves no doubt as to the efficacy of this modality of treatment in Burkitt's lymphoma. A number of problems still exist, however, in relation to the indications for and techniques of ABMT in Burkitt's lymphoma: (1) what is the optimum ablative regimen and should this include total body irradiation? (2) which patients should be considered for ABMT and, in particular, should patients in first complete response be considered?

For a variety of biological reasons, Burkitt's lymphoma has shown itself to be a particularly appropriate model for the study of these questions, most of which also apply to ABMT for other childhood lymphomas. In this review, we consider these problems within the context of the experience with over 50 autografts performed for Burkitt's lymphoma over the last five years at Centre Leon Berard.[51–53]

Nature of massive therapy

The most commonly used regimens were previously reported in detail[51] and are summarized in Table 24.5. The original BACT regimen described by Appelbaum was subsequently further intensified with a three-fold increase in the dose of BCNU.[51] The BEAM regimen incorporated two agents (etoposide and melphalan) which had been demonstrated in phase I and II studies to be effective at high doses and were introduced in an attempt to reduce the toxicity of the BACT combination.[51] The use of total body irradiation (TBI) remains somewhat controversial. Its place in conditioning regimens in leukaemia is unquestioned by most, although not all, and some of the massive therapy regimens are undoubtedly not marrow-ablative.[51] However, in the case of Burkitt's lymphoma, TBI has never been shown to be necessary, and engraftment is not a problem with ABMT. The conditioning regimens shown in Table 24.5 were not associated with any difference in response or survival related to the addition of TBI.[51] There is little doubt that the addition of TBI enhances the toxicity by increasing the frequency of interstitial pneumonitis and encephalopathy; moreover, in young children, the long-term sequelae must be taken into consideration.

Table 24.5 Massive therapy regimens, with and without total body irradiation, that have been used in Burkitt's lymphoma

Chemotherapy regimen

BACT Appelbaum
BACT IGR
BEAM
Cyclophosphamide + carmustine
Cyclophosphamide
Cyclophosphamide + doxorubicin + vinblastine + cytarabine + methotrexate

With additional TBI:
Cyclophosphamide + TBI
BACT + TBI
Cyclophosphamide + vinblastine + TBI
Cyclophosphamide + vinblastine + doxorubicin + TBI
Cyclophosphamide + doxorubicin + TBI

BACT = carmustine, cytarabine, cyclophosphamide, thioguanine
BEAM = carmustine, etoposide, cytarabine, melphalan
Carmustine (BCNU) = 1,3-bis(2-chloroethyl)-1-nitrosurea
Cytarabine (Aracytosine) = cytosine arabinoside
Etoposide = VP-16-213
Doxorubicin = Adriamycin
TBI = total body irradiation
IGR = Institut Gustave Roussy

Selection of patients

In the early clinical studies of ABMT in Burkitt's lymphoma, the patients selected were those with relapsed disease in whom conventional therapy had clearly failed. With the clinical experience gained and the broadening of indications to include patients at an earlier stage in their disease, it has become clear that certain parameters exist which predict the likely outcome of ABMT. A rational decision can, therefore, be made in the majority of cases before subjecting patients to expensive, labour-intensive and, most importantly, high-morbidity procedures.

Although massive therapy was 'effective' in

relapsed patients in terms of achieving complete response in up to 80 per cent, this response was almost invariably shortlived.[51] In Fig. 24.1, clear differences in survival are shown between patients with resistant relapse and those with sensitive relapse. With current regimens, there seems to be little justification for using massive therapy in the patients with resistant relapse. However, they remain an important group in which to consider phase I and II studies of new combinations of high dose therapy, as mentioned earlier. The trend in transplants for leukaemia has been to extend the procedure from second to first remission 'high risk' patients. The problem with such an approach is defining the criteria for high risk. In childhood acute lymphoblastic leukaemia (ALL) a number of features at diagnosis may enable an accurate scoring system of 'risk' to be developed.[51] This is not the case in Burkitt's lymphoma, with the exception of CNS involvement, as will be discussed later. Moreover, the introduction of more intensive conventional chemotherapy has improved the outcome in patients previously considered as high risk and, therefore, possible candidates for massive therapy. Thus, many of the patients who would previously have been considered for transplant are now curable with conventional therapy.

This emphasizes the importance of parallel or comparative studies between new conventional regimens and massive therapy. Indeed, a similar problem is now emerging in the case of childhood acute lymphoblastic leukaemia (ALL) where the improved results with the Berlin-Frankfurt-Munster (BFM)-type protocols make decisions about transplanting in first complete response, with all its attendant risks and complications, more difficult.

Similarly, the group of patients who were slow to achieve a complete response traditionally had a bad prognosis, but this feature has now disappeared as an adverse factor.[51] On the other hand, those patients who, although responding to induction chemotherapy, fail to achieve complete response, appear to have a particularly good outcome when grafted in partial response (i.e. prior to disease progression) and are clearly a suitable group for such therapy (*see* Fig. 24.1).

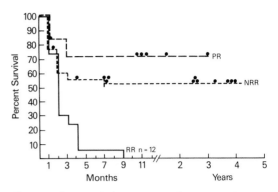

Fig. 24.1 Survival after massive therapy and ABMT in relation to disease status at time of procedure. PR, partial response to initial therapy; NRR, non-resistant relapse (responsive to salvage treatment); RR, resistant relapse.[42]

B-cell ALL of Burkitt type is very rare and has in the past been defined as more than 25 per cent L_3 blasts in the marrow, irrespective of the primary site of disease. Such patients were considered to have a worse outcome than those with stage IV lymphoma (< 25 per cent L_3 blasts). This, however, may only be the case when there is also CNS disease. With marrow involvement alone, disease-free survival is 80 per cent versus 30 per cent with CNS and bone marrow involvement simultaneously.[44] However, patients with a classical leukaemic picture and no extramedullary lymphomatous masses tend to fare badly and should, therefore, be considered for massive therapy in first complete response.[44,51]

Central nervous system disease in Burkitt's lymphoma remains one of the major therapeutic problems. This may occur in two situations: it may be present at diagnosis (13 per cent), usually in combination with another primary site or it may be a site of disease relapse, either in isolation or combined with other sites. With the Lymphome Malin B (LMB) regimen, where more intensive treatment is given to the CNS, including five courses of high dose methotrexate (MTX) (3 g/m²), the incidence of CNS relapse has declined markedly and is currently less than 5 per cent. In patients with CNS relapse, the response to massive therapy has been impressive and the role of high dose BCNU has been emphasized.[51] In our experience with 10 patients who had CNS relapse, five are long-term survivors.[51] In contrast, CNS disease at presentation may reflect a more aggressive biological variant and the relapse rate is high. Current survival in the LMB study for such patients is only 30 per cent, and, moreover, concurrent marrow involvement is a major adverse prognostic factor.

To date, we have treated 14 patients with CNS disease at presentation, and the preliminary results are encouraging; eight remain disease-free at over 10–27 months. This small group of patients requires further study and the use of other agents at higher doses, particularly those which cross the blood–brain barrier, such as very high dose cytarabine (cytosine arabinoside), VP-16 or possibly cisplatin should be investigated.

In conclusion, we feel that about 20 per cent of all patients with Burkitt's lymphoma are potential candidates for salvage therapy namely:

1. those who fail to achieve complete response with initial treatment
2. relapsed patients who are still responsive to salvage therapy
3. patients with CNS involvement at diagnosis, especially where there is more than 25 per cent marrow involvement.

Children with relapsed lymphoblastic lymphoma are also appropriate candidates for bone marrow transplantation while still sensitive to a salvage protocol. The majority of patients treated with cyclophosphamide-TBI seem to show better survival than those treated with non-TBI regimens. The strategy for this group of patients should be similar to that used for leukaemia at relapse.

Phase I and II studies in patients with 'resistant relapse' are being conducted to investigate the use of sequential high dose alkylating agents and the role of TBI. It is of particular importance to develop effective conventional 'salvage' regimens. Purging techniques in Burkitt's lymphoma are now at an advanced stage and the combination of immunological and chemical treatments, once of proven efficacy in individual patients at the laboratory level, should be the subject of randomized studies. Finally, it is expected that

as we learn more about the multidrug resistance phenotype this will enable us to determine whether the use of high dose chemotherapy can overcome resistance in these disorders.

References

1. Cabanillas F. In: Ford RJ, Fuller LM, Hagemeister FB (eds). *UT M.D. Anderson Clinical Conference on Cancer, vol. 27.* New York, Raven Press, 1984: 391–6.
2. Rodriguez V, Cabanillas F, Bodey GP. *Seminars in Oncology.* 1982; **9**, 87–92.
3. Spitzer G, Jagannath S, Dicke Z, et al. In: Ford, RJ, Fuller LM, Hagemeister FB, et al. *UT M.D. Anderson Clinical Conference on Cancer, vol. 27,* New York: Raven Press, 1984: 407–25.
4. Cabanillas F, Hagemeister FB, McLaughlin P, et al. *Journal of Clinical Oncology.* 1987; **5**, 407–12.
5. Spinolo J, McLaughlin P, Hagemeister FB, et al. *Third International Conference on Malignant Lymphoma,* Lugano, Switzerland, 1987 (abstract).
6. Cecil JW, Quagliana JM, Coltman CA, Al-Sarraf M, Thigpen T, Groppe CW. *Cancer Treatment Reports.* 1978; **62**, 801–3.
7. Jacobs P, King HS, Cassidy F, Dent DM, Harrison T. *Cancer Treatment Reports.* 1981; **65**, 987–93.
8. Bender RA, Anderson T, Fisher RI, Young RC. *American Journal of Hematology.* 1978; 203–9.
9. Dombernowsky P, Nissen NI, Larsen V. *Cancer Chemotherapy Reports.* 1972; **56**, 71–82.
10. Gams RA, Keller J, Case DC, et al. *Projects in Medicine, New York.* 1985; 75–8.
11. Brade WP, Herdrich K, Varini M. *Cancer Treatment Review.* 1985; **12**, 1–47.
12. Cavalli F, Jungi WF, Nissen NI, Pajak TF, Coleman M, Holland JF. *Cancer.* 1981; **48**, 1927–30.
13. Frei E, Blum R, Pitman SW, et al. *American Journal of Medicine.* 1980; **68**, 370–6.
14. Kantarjian H, Barlogie B, Plunkett W, et al. *Journal of Clinical Oncology.* 1983; **1**, 689–94.
15. Agre KA. In: Soper WT, Glott AB (eds). *Proceedings of the Drug Seminar on Bleomycin,* Silver Spring, MD: Automation Industries Inc. Vitro Laboratories Division. 1974; 66–82.
16. Haas CD, Coltman CA Jr, Gottlieb JA, et al. *Cancer.* 1976; **38**, 8–12.
17. Rudders RA. *Blood.* 1972; **40**, 317–32.
18. Terjanian T. Personal communication.
19. Olson K, Greene J. *Journal of the National Cancer Institute.* 1960; **25**, 133.
20. Krivit W, Bentley H. *American Journal of Diseases of Children.* 1960; **100**, 217.

21. Kennedy B, Theologides A. *Annals of Internal Medicine.* 1961; **55**, 719.
22. Weiss A, Jackson L, Carabasi R. *Annals of Internal Medicine.* 1961; **55**, 731.
23. Ansfield F, Schroeder J, Curreri A. *Journal of the American Medical Association.* 1962; **181**, 295.
24. Moore G, Bross I, Ausman R, *et al. Cancer Chemotherapy Reports.* 1968; **52**, 641.
25. Clarkson B, Krakoff I, Burchenal J, *et al. Cancer.* 1970; **25**, 279.
26. Whitecar JP, Bodey G, Harris J, *et al. New Journal of Medicine.* 1970; **282**, 732.
27. Goldhirsch A, Pirovino M, Sonntag RW, Tschopp L, Ryssel HJ, Brunner KW. *Cancer Treatment Reports.* 1980; **64**, 335–7.
28. Lachant NA, Cooper MR, Bloomfield CD, Ginsberg SJ, Gottlieb AJ, Pajak TF. *Proceedings of the American Society of Clinical Oncology.* 1981; **22**, 518.
29. Cabanillas F, Hagemeister FB, Bodey GP, Freireich EJ. *Blood.* 1982; **60**, 693–7.
30. Cabanallas F, Bodey GP. *Amsacrine Current Perspectives and Clinical Results with a New Anticancer Agent.* Proceedings of International Symposium. Princeton Junction, NJ: Communications Media for Education. 1982, 55–62.
31. Ifosfamide Symposium. *Cancer Research and Clinical Oncology.* vol. III: 1986; 537–8.
32. Segal ML, Grever MR, Ungerleider J, Balcerzak SP. *Proceedings of the American Society of Clinical Oncology.* 1982; **1**, 159.
33. Velasquez W, Cabanillas F, McLaughlin P, *et al. Proceedings of the American Society of Clinical Oncology.* 1986; **5**, 191 (abstract).
34. Frei E, Canellos GP. *American Journal of Medicine.* 1980; **69**, 585–94.
35. Appelbaum FR, Herzig GP, Ziegler JL, *et al. Blood.* 1978; **52**, 85–95.
36. Singer CRJ, Goldstone AH. *Clinical Haematology.* 1986; **15**, 105–150.
37. Appelbaum FR, Thomas ED. *Journal of Clinical Oncology.* 1983; **1**, 440–7.
38. Gorin NC, David R, Stachowiak J, *et al. European Journal of Cancer and Clinical Oncology.* 1981; **17**, 557–68.
39. Philip T, Armitage JO, Spitzer G, *et al. New England Journal of Medicine.* 1987; **36**, 1493–8.
40. Takvorian T, Nadler LM, Anderson KC, *et al. Blood.* 1984; **64**, 222a.
41. Yeager A, Braine H, Kaizer H, *et al. Proceedings of the American Society of Clinical Oncology.* 1984; **3**, 239 (abstract).
42. Santos GW, Kaizer H. In: Lowenberg B, Hagenbeek A (eds). *Minimal Residual Disease in Acute Leukemia.* Boston: Martinus Nijhoff, 1984, 165.
43. Bernard A, Boumsell L, Patte C, Lemerle J. *Medical and Pediatric Oncology.* 1986; **14**, 148–57.
44. Patte C, Philip T, Rodary C, *et al. Journal of Clinical Oncology.* 1986; **4**, 1219–26.
45. Wollner N, Watchel AE, Exelby P, Centore D. *Cancer,* 1980; **45**, 3034–9.
46. Philip T, Lenoir GM, Bryon PA, *et al. British Journal of Cancer.* 1982; **45**, 670–8.
47. Weinstein HJ, Lack E, Cassady JR. *Blood.* 1984; **2**, 422–6.
48. Patte C, Bernard A, Hartmann O, Lemerle J. *Pediatric Hematology and Oncology.* 1986; **3**, 11–18.
49. Hartmann O, Pein F, Beaujean F, *et al. Journal of Clinical Oncology.* 1984; **2**, 978–85.
50. Philip T, Biron P, Herve P, *et al. European Journal of Cancer and Clinical Oncology.* 1983; **19**, 1371–9.
51. Philip T, Pinkerton R, Hartmann O, *et al. Clinical Haematology.* 1986; **15**, 205–17.
52. Philip T, Biron P, Philip I, *et al. European Journal of Cancer and Clinical Oncology.* 1986; **22**, 1015–27.
53. Philip T, Biron P, Philip I, *et al.* In: Dicke K, Spitzer G, Zander AR (eds). *Autologous Bone Marrow Transplantation: Proceedings of the Third International Symposium.* UT M.D. Anderson Hospital and Tumour Institute, Houston, Texas. 1987.

CHAPTER 25

BONE MARROW TRANSPLANTATION IN NON-HODGKIN'S LYMPHOMAS

Augusto Pedrazzini, Arnold S Freedman and Lee M Nadler

Although significant advances have been achieved with conventional doses of chemotherapy and radiation therapy, most patients with non-Hodgkin's lymphoma (NHL) still succumb to their disease.[1,2] However, the majority of patients with low, intermediate, and high grade NHL[3] treated with aggressive combination chemotherapy achieve a complete remission.[4,5] Between 30 and 50 per cent of patients with intermediate or aggressive NHL achieve long-term disease-free survival[6] but patients with low grade histology are rarely cured. During the past decade treatment has been intensified by increasing the number of drugs, as well as their dosage and schedule, but the cure rate for both favourable and unfavourable histologies has probably not been improved. Although at least 50 per cent of relapsed NHLs are still sensitive to treatment[7], less than 15 per cent of patients with relapsed intermediate or high grade NHL achieve a long-term disease-free remission with any second line conventional treatment regimen.[8]

It has become clear that once primary conventional treatment has failed the only potentially curative approach for relapsed NHL entails supralethal doses of chemotherapy, with or without radiation therapy. These very high dose regimens have been developed by combining therapeutic modalities (cytotoxic drugs and total body irradiation) which share myelosuppression as the dose-limiting toxicity. In an attempt to minimize the attendant myelosuppression, bone marrow support from an identical twin (syngeneic)[9], a sibling (allogeneic)[10] or from the patient (autologous)[11,12] has been employed. The use of high dose chemotherapy and radiotherapy with bone marrow support has produced complete remission in the majority of patients with relapsed NHL whose tumour cells were still sensitive to conventional chemotherapy.[13] More importantly, this treatment has resulted in the cure of some patients.[14] Therefore, bone marrow transplantation has an established role in the treatment of patients with relapsed NHL.[15] In this chapter we review the indications for bone marrow transplantation in NHL, provide a summary of reported studies and identify questions which are presently under intensive investigation.

Who is cured with conventional treatment regimens?

Low grade non-Hodgkin's lymphoma

The favourable histologies include most of the nodular lymphomas as well as the diffuse well differentiated lymphomas (Group A to C in The Working Formulation) (*see* ref. 3 and Chapter 4). Although widely disseminated at diagnosis, patients with low grade lymphomas have median survival rates which may be as long as 8–10 years.[1,4] Although diagnosed in less than 10 per cent of patients, stages I and II low grade NHL can frequently be cured with local radiation therapy.[16] However, the prognosis of patients with advanced low grade NHL has not been significantly altered by single agent or combination chemotherapy, and very few such patients are cured (*see* refs. 17, 18, 19 and Chapter 19). Therefore, a number of different therapeutic strategies are presently under investigation, ranging from a 'watch and wait' policy to intensive chemotherapy.[20]

Intermediate and high grade non-Hodgkin's lymphomas

The poor prognosis NHL includes both diffuse and nodular large cell lymphomas, diffuse poorly differentiated and mixed lymphomas and undifferentiated lymphomas, i.e. intermediate (groups D to G) and high grade histologies (groups H to J) in the Working Formulation.[3] Without treatment these patients usually survive less than two years.[21] In contrast to the favourable lymphomas, the unfavourable lymphomas demonstrate a definite cure rate with combination chemotherapy. With the development of increasingly aggressive chemotherapeutic regimens the majority of patients now experience complete remission and long-term disease-free survival (*see* Chapters 16–18, 21). Prognostic variables include sites of disease, bulk of disease, stage of disease, extranodal disease, bone marrow infiltration and performance status. Depending on the treatment regimen, these prognostic factors correlate to a greater or lesser extent, with the likelihood of complete response (CR) and cure in poor prognosis lymphomas. In spite of these findings selection of treatment has, in general, not been based upon prognostic categories, and histology has remained as the primary criterion used to determine clinical management.

The results of more recent studies have suggested that response to therapy may be a more sensitive indicator of prognosis. Armitage *et al.*[22] demonstrated that patients who have not achieved a CR after three cycles of treatment have only a 25 per cent probability of cure, whereas patients who have achieved a CR after 3 cycles have a 75 per cent chance of cure. Therefore, patients with high grade NHL who do not achieve a rapid CR, or those with

significant bulk disease,[23,24] are much less likely to be cured by conventional combination chemotherapy. Biological markers such as immunological cell surface phenotype,[25] immunoglobulin and T-cell receptor gene rearrangements,[26,27] karyotypic analysis[27] and oncogene rearrangements[28,29] have yet to make a significant impact upon the determination of prognosis or upon treatment selection.

Salvage chemotherapy

Patients with relapsed or refractory NHL demonstrate minimal long-term benefit when treated with conventional second line treatment regimens. Patients with refractory lymphomas (i.e. those patients who do not achieve a CR with primary therapy) rarely achieve complete response with alternative non-cross-resistant chemotherapeutic regimens at standard dosage.[30] NHLs that have relapsed following the achievement of CR can be subdivided into lymphomas which remain sensitive to standard dose chemotherapy (i.e. sensitive relapses) and lymphomas resistant to reinduction treatment with a non-cross-resistant cytotoxic combination (i.e. resistant relapse).[12,13] Although lymphomas in the former group often demonstrate partial responses to conventional dose therapy, a second complete remission occurs only in a minority of patients, and cure is a rare event.[6,31,32,33,34] In a review of 16 studies, Singer and Goldstone[7] found that only 12 of 398 relapsed patients treated with a variety of different chemotherapeutic programmes were in continuous complete remission at two years.

In view of the failure of conventional dose chemotherapy to render these patients long-term survivors, a number of salvage regimens based upon non-cross-resistant drugs employed at significantly higher doses have been developed.[35,36] These regimens contain drugs which are not commonly employed in the same schedule and dosage in standard induction treatment. Cis-platinum,[35,37–40] ifosfamide,[42] etoposide[38,39,41,42] and cytosine arabinoside[44,45] have emerged as effective, non-cross-resistant drugs with synergistic potential and non-overlapping toxicities. Cabanillas and his colleagues have developed three combination chemotherapies[8,45,46] based upon the synergism observed *in vitro* and *in vivo* between these drugs. Overall, however, the results of salvage regimens with both primary refractory and relapsed NHL are very disappointing, and cure with these intensive salvage regimens remains infrequent. The major obstacle to the development of effective salvage treatment regimens for refractory and relapsed NHL is the inability of the available drugs to overcome intrinsic and secondary mechanisms of resistance when administered at non-marrow ablative dosages.

Rationale for high dose ablative therapy in non-Hodgkin's lymphoma

The rationale for high dose ablative therapy and bone marrow support in the treatment of NHL was largely based upon the extensive allogeneic transplant experience in the treatment of leukaemia.[47–54] Like leukaemias, lymphomas demonstrate a steep dose–response curve to chemotherapy and radiotherapy in animal[55] and human systems.[56] It was, therefore, likely that NHL would show a significant response to very high dose, ablative therapy.

The first important question was the nature of the ablative treatment regimen. The treatment regimen for relapsed leukaemias was based upon two principles; first, high dose alkylating agents were effective in eradicating resistant leukaemic cells; second, total body irradiation (TBI) would induce sufficient immunosuppression to permit allogeneic transplantation. The combination of high dose cyclophosphamide and TBI produced a highly effective and well tolerated treatment regimen.[57] Few patients died from early acute drug related toxicity[58] and the majority of patients who succumbed did so to infection,[59] graft versus host disease[60] or relapse.[61] Other regimens, including higher doses of cyclophosphamide and second alkylating agents (busulfan, BNCU, melphalan, etoposide, etc.) were also investigated with similar results.[62] Initially, only relapsed patients

with refractory NHL were treated and only a limited number of patients were cured. However, treatment of patients in sensitive relapse or earlier in first remission has resulted in less toxicity and has led to improved survival rates in comparison to standard treatment regimens.

The second important consideration was the bone marrow source. Three sources of bone marrow can be identified; each has its advantages and disadvantages.[10,15,60] In this section we will only briefly consider each bone marrow source, as they will be dealt with in more detail in later sections.

The ideal source of bone marrow is from an identical twin.[9] Sygeneic marrow is perfectly histocompatible, is not contaminated by tumour cells, has not been exposed to chemotherapy and will engraft rapidly and without graft-versus-host disease (GVHD) in virtually every individual. The major disadvantages of syngeneic transplantation are that only 1 in 80 individuals has an identical twin and that, since patient and donor are perfectly matched, no theoretical graft-versus-leukaemia effect can occur.[3–5]

The second source is from an HLA-matched sibling (i.e. allogeneic). The major advantage of this marrow source is that it is not contaminated by tumour cells, nor has it been previously exposed to treatment. The disadvantages are protean. GVHD has limited the use of bone marrow from mismatched or partially matched family members.[66,67] Moreover, a matched donor is available to less than 25 per cent of patients. Newer immunosuppressive therapies with either cyclosporine[66] or T-cell depletion with monoclonal antibodies[68,69] have not provided the expected breakthrough in preventing GVHD. Until recently 50 per cent of patients over the age of 20 years developed significant, often fatal GVHD.[60] In recent years, with the development of T-cell depletion using monoclonal antibodies, fewer patients develop GVHD, even up to the age of 50.[68] However, graft failure, and a higher proportion of leukaemic relapses, have been observed in some trials.[70]

The third source of bone marrow is from the patients themselves (i.e. autologous). The major advantage to this approach is that every patient has a donor. However, this bone marrow may previously have been exposed to extensive chemotherapy and may be contaminated by tumour cells.[71,72] Therefore, clinical trials involving bone marrow transplantation in NHL have examined each source of bone marrow with regard to availability, attendant complications and patterns of relapse.

Clinical studies of bone marrow transplantation in NHL

Considering the multitude of publications in this field we shall confine our analysis to a limited number of parameters for each study. These parameters have been chosen according to their relative importance in predicting which patients will benefit from bone marrow transplantation with regard to both response and toxicity.

Patient selection

It is now generally accepted that patient selection is a major factor in determining the disease-free survival achieved in trials of high dose, ablative chemotherapy and bone marrow rescue. This is consistent with earlier studies, which demonstrated that patients in the chronic stage of chronic myelogenous leukaemia (CML) have a significantly greater disease-free survival rate with bone marrow transplantation (BMT) than patients with more advanced stages (accelerated or blastic phase).[74] It is the experience of the European Bone Marrow Transplantation Group (EBMTG) that the responsiveness of the lymphoma to chemotherapy at a standard dosage is a very important prognostic factor for these patients.[31] The status of the disease at the time of transplantation can be categorized as follows (see also ref. 12):

a) *First Remission*: Which can be either complete or partial (at least 50 per cent reduction of all measurable disease). This is a group of patients whose disease has not developed significant resistance. Such patients have usually experienced minimal treatment-related toxicity and have a good performance status.

b) *Sensitive Relapse (SR)*: These patients have achieved a prior CR (or for some low grade lymphomas, a good PR) and subsequently relapsed. The disease is still responsive to standard salvage therapy, regardless of the number of prior remissions. A relapse is considered sensitive by any significant response to reinduction chemotherapy (or radiation therapy); generally more than a 50 per cent reduction in tumour bulk. For this subgroup the length of the prior disease-free interval may be very important for predicting sensitivity to, and outcome of, high dose therapy.

c) *Resistant Relapse (RR)*: Patients in relapse who are not responsive to chemotherapy. This group can be further subdivided into those patients who are not responsive to standard dose chemotherapy and those who are not responsive to more intensive salvage regimens. This difference is often difficult to evaluate in published series. Patients with RR generally have disseminated disease and also frequently have a poor performance status.

d) *Refractory to Induction Chemotherapy (RI)*: These patients have not achieved a clinically significant remission with primary aggressive combination chemotherapy.

For the purposes of analysis, patients will be categorized according to these subgroups whenever possible.

Ablative regimens

The ideal ablative regimen combines maximal tumour cell kill and minimal systemic toxicity, with the major dose-limiting toxicity being bone marrow aplasia. The 'standard' regimen of cyclophosphamide and TBI was empirically derived in an attempt to develop an immunosuppressive treatment regimen for patients with relapsed acute leukaemias undergoing allogeneic transplantation.[57] This regimen appeared to be effective in animal studies, with a tumour cell cytoreduction of 4 logs for TBI[74] and 3–4 logs for cyclophosphamide.[75] Initially the regimen consisted of cyclophosphamide 120 mg/kg (60 mg/kg daily for two days) and TBI of 850 cGy given on a single day.[76] This regimen was first used for syngeneic and allogeneic transplantation in relapsed acute leukaemias, and has since been used in CML and NHL. Subsequently, the irradiation has been fractionated; usually twice daily over three days.[78,79] Attempts to add additional chemotherapeutic drugs to cyclophosphamide and TBI have been complicated by increasing toxicity.[79]

With improvements in supportive care, and with better patient selection, it became clear that cure was possible following BMT. It was therefore important to consider the possible long-term sequelae of this procedure. In young patients, TBI was considered toxic at doses over 500 cGy, as the growth of the skeleton might be impaired;[80] cataracts also appeared to be a common side effect of radiotherapy. As a result of these side effects a number of centres attempted to develop ablative regimens based on combination chemotherapy alone, without radiation therapy. These regimens were based upon selecting drugs with non-overlapping toxicities, apart from their induction of marrow aplasia.

One combination, called BACT, first published by Appelbaum,[81] consists of BCNU 200 mg/m^2 on day 1, followed over the course of four days by a combination of cyclophosphamide 6400 mg/m^2 total dose, cytosine arabinoside 800 mg/m^2 and 6-thioguanine 800 mg/m^2 (Table 25.1). A similar programme with an increased dose of BCNU, to a total of 600 mg/m^2, has been studied at the Institut Gustave Roussy.[82] In the TACC protocol, CCNU is substituted for BCNU at a dose of 200–250 mg/m^2.[83] The BEAM programme is a combination of BCNU 300 mg/m^2 cytosine arabinoside and etoposide, both at 800 mg/m^2 and 140 mg/m^2 of melphalan.[84] In the BAVM regimen, etoposide is substituted by 5.2 mg/m^2 vindesine, which is given by continuous infusion over four days.[85]

There are also a number of combinations consisting of only three cytotoxic drugs. The M.D. Anderson Hospital in Houston, Texas, developed the CBNV regimen which combines cyclophosphamide 1.5 g/m^2/day over four days, with 300 mg/m^2 of BCNU and 1000 mg/m^2 of etoposide given over four days.[86,87] In the ABV combination cyclophosphamide is substituted

for by cytosine arabinoside at a dose of 800 mg/m^2 and in the BAC regimen the combination consists of BCNU and cyclophosphamide with cytosine arabinoside at the same doses as in the above protocols.[12]

There is no evidence to date that any one of these combinations is better than another. No study has shown any major advantage to a programme without irradiation. Moreover, there have been no comparative studies evaluating the ablative regimens in patients with SR, RR, and RI. Although it has not been formally studied, it seems that similar response rates are observed for most regimens when SR patients are treated. The ultimate selection of an ablative regimen, if all actually induce similar complete response rates, will depend on long-term complications as well as the availability of facilities to deliver TBI. The decision as to which ablative regimen should be used remains empirical, and serious consideration must be given to the side effects. Philip *et al.*[12] noted more early deaths in conditioning regimens combining radiation and chemotherapy. However, Armitage *et al.* noted better responses with TBI combinations.[88]

Syngeneic bone marrow transplantation in NHL

Appelbaum *et al.* published their first report of identical twin bone marrow transplantation for NHL in 1981.[89] This study was a retrospective analysis of 13 patients, 11 with intermediate and high grade NHL and two with Hodgkin's disease. All were treated with high dose, ablative therapy and bone marrow support from an identical twin. Six patients were given cyclophosphamide and 1000 cGy unfractionated TBI; in the remaining seven TBI was delivered over a 6–7 day period. Of 13 patients, ten were in RR, two in first untreated relapse and one in CR. Nine of the 11 NHL patients achieved CR and eight of the entire group of 13 patients died of progressive disease. One patient died because of septicaemia and four patients remain disease-free between 1½ and 16 years post-transplant (*see* ref. 10 and Table 25.2).

Table 25.1 Table of dosage in ablative programmes for non-Hodgkin's lymphoma

Protocol	TBI cGy/day	BCNU (carmustine) mg/m²/day	Cyclophosphamide mg/kg/day	Cytosine arabinoside mg/m²/day	6-thioguanine mg/m²/day	CCNU (lomustine) mg/m²	Melphalan mg/m²	Etoposide mg/m²/day	Vindesine mg/m²/day
CTX-TBI	400/d3–5		60/d1–2						
BACT		200/d1	50/d2–5	200/d2–5	200/d2–5				
BACT-IGR		200/d1–3	50/d2–5	200/d2–5	200/d2–5				
TACC			50/d2–5	200/d2–5	200/d2–5	250/d1			
BEAM		300/d1		200/d2–5			140/d1	200/d2–5	
BAVM		300/d1		200/d2–5				200/d2–5	5.2/d5
CBV		300/d1	1.5 g/m²/d2–5					250/d2–5	
ABV		300/d1						250/d2–5	
BAC		300/d1	1.5 g/m²/d2–5						

Table 25.2 Syngeneic and allogeneic transplantation in non-Hodgkin's lymphoma

Study	Ref.	No. patients	RI	RR	SR	1st	TD	CR	REL	No. CCR	Median (months)	Range (months)
Syngeneic:												
Appelbaum	10	13		10	3		1	12	8	4	–	18–196
Allogeneic:												
Appelbaum	10	60		42	16	2	17	37	23	14	–	12–72
Phillips	90	14	2	4	5	3	8	12	4	2	–	11+14+
O'Leary	91	10		3	4	3	1	9	4	5	29	18–73

RI, refractory to induction chemotherapy; RR, resistant relapse; SR, sensitive relapse; 1st, first remission (partial or complete); TD, toxic deaths; CR, in complete remission; REL, relapses; No. CCR, number of patients in continuous complete remission; TBI, total-body irradiation.

Allogeneic bone marrow transplantation in NHL

Sixty patients with NHL received bone marrow transplantation from an HLA matched sibling.[10] Forty-two had resistant relapse, 11 were in CR, two in RR and five in untreated relapse at the time of high dose therapy. Seventeen patients died of transplant-related complications and 37 of the 60 achieved a CR, including the 11 who were already in complete remission prior to ablative therapy. Of the 37 achieving CR, 14 survive in continuous complete remission between one and six years post-treatment (Table 25.2). All patients who did not achieve a complete remission died of progressive lymphoma.

Phillips[90] reported 14 patients with intermediate and high grade NHL treated with high dose cyclophosphamide and TBI followed by allogeneic bone marrow transplantation. At the time of harvest, two patients had refractory disease, four were in resistant relapse (RR) and four in untreated relapse; only three were in first CR. All patients engrafted with a median of 18 days (range 12–29) to 1000 WBCs. Only two did not achieve CR with ablative treatment and both died of progressive lymphoma. Eight patients died of interstitial pneumonitis and were without malignant disease clinically or, in five cases, at necropsy. Two patients died of acute GVHD and two relapsed. Two survive at 11 and 41 months after transplantation without evidence of disease (Table 25.2).

Ten relapsed patients treated with cyclophosphamide, BCNU, cytosine arabinoside and TBI followed by allogeneic bone marrow transplantation have been reported by O'Leary *et al.*[91] All had high grade histology (six Burkitt's and four lymphoblastic lymphoma) three were in first remission, four in later remission and three were in relapse at the time of transplantation. Four of the seven transplanted with disease sensitive to conventional treatment and one of the three treated with resistant disease survive, disease-free, at 29 months (range 18–73) after bone marrow transplantation (Table 25.2).

Autologous bone marrow transplantation (ABMT) in NHL

Ten years ago the first series of 22 NHL patients treated with autologous bone marrow rescue was published.[81] All patients were considered resistant to standard therapy and received the BACT ablative regimen. Few early treatment-related deaths were observed. Of the 18 evaluable patients, nine received autologous bone marrow and nine did not receive any marrow support. Patients receiving bone marrow support demonstrated significant earlier haematological reconstitution. Of all the patients treated, ten achieved a CR and eight a partial remission. Three patients who achieved CR survive disease-free today. This study demonstrated that ablative therapy could induce CR in resistant patients (although prior therapy was not very aggressive in comparison to present treatment regimens) and that autologous bone marrow support was feasible and hastened engraftment.

During the past decade an increasing number of centres have treated incurable NHL patients with high dose ablative therapy and autologous bone marrow support. In a report summarizing 2570 patients with haematological malignancies and solid tumours, receiving autotransplants at 43 centres worldwide, it was found that lymphoma was the disease most commonly treated by high dose ablative therapy and ABMT; this represented 935 transplants, or 36 per cent of the total.[13]

Although the experience of autologous bone marrow transplantation in patients with non-Hodgkin's lymphoma has exponentially increased, the interpretation of the published studies is often difficult because of variable patient selection, and differences between series with respect to histological subclassification, stage of the disease and the type of ablative therapy chosen. These characteristics are often poorly defined, and so comparison among studies is problematic.

There are obvious restrictions to autologous bone marrow transplantation. Bone marrow may be contaminated with malignant cells,[71,72] and therefore most centres have chosen not to transplant patients with bone marrow involvement at the time of transplantation. More recently, with the advent of monoclonal antibodies defining antigens on tumour cells but not on pluripotent stem cells, techniques have been developed to purge tumour cells from infiltrated bone marrow.[11,87]

Clinical trials with unpurged bone marrow

Intermediate and high grade lymphomas

Goldstone *et al.* have recently summarized the data on NHL patients transplanted by the European Bone Marrow Transplantation Group (Table 25.3).[31] Five hundred and eleven patients, of which 393 were adults with intermediate and high grade lymphoma, were reported. The study represents the experience of 41 centres and the large number of patients permits analysis of several variables. All bone marrows

were uninvolved at harvest. The conditioning was not uniform, with 59 per cent of the patients receiving only combination chemotherapy and the remaining 41 per cent TBI plus cytotoxic drugs. Purging was applied in 27 per cent. One hundred and thirty-five of the patients (26 per cent) treated were in first remission, 82 (16 per cent) were refractory to induction, 94 (18 per cent) were transplanted in resistant relapse and 159 (32 per cent) in sensitive relapse. A CR was obtained in 53 per cent of evaluable patients. Two hundred and two patients are still in CR. For patients in CR after ABMT, the likelihood of being disease-free at five years was 56 per cent. In multivariate analyses, the only significant prognostic factor was the disease status at the time of ABMT. For patients treated in first CR the risk of a toxic death was 9 per cent, for patients in relapse it was 20 per cent. Relapse occurred in 67 per cent of the cases in sites of

Table 25.3   Autologous transplantation in NHL with *unpurged* bone marrow

Study	Ref.	No. patients	RI	RR	SR	1st	TD	CR	REL	No. CCR	Median (months)	Range (months)
General												
Goldstone	31	511	82	94	159	135	87	30	254	202	>24+	–
Unpurged												
Philip	12	100					21			19	32+	21–35
			34				7	9	9	0		
				22			4	10	7	3		37–53
					44		10	38	15	16	33+	21–75
Philip	93	17	–	–	–	17	2	13		13	24+	9–83
Appelbaum	10	27	22	5			11	14	8	6	–	12–170
Armitage	88	29	27	2			2		21	6	12+	5–25
Armitage	95	19	3	16			9	12	4	3*	27+	22–34
Schouten	96	18		4	14		7	12	3	7	12+	3–60
Phillips	97	27		22	5	0	6		16	5	40+	19–71
Gribben	98	44		32	12	0	5		28	7	32+	–
Gulati	99	31					5	25	9	15	48+	
					17		5	11	6	4	45+	36–48
						14		14	3	11	49+	

RI, refractory to induction chemotherapy; RR, resistant relapse; SR, sensitive relapse; 1st, first remission (partial or complete); TD, toxic deaths, CR, in complete remission after BMT; REL relapses; No. CRR, number of patients in continuous complete remission. * Two additional patients were salvaged after relapse.

prior disease. Twenty per cent of the relapses were observed in the bone marrow or in the blood of patients who did not have bone marrow involvement prior to high dose ablative therapy and bone marrow reinfusion. The number of neutrophils reached 500 after a median of 18 days (range 7–95). In the previous analysis of the EBMT–NHL experience with 393 patients, it was shown that 70 per cent of the patients transplanted in first remission survived disease-free at two years. However, 50 per cent of those treated as responding relapse and only 20 per cent of those resistant to conventional salvage chemotherapy did as well.[92]

Philip *et al.*[12] analysed the results of 100 NHL patients transplanted at eleven centres in Europe and in the United States (Table 25.3). Patients were all adult with intermediate and high grade histological subtypes. Sixty-one received high dose chemotherapy only (BEAM, BACT or TACC) and 39 received high dose chemotherapy (17 melphalan, 13 cytosine arabinoside and cyclophosphamide, 5 cyclophosphamide and 4 BACT) plus TBI at different schedules. Thirty-four patients were refractory to induction chemotherapy. Of the 66 who relapsed after achieving complete remission with conventional therapy, 22 were in RR and 44 had SR. The disease-free survival at three years was zero for the refractory group, 14 per cent in the RR group and 36 per cent for patients responding to salvage chemotherapy. The morbidity and mortality rates were high. Twenty-one patients died from toxic complications, including ten from septicaemia and five from interstitial pneumonitis. The transplantation-related mortality was higher in the irradiated group (28 per cent) than in patients conditioned with chemotherapy only (16 per cent). In spite of this, the survival at three years was 19 per cent in both groups. Although all patients had histologically uninvolved bone marrow, eight patients relapsed in the marrow.

Philip *et al.* recently reported on 17 patients (five with intermediate, 12 with high grade histology) treated in France with ABMT while in partial remission after induction chemotherapy (Table 25.3).[93] As stated before, such patients have a short survival if treated with standard salvage chemotherapy. Two patients died of transplant-related complications and two did not reach CR with ablative chemotherapy. The remaining 13 are disease-free at a median of 24 months (range 3–86) after transplantation.

Appelbaum *et al.* described 27 patients who underwent ABMT (Table 25.3)[10]: 22 had intermediate and high grade NHL and five had Hodgkin's disease. All but four patients were in RR at the time of ABMT. Bone marrow was histologically negative in all patients,[94] and the last three patients underwent bone marrow purging with monoclonal antibodies and complement. Standard conditioning with cyclophosphamide and total body irradiation was used. Eleven patients died of transplant-related complications, 14 achieved CR and eight subsequently relapsed. Six of the 27, or 15 per cent, survive disease-free at two years.

Diffuse large cell lymphoma

Armitage *et al.* published a series on patients with diffuse large cell lymphoma (Table 25.3).[88] Eleven of the patients were refractory to induction chemotherapy, 16 were in resistant relapse and only two were sensitive to reinduction chemotherapy. Twenty-one received TBI and cytotoxic drugs and eight were conditioned with combination chemotherapy alone (CTX, CCNU, VP-16 and Ara-C). None of the patients in the latter group reached CR, but six out of 11 who entered CR after a TBI-containing regimen are in CCR at 9 months range. As well as TBI, good performance status and previous CR are considered to be favourable prognostic features. Four patients died of sepsis and in the remaining patients a blood cell count of 500 granulocytes per mm^3 was reached after a median of 23 days. Three patients who had never had bone marrow involvement relapsed in the marrow. This was associated with circulating lymphoma cells and occurred at the same time as the reappearance of normal haematopoiesis, suggesting possible contamination of the reinfused bone marrow.

Relapsed lymphoma

Armitage *et al*. summarized their experience of ABMT for relapsed lymphoma (Table 25.3);[95] a number of the patients in this study were included in the previous report.[89] Nineteen patients with progressing tumours received cytosine arabinoside, cyclophosphamide and TBI. Three were refractory to induction chemotherapy because they did not respond to CHOP and the other 16 were in resistant relapse. Twelve achieved complete response but only three remain in CCR at 566+, 604+ and 1035+ days. Two others have been successfully salvaged and are disease-free two and three years after relapse. There were nine toxic deaths among these patients: five from sepsis, three from interstitial pneumonitis and one as a result of haemorrhage.

Follicular lymphoma

Schouten *et al*. treated 18 patients with follicular lymphomas (Table 25.3).[96] Nine had converted to high grade lymphomas at the time of transplant, five of whom were considered to be in SR and four in RR. In nine others histological conversion had not occurred at the time of transplantation: two had follicular small cell NHL (group B in the working formulation), one follicular mixed (group C) and five had follicular large cell (group D, usually considered as intermediate grade histology); all were in SR. Among the patients who experienced conversion, three achieved CR, but only one remained disease-free at day 99; all of the patients with unconverted follicular histologies achieved CR. In the conversion group six patients died of transplant-related problems and two of progressive disease. Of the patients with follicular histology, one died of septicaemia and one relapsed one year later. In all, seven patients survive disease-free at 8–60 months.

Other studies

Phillips *et al*. have reported their experiences of ABMT in NHL (Table 25.3).[97] Twenty-four patients are reported, mostly non-responsive to conventional salvage regimens, together with an additional three patients with resistant Hodgkin's disease. All patients had relapsed: twenty two were in RR but five had responded to salvage chemotherapy. The preparative regimen consisted of cyclophosphamide and TBI. Complete remission after ABMT was observed in 15 patients, five of whom were in complete remission at 19+ to 71+ months. Fifteen relapsed or did not respond to treatment and six died of complications.

Gribben *et al*. reported on 44 NHL patients who were transplanted by the Bloomsbury Transplant Group (Table 25.3).[98] Twelve were refractory to induction chemotherapy, 32 received the ABMT after relapse and only 12 were responding to standard salvage chemotherapy at the time of transplant. Of these 12, five are in CCR with a median follow up of 26 months, whereas only two out of the 20 treated in RR are disease-free at 40+ and 54+ months. All but one were conditioned with chemotherapy alone, consisting of BCNU, etoposide, cytosine arabinoside and cyclophosphamide or melphalan (BEAM/BVAC). In the refractory group only five reached CR and the follow-up at time of publication was too short to draw meaningful conclusions.

Gulati *et al*. have recently published the results of 31 patients who had poor prognostic features at diagnosis (such as high LDH and bulky disease) or had relapsed (Table 25.3). Twenty-three had a histological diagnosis of diffuse large cell NHL and eight had diffuse mixed cell lymphoma. Fourteen patients were randomized to receive cyclophosphamide (120 mg/kg) and fractionated TBI (1320 cGy) plus ABMT immediately after achieving partial or complete remission with induction treatment (L 17M protocol).[101] They show a survival of 79 per cent (11/14) at a median follow-up of four years. Thirteen patients treated with the same induction protocol were randomized to continue treatment with the same combination chemotherapy; four are still in CR at 36–80 months. The remaining nine relapsed, and of those, six received ABMT. All six died, two of progressive disease and four of therapy-related complications. An additional 11 patients who relapsed after different induction regimens underwent ABMT. All responded to the treatment but six relapsed, one died of thrombotic complications and only four are in DFS at 3–5 years. The difference in DFS between patients transplanted in first partial or complete remission, and those transplanted after relapse is striking: 11/14 versus 4/17.

Clinical trials with purged bone marrow

Elimination of malignant cells from bone marrow: ex vivo purging

The concept of purging tumour cells from bone marrow with monoclonal antibodies (MoAbs) in patients with NHL arose from studies of ABMT in patients with lymphoblastic leukaemia.[101,102] There are several requirements of a MoAb which is to be used for bone marrow purging. First, the antibody must be strongly reactive with an antigen on the tumour cell surface, but must not be reactive with pluripotent or committed haematopoetic progenitor cells.[103] Careful *in vitro* screening using stem cell assays must be undertaken prior to considering an antibody for purging. Second, the antibody must be suitable for the techniques being used for tumour cell removal.

A large number of techniques to deplete normal cells of contaminating tumour cells using monoclonal antibodies have been developed over the last decade.[104] Complement and immunotoxins can be used to destroy tumour cells. Physical methods include the use of antibodies coupled to magnetic beads which can then be removed, along with attached tumour cells, from the marrow. Each method has advantages and disadvantages but, to date, it is not clear which is the most efficacious.[105] There is increasing evidence that purging with multiple antibodies, all directed at different antigens, is more effective than purging with a single antibody.[102] Similarly, the use of monoclonal antibodies directed against several epitopes present on a single antigen may also increase the efficiency of cytoreduction.

Most methods of purging appear to deplete between 2 and 5 logs of tumour cells, the precise number varies according to the antibody selected and the intensity of antigen expression.[106] However, at present it is unclear which

bone marrows need to be purged, and also whether purging is essential to prevent relapse from reinfusion of contaminating tumour cells with the bone marrow. It is known that tumour cells can be cultured from the bone marrow of histologically negative lymphoma patients.[71] Moreover, more sensitive techniques to identify tumour cells in bone marrow are likely to be positive in the majority of patients.[107] (These techniques include the detection of clonal immunoglobulin gene rearrangements or the use of the polymerase chain reaction to identify translocations, e.g. the 14;18 translocation which involves the *bcl*-2 oncogene and which can be identified with a markedly increased sensitivity by PCR than by cytogenetics.) Therefore, the necessity of purging can only be determined by performing well designed, randomized trials. These will be difficult to undertake in patients with overt tumour cell infiltration of the marrow, in whom reinfusion of unpurged marrow could be questioned on scientific and ethical grounds. Conversely, such trials may be difficult to interpret and to perform in patients with histologically normal marrow, since such patients are less likely to relapse. Because of this, very large numbers of patients in each arm of the trial would be required. This field of investigation is young, however, and at present it would seem more important to address issues such as the choice of ablative therapy and the selection of patients for ABMT.

Clinical studies

In 1982 a protocol using an anti-B1 MoAb was initiated at the Dana Farber Cancer Institute (DFCI) for *in vitro* treatment of bone marrow in patients with relapsed B-cell NHL (Table 25.4).[11] Patients below the age of 65 were included if their tumour cells expressed the CD 20 (B1) cell surface antigen. In addition, the patients had to attain a near complete remission prior to ABMT, a situation referred to as 'minimal disease' (no masses greater than 2 cm^2 and less than 5 per cent bone marrow involvement, both determined histologically and by flow cytometric analysis) with either chemotherapy or local radiotherapy.[108] Up to December 1987, 64 patients with a median age of 44, and with

Table 25.4 Autologous transplantation in NHL using *purged* bone marrow

Study	Ref.	No. patients	RI	RR	SR	1st	MAb*	TD	CR	REL	No. CCR	Median (months)	Range (months)
DFCI	109	73		0	64	9	B1+ MMA	4	71	19	50	24+	1–60
Philip	111	28		3	13	12	Y29/55	4 4		11 3 2 6	13 7 6	22+	2–52
Rohatiner	112	12			12		B1	1	11	0	11	NR	14–60
Hurd	113	16	8	5	3		BA-1 BA-2 BA-3	4	10		9	NR 55% at 32	NR
Baumgartner	114	7		0		6	Y29/55	1	6	1	5	27+	8–34
Braine	115	14			14	0	4-HC	2		5	7	20+	6–48

*MAb, monoclonal antibodies; MMA, multiple monoclonal antibodies; BA-1, BA-2, BA-3, antibodies against epitopes CD9, CD10, CD24; 4-HC, 4 hydroperoxycyclophosphamide; RI, refractory to induction chemotherapy; RR, resistant relapse; SR, sensitive relapse; 1st, first remission (partial or complete); TD, toxic deaths; CR, in complete remission after BMT; REL, relapses; No. CCR, number of patients in continuous complete remission

recurrent B-cell NHL had been treated on this protocol.[109] Essentially all of the patients presented with unfavourable histological subtypes and all had advanced stage disease (III/IV). All patients were induced into either a disease-free or minimal disease state. Nine additional patients received ABMT as consolidation in first remission. The bone marrows from an additional 11 patients with greater than 5 per cent tumour cells in the bone marrow were treated with anti-B1 and one or more monoclonal antibodies (including anti-B5, J5, and J2). Following bone marrow harvest, patients were treated with 60/mg/kg of cyclophosphamide over two days followed by 1200 cGy TBI fractionated over a three day period. A complete response was achieved in all 64 patients with no bone marrow involvement. Nineteen patients relapsed, most of these within the first six months. Essentially, all relapses occurred in sites of previous bulk disease and most of these patients died. Fifty patients are alive in unmaintained remission with a median disease free survival of 24+ months (range 1–60+).

The conditioning regimen was well tolerated by all patients. Nausea, vomiting, mucositis, weight loss and fever were frequently seen. One patient died of veno-occlusive disease of the liver on day 20 following bone marrow infusion and one died of intracerebral hemorrhage secondary to refractory thrombocytopenia on day 36.

The first evidence of WBC recovery was seen by days 10–12, with a granulocyte count reaching more than 500/mm³ between days 10–80 (median of 26 days). A stable platelet count above 20 000/mm³ was seen between days 14–180 (median of 29).

The reconstitution of B-cells in these patients was of interest in view of the presence of the CD20 antigen on 50 per cent of pre-B-cells and all mature normal B-cells. CD20-positive cells were first detected in the peripheral blood during the second month after autologous BMT, and 53 of 68 patients recovered to a level of at least 5 per cent of peripheral blood lymphocytes reactive with the CD20 monoclonal antibody at a median of three months. Normal percentages of monocytes, natural killer cells, T lymphocytes

and T8 lymphocytes (representing suppressor and cytotoxic populations) were observed after one month. However the T-helper lymphocytes (T4) and the T4/T8 ratio did not return to normal for a period of well over one year. Serum IgM had returned to normal by six months after ABMT, but in the majority of patients it took up to one year for levels of IgG and IgA to return to near normality.[110]

In summary, the preparative regimen used in these multiply relapsed patients with B-cell non-Hodgkin's lymphoma was able to induce a complete response in all patients. Anti-B1-treated bone marrow was able to fully reconstitute the patients both haematologically and immunologically. The toxicity of this programme was acceptable, with only two treatment-related deaths. Currently, 39 of 63 (62 per cent) patients remain in unmaintained remission with a median disease-free survival of 24+ months (range 9–54).

Fourteen patients with Burkitt's lymphoma who received anti-Y29/55-treated marrow have been reported by Philip *et al.*[111] along with an additional 14 patients treated with unpurged bone marrow (Table 25.4). Seventeen patients received BACT, 10 BEAM and one cyclophosphamide alone as ablative therapy. Of the 14 patients in the Y29/55 purged group, nine were in first partial or complete remission at the time of transplant and six of these had a positive bone marrow at disease presentation. Reasons for treatment included CNS involvement at diagnosis (five patients), a long interval to the time of achieving CR, or achievement of PR only with induction chemotherapy. After autologous BMT, six of the 12 patients transplanted in first partial or complete remission were reported alive after between 14 and 60 months.

The survival curves of relapsed patients treated with purged or unpurged marrow were comparable. The haematologic recovery of the two groups did not differ, and was similar to that observed at the DFCI.

Rohatiner *et al.* have reported 12 patients with relapsed NHL, ten with follicular lymphoma and two with high grade histology who received anti-B1-purged marrow following ablative high dose cyclophosphamide and TBI (Table 25.4).[112] One patient died of infection during aplasia.

Eleven of the patients remain in continuous complete remission with similar toxicity and haematological and immunological reconstitution to that seen at the DFCI. Recovery to 500 neutrophils/mm^3 occurred after a median of 25 days (range 15–45). With the predominant histological subtype of nodular lymphoma, this series of patients will require longer follow-up to determine the therapeutic efficacy of this treatment.

Hurd, at the University of Minnesota, reported twelve patients with B-cell lymphomas, of a variety of histological subtypes but mostly intermediate grade histology, who received autologous bone marrow treated *in vitro* with anti-CD9, anti-CD10 and anti-CD24 MoAb, plus complement (Table 25.4).[113]Engraftment was apparent at a median of 23 days (15–59). Three patients died of therapy-related deaths and three patients died of progressive lymphoma. The Kaplan–Meier projected survival at 32 months is 55±30 per cent and none of the patients relapsed after achieving CR with ABMT.

A study initiated by Baumgartner *et al.*[114] used anti-Y29/55 and rabbit complement to treat the bone marrow of paediatric patients with Burkitt's lymphoma or other B-cell type NHL prior to ABMT (Table 25.4). To date, seven patients with advanced stage disease were treated after remission induction with vincristine, doxorubicin (Adriamycin), cyclophosphamide and 600 cGy TBI followed by infusion of anti-Y29/55-treated marrow. Six of the seven patients were in complete remission at the time of the ABMT. Of the six patients in first remission, five were reported to be in continuous complete remission from 8+ to 34+ months (median 27+ months) post-BMT. The remaining patient, who was transplanted in first remission, had marrow involvement at diagnosis, and subsequently relapsed in the marrow at six weeks. One additional patient, who was in second partial remission at the time of transplant, subsequently relapsed in the abdomen. Haematological engraftmen of anti-Y29/55-purged marrow was similar to unpurged marrow. The median time required to achieve a white blood count of 1000/mm^3 was 13 days, while the median time required to achieve a platelet count greater than 50 000/mm^3 was 27 days.

Braine *et al.* reported the John Hopkins experience in 14 patients whose marrow had been purged with 4-hydroperoxycyclophosphamide (4-HC). No patient had bone marrow involvement or poor performance status and most had aggressive histology. The conditioning used was the standard combination of TBI and cyclophosphamide. All patients who were not in remission at the time of harvesting reached complete remission after high dose therapy. The median time required to reach a count of 500 granulocytes/mm^3 was 21 days (12–40). One patient died of infection. At a median observation time of 3.5 years, seven patients are in CCR. No significant delay in immunological reconstitution was observed.

Two groups have examined the use of anti-T-cell MoAbs defining pan T-cell antigens and complement as well as T101-ricin A chain for purging marrow of patients with T-cell lymphoblastic lymphoma prior to autologous BMT.

Seven patients have been reported from Johns Hopkins University (ages 5–39), who received marrow treated with either Leu-1 (anti-CD5) alone or in combination with Leu-9 (anti-CD7); both regimens included complement.[116] Three of these patients were in continuous complete remission at 131+ to 1,320+ days and four relapsed.

Gorin *et al.*[116] have reported three patients with advanced stage, T lymphoblastic lymphoma whose marrow was purged with T101-ricin A chain as a means of depleting neoplastic T lymphoblasts. All three patients engrafted required a similar period of time for the development of adequate numbers of granulocytes and platelets as was required in the previously reported trials of ABMT which included bone marrow purging. At the time of the report, only one patient remained disease-free at 11+ months.

Although it is difficult to know whether marrow purging had a significant effect in these studies, anti-T-cell MoAb with complement and immunotoxin T-101-treated marrow was clearly capable of reconstituting the bone marrow.

Conclusions

Following relapse from conventional salvage treatment, fewer than 10 per cent of patients survive disease-free for longer than a few months. Therefore, to date, bone marrow transplantation has been the only effective salvage regimen. Unfortunately, most physicians only refer patients for consideration of BMT after one or more relapses. In this setting, it is not surprising that the majority of early BMT trials[10,88,95] were associated with prohibitive toxicity and a high relapse rate. Examination of these studies revealed that the majority of patients had tumours which were resistant to treatment, a poor performance status and, in most cases, were transplanted in the presence of a significant tumour burden. Although only a small percentage of patients were long-term survivors, these early studies demonstrated the feasibility of the procedure and suggested that small numbers of patients could be cured.

Several groups have found a correlation between sensitivity of relapsed NHL to standard or high (salvage) dose therapy and the disease-free survival subsequently achieved with transplantation. It therefore appears possible to identify the patients who are likely to become long-term survivors, i.e. patients transplanted in sensitive relapse. Analysis of the data summarized in Tables 25.2, 25.3 and 25.4 showed a DFS of 36 per cent and 60 per cent for patients transplanted while responding to salvage chemotherapy, whereas those transplanted in RR had a DFS of 20 per cent. Patients who never responded to treatment, i.e. who were refractory to induction chemotherapy, were not salvaged.

In examining these results three major questions appear to be unanswered. First, which ablative regimen is most efficacious; second, what is the optimal source of bone marrow; finally, what is the impact of high dose chemotherapy and bone marrow rescue on the natural history of NHL? Each of these points will be addressed separately.

The choice of the ablative regimen continues to be a matter of significant debate. To date, no preparative regimen has been shown to be superior to any other. A successful regimen must balance dose intensity, tumour cell sensitivity and toxicity. It must be remembered that the dose-limiting toxicity of virtually every antineoplastic agent is non-haematological. Moreover, as agents are combined, new toxicities are described (e.g. veno-occlusive disease). The standard preparative regimen, consisting of high dose cyclophosphamide and TBI, was developed with the aim of combining immunosuppression with an antineoplastic effect. There are, however, several concerns about the use of TBI in patients receiving ABMT, since TBI contributes unique toxicities and its efficacy in certain histological subtypes of NHL is questionable. On the other hand, TBI is effective in eliminating both neoplastic cells in the sanctuary sites (CNS and testes) and cells resistant to drugs. A number of preparative regimens without TBI have been developed with both increased and decreased toxicity. However, the EBMTG has noted no differences in DFS between ablative regimens which contain TBI and those which do not.[31] Clearly a prospective randomized trial will be necessary, in which cyclophosphamide and TBI are compared with a drug regimen and no TBI, to determine their relative efficacy. Each arm of such a study would need to be stratified for the major histological subgroups.

The optimal source of bone marrow also remains undecided. The major difficulty in comparing the efficacy and toxicity of syngeneic and allogeneic BMT is the small number of reported cases. The theoretical advantage of graft-versus-leukaemia effect observed with allogeneic marrow has not been assessed for NHL. Moreover, very few patients with overt bone marrow infiltration have been treated with allogeneic transplantation to determine whether they will subsequently relapse in the marrow.

In contrast to the small numbers of patients treated with syngeneic and allogenic bone marrow transplantation, several thousand cases of autologous bone marrow transplantation for NHL have been reported. Although autologous bone marrow is the most frequently used source of bone marrow, several basic issues remain unresolved. It is presently unknown, for example, whether clonogenic lymphoma cells exist. Moreover, if they do exist it is not known whether they are removed during harvesting of the marrow or whether they survive the harvest and freezing procedure.

Virtually all patients who have undergone ABMT to date have had histologically normal bone marrows. It is, therefore, not known whether grossly involved bone marrow could be harvested and whether the contaminated bone marrow would lead to relapse.

During the past six years, several groups have attempted to deplete tumour cells from the marrow using monoclonal antibodies. *In vitro* studies suggest that 2 to 5 logs of tumour cells can be purged depending upon the antibody, or the combination of antibodies used. From published clinical trials, two conclusions can be thus far drawn. First, purged bone marrow has successfully engrafted. Second, there is no significant apparent prolongation of engraftment with purging. However, no controlled clinical trials addressing the efficacy for marrow purging have been reported. Since large numbers of patients will need to be randomized to determine the efficacy of bone marrow purging, this question will be difficult to address. Moreover, most investigators would argue that selection of patients and the nature of the ablative regimen are more important questions to consider before embarking on a randomized trial concerning purging.

The last important question is whether BMT has changed the natural history of NHL. The answer, so far, is no. Since the majority of patients are referred for BMT with resistant disease, at best 20 per cent of all relapsed patients may be cured. Considering the advanced age of many patients and the incidence of co-morbid disease, the impact of BMT on relapsed patients in reported series is at best modest. If BMT is to have an effect on the natural history of NHL it must be used when patients have sensitive disease. The precise timing of BMT in relationship to the patient's disease status may differ, depending on the histological subtype as well as prognostic factors. This is clearly the most important question to be addressed in the next decade.

Finally, it is important to examine the long-term sequelae of BMT. If this procedure is to be used much earlier, it is crucial to consider its long-term impact. In children, TBI can impair growth.[117] Other long-term side effects are restrictive and obstructive pulmonary diseases,

endocrine dysfunctions (hypothyroidism), infertility and cataract formation.[118] Infertility is generally the rule following TBI, whereas conditioning with drugs alone permits the recovery of normal levels of hormones as well as ovulatory cycles and sperm production.[119,120] Cataracts developed in 80 per cent of patients treated with single dose TBI whereas an incidence of 20 per cent was observed after fractionated TBI and with chemotherapy regimens only.[122] A major concern is the possibility of inducing secondary malignancies, as this is more frequently observed after curative treatment of other haematological malignancies. Solid tumours have been associated with irradiation after allogeneic BMT, but the overall incidence of secondary malignancies has been found to be low (less than 1 per cent).[122]

It is important to stress that the most important issue is the impact of BMT on the natural history of the NHL. From all the data reviewed in this chapter it is clear that if BMT is to cure patients with NHL, it has to be used much earlier in the course of the disease. Patients who are transplanted in first partial or complete remission appear, although their numbers are small, to have a 75 per cent chance of long-term, disease-free survival. This is true both for CR patients with bad prognostic features at presentation and for patients achieving only partial remission with induction treatment. Therefore, these preliminary data suggest that if patients with poor prognostic characteristics are treated with BMT in first remission, the natural history of the disease may be changed. It will eventually be important to compare marrow sources and ablative regimens in prospective trials. We believe that the answers to these questions will only be relevant if examined in patients responding to standard therapy. The efficacy of different ablative regimens may differ in different histological subtypes, but the likelihood of detecting these differences in relapsed patients will be small. Similarly, purging will be difficult to assess in patients who have already relapsed at sites of bulk disease. Therefore, the answers to these questions must await the inclusion of less advanced patients in clinical studies.

New technologies may have an impact upon the acute toxicity of high dose chemoradiotherapy. Preliminary evidence using colony stimulating factors (CSFs) to reverse the blood counts more rapidly after BMT[123] suggest that myeloid engraftment may be hastened by such factors. Such treatment could, therefore, lead to fewer toxic deaths and possibly to shorter hospital stays. Similarly, the availability of peripheral blood stem cells[124] and the possibility of increasing their numbers with CSFs may obviate the need for bone marrow harvest. Other biological response modifiers to stimulate endogenous host immune response of T-cell mediated functions and of NK cells also have potential for improving long-term survival. These studies are just beginning, but one should bear in mind that their impact on the natural history of NHL can only be assessed when BMT is undertaken in chemotherapy-sensitive patients.

References

1. Portlock CS. *Seminars in Hematology*. 1983; **20**, 25–34.
2. Skarin AT. *Seminars in Oncology*. 1986; **13**, 10–25, (suppl 5)
3. Non-Hodgkin's lymphoma pathologic classification project. National Cancer Institute sponsored study of classifications of non-Hodgkin's lymphomas: Summary and description of a working formulation for clinical usage. *Cancer*. 1982; **49**, 2112–354.
4. Rosenberg SA. *Journal of Clinical Oncology*. 1985; **3**, 299–310.
5. Horwich A, Peckham M. *Seminars in Hematology*. 1983; **20**, 35–58.
6. Skarin AT, Canellos GP, Rosenthal DS, *et al. Journal of Clinical Oncology*. 1983; **1**, 91–8.
7. Singer CRJ, Goldstone AH. *Clinical Hematology*. 1986; **15**, 105–50.
8. Cabanillas F, Velasquez WS, McLaughlin P, Jagannath S, *et al. Seminars in Hematology*. 1988; **25**, 47–50.
9. Fefer A. *Clinical Hematology*. 1986; **15**, 49–65.
10. Appelbaum FR, Sullivan KM, Buckner CD, *et al. Journal of Clinical Oncology*. 1987; **5**, 1340–47.
11. Nadler LM, Takvorian T, Botnick L, Bast RC, Finberg R, Hellman S, Canellos GP, Schlossman SF. *Lancet* ii. 1984; 427–31.
12. Philip T, Armitage JO, Spitzer G, Chauvin F, et al. *New England Journal of Medicine*. 1987; **316**, 1493–8.
13. Armitage JO, Gale RP. *Lancet*. ii, 1986; 960–2.
14. Appelbaum FR. *Bone Marrow Transplantation*. 1987; **2**, 227–31.
15. Petersen FB, Buckner CD. *Hematological Oncology*. 1987; **5**, 233–43.
16. Rudders RA, Kaddis M, DeLellis RA, Casey H Jr. *Cancer*. 1979; **43**, 1643–51.
17. Horning SJ, Rosenberg SA. *New England Journal of Medicine*. 1984; **311**, 1471–5.
18. Gospodarowicz MK, Bush RS, Brown TC, Chua T. *International Journal of Radiation Oncology, Biology and Physics*. 1984; **10**, 489–97.
19. Kalter S, Holmes L, Cabanillas F. *Hematological Oncology*. 1987; **5**, 127–38.
20. Young RC, Longo DL, Glatstein E, Ihde DC, Jaffe ES, DeVita VT Jr. *Seminars in Hematology*. 1988; **25**, 11–16.
21. Miller TP, Dana BW, Weick JK, Jones SE, Coltman CC, Dahlberg S, Fisher RI. *Seminars in Hematology*. 1988; **25**, 17–22.
22. Armitage JO, Weisenburger DD, Hutchins M, *et al. Journal of Clinical Oncology*. 1986; **4**, 160–4.
23. Fisher RI, Hubbard SM, DeVita VT, Jr. *et al. Blood*. 1981; **58**, 45–51.
24. Fisher RI, DeVita VT Jr, Johnson BL, *et al. American Journal of Medicine*. 1977; **63**, 177–82.
25. Freedman AS, Nadler LM. *Seminars in Oncology*. 1987; **14**, 193–212.
26. Yunis JJ. In: DeVita VT, Hellman S, Rosenberg S (eds). *Important Advances in Oncology*. 1986; 93–114.
27. Korsmeyer SJ. In: DeVita VT, Jr., Hellman S, Rosenberg S, (eds). *Important Advances in Oncology*. 1987; 3–25.
28. Israel MA, Helman LJ, Miser J. In: DeVita VT, Jr., Hellman S, Rosenberg S (eds). *Important Advances in Oncology*. 1987; 87–103.
29. Merkel DE, McGuire WL. In: DeVita VT, Jr., Hellman S, Rosenberg S, (eds). *Important Advances in Oncology*. 1988; 103–19.
30. Cabinallas F, Hagemeister FB, Bodey GP, Freireich EJ. *Blood*. 1982; **60**, 693.
31. Goldstone AH, Singer CRJ, Gribben JG, Jarrett M. *Bone Marrow Transplantation*. 1988; **3** (suppl 1), 33–6.
32. Cabanillas F, Hagemeister FB, Bodey GP, Freireich EJ. *Blood*. 1982; **60**, 693–7.
33. Laurence J, Coleman M, Allen SL, Silver RT, Pasmantier M. *Annals of Internal Medicine*. 1982; **97**, 190–95.
34. Coleman M, Boyd DB, Bernhardt B, *et al. Proceedings of the American Society Society for Clinical Oncology*. 1984; Abs. No. **246**.
35. Corder MP, Clamon GH. *Cancer*. 1984; **54**, 202.
36. Weich JK, Jones SE, Grozea PN, Fabian CJ, Dixon DO. *Cancer Treatment Reports*. 1984; **68**, 963.

37. Cavalli F, Jungi WF, Sonntag W, Nissen NI, Holland JH. *Schweizerische Medizinische Wochenschrift.* 1980; **110**, 1067.
38. Judson IR, Wiltshaw E. *Chemotherapy and Pharmacology.* 1985; **14**, 258.
39. Von Heyden HW, Scherfe A, Nagel GA. *Cancer Treatment Reports.* 1982; **9**, 45.
40. Bergerat JP, Drewinko B, Corry P, Barlogie B, Ho DH. *Cancer Research.* 1981; **41**, 25–30.
41. Hagberg H, Cavallin-Stahl E, Lind J. *Scandinavian Journal of Haematology.* 1986; **36**, 61.
42. Kroner T, Obrecht JP, Jungi WF. *Cancer Treatment Reviews.* 1982; **9**, 39.
43. Adelstein DJ, Lazarus HM, Hines JD, Herzig RH. *Cancer.* 1985; **56**, 1493.
44. Kantarjian H, Barlogie B, Plunkett W, Velasquez WS, McLaughlin P, Riggs S, Cabanillas F. *Journal of Clinical Oncology.* 1983; **1**, 689.
45. Cabanillas F, Hagemeister FB, McLaughlin P, et al. *Journal of Clinical Oncology.* 1987; **5**, 407–9.
46. Velasquez WS, Cabanillas F, Salvador P, et al. *Blood.* 1988; **71**, 117–22.
47. Thomas ED. *Cancer.* 1982; **49**, 1963–69.
48. Thomas ED. *Journal of Clinical Oncology.* 1983; **1**, 517–31.
49. Champlin RE, Gale RP. *Cancer Treatment Reports.* 1984; **68**, 145–61.
50. O'Reilly RJ. *Blood.* 1983; **62**, 941–64.
51. Goldman JM. *Hematological Oncology.* 1987; **5**, 265–79.
52. Santos GW, Tutschka PJ, Brookmeyer R, et al. *New England Journal of Medicine.* 1983; **309**, 1347–53.
53. Gale RP, Champlin RE. In: Gale RP (ed). *Recent Advances in Bone Marrow Transplantation.* New York: Alan R. Liss, 71–94.
54. Weisdorf D, Nestbit ME, Ramsay NKC, et al. *Journal of Clinical Oncology.* 1987; **5**, 1348–52.
55. Bruce WB, Meeker BE, Valeriote FA. *Journal of the National Cancer Institute.* 1966; **36**, 233–45.
56. Frei E III, Canellos GP. *American Journal of Medicine.* 1980; **69**, 585–94.
57. van Bekkum DW. *Seminars in Hematology.* 1984; **21**, 81–90.
58. Champlin RE, Gale RP. *Seminars in Hematology.* 1984; **21**, 101–8.
59. Meyers JD, Flourmoy N, Thomas ED. *Review of Infective Diseases.* 1982; **4**, 1119–32.
60. Storb R, Deeg HJ, Witehead J. et al. *New England Journal of Medicine.* 1986; **314**, 729–35.
61. Speck B, Bortin M, Champlin RE, et al. *Lancet.* **i**, 1984; 665–8.
62. Tutcshka PJ, Copelan EA, Klein JP. *Blood.* 1987; **70**, 1382–8.
63. Bortin MM, Truitt RL, Rimm A, Bach FH. *Nature,* 1979; **281**, 490–1.
64. Weiden PL, Flournoy N, Thomas ED, et al. *New England Journal of Medicine.* 1979; **300**, 1068–73.
65. Weiden PL, Sullivan KM, Flournoy N, et al. *New England Journal of Medicine.* 1981; **304**, 1529–33.
66. Powles RK, Pedrazzini A, Krofts M, et al. *Seminars in Hematology.* 1984; **21**, 182–7.
67. Beatty PG, Clift RA, Michelson EM, et al. *New England Journal of Medicine.* 1985; **313**, 765–71.
68. Apperley JF, Jones L, Hale G, et al. *Bone Marrow Transplantation.* 1986a; **1**, 53–68.
69. Arthur CK, Hows JM, Jones L, et al. *Bone Marrow Transplantation.* 1987; **2** (suppl. 1), 137.
70. Papa G, Arcese W, Mauro FR, et al. *Leukemia Research.* 1986; **10**, 1469–75.
71. Benjamin D, Magrath IT, Douglass EC, Corash LM. *Blood.* 1983; **61**, 1017–9.
72. Hu E, Trela M, Thompson J, Lowder J, Horning S, Levy R, Sklar J. *Lancet.* **ii**, 1985; 1092–5.
73. Segal GB, Simmon W, Lichiman MA. *Blood.* 1986; **68**, 1055–64.
74. Aget H, van Dyk J, I cung PMK. *Radiology.* 1977; **123**, 747.
75. Barbasch A, Higby DJ, Brass C, et al. *Cancer Treatment Reports.* 1983; **67**, 143.
76. Kim TH, Khan FM, Galvin JM. *International Journal of Radiation, Oncology, Biology and Physics.* 1980; **6**, 779.
77. Bacigalupo A, Vitale V, Frassoni F, et al. *Experimental Hematology.* 1983; **11**, 13.
78. Goolden AWG, Goldman JM, Kam KC, et al. *British Journal of Radiology.* 1983; **56**, 245.
79. Gale RP, Kersey JH, Bortin MM, Dicke KA, Good RA, Zwa N, Rimm AA. *Lancet.* 1983; **ii**. 663.
80. Sonneveld P, Van Bekkum DW. *Radiology.* 1979; **130**, 789.
81. Appelbaum FR, Herzig GP, Ziegler JL et al. *Blood.* 1978; **52**, 85–95.
82. Philip T, Biron P, Herve L, et al. *European Journal of Cancer and Clinical Oncology.* 1983; **19**, 1371–9.
83. Gorin NC, Najman A, Douay L, et al. *European Journal of Cancer and Clinical Oncology.* 1984; **20**, 217–25.
84. Biron P, Maraninchi D, Laporte JP, et al. *Cancer Treatment Reports.* 1986.
85. Philip T, Biron P, Maraninchi D, et al. In: Dicke KA, Spitzer G, Zander AR, Gorin NC (eds). *Autologous Bone Marrow Transplantation. Proceedings of the First International Symposium* 89–107, Houston: University of Texas.
86. Spitzer G, Dicke KA, Litam J, et al. *Cancer.* 1980; **45**, 3075–85.
87. Tannir NM, Spitzer G, Zander AR, et al. *European Journal of Cancer and Clinical Oncology.* 1983; 1091–6.
88. Armitage JO, Jagannath S, Spitzer G, et al.

European Journal of Cancer and Clinical Oncology. 1986; **22**, 871–7.

89. Appelbaum FR, Fefer A, Cheever MA, *et al. Blood*. 1981; **58**, 509–13.

90. Phillips GL, Herzig RH, Lazarus HM, *et al. Journal of Clinical Oncology*. 1986; **4**, 480–8.

91. O'Leary M, Ramsay MKC, Nesbit ME Jr, *et al. American Journal of Medicine*. 1983; **75**, 497–501.

92. Goldstone AH, Gribben J, Dones L. *Bone Marrow Transplantation*. 1987; **2** (suppl 1), 200–3.

93. Philip T, Hartmann O, Biron P, *et al. Journal of Clinical Oncology*. 1988; **6**, 1118–24.

94. Appelbaum FR, Sullivan KM, Thomas ED, *et al. International Journal of Cell Cloning*. 1985; **3**, 216–17.

95. Armitage JO, Gingrigh RD, Klassen LW, *et al. Cancer Treatment Reports*. 1986; **70**, 871–5.

96. Schouten HC, Bierman PH, Vaughan WP, *et al.* submitted for publication.

97. Phillips GL, Herzig RH, Lazarus HM, *et al. New England Journal of Medicine*. 1984; **310**, 1557–61.

98. Gribben JG, Vaughan Hudson B, Linch DC. *Hematological Oncology*. 1987; **5**, 281–93.

99. Gulati SC, Shank B, Black P, *et al. Journal of Clinical Oncology*. 1988; **6**, 1303–13.

100. Clarkson B, Ellis S, Little C, *et al. Seminars in Oncology*. 1985; **12**, 160–79.

101. Anderson KC, Sallan S, Takvorian T, *et al. International Journal of Cell Cloning*. 1985; **3**, 239–40.

102. Ritz J, Pesando M, Notis-McConarty J, Lazarus H, Schlossman S. *Nature*. 1980; **283**, 583.

103. Bast RC Jr, Ritz J, Lipton J, *et al. Cancer Research*. 1983; **43**, 1389–94.

104. Jansen J, Falkenburg JHF, Stephan DE, LeBien TW. *Seminars in Hematology*. 1984; **21**, 164–81.

105. Reading CL, Takaue Y. *Biochemica Biophysica Acta*. 1986; **865**, 141–70.

106. Treleaven JG, Kemshead JT. *Hematological Oncology*. 1984; **3**, 65–75.

107. Weiss LM, Warnke RA, Sklar J, Cleary ML. *New England Journal of Medicine*. 1987; **317**, 1185–9.

108. Takvorian T, Canellos GP, Ritz J, *et al. New England Journal of Medicine*. 1987; **316**, 1499–1505.

109. Takvorian T, Anderson K, Freedman A, *et al. Proceedings of the American Association for Cancer Research*. 1988; Abs. 726.

110. Pedrazzini A, Freedman A, Whitman J, Heflin L, Anderson K, Coral F, Nadler L. *Proceedings of the American Society of Hematology, Blood*. 1988; Suppl. Abs. No. BM 0095, (in press).

111. Philip T, Biron P, Philip I, *et al. European Journal of Cancer and Clinical Oncology*. 1986; **22**, 1015–27.

112. Rohatiner AZS, Barnett MJ, Arnott S, *et al. Blood*. 1986; **68**, 241a.

113. Hurd D, LeBien TW, Peterson B, *et al. Proceedings of the American Society of Clinical Oncology*. 1986; **5**, 193.

114. Baumgartner C, Brundel REG, Forster HK, *et al. Autologous Bone Marrow Transplantation, Proceedings of the First International Symposium*. 1985; 377–81.

115. Braine HG, Santos GW, Kaizer H, *et al. Bone Marrow Transplantation*. 1987; **2**, 7–14.

116. Gorin NC, Douay L, Laporte JP, *et al. Cancer Treatment Reports*. 1985; **69**, 953.

117. Sanders JE, Pritchard S, Mahoney P, *et al. American Journal of Medicine*. 1982; **73**, 688–92.

118. Tichelli A, Gratwohl A, Speck B, *et al. Schweizerische Medizinische Wochenschrift*. 1986; **116**, 1560–4.

119. Sklar CA, Kim YH, Williamson JF, Ramsay NK. *Medical Pediatric Oncology* 1982; **11**, 361–6.

120. Sanders JE, Buckner CD, Leonard JM. *Transplantation*. 1983; **36**, 252.

121. Deeg HJ, Flournoy N, Sullivan KM, *et al. International Journal of Radiation, Oncology, Biology and Physics*. 1984; **10**, 957.

122. Deeg HJ. In: Deeg HJ, Klingemann HG, Phillips GL (eds). *Bone Marrow Transplantation*. Berlin: Springer Verlag, 1988.

123. Appelbaum FR, Nemunaitis J, Singer J, *et al. Proceedings of ASCO*. 1988; **7** Abs. 892.

124. Kessinger A, Armitage JO, Landmark JD, Smith DM, Weisenburger DD. *Blood*. 1988; **71**, 723–7.

CHAPTER 26

IMMUNOLOGICAL APPROACHES TO THE THERAPY OF LYMPHOID NEOPLASMS

Kenneth A Foon, Mark S Roth, Mark S Kaminski and Lee M Nadler

In this chapter we include a discussion of immunological approaches to a variety of haematological malignances in addition to non-Hodgkin's lymphoma. This is important in order to give an overall perspective of the biological agents and their role in cancer therapy and to emphasize certain principles that may be applicable to the non-Hodgkin's lymphomas.

Interferons

Interferon was the term originally applied to a soluble factor that was recognized by its ability to induce interference against viral infection of chick chorioallantoic membrane by influenza A virus.[1] It has subsequently been shown to be a family of closely related proteins and glycoproteins which, in addition to antiviral activity, are potent regulators of cellular function and structure and possess direct antiproliferative activities. These latter properties underlie the current interest in interferon as an anticancer agent.

Three major species of human interferon are recognized and designated α-interferon, β-interferon, and γ-interferon[2] (Table 26.1). Alpha interferon is produced by leucocytes (B-cells, T-cells, null cells and macrophages) upon exposure to B-cell mitogens, viruses, foreign cells or tumour cells. Beta interferon is produced by fibroblasts upon exposure to viruses or foreign nucleic acids. Gamma interferon is produced by T lymphocytes upon stimulation with T-cell mitogens, specific antigens, or interleukin-2.[3] By use of recombinant DNA techniques, complete nucleotide sequences for α-, β, and γ-interferons have been defined and amino acid sequences derived.

The genes recognized to code for α-interferon have been assigned to chromosome 9.[4] Sixteen distinct sequences for α-interferon have been described.[4] Each is approximately 166 amino acids in length with an additional 20 amino acid secretory peptide present on the amino-terminal end. The human genes differ by approximately 10 per cent in nucleotide sequence and 15–20 per cent in amino acid sequence.[5] Two recombinant human interferons, α-A and α-D, make up more than 60 per cent of interferons present after buffy coat stimulation and have been extensively studied.[6] While they possess different antiviral and antiproliferative activity *in vitro*, similar effects *in vivo* on immune effector cells have been observed.[6] The α-interferon used in the first human clinical trials was obtained from Sendai virus-stimulated buffy coat leucocytes and represented 1 per cent purity (10^6 units/mg protein).[7] One unit of interferon reduces viral replication by about one-half. Refinement in purification methods by use of high performance liquid chromatography, two-dimensional polyacrylamide gel electrophoresis, and immunoaffinity chromatography has allowed purification to homogeneity (10^8 units/mg protein).[8–10] The use of recombinant DNA techniques with splicing of the α-interferon gene into *Escherichia coli* has made available pure

Table 26.1 Interferons in clinical use

Type	Subtype* (new nomenclature)	Source	Purity (%)	Amino acid differences
α	Leucocyte (IFN-α (LE))	Leucocytes from normal blood	<1†	
	Lymphoblastoid (IFN-α-N1) Wellferon (Burroughs Wellcome)	Lymphoblastoid (Namalva) cells in culture	<1†	
	Recombinant α-2 (IFN-α-2b) Intron-A (Schering)	Transformed *E. coli*	>95	Arginine at position 23, deletion at position 44 when compared to other α-subtypes.
	Recombinant α-A (IFN-α2a) Roferon-A (Hoffman-La Roche)	Transformed *E. coli*	>95	Lysine at position 23, deletion at position 44.
	Recombinant α-D (IFN-αD)	Transformed *E. coli*	>95	29 variations from α-A
	Recombinant α-2 arg (IFN-α2c)	Transformed *E. coli*	>95	Arginine at position 23, arginine at position 34
β	Fibroblast (IFN-β)	Fetal foreskin fibroblast in culture	<1†	
	Recombinant β-cys (rIFN-β-cys)	Transformed *E. coli*	<95	Cysteine at position 17
	Recombinant β-ser (rIFN-β-ser)	Transformed *E. coli*	<95	Serine at position 17
γ	Immune (IFN-γ)	T lymphocytes from normal blood	<1†	
	Recombinant γ (rIFN-γ)	Transformed *E. coli*	>95	

*New nomenclature was proposed at a joint meeting of the World Health Organization and USAN council in May 1985.
†These crude preparations can be purified to near homogeneity (*see* text).

single-species α-interferon in larger quantities.

Unlike α-interferon, only a single protein species has been identified for both β and γ.[5] Beta interferon consists of 166 amino acids and has 45 per cent homology of nucleotide sequence and 29 per cent homology of amino acid sequence with α-interferon.[5] Gamma interferon consists of 146 amino acids and has approximately 12 per cent amino acid sequence homology with α-interferon.[11] Gamma interferon may exist in biological fluids in a dimeric form.[12]

Industrial-scale production of β- and γ-interferon has only recently been accomplished, and clinical trials are limited in number. Alpha interferon, however, has been extensively studied for the past decade in both basic science and clinical research, and it is among the most potent biological agents ever administered to man. Although antitumour activity has been seen both *in vitro* and *in vivo* in some solid malignancies (breast cancer, renal cell cancer, Kaposi's sarcoma, bladder cancer, ovarian cancer, and melanoma),[13,14] the most impressive responses have occurred in the haematological malignancies.

Clinical experience

A summary of clinical trials using α-interferon for the lymphoid malignancies is presented in Table 26.2. Some reported trials have used highly purified preparations (10^8 units/mg protein). Impurities in the latter include albumin, transferrin and additional lymphokines. Despite these contaminants, the toxicities and antitumour responses seen with both the highly purified material extracted from leucocytes and the recombinant DNA preparations have been similar. The major side-effects have involved a 'flu-like illness (fever, chills, muscle aches, headache, gastrointestinal upset and fatigue). The onset of fever is generally 4–8 hours after administration, tachyphylaxis to fever usually occurs, but fatigue and anorexia increase with dosage and duration of treatment and remain the usual dose-limiting toxicities. Other reported side-effects include dose-related myelosuppression, elevated transaminase concentrations, paraesthesias,

anosmia, somnolence, confusion, and impotence in men. One occurrence of interstitial nephritis has been reported,[15] and elevation of hepatic transaminase levels was the dose-limiting toxicity in another study.[16] All of these toxicities are reversible upon cessation of the drug.

Non-Hodgkin's lymphoma

The histological classification of non-Hodgkin's lymphoma has recently been reformulated as described in detail in Chapter 4. On the basis of prognosis and morphology, the histological types of malignant lymphoma were grouped into low, intermediate, and high grade malignancy in the Working Formulation.[17] Although many chemotherapeutic agents produce responses, most patients with low grade non-Hodgkin's lymphoma are not curable with currently available treatment. This, in combination with the indolent nature and maintenance of responsiveness of the included diseases, leads to repeated episodes of treatment and relapse; eventually the patient dies from unrelated causes, toxicity of therapy, progressive disease, or emergence of a more aggressive histological subtype. The low grade non-Hodgkin's lymphomas have shown responses to α-interferon.[18–24] In trials with crude α-interferon preparations, responses were reported in four of seven patients.[18,19] In the largest series reported to date,[20] previously treated patients received recombinant leucocyte α-interferon at a dose of 50×10^6 units/m² of body surface area intramuscularly three times a week. Thirteen responses were served (four complete and nine partial responses) among 24 evaluable patients, with a median duration of response of 8 months. Alpha interferon in combination with standard cytotoxic agents is currently under investigation as first-line therapy.

Alpha interferon has shown less effectiveness in the intermediate and high grade lymphomas. Thirty-six patients have been treated with both crude and recombinant α-interferon and five responses reported.[18,20,22,24,25] Further study of α-interferon in unfavourable non-Hodgkin's lymphomas may be warranted

Table 26.2 Clinical trials with α-interferon in haematological malignancies

Tumour	Number of evaluable patients	Response rates			Total response* (%)	Reference
		Complete	Partial	Minor		
Hairy cell leukaemia†	158	22	86	44	96	36-45
Non-Hodgkin's lymphoma						
Low grade	92	9	30	6	42	18-24
Intermediate and high grade	36	1	4	2	14	18, 20, 22, 24, 25
Hodgkin's disease	8	0	0	2	0	22
Cutaneous T-cell lymphoma	20	2	7	2	45	26, 27
Chronic lymphocytic leukaemia	67	0	12	0	18	24, 29-33

*Total response (%) = complete response + partial responses divided by the number of evaluable patients.
†Complete response means absence of hairy cells in the bone marrow and normalization of peripheral blood white cells, platelets, and erythrocytes. Partial response means a normalization of peripheral blood white cells, platelets, and erythrocyte counts and greater than 50 per cent reduction in hairy cells in the bone marrow. Minor response generally means improvement in haemoglobin to more than 1.55 mmol/l 10 (g/dl) or improvement in platelets to more than 100 000 cells/l or improvement in neutrophils to more than 1000 cells/l. Total response (%) for hairy cell leukaemia includes minor responses.

to establish which patient subgroups might benefit from treatment.

Cutaneous T-cell lymphoma (mycosis fungoides and Sezary syndrome) is a subtype of non-Hodgkin's lymphoma and is characterized by a malignant proliferation of mature helper-T lymphocytes that presents with skin infiltration and an indolent clinical course. Effective therapies include topical mechlorethamine, psoralen plus ultraviolet light, total skin electron-beam irradiation, and systemic chemotherapy. Unfortunately, prolonged disease-free survival has been reported only rarely with these therapies; at best, only 25 per cent of patients with advanced disease respond and remission duration is short.[26] Responses in nine of 20 patients (two complete and seven partial) with advanced stages of disease refractory to prior therapy were observed[27] using recombinant α-interferon at an intramuscular dosage of 50×10^6 units/m² body surface area three times a week. Responses, defined as at least a 50 per cent decrease in the sum of perpendicular measurements of malignant lesions lasting at least one month, occurred within four weeks of therapy and lasted from three months to more than 25 months. Extracutaneous responses also occurred. A decrease in the size of large lesions by more than 90 per cent was observed in a number of patients, suggesting that α-interferon is the best single agent for cutaneous T-cell lymphoma.

Chronic lymphocytic leukaemia

Chronic lymphocytic leukaemia is a haematological malignancy characterized by proliferation and accumulation of relatively mature-appearing lymphocytes. The non-Hodgkin's lymphoma phase of chronic lymphocytic leukaemia is diffuse small cell lymphoma which is a low grade malignancy. Most patients have a clonal proliferation of B lymphocytes.[28] Chronic lymphocytic leukaemia and diffuse small cell lymphoma typically occur in persons over 50 years (median age, 60 years) and affect men more than women at a ratio of 2:1.[28] These diseases are usually stable over months to years, but transformation to a more aggressive disease state does occur. Alkylating agents, radiation

therapy, and corticosteroids are commonly used to treat patients, although few data show that survival is substantially improved. In a number of early studies, crude α-interferon preparations were reported to be effective in patients with advanced chronic lymphocytic leukaemia and diffuse small cell lymphoma.[24,29,30] In a phase II trial of recombinant α-interferon, 18 patients were treated with both high-dose (50×10^6 units/m² intramuscularly) and low-dose (5×10^6 units/m² intramuscularly) recombinant α-interferon three times a week;[31] only two brief responses were reported. Five patients appeared to have an acceleration of disease while receiving recombinant α-interferon. This low response rate was confirmed by a number of investigators.[21,22,30,32,33] A recent preliminary report suggests that patients with early stage disease treated with low doses of interferon may respond.[34]

Hodgkin's disease

Eight patients with advanced refractory Hodgkin's disease have been treated with crude α-interferon.[22] Only two brief, minor responses were reported. In a recent study with recombinant α-interferon, however, approximately 30 per cent of patients with advanced refractory Hodgkin's disease have shown a response.(E. Bonnem, personal communication). Additional clinical trials in Hodgkin's disease will clearly be needed.

Hairy cell leukaemia

Hairy cell leukaemia is a well-characterized lymphoproliferative disorder in which cells with lymphoid morphology and villous cytoplasmic projections infiltrate the bone marrow, blood and retriculoendothelial system. It is of B-cell origin and usually presents with cytopenias.[35] The disease is often indolent, with median age of onset age 50 years and 5:1 male-to-female ratio. Standard initial therapy is splenectomy, which often restores haematological parameters to normal; however, most of these patients have a relapse weeks to years after splenectomy. Treatment of relapses has been generally poor with standard cytotoxic agents, but excellent responses were reported[36] in seven patients with hairy cell leukaemia (three complete and four partial responses) treated with crude α-interferon. Similar data have been reported by a number of investigators using recombinant α-interferon. Response rates have been comparable with recombinant preparations after therapy three times a week or daily with doses ranging from 3 to 6 × 10⁶ units intramuscularly or subcutaneously.[36–45]

Although the initial report suggested that complete responses were frequent, this has not been confirmed with only 22 complete responses among 158 responses reported in the literature.[36–45] More important, however, is that virtually all of the patients who responded demonstrated normalization of peripheral blood cell counts, which was maintained while they were receiving interferon therapy. Many of these patients had had no prior therapy including splenectomy. In patients with response, disease has rarely been reported to become refractory to α-interferon; many patients have been followed for more than 4 years. In addition, improvement in natural killer activity and immunological surface markers parallels the haematological recovery.[42] In a recent study,[38] interferon treatment was discontinued in 25 patients after 12 months of treatment. In eight of the 25 patients, a relapse occurred at a median of 6 months after cessation of treatment and remission was re-induced in five of the eight patients who had completed 3 months of therapy.

Studies to assess low-dose (3–4 × 10⁶ units) α-interferon are currently underway. Phase III trials in which patients with newly diagnosed hairy cell leukaemia are randomly assigned to undergo splenectomy or receive α-interferon treatment are also underway. Pentostatin or 2′-deoxycoformycin,[46] an adenosine deaminase inhibitor, may be even more effective than interferon and phase III trials to address this issue have recently been initiated. Although hairy cell leukaemia accounts for less than 2 per cent of all cases of leukaemia, its response to α-interferon makes it an ideal disease to study the putative mechanisms of activity that are addressed below.

Mode of interferon action

The effect of interferon at the cellular level is initiated by binding of the interferon molecule to a cell surface membrane receptor.[47] Competitive binding studies indicate that α- and β-interferon interact with one cell surface receptor, whereas γ-interferon may interact with another receptor.[47] After binding to the cell surface membrane, human interferon is rapidly internalized and degraded.[48] Whether this internalization is required for the biological responses to interferon has not been resolved. It occurs after the binding of several polypeptide hormones to their target cells. A down-regulation of interferon receptors after exposure of cells has been reported.[48]

Direct and indirect anticancer activity of interferon probably results from a number of different mechanisms, including induction of several intracellular proteins, enhancement of immune effector cells, and changes in cellular surface structure (Table 26.3). Two enzymes appear to play a major role in interferon activity. Treatment of cells in culture with interferon results in an increase in 2′-5′-oligoadenylate synthetase;[49,50] there is evidence that this response represents the induction of a gene that is subject to control by interferon.[51] 2′-5′-Oligoadenylate synthetase is capable of synthesizing a novel series of oligonucleotides, 2′-5′-oligoadenylates, in the presence of double-stranded RNA and ATP. These oligonucleotides range from two to 15 nucleotides in length and are collectively referred to as 2′-5′A. 2′-5′A in turn activates a latent endoribonuclease that is capable of cleaving both viral and host cell RNA, (messenger RNA and ribosomal RNA) effectively inhibiting transcription and translation.[47] 2′-5′A introduced into normal and neoplastic cells appears to inhibit both protein and DNA synthesis.[52] The second enzyme activated by exposure of cells to interferon is a protein kinase capable of phosphorylating peptide eukaryotic initiation factor (e1F-2α) and ribosome-associated protein P1.[47,53] Recent observations suggest that the interferon-induced protein kinase is protein P1.[53] The net result of the kinase activation is the inhibition of peptide chain initiation. The exact role of these observations in relation to anticancer activity remains undetermined. Preliminary data exist correlating the levels of induced 2'-5'-oligoadenylate synthetase with interferon administration,[54] although correlation with antitumour activity has not been made.[55]

Antiproliferative effect

Alpha interferon has antiproliferative activity on some malignant tumour cells. Dose-dependent inhibition *in vitro* of haematological cell lines using α-interferon has been shown in Burkitt's lymphoma, lymphocytic lymphoma, acute myelogenous leukaemia, chronic myelogenous leukaemia, chronic lymphocytic leukaemia and multiple myeloma.[56–60] Interestingly in comparative antiproliferative studies, α-interferon has shown a greater inhibitory effect in cells of haematopoietic origin than either β-interferon or γ-interferon, using both crude and recombinant interferons.[57,58,61] Of note is the observation that non-cycling tumour cells (G_0–G_1) appear to be a more sensitive target for the antiproliferative activity of human interferon.[62,63]

Crude murine α-interferon preparations have been shown to inhibit the growth of transplantable tumours of diverse origins (melanoma, Friend leukaemia, osteogenic sarcoma, Lewis lung, Ehrlich ascites).[64–67] In support of a direct antiproliferative effect are studies of transplanted human tumours in immunodeficient nude mice in which immunomodulatory effects of administered human α-interferon are minimal.[68,69] Dose-dependent growth inhibition is observed in these models and persists only for the duration of treatment.[68,69] Evidence for direct antiproliferative effect in human trials is suggested in cutaneous T-cell lymphoma. Four of 10 patients who had had a relapse while receiving a 10 per cent maintenance dosage demonstrated responses after re-escalation to a 100 per cent dosage.[38] This would suggest a 'dose-dependent' direct antitumour effect rather than an indirect effect via the immune system as we have not been able to document enhancement of the immune system at high doses of α-interferon.

Mechanisms of interferon activity in specific diseases

Hairy cell leukaemia is the model disease for studying the effects of α-interferon. Patients with hairy cell leukaemia have a severe deficiency in natural killer cell activity. Recovery of natural killer activity has been reported[42,70] in most patients with hairy cell leukaemia after α-

Table 26.3   Cellular events after treatment with α-interferon

---

Intracellular protein changes
Increased 2'-5'-oligoadenylate synthetase
Increased protein kinase activity

Direct antiproliferative effects
Antiproliferative effect on tumour cell lines
Antiproliferative effect on murine tumours *in vivo*
Antiproliferative effects on transplanted tumours in nude mice

Immunomodulatory activities
Enhancement (low dose) or suppression (high dose) of natural killer activity
Augmentation of antibody dependent cellular cytotoxicity
Enhancement of tumoricidal activity of macrophages
Regulation of antibody production in B-cells
Enhancement of cytotoxic phase of mixed lymphocyte culture
Depressed lymphoproliferative phase of mixed lymphocyte culture
Increased expression of cell surface antigens, HLA-A, B, C and β_2 microglobulin
Decreased oncogene expression

---

interferon therapy. The recovery of natural killer cells paralleled haematological recovery. It remains unclear whether the natural killer cells played a direct role in haematological recovery or were simply a byproduct of interferon-induced haematological recovery. However, it was of interest that the low natural killer activity in cells from untreated patients was not really attributable to a relative deficiency or dilution of the effector cells because the percentage of Leu 11-positive cells (Leu-11 identifies natural killer cells) was within the normal range. This suggests that α-interferon activated these cells into functional effector cells.[42] In addition to natural killer cell recovery, improvement in the total numbers of T lymphocytes, including both helper and suppressor populations, and monocytes paralleled the improvement in the other haematological parameters following α-interferon therapy.

Hairy cell leukaemia and low grade lymphoma are indolent diseases of B-cell origin in which α-interferon has a high degree of activity.[18–24,36–45] The lack of responsiveness of another indolent B-cell malignancy, chronic lymphocytic leukaemia, has as yet been unexplained.[24,29–33] A comparison of binding of iodinated recombinant α interferon to normal peripheral blood mononuclear cells, hairy cell leukaemia cells, and chronic lymphocytic leukaemia cells demonstrated that hairy cells bound approximately twice as much iodinated interferon as chronic lymphocytic leukaemia and normal cells; however, the hairy cells had twice the surface area, which may explain the greater number of receptors.[71]

Alpha interferon has been reported to induce cell surface and intracellular proteins in patients with hairy cell leukaemia.[72] Autoradiographic analysis of one-dimensional polyacrylamide gels showed induction of at least six proteins in nine patients treated with recombinant α-interferon. Overall protein synthesis was not significantly altered. Some of these proteins were in the cell membrane, leading the investigators to suggest that interferon induces a protein signal in the hairy cell which leads to their destruction.[72]

Most recently Baldini *et al.*[73] isolated hairy cells from the spleens of previously untreated patients and cultured them in the presence of recombinant human α-interferon. Monoclonal antibody surface marker studies revealed a significant enhancement of class II HLA antigen (HLA-DR). Because HLA antigens have been shown to be involved in cell-mediated cytotoxicity,[74] they speculated that selected enhancement of class II HLA antigen may be another *in vivo* therapeutic mechanism of α-interferon action.

Monoclonal antibodies

Passive immunotherapy using heteroantisera for the treatment of cancer in animals and humans has been studied for over 50 years. Attempts have been made to treat animal tumours with sera from immunized syngeneic, allogeneic, or xenogeneic animals. A number of studies of passive immunotherapy using heterologous antisera in humans have also been performed.[75] These studies have generally been attempted in patients with large tumour burdens and, as would be expected, responses have been transient at best. A wide variety of patients with leukaemias and lymphomas has been treated with antisera raised in sheep, horses, rabbits and goats. Problems such as anaphylaxis, serum sickness, and severe cytopenias have been encountered with these antisera.

There are a number of potential mechanisms by which unconjugated antibodies might be cytotoxic to tumour cells. Antibodies bound to the cell surface membrane of tumour cells may lead to cell lysis by complement-dependent or antibody-dependent cellular cytotoxicity. Circulating tumour cells bound by antibody may be more susceptible to phagocytosis by the reticuloendothelial system. Antibody bound to the cell surface membrane of tumour cells may enhance immunogenicity of the tumour cell leading to activation of the host's immune system. In any of these cases, successful therapy with antibodies is dependent on the accessibility of the antibody to the tumour, the immunity of the host, the degree of specificity of the antibodies used for targeting, and the class of antibody injected.

Due to the potential therapeutic advantage of targeting of cytotoxic agents to antigen expressed by tumour cells, attempts have been made to link tumour-specific heteroantisera to drugs such as methotrexate, chlorambucil, and doxorubicin. Other agents such as radio-isotopes, toxins, and enzymes have also been conjugated to antibody. One of the major problems encountered in these initial attempts at immunoconjugate preparation has been the inability to develop tumour-specific antibodies with sufficient specificity and in sufficient amounts suitable for *in vivo* therapy.

Monoclonal antibodies have created a new wave of enthusiasm for using antibodies for the treatment of cancer. Monoclonal antibodies are specific for a single target antigen, can be produced in large quantities with high degrees of purity, and can be uniformly coupled to drugs, toxins, and radionuclides. The specificity of monoclonal antibodies should theoretically reduce toxicity to normal tissues that are non-reactive with the antibody conjugate. Unlike crude heteroanatisera, the monoclonal antibodies require no absorption with normal tissues to remove unwanted reactivities, and are of a single immunoglobulin subclass. Monoclonal antibodies can be produced in large quantities from ascites fluid or by tissue culture production techniques with a purity ranging from 95 to 99 per cent.

Results of clinical trials with unlabelled antibodies

Some investigators[76–91] have attempted to treat lymphoid or myeloid leukaemias with unlabelled monoclonal antibodies (Table 26.4). In some studies, patients with advanced B-cell-derived chronic lymphocytic leukaemia (CLL) received T101 monoclonal antibody (anti-CD5).[82–85] T101 recognizes the CD5 antigen which is a 65 kilodalton glycoprotein antigen found on normal and malignant T cells and B-cell chronic lymphocytic leukaemia cells. T101 could be safely infused and led to transient reductions in circulating leukaemia cells; there was no sustained effect on the bone marrow, involved lymph nodes or other organs. This therapy resulted in some intravascular leukaemia cell injury, but destruction in the spleen, liver, and lungs was probably more important. Similar results have been reported in patients with adult

T-cell leukaemia/lymphoma, acute lymphoblas-tic leukaemia (ALL), and acute myelogenous leukaemia (AML) treated with other monoclonal antibodies.[86,89,90] Patients with cutaneous T-cell lymphoma who received (anti-CD5) antibody have had only transient improvement in skin lesions and lymphadenopathy.[84–88]

Results of clinical trials with anti-idiotype antibodies

One particular therapeutic approach with monoclonal antibodies which merits more extensive discussion involves the use of monoclonal anti-idiotype antibodies in B-cell malignancies. Unlike the antibodies used for therapy discussed above, in which the target antigen is tumour-related or associated, anti-idiotype antibodies have as their target a tumour-specific antigen, the idiotype of the cell surface immunoglobulin present on B-cells. Indeed, this antigen is the closest we have come to identifying a tumour-specific antigen in man. This specificity is based on the fact that individual B-cells are committed to the synthesis of only one immunoglobulin species with a unique variable region structure (idiotype). Moreover, since B-cell lymphomas and leukaemias are clonal in nature, members of the malignant clone should express the same im-munoglobulin molecule, and hence the same idiotype. This feature thus represents a marker by which these tumour cells can be distin-guished from normal cells of the host. These facts also imply that an individual patient's tumour cell idiotype will be different from that of other patients, hence anti-idiotype antibodies must be 'tailor-made' for the individual patient. Because of the highly specific nature of these antibodies, treatment with these antibodies have yielded important results regarding the ultimate potential of monoclonal antibody therapy.

The largest experience reported with anti-idiotype therapy is the work of Levy and coworkers. Their first attempt at this therapy was in a patient originally diagnosed as having a malignant lymphoma of the nodular, poorly differentiated, lymphocytic type (follicular small cleaved cell lymphoma).[77] At the time of treatment, the patient had evidence of rapidly

Table 26.4 Clinical trials with unlabelled monoclonal antibodies

Disease	Antibody/class	No. patients	Toxicity	Effect	References
B lymphoma	A689/IgG$_{2a}$	1	Renal	Transient reduction in circulating cells	76
B lymphoma	Anti-idiotype/IgG$_1$ IgG$_{2a}$ or IgG$_{2b}$	11	Fever, chills, nausea, vomiting, headache, diarrhoea, transient dyspnoea	1 complete and 5 partial responses	77, 78
B-lymphoma	1F5/IgG$_{2a}$	4	Fever, myelosuppression	1 partial and 1 minor response	81
B-CLL	Anti-idiotype/IgG$_{2b}$ and IgG$_1$	1	Fever, urticaria	Transient reduction in circulating cells	80
B-CLL	T101/IgG$_{2a}$	18	Dyspnoea, fever, malaise, urticaria, hypotension	Transient reduction in circulating cells	82–85
CTCL	T101/IgG$_{2a}$ Anti-Leu-1/IgG$_{2a}$	30	Dyspnoea, urticaria, fever, cutaneous pain	10 minor remissions	84–88
cALL	Anti-J5/IgG$_{2a}$	4	Fever	Transient reduction in circulating cells	89
AML	PM/81/IgM AML-2-23/IgG$_{2b}$ PMN 29/IgM PMN 6/IgM	3	Fever, back pain, arthralgia, myalgia	Transient reduction in circulating cells	90
ATL	Anti-Tac/IgG$_{2a}$	2	None	1 partial response	91

B-CLL, B-chronic lymphocytic leukaemia; CTCL, cutaneous T-cell lymphoma; cALL, common acute lymphoblastic leukaemia; AML, acute myelogenous leukaemia; ATL, adult T-cell leukaemia/lymphoma progressive systemic disease which was resistant to chemotherapy and interferon. Following eight continuous six-hour intravenous infusions spaced over the period of one month, the patient entered a complete clinical remission that has been sustained for more than 5 years without further treatment (R. Levy, personal communication). The mechanisms accounting for this dramatic response are not clear. Because it was noted that the patient's antitumour response continued after the period of passive antibody administration, evidence of an anti-idiotype antibody response by the patient himself was looked for, but none was detected. It is still possible that indirect mechanisms could have been involved. Since the immune system may be regulated in part by networks of interactions between idiotypes and anti-idiotypes,[92] the administered anti-idiotype could have altered the balance of such a network of interactions resulting in an antiproliferative response against the patient's tumour.

Encouraged by the above result, Levy *et al.* have now treated an additional 13 patients with individually tailored anti-idiotype antibodies of varying antibody subclasses.[78] Some patients have been treated with more than one antibody (differing in isotype or epitope specificity) during the course of an individual treatment period. The dramatic result of the first patient has not been reproduced so far. Instead, significant tumour responses have been demonstrated in 50 per cent of the patients, but these have not been complete responses and have not lasted for longer than a few months.

Nevertheless, several important lessons have been learned from these studies. It was found that up to 900 mg of monoclonal anti-idiotype antibody could be infused safely as a single dose provided the level of circulating free antigen (idiotype) was low or non-detectable and if no immune response by the host against the infused mouse protein (human antimouse antibodies) was present. The presence of both serum idiotype and human antimouse antibodies was correlated with acute toxicity during infusions which consisted of fever, rigor with dyspnoea, arthralgias, and headache. Thrombocytopenia occurred less commonly.

This suggests that the toxicity was due to immune complex formation. The presence of significant levels of serum idiotype was found to be a barrier to antibody penetration to tumour sites and thus to a clinical response. Plasmapheresis was shown to reduce transiently serum idiotype levels but not to a degree sufficient to eliminate this barrier. The effect of the presence of an antimouse response by the host was similar in that tissue penetration and clinical response were prevented by these antibodies.

Another means by which patients' tumours could evade the therapeutic effects of anti-idiotype antibodies was by the emergence of idiotype variants within tumours during treatment.[93] This phenomenon was recognized when tumours of two patients lost reactivity with the anti-idiotype antibody generated against the respective original tumours during treatment. Subsequent studies showed that this loss of reactivity was not due to antigenic modulation. Comparison of immunoglobulin gene rearrangements by Southern blot analysis in pretherapy and post-therapy tumours from each patient revealed identical rearrangements in each case. This strongly suggests that all cell populations studied were part of a single monoclonal lymphoma in each patient. In one of these cases the anti-idiotype antibody was known to react with only the heavy chain variable region of the surface IgM protein of the pretherapy tumour and not with light chain regions. Eight independent heavy chain variable region isolates from tumours prior to and after treatment were subjected to nucleotide sequence analyses.[94] Extensive point mutations were demonstrated in all isolates and no two sequences were identical. A clustering of mutations encoding for amino acid changes was observed in the CDR2 region.

Comparison of pretherapy and post-therapy sequences implicated a single amino acid in CDR2 at position 54 as being important in determining reactivity with the anti-idiotype antibody. Three of the post-therapy sequences had a common substitution at that position, and a fourth post-therapy sequence had other substitutes in a neighbouring position. Thus, clones with mutations in this region apparently escaped the antibody's strong negative selection pressure *in vivo*. Further analysis indicated that there was a significant bias against mutations resulting in amino acid changes in portions of the V- region gene other than CDR2, even in the absence of any selection by antibody treatment. Thus the non-random clustering in CDR2 may have been due to endogenous selective forces interacting with tumour cell-surface immunoglobulin. Such selective forces are presumably the same ones which operate upon normal B-cells during the process of somatic mutation of V-regions: one of the components of the process of generation of antibody diversity. The generality of these concepts is being explored in other patients' tumour samples. It is now believed that somatic mutation accounted for tumour escape in additional patients and that somatic mutation prior to any therapy may be the rule rather than the exception.[95,96] This poses an additional problem for anti-idiotype antibody therapy in that more than one antibody may need to be developed for each individual patient, possibly over a period of time, so that idiotypic variants already present within the tumour or subsequently developing within it can be recognized.

It is still unclear why the excellent response in the first treated patient has not been reproduced. Various factors have been examined for their ability to predict response to this therapy,[97] including the isotype of the anti-idiotype antibody used, the density of cell surface idiotype, the epitope recognized by the anti-idiotype antibody, the affinity of anti-idiotype antibody for antigen, the relative ability of the anti-idiotype antibody to modulate surface antigen, the direct effect of antibody on tumour cell proliferation *in vitro*, and the degree of T-cell infiltration present in pretherapy tumour specimens. None of these factors has been positively correlated with good clinical outcome except the number of T-cells present in pretherapy tumour tissue.[97,98] In the two best responding cases the T-cells actually outnumbered the tumour cells. The majority of these T-cells were of the helper-inducer phenotype (CD4). Whether the anti-idiotype antibodies given to these patients augmented an ongoing cell-mediated cytotoxic response by the

host against the tumour is not clear. Certainly more observations on pretherapy T-cell infiltration must be made before the significance of this observation becomes apparent. However, these findings raise the possibility that adoptive immunotherapy with cloned T-cell populations could be of value when coupled with anti-idiotype therapy. Another factor which has yet to be fully explored is the nature of somatic mutation in the immunoglobulin genes of the various tumours of patients undergoing treatment. Such studies may more fully define endogenous host responses which may regulate tumour growth and be relevant to the response to therapy.

While anti-idiotype therapy remains an interesting area of investigation, its general applicability to the treatment of B-cell lymphoma still remains to be defined. Certainly, the time-consuming nature of the isolation of individually tailored antibodies limits the availability of these reagents for therapy. This latter problem is compounded by the finding of the emergence of idiotypic variants which might require the isolation of additional antibodies for the treatment of individual patients. Overcoming these shortcomings will go a long way towards increasing the feasibility of this approach.

Problems with unlabelled monoclonal antibody therapy

Monoclonal antibody therapy has several shortcomings that must be addressed. First, with few exceptions unlabelled antibodies are clearly not very effective in destroying tumour cells. While they target quite well to tumour cells *in vivo*, most murine antibodies do not fix human complement and do not effectively mediate tumour lysis through human effector cells. By conjugating toxins, drugs and/or isotopes to antibodies, the limited cytotoxicity inherent in the use of antibody alone may be overcome. Treatment with antibodies such as (anti-CD5 and anti-CD10 (anti-common acute lymphoblastic leukaemia antigen)) results in modulation of the antigen from the cell surface which prevents further antibody from binding to the tumour cells. The antigen–antibody complex is pinocytosed into the cytoplasm,[99] a phenomenon that might be advantageous when drugs or toxins are linked to the antibody to enhance the cytoxicity. Antigen in the circulation poses another potential problem because it may prevent the antibody from reaching the tumour cells. This was clearly a major problem with anti-idiotype antibodies. Plasmapheresis was not very effective in reducing the circulating idiotype. Furthermore, murine antibodies can stimulate production of human antimouse antibodies which lead to antibody neutralization. This situation may be correctable by treatment with high initial doses of antibody (> 500 mg) to induce tolerance or by simultaneous treatment with immunosuppressive drugs. Another potential problem is that the heterogeneity of antigen expression on tumour cells may necessitate therapy with more than one antibody.

Imaging and therapy trials with labelled monoclonal antibodies

Antisera and monoclonal antibodies conjugated to radionuclides for tumour imaging have been extensively studied.[100] The T101 antibody conjugated to indium-111 has been used for imaging in 12 patients with cutaneous T-cell lymphoma.[101,102] Tumours as small as 0.5 cm have been localized; however, non-specific uptake of the immunoconjugate in the liver and spleen has prevented critical evaluation of these organs. This problem has been partially circumvented by the administration of intracutaneous injections of the immunoconjugate so that it is taken up by the lymphatics leading directly to lymph node sites of disease.[103] This procedure does not, of course, facilitate visualization of extralymphatic disease.

Recent results have demonstrated that when 100–300 mCi of iodine-131 were linked to the T101 or the Lym-1 antibodies and injected intravenously into patients with T- and B-cell non-Hodgkin's lymphoma respectively, excellent antitumour responses resulted[104,105] (Table 26.5). Antitumour activity has also been reported using anti-ferritin heteroantisera labelled with iodine-131 in patients with advanced Hodgkin's disease.[106] A number of centres are studying toxin and drug conjugates with murine antibodies; clinical trials have just begun and while favourable responses have not yet been reported, this remains an important avenue of investigation.[107,108]

Table 26.5   Clinical trials with labelled monoclonal antibodies

Disease	Antibody/class	Label	No. patients	Toxicity	Effect	References
B lymphoma	Lym-1/IgG$_{2a}$	[131]I	9	None	3 complete 1 partial, and 3 minor responses	104
CTCL	T101/IgG$_{2a}$	[131]I	6	Dyspnoea, fever, urticaria, myelosuppression	2 partial and 3 minor responses	105
Hodgkin's disease	Antiferritin/ heteroantisera	[131]I	38	Myelosuppression	40% partial responses	106
B-CLL	T101/IgG$_{2a}$	Ricin-A	5	None	Transient reduction in circulating cells	107, 108

CTCL, cutaneous T-cell lymphoma; B-CLL, B-chronic lymphocytic leukaemia

Toxicity

Side-effects of unlabelled monoclonal antibody therapy are usually minor. Respiratory distress following the rapid infusion of monoclonal antibody has been described,[83,84] and some patients have demonstrated transient elevation of creatinine and hepatic enzymes.[76,86] Fever and urticaria are common but are rarely dose limiting. Nausea and vomiting have also been reported.[78]

The major dose-limiting toxicity with radiolabelled antibodies has been myelosuppression.[102,103] This is secondary to both specific localization of antibody in the bone marrow as well as the non-specific effects of total body irradiation.

Conclusion

The importance of interferon as a direct antitumour agent or a biological response-modifier remains an unanswered question in the treatment of malignant diseases. Although it is clear that interferon will not be effective in most cancers, we have reviewed interferon's effectiveness in managing some of the haematological malignancies. Even in these diseases, the optimal dose of interferon is uncertain. High doses may have greater direct antiproliferative activity, yet they may also suppress the immune system. Low doses may be more effective in enhancing the immune system. Interferon's role as a first-line treatment or in combination with standard cytotoxic drugs or other biological response-modifiers is an area of ongoing research. Regardless of the eventual role of α-interferon in the treatment of cancer, it is an important first member of a family of biological response-modifiers used in treating human malignancies, and as such has provided important information which will contribute to the development of treatment with other cytokines. A variety of additional lymphokines are currently under investigation. Interleukin-2 with or without lymphokine-activated killer cells has been shown to have some activity in non-Hodgkin's lymphoma patients in preliminary studies.[109] Combination therapy of interleukin-2 and interferon is currently planned. Other lymphokines such as tumour necrosis factor have not been evaluated sufficiently in non-Hodgkin's lymphoma.

The use of monoclonal antibodies and antibody immunoconjugates in the treatment and radioimaging of cancer is in its infancy. Although much work remains to clarify the issues surrounding the use of monoclonal antibodies, studies in animal tumour models and humans have clearly demonstrated that antibodies alone or antibody conjugates can be safely administered with minimal adverse effects; in selected cases they may have diagnostic and therapeutic value. Non-specific localization of antibody in the reticuloendothelial system, host antibody response, and antigenic heterogeneity are major obstacles to safe and effective treatment with monoclonal antibodies. These issues are under investigation in animal models and humans. Although anti-idiotype antibodies are highly specific and have produced excellent responses in a small number of patients, problems such as instability of the idiotype, and the difficulty of tailoring antibodies to individual patients clearly limit the role of anti-idiotype therapy. Perhaps the most important future role for monoclonal antibody therapy will be in patients with minimal disease in the 'adjuvant' setting, in whom antibody conjugates might eliminate micrometastatic deposits of tumour cells. This remains to be addressed in controlled trials.

References

1. Isaacs A, Linderman J. *Proceedings of the Royal Society of London Biologists.* 1957; **147**, 258–67.
2. Stewart WE II, Blalock JE, Burke DC, *et al. Journal of Immunology.* 1980; **125**, 2353.
3. Fleischmann WR, Klimpel GR, Tyring SK, Voss WR, Baron S. In: Sunkara PS (ed). *Novel Approaches to Cancer Chemotherapy.* Orlando, Florida: Academic Press, 1984: 1–22.
4. Sehgal PB. *Biochemica Biophysica Acta.* 1982; **695**, 17–33.
5. Borden EC. *Cancer.* 1984; **54**, 2770–6.
6. Hawkins MJ, Borden EC, Merritt JA, *et al. Journal of Clinical Oncology.* 1984; **2**, 221–6.
7. Cantell K, Hirvonen S. *Texas Reports in Biology and Medicine.* 1977; **35**, 138–44.

8. Pestka S. *Scientific American*. 1983; **249**, 37–43.
9. Lin LS, Stewart WE II. *Methods in Enzymology*. 1981; **78**, 481–7.
10. Berg K, Heron I. *Methods in Enzymology*. 1981; **78**, 487–99.
11. Epstein LB. *Nature*. 1982; **295**, 453–4.
12. Yip YK, Pang RHL, Urban C, Vilcek J. *Proceedings of the National Academy of Sciences USA*. 1981; **78**, 1601–5.
13. Kirkwood JM, Ernstoff MS. *Journal of Clinical Oncology*. 1984; **2**, 336–52.
14. Bonnem EM, Spiegel RJ. *Journal of Biological Response Modifiers*. 1984; **3**, 580–98.
15. Auerbuch SD, Austin HA, Sherwin SA, *et al*. *New England Journal of Medicine*. 1984; **301**, 32–5.
16. Sherwin SA, Knost JA, Fein S, *et al*. *Journal of the American Medical Association*. 1982; **248**, 2461–6.
17. The Non-Hodgkin's Lymphoma Pathological Classification Project. *Cancer*. 1982; **49**, 2112–35.
18. Merigan TC, Sikora K, Bredden JH, Levy R, Rosenberg SA. *New England Journal of Medicine*. 1978; **299**, 1449–53.
19. Louie AC, Gallagher JG, Sikora K, Levy R, Rosenberg SA, Merigan TC. *Blood*. 1981; **58**, 712–18.
20. Foon KA, Sherwin SA, Abrams PG. *New England Journal of Medicine*. 1984; **311**, 1148–52.
21. O'Connell MJ, Colgan JP, Oken MM, Ritts RE, Kay NE, Itri LM. *Journal of Clinical Oncology*. 1986; **4**, 128–36.
22. Horning SJ, Merigan TC, Krown SE, *et al*. *Cancer*. 1985; **56**, 1305–10.
23. Leavitt RD, Kaplan R, Ozer H. *Blood*. 1984; **64** (suppl. I), 182a.
24. Gutterman JU, Blumenschein GR, Alexanian R. *Annals of Internal Medicine*. 1980; **93**, 399–406.
25. Leavitt RD, Ratanatharathorn V, Ozer H, Rudnick S, Ferraresi R. *Proceedings of the American Society of Clinical Oncology*. 1983; **2**, 54.
26. Bunn PA, Foon KA, Ihde DC. *Annals of Internal Medicine*. 1984; **101**, 484–7.
27. Bunn PA, Ihde DC, Foon KA. *Cancer*, 1986; **57**, 1689–95.
28. Gale RP, Foon KA. *Annals of Internal Medicine*. 1985; **103**, 101–120.
29. Misset JL, Mythe G, Gastiaburu J, *et al*. *Biomedicine*. 1982; **36**, 112–16.
30. Huang A, Laszlo J, Brenchman W. *Proceedings of the American Association of Cancer Research*. 1982; **23**, 113.
31. Foon KA, Bottino G, Abrams PG. *American Journal of Medicine*. 1985; **78**, 216–20.
32. Ozer H, Leavit R, Ratanatharathorn V. *American Society of Hematology*. 1983; **62**, 211a.
33. Schulof RS, Lloyd MI, Stallings JJ, *et al*. *Journal of Biological Response Modifiers*. 1985; **4**, 310–23.
34. Montserrat E, Vinolas N, Urbano-Ispizva A, Ribera JM, Gallert J, Rozman C. *Blood*. 1986; **68** (suppl. 1), 227a.
35. Golomb HM. *Cancer*. 1978; **42**, 946–56.
36. Quesada JR, Reuben J, Manning JT, Hirsch EM, Gutterman JU. *New England of Medicine*. 1984; **310**, 15–18.
37. Quesada JR, Hersh EM, Gutterman JU. *Proceedings of the American Society of Clinical Oncology*. 1984; **3**, 207.
38. Quesada JR, Hersh EM, Manning JT, *et al*. *Blood*. 1986; **68**, 493–7.
39. Ratain MJ, Golomb HM, Vardiman JW, Vokes EE, Jacobs RH, Daly K. *Blood*. 1985; **65**, 644–8.
40. Jacobs AD, Champlin RE, Golde DW. *Blood*. 1985; **65**, 1017–20.
41. Golomb HM, Jacobs A, Fefer A, *et al*. *Journal of Clinical Oncology*. 1986; **4**, 900–5.
42. Foon KA, Maluish AE, Abrams PG, *et al*. *American Journal of Medicine*. 1986; **80**, 351–6.
43. Worman CP, Catovsky D, Bevan PC, *et al*. *British Journal of Haematology*. 1985; **60**, 759–63.
44. Habermann T, Hoagland H, Chang M, Phylidy R. *Blood*. 1985; **66** (suppl. 1), 2009.
45. Castaigne S, Sigaux F, Cantell K, *et al*. *Cancer*. 1986; **57**, 1681–4.
46. Spiers ASD, Moore D, Cassileth PA, *et al*. *New England Journal of Medicine*. 1987; **316**, 825–30.
47. Williams BRG. In: Sikora K (ed). *Interferon and Cancer*. New York: Plenum Press, 1983: 33–52.
48. Feinstein S, Traub A, LaZar A, Mizrahi A, Teitz Y. *Journal of Interferon Research*. 1985; **5**, 65–7.
49. Ball LA. *Virology*. 1979; **94**, 282–96.
50. Ball LA. In: Boyer PD (ed). *The Enzymes*, vol. XV. New York: Academic Press, 1982: 281–313.
51. Merlin G, Chebath J, Benech P, Metz R, Revel M. *Proceedings of the National Academy of Sciences USA*. 1983; **80**, 4904–8.
52. Revel M, Kimchi A, Schulman L, *et al*. *Annals of the New York Academy of Science*. 1980; **350**, 349–472.
53. Bischoff JR, Samuel CE. *Journal of Biological Chemistry*. 1985; **260**, 8237–9.
54. Schattner A, Merlin G, Wallach D, *et al*. *Journal of Interferon Research*. 1981; **1**, 587–94.
55. Merritt JA, Borden EC, Ball LA. *Journal of Interferon Research*. 1985; **5**, 191–8.
56. Balkwill FR, Oliver RTD. *International Journal of Cancer*. 1977; **20**, 500–5.
57. Borden EC, Hogan TF, Voelkel JG. *Cancer Research*. 1982; **42**, 4948–53.
58. Chadha KC, Srivastava BI. *Journal of Clinical Hematology and Oncology*. 1981; **11**, 55–60.

59. Salmon SE, Durie BGM, Young L, Liu RM, Trown P, Stebbing N. *Journal of Clinical Oncology.* 1983; **1**, 217–25.

60. Denz H, Lechleitner M, Marth CH, Daxenbichler G, Gastl G, Braunsteiner H. *Journal of Interferon Research.* 1985; **5**, 147–57.

61. Blalock J, Georgiades JE, Langford MP, Johnson HM. *Cell Immunology.* 1980; **49**, 390–4.

62. Horoszewicz JS, Leong SS, Carter SW. *Science.* 1979; **206**, 1091–3.

63. Creasey AA, Batholomew JC, Merigan TC. *Proceedings of the National Academy of Sciences USA.* 1980; **77**, 1471–5.

64. Bart RS, Porzio NR, Kopf AW, Vilcek JT, Cheng EH, Farcet Y. *Cancer Research.* 1980; **40**, 614–19.

65. Rososi GB, Marchegiani M, Matarese GP, Gresser I. *Journal of the National Cancer Institute.* 1975; **54**, 993–6.

66. Crane JL, Glasgow LA, Kern ER, Younger JS. *Journal of the National Cancer Institute.* 1978; **61**, 871–4.

67. Greseer I, Tovey M. *Biochemica Biophysica Acta.* 1978; **526**, 231–47.

68. Yoshitake Y, Kishida T, Esaki K, Kawamata J. *Giken Journal.* 1976; **19**, 125–7.

69. Balkwill FR, Moodie EM, Freedman V, Fantes KH. *International Journal of Cancer.* 1982; **30**, 231–5.

70. Semenzato G, Pizzolo G, Agostini C, *et al. Blood.* 1986; **68**, 293–6.

71. Faltynek DR, Princler GL, Rusetti FW, Maluish AE, Abrams PG, Foon KA. *Blood.* 1986; **67**, 1077–82.

72. Samuels BL, Brownstein BH, Golomb HM. *Proceedings of the American Association of Cancer Research.* 1985; **26**, 20.

73. Baldini L, Cortelezzi A, Polli N, *et al. Blood.* 1986; **67**, 458–64.

74. Meur SC, Schlossman SF, Reinherz EL. *Proceedings of the National Academy of Sciences USA.* 1982; **79**, 4395–9.

75. Rosenberg SA, Terry WD. *Advances in Cancer Research.* 1977; **25**, 323–88.

76. Nadler LM, Stashenko P, Hardy R, *et al. Cancer Research.* 1980; **40**, 3147.

77. Miller RA, Maloney DG, Warnke R, Levy R. *New England Journal of Medicine.* 1982; **306**, 517.

78. Meeker TC, Lowder J, Maloney DG, *et al. Blood.* 1985; **65**, 1349.

79. Rankin EM, Hekman A, Somers R, Huinink B. *Blood.* 1985; **65**, 1373.

80. Giardina SL, Schroff RW, Woodhouse CS, *et al. Journal of Immunology.* 1985; **135**, 653.

81. Press OW, Appelbaum F, Ledbetter JA, *et al. Blood.* 1987; **69**, 584.

82. Dillman RO, Shawler DL, Sobol RE, *et al. Blood.* 1982; **59**, 1036.

83. Foon KA, Schroff RW, Bunn RA, *et al. Blood.* 1984; **64**, 1085.

84. Dillman RO, Shawler DL, Dillman JB, Royston R. *Journal of Clinical Oncology.* 1984; **2**, 881.

85. Bertram JH, Gills PS, Levine AM, *et al. Blood.* 1986; **67**, 1680.

86. Foon KA, Schroff RW, Bunn RA. In: Foon KA, Morgan AC (eds). *Monoclonal Antibody Therapy of Human Cancer.* Boston: Martinus Nijhoff Publishing. 1985: 85.

87. Miller RA, Oseroff AR, Stratte PT, Levy R. *Blood.* 1983; **62**, 988.

88. Miller RA, Levy R. *Lancet.* 1981; **ii**, 226.

89. Ritz J, Pesando JM, Sallan SE, *et al. Blood.* 1981; **58**, 141.

90. Ball ED, Bernier GM, Cornwell GG, McIntyre OR, O'Donnell JF, Fanger MW. *Blood.* 1983; **62**, 1203–10.

91. Waldmann TA, Longo DL, Leonard WJ, *et al. Cancer Research.* 1985; **45**, 4559s–62s.

92. Jerne NK. *Annals of Immunology.* 1974; **125C**, 373.

93. Meeker T, Lowder J, Cleary ML, *et al. New England Journal of Medicine.* 1985; **312**, 1658.

94. Cleary ML, Meeker TC, Levy S, *et al. Cell.* 1986; **44**, 97.

95. Raffeld M, Neckers L, Longo DL, Cossman J. *New England Journal of Medicine.* 1985; **312**, 1653.

96. Carroll WL, Lowder J, Streifer R, Warnke R, Levy S, Levy R. *Journal of Experimental Medicine.* 1986; **164**, 1566.

97. Lowder JN, Meeker TC, Campbell M, *et al. Blood.* 1987; **69**, 199.

98. Garcia CF, Lowder J, Meeker TC, Bindl J, Levy R, Warnke RA. *Journal of Immunology.* 1985; **135**, 4252.

99. Schroff RW, Farrell MM, Klein RA, Oldham RK, Foon KA. *Journal of Immunology.* 1984; **133**, 1641.

100. Goldenberg DM, DeLand FH. *Journal of Biological Response Modifiers.* 1982; **1**, 121.

101. Bunn PA, Carrasquillo JA, Keenan AM, *et al. Lancet.* 1984; **ii**, 1219.

102. Carrasquillo JA, Bunn PA, Keenan AM, *et al. New England Journal of Medicine.* 1986; **315**, 673.

103. Mulshine J, Keenan A, Carrasquillo J, *et al. Proceedings of the American Society of Clinical Oncology.* 1985; **4**, 205 (abstract).

104. DeNardo SJ, DeNardo GL, O'Grady LF, *et al. Journal of Nuclear Medicine.* 1986; **27**, 903 (abstract).

105. Rosen ST, Zimmer AM, Goldman-Leikin R, *et al. Journal of Clinical Oncology.* 1987; **5**, 562–73.

106. Lenhard RE, Order SE Jr, Spunberg JJ, Asbell SO, Leibel SA. *Journal of Clinical Oncology.* 1985;

3, 1296–1300.

107. Laurent G, Pris J, Farcet JP, *et al. Blood.* 1986; **68**, 752.

108. Hertler AA, Schlossman DM, Borowitz MJ,

Frankel AE. *Blood.* 1986; **68** (suppl. 1), 223a.

109. Rosenberg SA, Lotze MT, Muul LM. *et al. New England Journal of Medicine.* 1987; **316**, 889–97.

CHAPTER 27

FUTURE PROSPECTS FOR TREATMENT

Ian Magrath

At the present time, approximately 60 per cent of all patients with intermediate and high grade non-Hodgkin's lymphomas (NHL), if treated optimally, are cured – a result which is largely due to the empirical development of effective combination chemotherapy regimens. This figure represents a substantial improvement over the treatment results of 20 years ago, when perhaps 10 per cent of a similar group of patients could be expected to achieve prolonged, disease-free survival. In the USA alone, where the American Cancer Society estimated that in 1987 almost 30 000 patients would be diagnosed with NHL, of whom some 68 per cent would be of intermediate or high grade (see Chapter 1), this improvement could result in the saving of some 10 200 lives each year. By any standards, and particularly, perhaps, by the standards of the oncologists of yesteryear, this accomplishment is truly remarkable. Yet in the USA, it was estimated that 15 700 patients would die from NHL in 1987. This figure is composed of patients with low grade lymphomas – almost all of whom eventually die from their disease – and patients with intermediate and high grade lymphomas whom modern treatment protocols fail to cure. In the developing countries, which account for approximately 80 per cent of the world's population, the vast majority of patients with NHL ultimately die from their disease, since few receive optimal therapy. In the USA, the relative five-year survival of patients with intermediate grade lymphoma who presented in 1979–80 was estimated, from data in the National Cancer

Institute Surveillance, Epidemiology and End Results programme to be 42 per cent. This does not take into account the possible influence of regimens such as M-BACOD and ProMACE-MOPP (see Chapter 21 for details of these drug regimens) which were introduced in 1983, and it remains to be seen whether such protocols will significantly improve the survival of all patients with intermediate grade NHL.

It is in any event likely that a high proportion of patients will not be treated optimally, or that there may be an unrecognized selection process with respect to patients treated in research centres. In any event, there is considerable room for improvement in survival rates. Even without further improvements in therapy, one means of improving survival is to ensure that optimal therapy is provided to as many patients as possible, whether in the more or less developed countries. But even if this could be accomplished, current optimal therapy suffers from a number of disadvantages which will become of greater importance as treatment results improve still further. In contrast to the curative treatment of other once fatal diseases, such as serious bacterial infections, the cure of patients with NHL is presently obtained only at the expense of considerable patient discomfort and inconvenience. Chemotherapy is associated with a broad spectrum of acute and late toxicities, some of which may (rarely) be fatal, and requires the employment of a skilled team of medical, nursing and ancillary health professionals for its safe administration. In spite of these drawbacks, the achievements of recent years provide powerful reasons for optimism – it now appears to be entirely possible that eventually the majority of patients with NHL will be cured. But how will this be accomplished? Are there prospects for improving the efficacy of chemotherapy, while at the same time lessening toxicity? And does chemotherapy, supplemented in a small proportion of patients by surgery or radiotherapy, represent the ultimate therapeutic approach to NHL; or are there prospects for the development of new approaches to treatment based on completely different principles?

Today, because of the dramatic advances that have been made in understanding the pathogenesis of the NHLs, there is every reason to believe that future treatment approaches will be directed towards the uniquely disturbed biochemical pathways of malignant lymphoid cells. This much more specific approach will hopefully avoid the inescapable side-effects of current chemotherapy, which must, because of its relatively non-specific nature, affect normal cells as well as neoplastic cells.

However, highly disease-specific therapies are not 'just around the corner', and much more basic and applied research is needed before such approaches can be explored in the clinical setting. Nevertheless, even with the limited information available today, it is possible to envisage approaches of this kind. In the meantime, it is probable that increased survival, and also lessened toxicity, will result from continued attempts to improve available treatment regimens. While empiricism will remain a large component of ongoing and future chemotherapy trials, it is also likely that greater knowledge of pharmacokinetics and the mechanisms of drug action, as well as an improved understanding of the reasons for failure, including drug resistance, will aid considerably in improving the therapeutic index of current treatment approaches.

Increasing the therapeutic index of chemotherapy

Intermediate and high grade lymphomas

At present, patients with intermediate and high grade lymphomas are treated with combinations of four to 10 drugs, which include the agents known to be most active in NHL. Improvements in survival are likely to be made by increasing the dose intensity ($mg/m^2/week$) of the most effective of these drugs, and eliminating agents which add nothing to the efficacy of the regimen. In drug combinations, however, it is difficult to determine the role of individual drugs without randomized trials designed to answer a specific question of this kind. Such trials are much less appealing than those designed to improve survival, although it is to be hoped that the information derived from them will lead to better design of future trials. Dose intensity analysis confined to a single type of malignant lymphoma may, in some circumstances, provide insights into the relative contribution of the component drugs without the need for randomized clinical trials, as long as there are sufficient differences in the administered dosage of individual drugs among the patients being treated with a single protocol (e.g. because of unacceptable myelosuppression) or sufficient similarity of the drug combinations used among different protocols. Unfortunately, most protocols require simultaneous reductions in several drugs, or delay in the commencement of the next round of therapy for unacceptable myelosuppression, so that the contribution of each drug may be difficult or impossible to discern, although the importance of the overall dose intensity of the protocol may be inferred. Interprotocol comparison faces the problem of the wide variety of drugs in use in different protocols. However, although both inter- and intraprotocol dose intensity may prove to be of limited value in determining the relative importance of the various components of a drug combination in a specific disease, analysis of this kind is warranted.

Increasing the dose intensity does not necessarily equate with increased toxicity. Smaller doses given more often may be less toxic to normal tissues, yet achieve a higher dose intensity, and hopefully, therapeutic efficacy. Moreover, the duration of therapy – of considerable importance with regard to cumulative toxicity and the likelihood of developing a serious unwanted consequence of treatment – may well be shortened with impunity. It appears that the rapidly growing neoplasms do not benefit from prolonged treatment, and survival rates which do not significantly differ from those achieved by protocols of much longer duration have been achieved with treatment durations as short as 2–3 months in both intermediate and high grade lymphomas.[1,2,3] There is therefore good reason to be optimistic that 'fine tuning' of current drug combination regimens will result in significant improvements in survival and a simultaneous decrease in toxicity. Beyond this, only the development of new agents with higher therapeutic indices, which can be incorporated into primary drug combinations, or the devising of methods of overcoming drug resistance, hold promise of an improvement in the results obtained with conventional chemotherapy approaches.

Low grade lymphomas

In the low grade lymphomas, standard treatment approaches, including single agent therapy and 'watch and wait' (also known as 'watchful waiting') are palliative, but research protocols in which very aggressive chemotherapy is used, including treatment sufficiently intensive to require marrow transplantation, could result in the cure of some patients. More data will be required before it will be possible to draw such a conclusion, but if this approach does prove successful, the same process of 'fine tuning' of chemotherapy regimens, as described for the intermediate and high risk lymphomas, will apply. In the absence of improvement in survival through such an approach, completely different methods of treatment will need to be developed for the low grade lymphomas, possibly taking advantage of their apparent greater retention of response to growth regulation (see below).

Colony stimulating factors (CSF)

An exciting development, which could have a profound impact on the therapeutic index of current chemotherapy protocols, is the molecular cloning of colony stimulating factors. These molecules, which can now be produced in large quantities in bacteria or yeasts and readily purified from this source, induce the proliferation and differentiation of haemopoietic cells. Recent clinical trials have demonstrated that both GM-CSF and G-CSF are able to induce a marked increase in the numbers of circulating, functional granulocytes, and can shorten the duration of neutropenia after chemotherapy and probably lessen the risk of fever and serious infection during a neutropenic period.[4,5,6] These agents do not appear to result in gradual depletion of bone marrow stem cells with repeated use, but more information is required before definitive statements in this regard can be made. GM-CSF also stimulates macrophages (and causes the release of numerous macrophage synthesized factors) and eosinophils, and inhibits granulocyte migration. G-CSF has a narrower effect – on granulocytes only – and also stimulates granulocyte migration. It seems likely that the CSFs will permit a significant increase in dose intensity, by permitting more frequent administration or higher doses of myelosuppressive drugs, and clinical trials designed to explore this possibility and to determine whether increased dose intensity will indeed result in increased survival rates are already in progress. The possibility that non-myelosuppressive toxicities may become dose limiting in this circumstance exists, but it is unlikely that this will be of sufficient magnitude to prevent a significant increase in dose intensity.

Biological approaches

Malignant lymphomas retain many of the characteristics of their normal counterpart cells, including the ability to respond to a variety of growth factors. Genetic changes associated with the malignant state may result in the constitutive expression of growth factors for which the cell also bears a receptor, and the establishment of an autocrine loop with perpetual self-stimulation of growth. Alternatively, genetic changes can result in the independence of a tumour cell from growth factors required by its counterpart normal cell, such that the malignant cell undergoes inappropriate proliferation in the absence of the growth factor. Genetic changes of this kind may entail the constitutive expression of a gene involved in cell proliferation, whose regulation is normally under the control of external signals. Chromosomal translocations involving the c-*myc* gene or *bcl*-2 may be of this kind (*see* Chapter 6). It is also easy to imagine that genetic changes could also result in failure of negative growth regulatory signals to be heeded by the cell. Clearly, an understanding of the pathogenetic mechanisms of growth deregulation in a given tumour may permit the development of novel therapeutic approaches directed towards the deregulated pathway. One possibility is the use of molecules (monoclonal antibodies or drugs) to block the binding of required, and possibly constitutively expressed growth factors, to the tumour cell. Another is to direct the therapeutic endeavour towards down-regulation of the constitutively expressed gene, or genes, whose expression has been increased as a result of the genetic lesion. However, until much more is known about the pathways involved, such approaches will remain theoretical.

Current clinical trials involving biological response modifiers are largely empirical, but have had some success in the low grade lymphomas. Interferons, for example, may be as effective as single drugs in the small cleaved cell follicular lymphomas (*see* Chapter 26). Such tumours may provide particularly good targets for such therapeutic attempts, since their behaviour strongly suggests that they retain considerable ability to respond to normal regulatory signals. The potential therapeutic role of cloned T-suppressor or cytotoxic cells specific for the tumour cell remains to be seen, but the molecular cloning of interleukin-2 has made such an approach technically feasible. Finally, a new area of considerable promise is the direction of therapeutic endeavours at oncogene proteins such as tyrosine kinases as present in the

cytoplasmic moieties of many membrane receptors, or signal transducers such as the *ras* G-binding proteins.[7] Much preliminary *in vitro* and animal investigation needs to be undertaken before such approaches can be explored in human tumours.

Tumour specific therapy

Use of anti-idiotypic antibodies

The need for normal B- and T-cells to react to specific antigens, and the clonal nature of neoplastic lymphoid cells, together result in the possession by most NHL cells of a clonally specific marker, namely the antigen receptor. In the case of B-cells, this is immunoglobulin; in T-cells, the antigen receptor complex is usually composed of Tα and Tβ chains coupled to the CD3 molecule. Antibodies directed against the antigen binding component of the antigen receptor are referred to as anti-idiotypic antibodies, and in monoclonal tumours they should be highly tumour specific. Therapeutic trials involving anti-idiotypic antibodies have so far met with limited success, and are discussed in Chapter 26. Reasons for failure include all of those relevant to monoclonal antibodies, but ultimately, since the antigen receptor is not essential to the malignant state, somatic mutation (which has been known to occur in B-cell neoplasms) or modulation may develop, with resultant removal of the therapeutic target, but without affecting the growth characteristics of the tumour. The possibility of coupling drugs, radioisotopes or toxins to anti-idiotypic antibodies could surmount this problem if essentially all tumour cells could be destroyed before modulation could occur, and anti-idiotypic antibodies could also be coupled to other biological response modifiers, but it seems unlikely that such a technically demanding treatment approach directed towards an antigen which can apparently be modulated with impunity by the malignant cell will become a major therapeutic approach in the future.

Antiviral therapy

The direct participation of viruses in the development of lymphoid neoplasia in man has not yet been unequivocally demonstrated. However, as discussed in Chapter 11, some viruses, including Epstein–Barr virus (EBV) and several human retroviruses appear to have at least indirect roles in tumorigenesis, and it remains possible that, in some cases, viral genes may be essential to the generation or maintenance of the neoplastic state. If this is so, viral genes represent a potential target for therapy. In the context of an established tumour, viral replication may have little relevance, or only indirect relevance to its tumorigenic role, so that the use of drugs designed to inhibit viral replication is unlikely to have an antitumour effect. There exists, however, another target worthy of consideration. It is probable that viral genes which regulate, by a process of transactivation, the expression of other virus genes (some of which may be involved in replication) also act on cellular genes. Such viral genes are usually 'early genes', i.e. genes expressed in the absence of, or shortly before viral replication. An effect on normal cellular genes has been clearly demonstrated in the case of the *tax* genes of the human T-lymphotrophic viruses which induce increased expression of interleukin-2 receptor (*see* Chapter 11). The use of molecules which prevent the transactivation of cellular genes could provide a non-toxic therapy for tumours in which such a phenomenon is relevant to pathogenesis. Although other cells in the patient may be infected with viral genomes, since the therapy is directed at viral rather than cellular genes, such toxicity should have little effect on normal tissues. In fact, in patients with human immunodeficiency virus (HIV) infection, a similar approach could be adopted to combat the profound immunosuppressive effects of HIV itself.

Molecules which could affect transactivator genes include drugs (possibly specifically designed, or screened for) which bind to the protein product, or anti-sense oligonucleotides which bind to the messenger RNA of the trans-activating gene and prevent its translation. The stability of anti-sense molecules and the assurance that these molecules will be able to enter tumour cells in sufficient concentration poses numerous problems, and treatment with such molecules may not prove feasible. Nonetheless, methods of surmounting this problem, including chemical modification, the use of liposome-encapsulated oligomer, or even the incorporation of anti-sense molecules, with a functional promoter, into defective virus particles capable of infecting the tumour cell, could ultimately prove possible, although there are numerous technical and ethical problems to surmount if such an approach is ever to become a reality.

If viruses could be proven to be relevant to the pathogenesis of NHL, whether or not they have an essential role, then the prevention of virus infection by means of vaccines is an approach worthy of consideration for the prevention of specific lymphomas. The development of vaccines to prevent EBV infection, and more recently, human retrovirus infection has been under exploration for some years.

Treatment directed at the molecular consequences of genetic abnormalities

For many years immunologists have sought tumour specific antigens. In man, however, with the exception of the special case of idiotype, tumour-specific antigens have not been demonstrated. More recently, with the demonstration that lymphoid neoplasms are often, and probably always, the consequence of highly specific genetic changes occurring in specific cell types (*see* Chapter 6), it has become aparent that the genetic lesion itself is tumour specific and, as such, provides a potential therapeutic target. For example, the most frequent non-random chromosomal translocations associated with NHL – 14;18 and 8;14 – have been shown to result in some cases in the production of mRNA molecules in the tumour cells which are not present in their normal counterpart cells. In tumours bearing 14;18 translocations, a fusion mRNA molecule consisting of the *bcl*-2 gene coupled to an immunoglobulin constant region (usually via the J or joining region) is synthesized (Fig. 27.1). It may well prove possible to synthesize molecules (including anti-sense oligomers) which specifically bind to this fusion transcript and prevent *bcl*-2 expression in tumour cells, but not in normal cells. In the case of the 8;14 translocation, when the breakpoint on chromosome 8 is within the first intron of the c-*myc* gene, sequences present in the first c-*myc* intron are found in the mRNA, since the position of the breakpoint prevents correct mRNA splicing, which normally leads to the excision of these sequences (Fig. 27.2). These intron sequences also provide a tumour-specific target, which is likely to be exploited in the future, either via anti-sense molecules, or other kinds of molecules which might bind specifically to the intron sequences present in tumour cell mRNA but not the mRNA of normal cells and prevent translation of c-*myc*. In the two examples given, the abnormal expression of the genes mentioned – *bcl*-2 and c-*myc* – is believed to play a critical role in tumorigenesis, so that the elimination of their protein products in the respective tumour cells is likely to have a profound therapeutic effect.

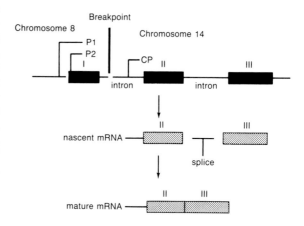

Fig. 26.2 Diagrammatic representation of the abnormal mature mRNA molecule which results from 8;14 translocations in which the breakpoint is in the first c-*myc* intron. The translocated gene is transcribed from a normally cryptic promoter site in the intron, and sequences between the promoter and the second exon are not spliced out of the nascent message since the upstream consensus splice sequence required for splicing is not present in the transcript.

MOLECULAR CONSEQUENCES OF 14;18 TRANSLOCATION

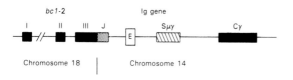

Fig. 26.1 Diagrammatic representation of the molecular consequences, at the DNA level, of the 14;18 chromosomal translocation which occurs in follicular lymphomas and some diffuse large cell and small non-cleaved cell lymphomas. A fusion transcript including the *bcl*-2 gene, translocated from chromosome 18, and a part of the immunoglobulin locus from chromosome 14 is produced.

Clearly, as more becomes known of the pathogenesis of the NHLs, more novel therapeutic aproaches will become practical realities. The appeal of such approaches is their absolute tumour specificity, but it is unlikely that approaches of this kind will soon be ready for clinical trial. If this does eventually come about, it is likely to be much simpler than current chemotherapeutic approaches to treatment. Although each tumour, or even tumour subtype, will require its own therapy, this may eventually be no more impractical than is the current use of highly specific antivenoms for individuals bitten by different species of poisonous snakes. Such a time is presumably a long way off at present. Nonetheless, even the theoretical possibilities – which could hardly be contemplated a decade or so ago – provide grounds for considerable optimism that in the future, simple, highly specific and minimally toxic treatments will be available for NHL. The lymphoid nature of the lymphomas has permitted the application of numerous techniques, developed initially for the study of normal lymphocyte characteristics and molecular changes occurring during lymphocyte differentiation and activation, to be applied to the study of the biology of the NHLs, including their cytogenetic and molecular genetic abnormalities. This makes it highly probable that the NHLs will be in the vanguard of this new era of cancer therapy, just as they have been, and remain, in the vanguard of the development of effective chemotherapeutic regimens.

References

1. Klimo P, Connors JM. *Annals of Internal Medicine.* 1985; **102**, 596.
2. Schwenn M, Blattner S, Weinstein H. *Proceedings of the American Society of Clinical Oncology.* 1988; **876**, 227.
3. Müller-Weihrich ST, Ludwig R, Reiter A, *et al. Proceedings of the Third International Conference on Malignant Lymphomas.* 1987; **62**, 83 (Abstract).
4. Brandt SJ, Peters WP, Atwater SK, *et al. New England Journal of Medicine.* 1988; **318**, 869.
5. Morstyn G, Campbell L, Souza LM, *et al. Lancet.* 1988; **i**, 667.
6. Bronchud MH, Scarffe JH, Thatcher N, *et al. British Journal of Cancer.* 1987; **56**, 809.
7. Magrath IT. In: Magrath IT (ed). *New Directions in Cancer Treatment.* Heidelberg: Springer, 1989, 399–427.

INDEX